CLINICAL ANATOMY

(A Problem Solving Approach)

Volume 1

Volume 2

 DVD Contents

Demonstration of Dissected Specimens in Anatomy

UPPER LIMB

- Brachial Plexus
- Quadrangular and Lower Triangular Space
- Cubital Fossa
- Radial Nerve in Radial Groove

LOWER LIMB

- Gluteal Region,
- Popliteal Fossa
- Interior of Knee Joint
- Dorsum of Foot

THORAX

- External Features of Heart
- Lungs
- Mediastinum

- Flexor Retinaculum of Hand
- Parotid Gland
- Cerebrum
- Hindbrain
- Spinal Cord

ABDOMEN

- Liver
- Kidney, Ureter and Urinary Bladder
- Sagittal Section of Female Pelvis
- Placenta

HEAD AND NECK

- Cranial Cavity
- Nasal Cavity
- Larynx

System requirement:
- **Windows XP or above**
- **Power DVD player (Software)**
- **Windows media player 11.0 version of above (Software)**

The accompanying DVD ROM is playable only in Computer and not in DVD player.

Kindly wait for a few seconds for DVD to autorun. If it does not autorun, then please do the following:
- Click on 'My Computer'
- Click the **DVD/CD drive labeled JAYPEE** and after opening the drive, kindly double-click the file named **Jaypee**

CLINICAL ANATOMY

(A Problem Solving Approach)

Third Edition

Volume 1

Neeta V Kulkarni MD

Retired Professor of Anatomy
Dr Somervell Memorial CSI Medical College
Karakonam, Thiruvananthapuram
Kerala, India

Formerly

Professor and Head, Department of Anatomy
Government Medical College
Thiruvananthapuram, Kerala, India

Foreword

YM Fazil Marickar

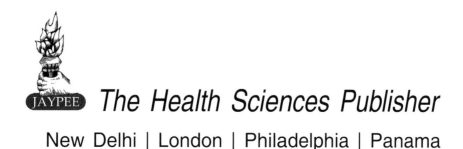

The Health Sciences Publisher

New Delhi | London | Philadelphia | Panama

Jaypee Brothers Medical Publishers (P) Ltd

Headquarters

Jaypee Brothers Medical Publishers (P) Ltd
4838/24, Ansari Road, Daryaganj
New Delhi 110 002, India
Phone: +91-11-43574357
Fax: +91-11-43574314
Email: jaypee@jaypeebrothers.com

Overseas Offices

J.P. Medical Ltd
83 Victoria Street, London
SW1H 0HW (UK)
Phone: +44-2031708910
Fax: +02-03-0086180
Email: info@jpmedpub.com

Jaypee Medical Inc.
The Bourse
111 South Independence Mall East
Suite 835, Philadelphia, PA 19106, USA
Phone: +1 267-519-9789
Email: joe.rusko@jaypeebrothers.com

Jaypee Brothers Medical Publishers (P) Ltd
Bhotahity, Kathmandu, Nepal
Phone: +977-9741283608
Email: kathmandu@jaypeebrothers.com

Jaypee-Highlights Medical Publishers Inc.
City of Knowledge, Bld. 237, Clayton
Panama City, Panama
Phone: +1 507-301-0496
Fax: +1 507-301-0499
Email: cservice@jphmedical.com

Jaypee Brothers Medical Publishers (P) Ltd
17/1-B Babar Road, Block-B, Shaymali
Mohammadpur, Dhaka-1207
Bangladesh
Mobile: +08801912003485
Email: jaypeedhaka@gmail.com

Website: www.jaypeebrothers.com
Website: www.jaypeedigital.com

Inquiries for bulk sales may be solicited at: jaypee@jaypeebrothers.com

Clinical Anatomy (A Problem Solving Approach)

Third Edition: **2016**

ISBN: 978-93-5152-966-8

Printed at Replika Press Pvt. Ltd.

An Inspirational Quote

Success in learning is not the property of the brilliants.
It is the reward for those who are motivated, dedicated and full of enthusiasm.
To put it simply, there is no short-cut to hard work for success in life.

In Memory of

My husband (Dr VP Kulkarni) who was a pillar of strength during the making of the first edition.

Dedicated to

The great anatomists of our country who have shown faith in the sincere attempts
for uplifting the discipline to newer scales.

Foreword to the Third Edition

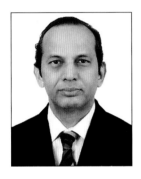

The book on Anatomy by Neeta V Kulkarni is quite different from the usual textbooks of Anatomy. A lot of clinical correlation of Anatomy is introduced to make the book interesting to the new Anatomy students. The layout is clear. The drawings are simple and reproducible. Osteology is made simple and understandable. The chapter with clinically related questions and explanations of the anatomical details is very useful for correlating anatomy with realistic clinical conditions. The boxes on *Clinical Correlation* and *Student Interest* are unique and make the book different from others. The language is good. I am sure the first-year MBBS students will benefit by reading this book.

YM Fazil Marickar
Principal
Mount Zion Medical College, Adoor, Kerala, India
Former Professor and Head of the Department of Surgery
Government Medical College
Thiruvananthapuram, Kerala, India

Preface to the Third Edition

It gives me immense pleasure to present the third edition of *Clinical Anatomy (A Problem Solving Approach) (Volumes 1 and 2)* for the benefit of the undergraduate medical students and postgraduates in addition to dental, nursing, pharmacy and physiotherapy students.

The basic theme of the first edition—*'Anatomical Thinking to Solve Clinical Problems'* is the backbone of this edition too. This theme emphasizes the fact that anatomy occupies the centerstage throughout the undergraduate medical curriculum and beyond, and is not restricted to the preclinical phase only.

The syllabus of Anatomy for the First MBBS Course of one-year duration is indeed very vast in spite of the attempts to trim it. As teachers, it is our duty to expose the undergraduate students to the basic knowledge (gross structure, microscopic structure and embryology of the entire human body). This has posed a huge challenge to the teachers and the students alike due to shortened duration of the course. The newly admitted medical students who strive to learn and grasp the three basic subjects and appear for the final examination at the end of one year are indeed comparable to the pathetic looking overburdened primary school students.

In an attempt to make learning anatomy less stressful for undergraduates, some new student-friendly ideas are introduced in the new edition:

1. Integration of Anatomy and its clinical relevance in all branches of Anatomy like gross anatomy, microanatomy, osteology, embryology, radiology, etc.

2. Developing student awareness that gross anatomy can be learnt from plain radiographs, CT and MRI scans and from intraoperative photographs taken during the operation on the patient.

3. Training of students in solving clinical problems by anatomical knowledge is undertaken by exposing the students to clinicoanatomical problems (case-based problems). In this way, the students become aware about the essentiality of anatomical knowledge during clinical training.

4. Thorough revision of all the chapters (especially, general embryology, general anatomy and osteology) and addition of new educative diagrams is undertaken, keeping in mind the difficulties of students in learning anatomical facts.

5. Introduction of the so-called *dialogue boxes (Student Interest)* throughout the text is a novel idea for giving practical hints on how to learn a topic. The important points are re-emphasized so that the students' interest in the topic is enhanced. The dialogue boxes also highlight *Must Know* topics in Anatomy and are useful before the commencement of theory and practical examinations.

6. *Embryologic Insight boxes* highlight the precise developmental sources of the structure or organ and *Clinical Correlation boxes* highlight the clinical importance of the structure or structures.

7. *Added Infromation boxes* are for the postgraduates and teachers. In this way, an undergraduate student is kept out of the extra burden.

The third edition of *Clinical Anatomy (A Problem Solving Approach) (Volumes 1 and 2)* caters to the present-day needs of the undergraduate students. I feel that if the students feel satisfied and relaxed while going through the text (and not overwhelmed and burdened), the objective of the textbook is achieved.

Neeta V Kulkarni

Foreword to the Second Edition

I am extremely happy to write a foreword for the second edition of the book titled *Clinical Anatomy (A Problem Solving Approach)* by Dr Neeta V Kulkarni. Generally, we observe that many books of Anatomy and Embryology are mainly based on description of structures. Like a born teacher, she has not only described structure but has also shown her talent and maturity of thought by stressing the main purpose of knowing gross anatomy and embryology.

In the book, the author has given considerable justice to the living anatomy by inclusion of images of plain radiographs, computed tomography (CT), magnetic resonance imaging (MRI), digital subtraction angiography (DSA) and three-dimensional reconstruction images using multidetector CT. Added to this, there are intraoperative photographic views of various internal organs in the body. She has shown how technology can be harnessed to convert this so-called static subject into a dynamic entity. She has been an Anatomy teacher throughout her career and has assimilated the subject well. Knowledge, when it becomes ripe, gives wisdom and she has used her experienced wisdom to innovate the presentation according to the need of the day. This edition covers general embryology, genetics, special embryology, gross anatomy and basic knowledge of the tissues of the body with emphasis on application.

The reduction in the time of teaching anatomy at preclinical level is a very unfortunate step. This exhaustive subject deserves ample time to learn and understand. Clinical anatomy for students with its problem-solving approach will minimize the hardships of learning to understand anatomy.

I often used to wonder if we should have separate anatomy texts catering to the needs of undergraduate curriculum, clinical postgraduate curriculum (as per the specialty chosen) and separate books for anatomists. But now I feel that books like *Clinical Anatomy* can build the bridges and provide a refreshing anatomical elixir to all involved in providing health care.

Let me wish a wholesome response to the new edition.

BR Kate MS FAMS FSAMS
Ex-Director of Medical Education and Research
Mumbai, Maharashtra, India

Preface to the Second Edition

Anatomy is the basis of medical profession as human body is the focus of examination, investigation and intervention for diagnosis and treatment of diseases. There is a reawakening of the importance of anatomy with the realization that sound knowledge of anatomy is the backbone of safe medical practice. A doctor with sound anatomical knowledge is well-equipped to perform safe procedure or surgery than the one who makes mistakes by cutting normal anatomical relations of the structure or organ, operated upon (for which the doctor is sued in the court of law for negligence). One must appreciate that application of anatomical knowledge is the ongoing process throughout the medical career. Therefore, clinical anatomy occupies the centerstage right from the outset of medical training. There are intentional efforts by health educationists over the world to bridge the gray zone between preclinical anatomy and clinical anatomy. Learning anatomy (which includes gross anatomy, microscopic anatomy, embryology and genetics) in a short span of time is a Herculean task. Therefore, though it is not conceptually difficult; its sheer bulk makes anatomy overwhelming. In this context, a shift towards teaching/learning basic anatomy alongside clinical anatomy is a progressive step. The key to successful and enjoyable learning lies in consciously integrating the basic and the clinical anatomy right from the entry point by initiating the trainees to identify normal anatomical structures in plain radiographs, CT scans, ultrasound scans, MRI, etc. Added to this, they may be exposed to patients presenting with typical deformities due to nerve injury, patients with hemiplegia, paraplegia, etc., patients with obvious congenital defects, and patients with thyroid swelling, parotid swelling, etc. This is bound to arouse their interest in learning. Another very interesting approach is to train the trainee in clinical problem-solving by using anatomical knowledge. This approach not only convinces the trainees that preclinical anatomy is an integral part of bedside medicine but also expands their thinking capacity (brain power). This approach is indispensable for concept clarity and retention (rather than rote learning).

Giving due regard to the constructive suggestions and comments from readers (both students and teachers) and bowing down to the request of Jaypee Brothers Medical Publishers (P) Ltd, New Delhi, India, the work on second edition of *Clinical Anatomy (A Problem Solving Approach)* was undertaken. The basic theme of the first edition of *developing skills in anatomical thinking for solving clinical problems* has been retained. New chapters have been added on general anatomy (for giving conceptual background about basic tissues), general embryology and genetics, besides osteology. All the chapters on regional anatomy have been extensively revised and enriched with plenty of new figures including photographs of clinical material (collected from various clinicians) and radiological images (collected from radiologists) to emphasize relevance of Anatomy in the practice of medicine. The solved examples on clinicoanatomical problems and multiple choice questions (MCQs) (given at the end of each section) not only aid in revising but also lend credence to the theme of the book. *Clinical Insight*, *Embryologic Insight* and *Know More* are displayed in boxes.

I am sure that this edition too will spread positive vibes towards this tough subject and will reiterate the fact that the subject is interesting only if looked through the mirror of its clinical relevance. Moreover, this text can be a good resource material in problem-based learning (PBL) curriculum in graduate medical education.

Neeta V Kulkarni

Acknowledgments

I shall fail in my duty if I do not extend my gratitude once again to all the clinical fraternity who were generous in giving the radiological images and the photographs of patients and of procedures on the patient (like lumbar puncture, brachial plexus block, venipuncture, etc.) in addition to the photographs of organs seen during the operation while making the first, second and third editions of *Clinical Anatomy (A Problem Solving Approach)*.

The names that come foremost to my mind during the making of first edition are Dr YM Fazil Marickar (Former Professor and Head of Surgery Department, Government Medical College and Hospital, Thiruvananthapuram, Kerala, India and currently Principal of Mount Zion Medical College, Adoor, Kerala), and Dr Ramanarayan (Former Professor and Head of Cardiothoracic Surgery, Medical College and Hospital, Thiruvananthapuram, Kerala, India). I would like to extend my special thanks to Dr N Vijayshankar (Former Director of Neuroanatomy in Old Westbury, New York and United States of America) for his valuable help in the chapters on Neuroanatomy. A special mention of gratitude is a must to the Department of Radiology, Christian Medical College, Vellore, Tamil Nadu, India) for providing high-quality images of Normal Anatomy and Altered Anatomy in disease state.

During the making of second edition, there was an overwhelming response from clinicians. I have great pleasure in extending my sincere thanks to my friend Dr Elezy MA (Former Professor and Head of Anatomy, Government Medical College, Trichur, Kerala, India) for sending a large collection of radiological images of anesthetic procedures and of operative procedures over a long period of time through her contacts with clinical fraternity in Trichur, Palaghat, Cochin and Calicut in Kerala, India. Not only Dr Elezy but her family and friends also deserve special mention (Dr VK Sreekumar, Professor of Surgery, Medical College, Trichur; Dr Raghushankar, Associate Professor of Surgery, Karuna Medical College, Palaghat; Dr Kesavan, Anesthesiologist, Medical College, Trichur; Dr NK Sanilkumar, Cochin; Dr R Vijayakumar, Orthopedic Surgeon, Medical College, Trichur; Dr Bejohn JK, Pediatric Surgeon, Medical College, Trichur; Dr Shameer VK, Medical College, Trichur; Dr Santhosh Nambiar, Medical College, Trichur; and Dr Jamal TM, Medical College, Calicut). Thanks are also due to Dr Girijamony (HOD, Anatomy, Medical College, Trichur) for providing the images of laparoscopic anatomy of abdominal and pelvic organs.

I am ever indebted to the clinical fraternity of Dr SMCSI Medical College, Karakonam, Kerala, India for their cooperation. The list includes Dr R Varma, Head of Pediatric Surgery; Dr Vimala, Head of Nephrology Department; Dr Punithen, Associate Professor of Surgery; Dr Jacob Thomas, Professor of Surgery; Dr Mariam Philip of Dermatology Department; Dr Regi Ebenezer of ENT Department; Dr Sara Ammu Chacko, HOD, Radiodiagnosis; Dr Nitta H and Dr Sebastian (Radiodiagnosis); Dr Aneesh Elias and Dr Sara Varghese of Plastic Surgery; and Dr Adeline Thankam of Obstetrics and Gynecology.

Special thanks are extended to Dr Paul Augustine from Regional Cancer Centre (RCC), Thiruvananthapuram, Kerala, India for providing the image of peau d'orange.

During the making of the third edition too, I depended a lot on the feedback of my former colleagues and well-wishers from Kerala, India. Dr Elezy MA was kind enough to send some photomicrographs.

I am thankful to Dr YM Fazil Marickar, a surgeon par excellence and an academician for having agreed to write a foreword for this edition. I cannot resist the temptation to mention that his better half, Dr VM Kurshid is the Professor of Anatomy working in Gokulam Medical College, Thiruvananthapuram, Kerala, India and my former colleague in Medical College, Thiruvananthapuram, Kerala, India.

The assistance of the graphic artists (Mr Vishal Soni and Mr Abhay Mangave) of Pune, Maharashtra, India in renovating the old figures and developing the new ones was most appreciable.

I will ever remain indebted to Shri Jitendar P Vij, Group Chairman of Jaypee Brothers Medical Publishers (P) Ltd., New Delhi, India for prompting me to take up this project. I place on record my thanks to Mr Tarun Duneja (Director-Publishing), Ms Samina Khan (Executive Assistant to Director-Publishing) and the entire staff of the Production Unit involved in the publishing of the third edition.

My son and daughter (and their respective spouses) remain my inspirational strength.

With all humility in my heart, I place the third edition at the lotus feet of the Almighty and pray that the book is beneficial to the entire student community of Medical Colleges.

Contents

Section 4: Lower Limb

Section 5: Thorax

Volume 2

Section 8: Vertebral Column and Spinal Cord, Cranial Cavity and Brain

Section 9: Cranial Nerves

Section 1

GENERAL ANATOMY

1

Anatomy—Past, Present and Future

Chapter Contents

ANATOMY IN BRIEF

Anatomy is a branch of medical science that deals with the study of structures inside the human body. Knowledge of the position of anatomical structures (organs, blood vessels, nerves, lymph nodes, endocrine and exocrine glands, bones, joints, etc.) helps the examining physician in understanding the affected anatomical structure in a particular disease or in locating the structure correctly while feeling or palpating it on the body surface or in correctly identifying the structure to be cut during surgery. This knowledge is equally essential in understanding and interpreting radiological images. The history of Anatomy throws ample light on the thirst of knowledge for this branch of medical sciences in the mind of the researchers of ancient era.

Greek Era

Hippocrates of Greece (469–399 BC) was the father of medicine and founder of Anatomy. He conceptualized that disease had a physical basis and hence he dissected animals and dead human bodies to learn the structures inside them.

Roman Era

Claudius Galen (130 to 200 AD) was the most accomplished Greek physician, surgeon and philosopher of Roman Empire. He was given the position of personal physician of several emperors. He wrote extensively on anatomy from observations of dissections on animals. Galen was so substantial that his observations remained unchallenged for several centuries.

Dark Ages

Dark ages included the period extending from the third to the thirteenth centuries. It was so called because of the lack of any progress in science and arts in Europe.

Fourteenth Century

Mondino, an Italian anatomist (1276 to 1326) was the restorer of human anatomy as he taught anatomy by doing dissections on human dead bodies and wrote his observations in a book called ***Anathomia***.

Renaissance

During fifteenth and sixteenth centuries both arts and science were revived and flourished. Leonardo da Vinci (1452 to 1519) was an artist, painter, mathematician, engineer and anatomist. Vitruvian man was his most famous anatomical drawing of a geometrically proportionate human male. Leonardo was the inventor of cross sectional and illustrative anatomy.

Andreas Vesalius, a Flemish anatomist and surgeon performed extensive dissections on executed criminals after obtaining permission from the Pope. Vesalius was the first to describe accurate human anatomy in his treatise in Latin called **de fabrica humani corporis**. Thus, it was Vesalius who truly challenged Galilean dogmas. Vesalius was aptly called the father of **modern anatomy** (Fig. 1.1).

Seventeenth Century

William Harvey was credited with discovery of blood circulation. To prove the role of heart as central pump in blood circulation, he had the valour to dissect his own freshly dead father and sister before burial.

Another discovery attributed to this century was the use of microscope to study microscopic structure of tissues obtained from bits of organs.

Eighteenth Century

As the chemical called **formaldehyde** was accepted as preservative of tissues, Medical Schools were started in England and Scotland. For doing dissections, executed criminals were used. To set up Anatomy Museums demand for more and more cadavers increased. This led to crimes like grave robbing even by medical students and professors. The famous Hunter brothers (John and William) set up well known anatomy museums in London and Glasgow.

Another epoch making discovery was the foundation of embryology or developmental anatomy credit for which goes to Von Baer.

Nineteenth Century

To cope with the increasing demand for dead human bodies, body snatchers were deployed by doctors in London and Scotland. Two very famous body snatchers were William Burke and William Hare who committed fifteen murders of boarders (for being late in paying the rent), in the year 1828. To put a stop to this illegal trade of body snatching, the parliament in Great Britain passed Warburton Anatomy Act under which dissections of human cadavers by medical students were compulsory and only unclaimed dead bodies were allowed for dissection in medical schools (apart from donated bodies). Nineteenth century saw the discovery of X-ray by Rontgen in 1895 and the beginning of radiological anatomy.

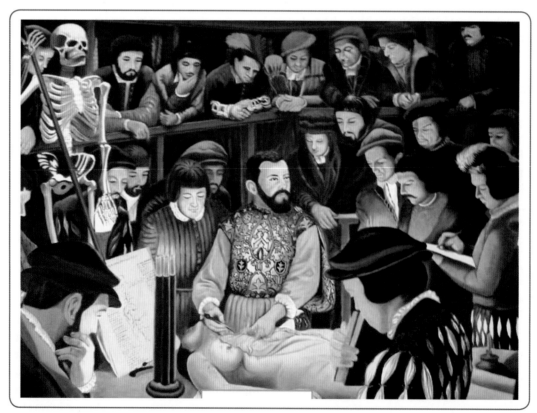

Fig. 1.1: Andreas Vesalius father of modern anatomy

Twentieth Century

With the advent of newer and newer technological advances newer approaches to learning structure and function of the organs and tissues were discovered. The newer imaging techniques like CT scan, ultrasound, MRI, PET, etc. radiological anatomy (living anatomy) achieved greater importance.

Twenty First Century

Visible Human Project (VHP) created by NLM-NIH USA (National Library of Medicine in National Institute of Health in USA) is an excellent digital image library highly useful in learning living anatomy. With introduction of integrative approaches in medical curriculum at the undergraduate level, there is a positive shift in the objectives of learning anatomy, physiology and biochemistry. The three preclinical basic subjects (Anatomy, Biochemistry and Physiology) are learnt in the context of their ability in clinical problem-solving right from the beginning of undergraduate medical course.

2

Basic Tissues of the Body

Chapter Contents

STRUCTURAL ORGANIZATION OF HUMAN BODY

The complex human body shows five levels of structural organization (Fig. 2.1) starting from the cells and basic tissues to the organs and organ systems.

- The cells are the structural and functional units of the body, e.g. the epithelial cells, muscle cells (myocytes), neurons (nerve cells), connective tissue cells (fibroblasts), special connective tissue cells (chondrocytes, osteocytes, etc.).
- The groups of cells with similar structure and functions comprise the basic tissues, e.g. epithelial tissue, connective tissue, muscular tissue and neural tissue.
- The different types of basic tissues make up the organs, e.g. heart, kidney, lung and skin.
- A group of organs work in unison to perform a specific function form the organ system.
- Various organ systems capable of carrying out the basic life processes comprise an entire human being.

The knowledge of the histological structure of the organs helps us to understand the functions. It is also necessary to understand the pathological changes in the normal tissues in diseases. This helps in histopathological diagnosis of the disease from a bit of tissue (taken from diseased organ or lymph node) to examine under the microscope after processing and staining.

BASIC TISSUES OF THE BODY

There are four basic tissues in the body as follows:
1. Epithelial tissue
2. Connective tissue
3. Muscular tissue
4. Neural tissue

EPITHELIAL TISSUE

The epithelium is a layer or layers of cells resting on the basement membrane. It lines the external surfaces of the body and internal surface of body cavities and of hollow viscera (except the synovial cavity of a joint). The epithelia also line the secretory units and ducts of exocrine glands, kidney tubules, lung alveoli, etc. The chief functions of the epithelial tissue are protection, absorption and secretion.

General Features of Epithelium

- The epithelial tissue is rich in cells and poor in extracellular matrix. The cells are closely aggregated to form cellular sheets.
- The cell-to-cell junctions or intercellular adhesions are well developed in epithelial cells. The cell junctions maintain cell harmony and cell-to-cell communications.

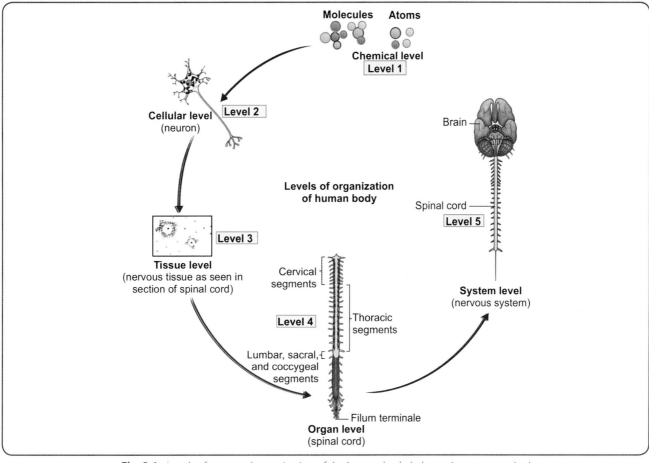

Fig. 2.1: Levels of structural organization of the human body (schematic representation)

- The basal surfaces of the epithelial cells rest on the basement membrane which separates the cells from the deeper vascular connective tissue. The luminal or apical surfaces of the cells may show structural specialization in response to the absorptive function.
- The epithelial tissue is avascular and hence receives nutrition by diffusion from blood capillaries of the connective tissue deeper to the basement membrane.
- The epithelium is capable of regeneration as exemplified by a very high rate of mitosis in intestinal epithelium and in the basal layer of the epidermis.

💡 **ADDED INFORMATION**

Details of Cell Junctions (Fig. 2.2)
The intercellular junctions contain specific structural proteins with glue-like properties.
- Cell junctions on lateral surface of epithelial cells.

Contd…

Contd…

💡 **ADDED INFORMATION**

- ***Tight junctions (zonula occludens)*** are located close to the luminal surface of the epithelial cells. In the tight junctions, the outer surfaces of the plasma membranes of the adjacent cells fuse thereby obliterating the intercellular space. The tight junctions occlude intercellular spaces for from the lumen of the viscus.
- ***Zonula adherens (adherens belt)*** is below the tight junction. The opposing plasma membranes show a gap of 20 nm and a dense plaque like material is present on the cytoplasmic surfaces of the plasma membranes at the junction. The microfilaments are embedded in this plaque. The zonula adherens provides rigidity to apical parts of the epithelial cells.
- ***Desmosomes (macula adherens)*** are punctate or spot-like in appearance on light microscopy. The attachment plaques contain adhesion molecules called ***cadherin***. The desmosomes provides firm adhesion to cells which are subject to friction as seen typically in stratum spinosum of the epidermis.

Contd…

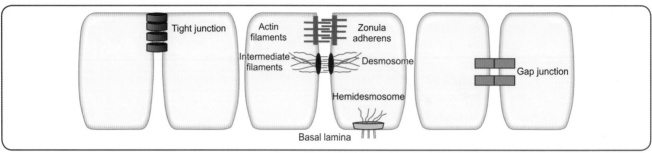

Fig. 2.2: Various types of specialized junctions

Contd…

 ADDED INFORMATION

> – **Gap junctions (nexus)** are visible only by electron microscope. They are located close to the basal side of lateral surfaces of the cells. They contain transmembrane protein channels (connexons) that allow passage of small molecules between neighboring cells and thus allow cell-to-cell communication (including metabolic and electric coupling of cells).
> • Cell junctions on the basal surface of epithelial cells:
> – **Hemidesmosomes** are half desmosomes that attach the basal surface of epithelial cell to the basal lamina of the basement membrane. The attachment plaque contains plenty of integrin molecules in the hemidesmosomes.

Surface Modifications of Epithelial Cells

• The **cilia** are long hair like projections of plasma membrane which serve the protective function in air conducting passages of respiratory system. The dust particles (inhaled from atmospheric air) and mucus (secreted by the goblet cells in the epithelium of air conducting passages) are driven upwards towards nasal cavity via nasopharynx by coordinated beating of the cilia lining the epithelium of bronchi, trachea, etc. Thus, cilia prevent the entry of dust particles into the bronchioles and the lung alveoli. Table 2.1 explains the differences between microvilli and cilia.
• **Microvilli** are the infoldings of apical plasma membrane (to increase the surface area). They are visible under electron microscope. Under the light microscope, microvilli appear as brush border or striated border, which is distinct when stained with special stains. They increase the surface area for absorption manifold. The microvilli are characteristic of epithelium of small intestine and of kidney tubules.
• **Stereocilia** represent long microvilli but are non-motile. They are found in sites where fluid secretion and resorption take place, e.g. in vas deferens and epididymis.

CLINICAL CORRELATION

Kartagener's Syndrome
This is a genetic disease, in which the person is born with immotile cilia. The patients suffer from respiratory symptoms caused by the accumulation of dust and other particulate matter (inhaled from atmospheric air), which normally are trapped by pseudostratified ciliated columnar epithelium.

TABLE 2.1: Differences between cilia and microvilli

Cilia	Microvilli
10 μm in length and 0.25 μm in diameter	1–2 mm in length and about 75–90 μm in diameter
Motile	Non-motile
Contains 9+2 pattern of microtubules	Contains numerous microfilaments (actin filaments)
Concerned with movement of ova through uterine tube and movement of secretions in trachea and bronchi towards pharynx	Concerned with absorptive functions
Seen over lining epithelium of respiratory tract and uterine tube	Seen over intestinal epithelium and proximal convulated tubule of kidney

Basement Membrane

The basement membrane is a structure that supports the epithelium. It consists of two distinct layers.

1. **Basal lamina:** The layer in contact with the epithelial cells. It is also produced by epithelial cells and is composed of type IV collagen fibers and laminin containing matrix.
2. **Reticular lamina:** It is the deeper layer and composed of reticular tissue, collagen fibers and matrix. It merges with surrounding connective tissue. It is synthesized by fibroblasts.

Functions of Basement Membrane

• It provides adhesion on one side to epithelial cells (or parenchyma); and on the other side to connective tissue (mainly collagen fibers).
• It acts as a barrier to the diffusion of molecules. The barrier function varies with location (because of variations in pore size). Large proteins are prevented from passing out of blood vessels, but (in the lung) diffusion of gases is allowed.

- Recent work suggests that basement membranes may play a role in cell organization, as molecules within the membrane interact with receptors on cell surfaces. Substances present in the membrane may influence morphogenesis of cells to which they are attached.
- The membranes may influence the regeneration of peripheral nerves after injury, and may play a role in re-establishment of neuromuscular junctions.

CLINICAL CORRELATION

- The **basement membrane thickens** in pathologic conditions like **nephropathies** (kidney diseases) and **vasculopathies** (diseases of blood vessels). A thickened basement membrane is visible under the light microscope with routine hematoxylin and eosin staining.
- While examining the tissue biopsy from primary site of cancer arising from the epithelium (**epithelioma**), the pathologist looks for the basement membrane. An intact basement membrane is an indication that the cancer is localized to the primary site. This is known as **carcinoma in situ** stage of cancer. If the basement membrane is broken, it is an indication that cancer cells have begun to spread from the primary site.

Nourishment of Epithelium

As the epithelium is avascular it is nourished by capillaries in reticular lamina of basement membrane by a process called **diffusion**.

Classification of Epithelium (Flowchart 2.1)

Based on the number of cell layers, the epithelium is classified as follows:
- **Simple epithelium:** It is composed of a single layer of cells resting on a basement membrane.
- **Stratified (compound) epithelium:** It is composed of more than one layer of cells stacked on each other, out of which only the basal cells rest on the basement membrane.

Based on the shape of cells in the surface layer, the simple and stratified epithelia are further classified as follows:

Simple Epithelium

Simple squamous epithelium (Pavement epithelium) (Fig. 2.3A)

Characteristics
- A single layer of flat squamous shaped cells rest on the basement membrane.

Flowchart 2.1: Classification of epithelia

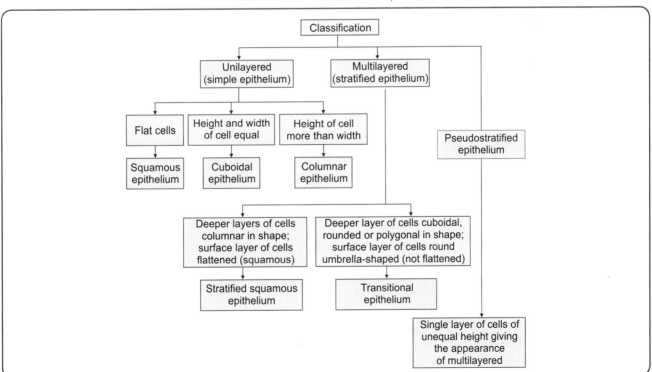

- The cytoplasm forms a thin film and flattened nuclei are visible.

Function: Active transport of gases and nutrients through the cells.

Distribution

- Endothelium of the blood vessels.
- Endocardium of the heart chambers.
- Mesothelium of the serous membranes (pericardium, pleura and peritoneum).
- Epithelium of loops of Henle and parietal layer of Bowman's capsule in kidneys.
- Epithelium of lung alveoli.

Simple cuboidal epithelium (Fig. 2.3B)

Characteristics

- A single layer of cuboidal cells resting on basement membrane.
- The cells have equal height and breadth and their nuclei are rounded.

Distribution

- Germinal epithelium covering the surface of ovary.
- Lining of thyroid follicles (where the cells secrete thyroid hormones).
- Pigment cell layer of retina.

Simple columnar epithelium (Fig. 2.3C)

Characteristics

- A single layer of tall columnar cells resting on the basement membrane.
- Nuclei of the cells are elongated and placed closer to the base.

Subtypes of simple columnar epithelium

- Unmodified *simple columnar* epithelium as seen in some ducts of exocrine glands.
- *Secretory simple columnar* mucus secreting cells are present in gastric mucosa.
- *Simple columnar epithelium with goblet cells* lines small and large intestines. The goblet cells are the modified simple columnar cells at places, for the purpose of secretion of mucus.
- Simple columnar epithelium showing surface modifications for increasing absorptive surface is found in small intestine, renal tubules and gall bladder. Each columnar cell shows numerous microvilli (Fig. 2.3D) at its apical surface. Ultramicroscopically, the microvilli are minute finger-like projections of plasma membrane. Under low power they appear as striated or brush border.

- Simple columnar epithelium with cilia (Fig. 2.3E) (ciliated columnar epithelium) lining the uterine tube and uterus serves the function of transport of gametes.
- ***Pseudostratified ciliated columnar epithelium*** (Fig. 2.3F) with goblet cells (also known as respiratory epithelium) lines the respiratory tract from nasal cavity to intrapulmonary bronchi. Here, all the cells rest on the basement membrane but the nuclei of the cells

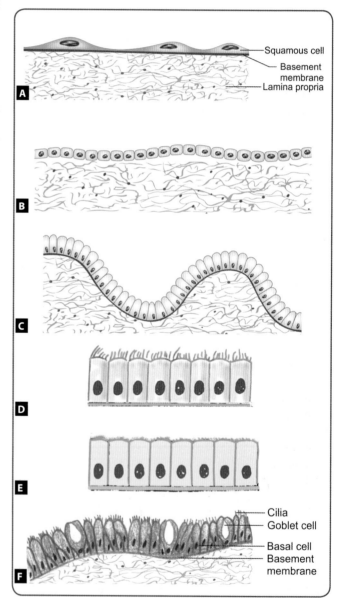

Figs 2.3A to F: Microscopic structure of **A.** Squamous epithelium; **B.** Cuboidal epithelium; **C.** Simple columnar epithelium; **D.** Columnar epithelium showing cilia; **E.** Columnar epithelium showing a striated border made up of microvilli; **F.** Pseudostratifed ciliated columnar epithelium

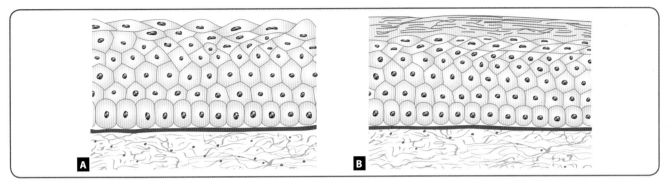

Figs 2.4A and B: Microscopic structure of stratifed squamous epithelium **A.** Non-keratinized; **B.** Keratinized

are at varying levels, thus creating false impression of stratification. This epithelium consists of shorter and taller cells. The taller cells bear cilia. The cilia dispel the foreign particles inhaled in the air towards nasal cavity and the mucus secreted by the goblet cells traps the foreign particles not dispelled by the cilia.

- ***Pseudostratified columnar epithelium*** with stereocilia (long, thick and non-motile microvilli) is found in vas deferens and epididymis, where the epithelium serves the functions of protection, absorption and secretion.

Stratified Epithelium

The stratified epithelium is multilayered where only the cells of basal layer rest on the basement membrane. It is divided into following types.

Stratified squamous non-keratinized epithelium (Fig. 2.4A)

- This epithelium is found in cornea, conjunctiva, oral mucosa, tongue, oropharynx, laryngopharynx, esophagus, ectocervix, vagina and male urethra inside the glans penis, etc.
- It forms the moist surfaces that are protective in function.
- It consists of multiple layers of cells of which superficial cells are flat (squamous) and basal cells are columnar. The intervening rows of cells are polyhedral. The basal cells are capable of mitosis to produce new cells. There is migration and gradual transformation of new cells into polyhedral cells and finally into flat cells, which are shed from the body periodically. The cells in all layers have nuclei.

Stratified squamous keratinized epithelium (Fig. 2.4B)

- This epithelium is found in epidermis of skin, lining of external auditory meatus, vestibule of nasal cavity, lining of the lowest part of anal canal, etc.

- It provides protection against abrasion, bacterial invasion and desiccation (drying).
- It is characterized by keratinization of superficial cells, which are dead and shed from the body surface. In the thick or glabrous skin of palms and soles, it is composed of five layers from basal to superficial aspect:
1. Stratum germinativum or basal layer with columnar cells having mitotic capacity.
2. Stratum spinosum of polygonal cells attached to each other by desmosomes.
3. Stratum granulosum of cells filled with keratohyalin granules.
4. Stratum lucidum, a layer with clear cells without distinct boundaries.
5. Stratum corneum having dead keratinized cells without nuclei.

Stratified cuboidal epithelium (Fig. 2.5A)

- This epithelium lines the ducts of sweat glands where it consists of two layers of cuboidal cells.
- The seminiferous epithelium in the testis is regarded as a special type of stratified cuboidal epithelium as a series of germ cells called ***spermatogonia***, ***primary spermatocytes***, ***secondary spermatocytes*** and ***spermatids*** are arranged from the basement membrane inwards.

Stratified columnar epithelium (Fig. 2.5B)

- This epithelium lines the spongy part of male urethra and the main ducts of large salivary glands and large ducts of mammary glands.
- There are several layers of columnar cells, which serve protective and secretory functions.

Transitional epithelium (Fig. 2.6)

This is a special type of epithelium lining the urinary passages. Hence it is called ***urothelium***.

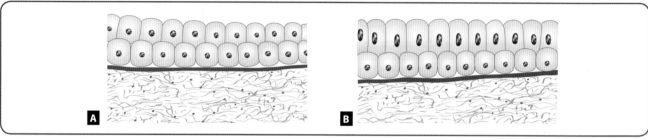

Figs 2.5A and B: Microscopic structure of **A.** Stratified cuboidal epithelium; **B.** Microscopic structure of stratified columnar epithelium

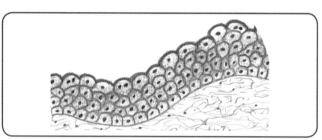

Fig. 2.6: Microscopic structure of transitional epithelium

It is found in renal calyces, renal pelvis, ureter, urinary bladder and proximal part of urethra.

It provides a permeability barrier to water and salts in urine.

When examined under light microscope it consists of:
- Cuboidal cells in basal layer, which are uninucleated and basophilic.
- Polygonal or rounded cells in middle layer.
- Large and facetted surface or umbrella cells (which are exposed to the urine).

Under electron microscope, the umbrella cells present modified plasma membrane on their luminal surface. Their apical cytoplasm contains microfilaments and fusiform membrane bound vesicles enclosing uroplakin plaques. In the distended state of the urinary bladder, the epithelium is stretched and the surface cells become flattened. The fusiform vesicles along with uroplakin plaques merge into the surface plasma membrane providing a reserve membrane during stretching.

 EMBRYOLOGIC INSIGHT

The epithelium is derived from endoderm, mesoderm and ectoderm as follows:
- **Endoderm forms:** The epithelium lining the gastrointestinal tract (with associated glands like liver and pancreas) and respiratory passages (and lung alveoli).
- **Mesoderm forms:** The endothelium lining blood vessels, mesothelium lining serous membranes, endocardium lining cardiac chambers, epithelium of kidney tubules and germinal epithelium of ovaries, etc.

Contd…

Contd…

 EMBRYOLOGIC INSIGHT

- **Ectoderm forms:** The epidermis of skin, oral mucosa, lining of ear canal and epithelium covering outer surface of tympanic membrane.

 STUDENT INTEREST

Basic tissues of the body are the foundation of **histology and pathology**. Epithelium is a layer or layers of cells resting on the basement membrane. Epithelium lines hollow organs like digestive tract, respiratory tract, genitourinary tracts, ducts, secretory units of exocrine glands, kidney tubules and external surface of the body like epidermis of the skin (to cite a few examples). Epithelia are divided in to simple and compound (or stratified). In simple epithelium, there is a single row of similar cells in which all cells rest on the basement membrane. In compound epithelium there are multiple layers of cells but only the cells of basal layer rest on the basement membrane. The cells of epithelium work in harmony for which they are connected to adjoining cells by junctional complexes. Do not forget to brush your knowledge of the junctional complexes, surface specializations and the basement membrane.

Glandular Epithelium

The glands may consist of a single cell or aggregations of epithelial cells specialized for secretory function. The endocrine glands release secretion (hormone) directly into blood capillaries. The exocrine glands consist of secretory units (which synthesize the secretion) and ducts (by which they let out their secretion).

Classification of Exocrine Glands (Flowchart 2.2)

According to number of cells:
- Unicellular (e.g. goblet cell)
- Multicellular (e.g. salivary glands, sweat glands, mammary glands, liver, pancreas, etc.). Subdivisions are shown in Figures 2.7A to F.

Flowchart 2.2: Classification of glands

```
                          ┌─────────┐
                          │ Glands  │
          Without ducts   └─────────┘   With ducts
      ┌─────────────┐                  ┌─────────┐
      │  Endocrine  │                  │ Exocrine│
      └─────────────┘                  └─────────┘
                            ┌──────────────┴──────────────┐
                      ┌─────────────┐              ┌──────────────┐
                      │ Unicellular │              │ Multicellular│
                      └─────────────┘              └──────────────┘
                      ┌─────────────┐
                      │ Goblet cell │
                      └─────────────┘
```

On the basis of number of ducts that drain the gland	On the basis of shape of the secretory unit	On the basis of nature of secretory product	On the basis of secretory mechanism
• Simple • Compound	• Tubular • Acinar • Alveolar	• Serous • Mucous • Mixed	• Merocrine • Apocrine • Holocrine

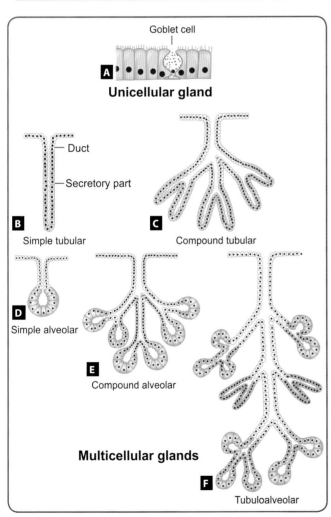

Goblet cell

A

Unicellular gland

— Duct

— Secretory part

B

Simple tubular

C

Compound tubular

D

Simple alveolar

E

Compound alveolar

Multicellular glands

F

Tubuloalveolar

Figs 2.7A To F: Scheme to show various ways in which the secretory elements of a gland may be organized **A.** Unicellular gland; **B.** to **D.** Multicellular glands with a single duct are simple glands; **E.** and **F.** Multicellular glands with branching duct system are compound glands

Subtypes of Multicellular Exocrine Glands

Depending on duct pattern:
- Simple, if one duct drains the gland.
- Compound, if there is branching pattern of the ducts.

Depending on the shape of the secretory units:
- Simple tubular or coiled tubular (when the secretory units are shaped like small tubes).
- Alveolar or acinar (if secretory units are shaped like small bags).
- Tubuloalveolar (combination of the above two shapes).

Depending on the type of secretion (Figs 2.8A to C):
- **Serous:** Watery fluid containing protein (examples; parotid and lacrimal glands).
- **Mucous:** Viscous secretion containing mucus (examples; esophageal glands, pyloric glands, sublingual salivary glands).
- **Mixed:** Example—submandibular salivary glands.
  Comparison of mucous and scours acini has been given in Table 2.2.

Note: Serous, mucous and mixed acini have distinctive histological features, which you have to draw in histology records.

Depending on the mode of their secretion (Figs 2.9A to C):
- **Merocrine (eccrine)** in which secretory product is expelled by exocytosis (e.g. sweat glands involved in thermoregulation and supplied by cholinergic sympathetic innervation) (Fig. 2.9A).
- **Apocrine** in which the secretory product accumulates in apical cytoplasm and is expelled by pinching of the apical plasma membrane (e.g. mammary gland and apocrine type of sweat glands that are active after puberty and are found in skin of axilla and around genital organ) (Fig. 2.9B).

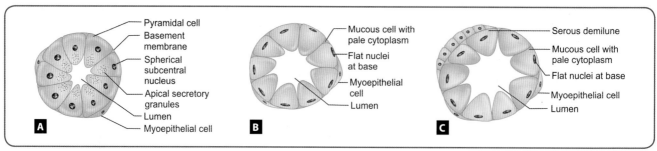

Figs 2.8A to C: Types of acini **A.** Serous; **B.** Mucous; **C.** Mixed

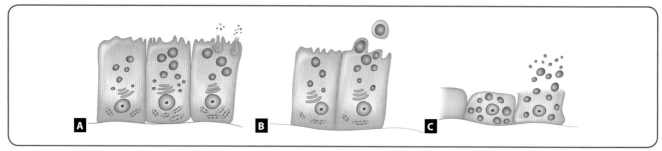

Figs 2.9A to C: Types of glands based on the manner in which their secretions are poured out of the cells **A.** Merocrine; **B.** Apocrine; **C.** Holocrine

Table 2.2: Comparison between serous and mucous acini	
Serous acini	**Mucous acini**
Triangular cells with rounded nucleus at the base. Cell boundaries are indistinct	Tall cells with flat nucleus at the base. Cell boundaries are distinct
Contain zymogen granules	Contain mucoid material
Darkly stained with H and E (because of the presence of zymogen granules, the color varies from pink to dark purple)	Lightly stained and appear empty with H and E
Thin watery secretion	Thick mucoid secretion
Example: Parotid gland	Example: Sublingual gland

- **Holocrine** in which the cell (after accumulation of secretory product) dies and is expelled along with its contents (e.g. sebaceous gland) (Fig. 2.9C).

CONNECTIVE TISSUE

The connective tissue serves the function of connecting and supporting the different basic tissues and organs of the body. It is widely distributed in the body. The impaired structure and function of the connective tissue is the cause of some disorders of connective tissue. In inflammation of any organ it is the connective tissue that acts as a battle ground for the fight between the infecting agents and immune cells in the connective tissue (macrophages, plasma cells, white blood corpuscles, etc.).

Basic Components

The connective tissue consists of the following three basic components (Fig. 2.10):
1. Connective tissue cells (both resident and wandering).
2. Intercellular material (or ground substance or matrix).
3. Fibers (collagen, elastic and reticular).

Cells of Connective Tissue (Fig. 2.11)

Connective tissue contains different types of cells with a wide spectrum of functions. The cells of connective tissue are divisible into two categories:
1. **Resident cells or fixed cells** arise from mesenchymal stem cells. Examples of resident cells are—fibroblasts, myofibroblasts, adipocytes and persistent mesenchymal stem cells.

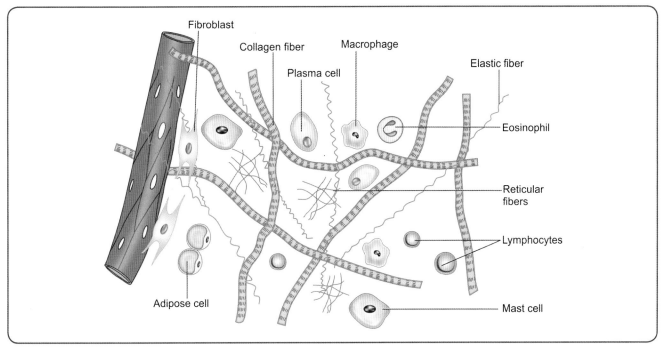

Fig. 2.10: Components of loose connective tissue

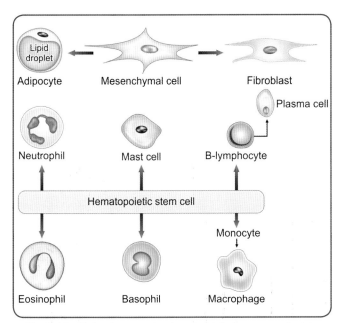

Fig. 2.11: Cells of connective tissue and their sources of origin

2. **Transient or wandering cells** arise from hemopoietic stem cells of bone marrow. Examples of transient cells are—macrophages, mast cells, plasma cells, monocytes, lymphocytes, eosinophils and neutrophils

(from blood circulation) in addition to pigment cells or melanocytes derived from neural crest.

Resident cells

- **Fibroblasts** are the most common type of cells in connective tissue. They are stellate or spindle-shaped cells with little cytoplasm. They are metabolically very active as they synthesize the connective tissue fibers and the ground substance. The electron microscopic appearance of fibroblasts reveals characteristics of protein secreting cells, like well developed rough endoplasmic reticulum, one or more Golgi zones and abundant mitochondria. Most abundant protein in the body is collagen and it is produced by fibroblasts. The surfaces of active fibroblasts show characteristic scalloping (coves). It is here that collagen fibrils are polymerized to form collagen fibers in the extracellular compartment. Figure 2.9 illustrates the steps in the process of intracellular synthesis of procollagen and extracellular formation and assembly of collagen fibers from tropocollagen.

- **Myofibroblasts** are special type of fibroblasts that possess properties of both fibroblast and smooth muscle cell. The myofibroblasts play a significant role in wound contraction during the process of healing.

- *Adipocytes* or *lipocytes* or *fat cells* are large in size (average size 50 microns). They store neutral fat (triglycerides) in the form of energy. Each cell contains a single lipid droplet in the cytoplasm. The lipid droplet is so large that it pushes the cytoplasm and the nucleus to the periphery. Thus, the cytoplasm is reduced to a rim containing cell organelles and a flattened nucleus. On routine staining the lipid droplet is dissolved. Therefore, the cell gives an empty appearance with a peripheral rim of stained cytoplasm containing a nucleus. This appearance is similar to the appearance of a signet ring.
- *Persistent mesenchymal stem cells* are capable of differentiating into fibroblasts, myofibroblasts and adipocytes of connective tissue.
- *Pigment cells* or *melanocytes* of connective tissue are found in dermis, choroid and iris of eyeball.

Migrant cells

- *Mast cells* are usually found in close relation to the blood capillaries. They are large in size. Their cytoplasm is filled with basophilic granules. The mast cell granules on staining, show metachromasia, i.e. they take up different color other than that of the color of the stain. For example, if stained with toluidine blue, the granules take up purple color. The granules contain histamine (vasoactive agent), heparin (anticoagulant) and eosinophilic chemotactic factor of anaphylaxis.
- *Macrophages* or *histiocytes* are part of the mononuclear phagocytic system (MPS) which develop from monocytes of the circulating blood. They are large cells with round nuclei and abundant acidophilic cytoplasm rich in lysosomes. They show irregular contours or ruffles of the plasma membrane. Their main function is phagocytosis by ingestion of foreign substances, cancer cells, worn out red blood cells, carbon particles in the lungs of heavy smokers, etc. Under pathological conditions several macrophages group around a large foreign body and may fuse together to form a multinuclear giant cell.
- *Plasma cells* or *plasmatocytes* are derived from B lymphocytes. They are responsible for production of antibodies (immunoglobulins) produced in response to penetration by antigens. The antibodies are generally released into the blood circulation but may be stored temporarily in the cytoplasm of the plasma cells as Russell bodies. The plasma cell is rounded with eccentrically placed nucleus which shows characteristic cart wheel or clock face appearance. This is due to radiating distribution of darkly stained heterochromatin (coiled inactive chromatin) alternating with empty spaces representing euchromatin (uncoiled active chromatin) in the periphery of the nucleus. The cytoplasm of plasma cells is highly basophilic due to abundant rough endoplasmic reticulum. The Golgi body appears pale on routine histological staining. This pale appearance is described as perinuclear halo or Golgi ghost or negative image of Golgi.
- *White blood cells* or *leukocytes* (B lymphocytes, T lymphocytes, neutrophils, basophils, eosinophils and monocytes) migrate to the connective tissue from blood capillaries by a process of diapedesis. They are found in large numbers during inflammation when they actively destroy the pathogens.

STUDENT INTEREST

Every student must know the three basic components of connective tissue (cells, fibers and matrix or ground substance). The structure and function of each cell of the connective tissue is a must know topic. Learn by drawing diagrams. Physical and chemical characters of three types of fibers (collagen, elastic and reticular) must be studied. Pay attention to the role of fibroblast in producing collagen and collagen fibers.

Intercellular material (Ground substance)

The connective tissue is composed of abundant ground substance. The connective tissue cells and fibers are embedded into it. The ground substance is amorphous and transparent. On light microscopy it is difficult to visualize the ground substance.

Chemically the ground substance is composed mainly of mucopolysaccharides or glycosaminoglycans (GAG) like hyaluronic acid, proteoglycans, etc. and structural glycoproteins or multiadhesive glycoproteins (like fibronectin, laminin, chondronectin, etc.).

The ground substance allows free exchange of nutrients and gases between the cells of the tissues and blood in the capillaries. Water or tissue fluid might accumulate in the ground substance in case of venous stasis or of lymphatic stasis causing edema.

Connective Tissue Fibers

The connective tissue fibers are of three types—collagen, elastic and reticular (Figs 2.12A to C).

Collagen Fibers

The collagen fibers are the white fibers of connective tissue. They are composed of the collagen, which is the most abundant structural protein in the body. They provide

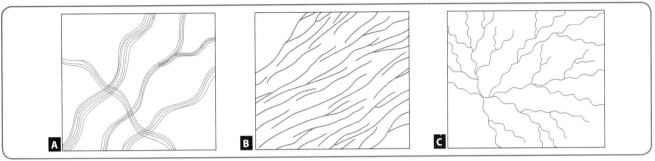

Figs 2.12A to C: Fibers of connective tissue **A.** Collagen fibers; **B.** Reticular fibers; **C.** Elastic fibers

tensile strength to the tissues. Their strength is comparable to that of steel cables. The collagen fibers aggregate into wavy bundles, which may branch. However, the individual fibers do not branch. They exhibit birefringence, which means when polarized light is thrown on the fibers the light is split into two beams that are refracted in two directions. The collagen fibers are secreted not only by fibroblasts but also by chondroblasts in cartilage, osteoblasts in bone and odontoblasts in teeth. The collagen fibers are visible on light microscopy. They appear pink on staining with eosin. However, the collagen fibrils (which make up the fibers) are visible only by electron microscopy.

 ADDED INFORMATION

Biosynthesis and Secretion of Collagen (Fig. 2.13)

The collagen is secreted by fibroblasts in connective tissue, by osteoblasts in bone, by chondroblasts in cartilage and by odontoblasts in tooth. The collagen is also secreted by non connective tissue cells like smooth muscle cells, Schwann cells and epithelial cells.

Intracellular Synthesis of Procollagen

- The proline, glycine and lysine form the alpha polypeptide chains, which reach the rough endoplasmic reticulum. Here the lysine and proline are hydroxylated for which vitamin C is an essential cofactor. The deficiency of vitamin C (scurvy) with resultant defective collagen leads to widespread effects like bleeding gums, loose teeth, weak bones and poor wound healing.
- The polypeptide chains coil around each other to form a triple helix except at the terminals where the chain remains uncoiled. This forms the soluble procollagen molecules.
- The packaging of procollagen molecules takes place in Golgi apparatus for transportation out of the cells.

Extracellular Synthesis of Collagen (Fig. 2.13)

- The soluble procollagen is converted into nonsoluble tropocollagen by cutting the uncoiled terminals.
- The tropocollagen molecules aggregate to form collagen fibrils, which are polymerized into collagen fibers on the surface coves.

CLINICAL CORRELATION

Genetic Disorders of Collagen Synthesis

Defective collagen encoding genes cause autoimmune disorders in which immune responses destroy the collagen fibers. Examples of autoimmune disorders are rheumatoid arthritis and osteogenesis imperfecta.

Types of collagen fibers

There are numerous types of collagen fibers that differ from each other genetically, immunologically and chemically. They are designated by Roman numerals according to their order of discovery. Type I, type II, type III and type IV fibers are very commonly seen. Type I fibers are found in fascia, tendons, ligaments, aponeuroses, capsules of glands, sclera, fibrocartilage, bone and dentin. Type II fibers are found in hyaline and elastic cartilages and cornea. Type III fibers are the reticular fibers which occur in spleen, lymph nodes etc. Type IV fibers are seen in basement membranes.

Elastic Fibers

The elastic fibers impart elasticity to the tissues. They are composed of an amorphous core of elastin surrounded by a glycoprotein named fibrillin. Unlike collagen fibers they do not form bundles. The individual fibers branch and anastomose. They are highly refractile when unstained and are yellow in color when fresh. The elastic fibers can be stretched like a rubber band. Relaxed elastic fibers do not show birefringence but stretched fibers are highly birefringent. They stain poorly with hematoxylin and eosin stains. They are produced by fibroblasts, epithelial cells and smooth muscle cells. The elastic fibers occur in loose areolar tissue, ligaments of joints, ligamenta flava, and ligamentum nuchae, dermis, and lung, and elastic cartilage, suspensory ligament of lens and as fenestrated membranes in elastic arteries.

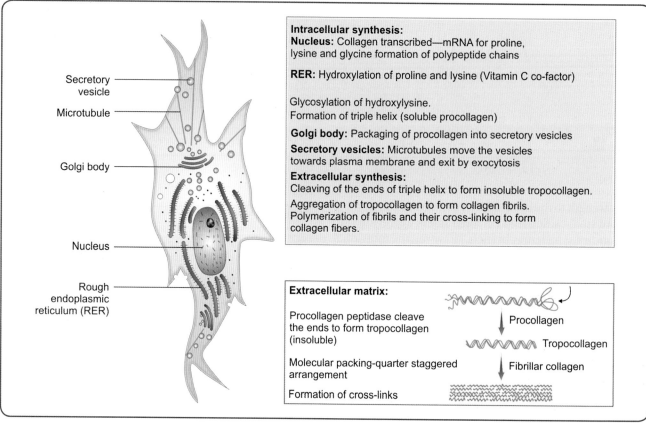

Fig. 2.13: Illustrates the steps in intracellular and extracellular synthesis of collagen by fibroblast

CLINICAL CORRELATION

Marfan's Syndrome
Marfan's syndrome results due to gene mutation causing defect in the production of elastic fibers (due to defective formation of fibrillin). The structures that are rich in elastic fibers (tunica media of aorta, suspensory ligaments of the lens in eyeball, periosteum and ligaments of the joints) are affected in Marfan's syndrome. The patients are liable to develop aortic aneurysm, lens dislocation, abnormally long limb bones and highly flexible joints.

Reticular Fibers

The reticular fibers are very thin and delicate type III collagen fibers. They are mainly produced by fibroblast but other cells like reticular cells in bone marrow and lymphoid tissues, smooth muscle cells and Schwann cells are also capable of producing them. The reticular fibers give support to the nerve fibers, muscle fibers, blood vessels and form stroma in the glands. The reticular fibers branch and anastomose to form a network or reticulum. They appear black when stained by silver stains. They are called *argyrophilic fibers* due to their affinity for silver stains. The reticular fibers provide supporting network in spleen, lymph nodes, thymus, bone marrow, endocrine and exocrine glands and liver. They are an integral part of the reticular lamina of basement membranes.

Classification of Connective Tissue Proper

- Loose or areolar connective tissue
- Dense connective tissue
- Yellow elastic tissue
- Reticular connective tissue
- Adipose tissue
- Myxomatous connective tissue (embryonic connective tissue).

Loose Connective Tissue

The loose connective tissue is rich in ground substance and poor in fibers and connective tissue cells. It is the most abundant connective as it forms the stroma of the organs and tunica adventitia of blood vessels. It lies underneath the epithelia forming lamina propria of mucous membranes and in submucosa of hollow organs.

Dense Connective Tissue

This type is composed predominantly of collagen fibers hence also called ***white fibrous tissue***. It is subdivided into two types, dense irregular and dense regular.

1. The dense irregular connective tissue (Fig. 2.14A) is characterized by collagen and elastic fibers (running in irregular orientation), few cells and moderate amount of ground substance. It is found in reticular layer of dermis, periosteum and perichondrium.
2. The dense regular connective tissue (Fig. 2.14B) is characterized by densely arranged fibers, fewer cells (mostly fibroblasts) and minimum ground substance. The collagen fibers are regularly oriented and are arranged in bundles. The regular dense connective tissue is found in tendons, ligaments, capsules, fasciae and aponeuroses. The tendons attach the muscle belly to the bone or cartilage. A tendon consists of parallel collagen fibers and fibroblasts. A longitudinal section of tendon consists of bundles of collagen fibers and parallel rows of elongated nuclei of fibroblasts that are compressed between collagen fibers.

Yellow Elastic Tissue

This type is composed predominantly of elastic fibers. The elastic tissue is found in ligamenta flava (which connect the laminae of adjacent vertebrae), cricovocal membrane of laryngeal skeleton, vocal ligaments, lung alveoli and in tunica media of the aorta.

Reticular Connective Tissue

The reticular tissue is a network of reticular fibers and reticular cells (subtype of fibroblasts). It provides a soft structural framework to support the cells of lymph nodes, spleen and bone marrow.

Adipose Tissue

The adipose or fatty tissue contains a collection of fat cells or adipocytes (Fig. 2.15). It provides warmth, cushioning effect and is also store house of energy reserve of the body. The adipose tissue is of two types. The white adipose tissue is found in adult and the brown adipose tissue is found in fetus and newborn.

1. ***White adipose cells*** (white adipocytes) are larger in size and are called ***unilocular*** because their cytoplasm is filled by a single large lipid droplet. The cell nucleus is flat and pushed by the lipid droplet to the periphery. The mitochondria are few in number and are dispersed in the peripheral rim of cytoplasm. The white fat is widely distributed in the subcutaneous tissue in the body in adults. In addition, it is found in yellow bone marrow and in abdominal cavity inside the peritoneal folds and around kidneys. It functions as store house of energy.

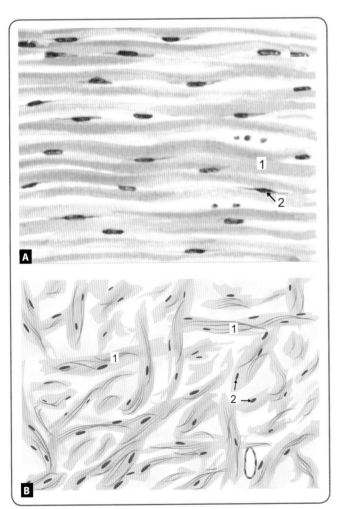

Figs 2.14A and B: Microscopic structure of **A.** Dense regular collagenous connective tissue (tendon); **B.** Dense irregular connective tissue (dermis of skin) **Key: 1.** Collagenous fibers **2.** Nuclei of fibroblast

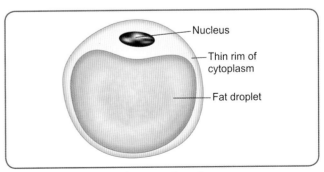

Fig. 2.15: Fat cell

2. **Brown adipose cells** (brown adipocytes) are small polygonal cells and are called **multilocular** because their cytoplasm is filled with multiple lipid droplets. The nucleus is in the cell center and cell organelles are spread out in the cytoplasm. There are numerous mitochondria, which contain large quantity of iron-containing pigments cytochromes (which impart brown color to adipocytes). The brown adipose tissue is more widely distributed in fetuses and newborn. In adult it is seen in the interscapular region and in the lumbar region behind the kidneys.

Myxomatous (Mucoid) Connective Tissue (Fig. 2.16)

This tissue is characterized by abundant ground substance, few cells and fewer fibers. In the fetus, it occurs as Wharton's jelly in the umbilical cord. The jelly like viscous ground substance is rich in hyaluronic acid. The fibers are hardly visible and fibroblasts assume star-shape, hence called **stellate cells**. The Wharton's jelly develops from extraembryonic mesoderm (primary mesoderm). In the adult, it is found in vitreous humor of eyeball.

MUSCULAR TISSUE

The muscular tissue is composed of elongated muscle cells called **myocytes** or **muscle fibers**. The muscle fibers are the basic units of the muscle. They aggregate to form a muscle. The main function of the muscle is contraction for performing mechanical work like locomotion, movements of hand, facial expressions, pumping action of heart and peristaltic movement of intestines to name

a few. The muscle fibers are equipped in their cytoplasm with contractile proteins called **actin** and **myosin**. These proteins are filamentous in nature and hence are called **myofilaments**.

Types of Muscle Tissue

There are three types of muscular tissue in the body that differ in distribution, microscopic structure and function:
1. Skeletal muscle
2. Cardiac muscle
3. Smooth muscle

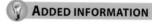 **ADDED INFORMATION**

There are other contractile cells in the body not belonging to muscular tissue but having actin and myosin filaments. They are myoepithelial cells, myofibroblasts and pericytes. The myoepithelial cells are found around the secretory units in salivary glands, mammary glands and sweat glands. The myofibroblasts are modified fibroblasts involved in wound healing. The pericytes are small fusiform cells around the capillaries and venules. They have the potential to differentiate into myofibroblasts and fibroblasts and can give rise to new blood vessels.

Skeletal Muscle

The skeletal muscles are so called because by and large they attach to the bones and cartilages. They are also known as striated because their cells show cross striations when examined under light microscope (Fig. 2.17). They

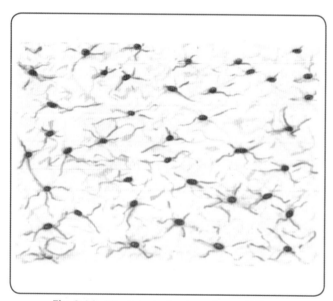

Fig. 2.16: Microscopic structure of mucoid tissue

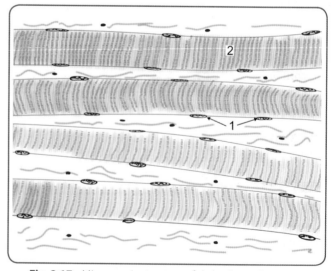

Fig. 2.17: Microscopic structure of skeletal muscle seen in longitudinal section **Key: 1.** Peripherally placed nuclei; **2.** Muscle fibers with transverse striations

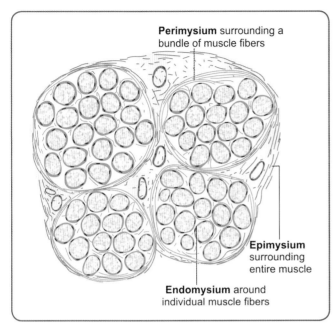

Fig. 2.18: Microscopic structure of connective tissue present in relation to skeletal muscle

are described as voluntary muscle as they contract under the influence of motor neurons of somatic nervous system and are supplied by axons of lower motor neurons (like neurons of ventral horn of spinal grey matter).

Organization of connective tissue framework in a skeletal muscle

The muscle fibers and their bundles are supported by a well defined connective tissue framework, which provides routes for the nerves and blood vessels to reach the individual muscle fiber (Fig. 2.18).

- Endomysium is a delicate connective tissue covering of each muscle fiber.
- Perimysium covers the muscle bundles or fascicles containing aggregations of muscle fibers.
- Epimysium is the common outer connective tissue covering of the all the muscle bundles.

Histology of Muscle Fiber (Fig. 2.19)

The muscle fiber is an elongated multinucleate syncytium. Its cytoplasm is called **sarcoplasm** and plasma membrane is called **sarcolemma**. The flattened nuclei are placed at the periphery and in a row parallel to the sarcolemma (Fig. 2.17). The sarcoplasm is filled with structural and functional subunits of muscle fibers called **myofibrils**, which are composed of bundles of thin actin and thick myosin filaments (the contractile proteins). The myofibrils are surrounded by special type of smooth endoplasmic reticulum (called **sarcoplasmic reticulum**) and the sarcoplasm contains mitochondria, glycogen and myoglobin (a red colored oxygen binding protein).

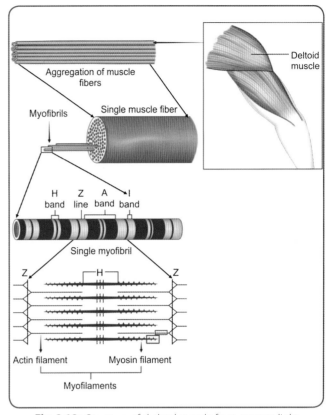

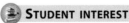

Fig. 2.19: Structure of skeletal muscle from gross to light microscopic and to ultramicroscopic levels at a glance

Cross striations

The characteristic cross striations of muscle fibers are due to presence of alternating light and dark bands (composed of above mentioned contractile proteins) arranged in regular pattern on the myofibrils. The dark bands are A (anisotropic) bands and the light bands are I (isotropic) bands. A bands show light area in the middle called **H band**, which is bisected by a transverse dark line called **M line**. I band is bisected by a thin dark line called **Z line**. A sarcomere is the segment of a myofibril between consecutive Z lines. It is the basic contractile unit of the striated muscle (Fig. 2.19).

🏛 STUDENT INTEREST

The skeletal muscle fiber is a single elongated multinucleate cell. It has very interesting features. It is covered by sarcolemma and its cytoplasm is called **sarcoplasm**, which contains several flattened nuclei (lying under the sarcolemma), sarcoplasmic reticulum, mitochondria, myoglobin, glycogen, etc. The myofibrils are the thread like contractile structures that fill the sarcoplasm. The dark or A bands and light or I bands of the myofibrils are in register. This is the reason why the muscle fiber appears striated. The light band is bisected by a dark line called **Z line** and dark band is bisected by a lighter H-band.

Contd...

Contd...

> The segment of the myofibril between two consecutive Z lines is called **sarcomere**, which is the basic contractile unit of striated muscle. On election microscope (EM) examination each myofibril is composed of actin and myosin filaments (which are called **myofilaments**) Actin and myosin are contractile proteins. Learn to draw a sarcomere. Easy trick to remember which band is A and which band is I: A is dark band (second letter in 'dark' is A and I is light band (second letter in 'light' is I).

Muscle triad

The electron microscope (EM) appearance of muscle fiber reveals that at A-I junctions of each myofibril there is a triad consisting of invaginated sarcolemma (T tubule) flanked on upper and lower sides by terminal cisternae of sarcoplasmic reticulum.

Functions of muscle triad

- T tubules carry the signals of depolarization from the surface sarcolemma into the deeper part of muscle fibers so that deeper and superficial myofibrils contract synchronously.
- T tubules transmit the wave of depolarization to membranes of terminal cisternae at triads. This triggers the release of calcium ions from the sarcoplasmic reticulum into the sarcoplasm. The calcium ions act on actin and myosin filaments causing contraction of muscle. When the contraction ceases, the released calcium is taken back inside the sarcoplasmic reticulum.

Nerve supply of skeletal muscle and motor unit

The nerve and the accompanying blood vessels supplying the skeletal muscle enter the muscle at a specific point called **neurovascular hilum**. For example, thoracodorsal nerve and thoracodorsal artery enter the neurovascular hilum on the latissimus dorsi muscle. The thoracodorsal nerve contains axons of anterior horn cells of C6, C7 and C8 segments of spinal cord, which supply the muscle fibers of latissimus dorsi via their numerous branches that pass through epimysium, perimysium and endomysium to reach the respective muscle fiber. From this we understand that one axon of anterior horn cell supplies several muscle fibers. One motor neuron and the muscle fibers supplied by it constitute one motor unit. The number of muscle fibers is smaller in motor units of muscles which are involved in fine and precise movements (for example in extraocular muscles, the ratio of motor neuron to muscle fiber is 1:4 to 10). Conversely, the number of muscle fibers is very large in motor units of muscles like latissimus dorsi and gastrocnemius, where force of contraction rather than precision is necessary.

> **Additional Features of Skeletal Muscles**
>
> - The arrangement of muscle fibers may be different according to the functional needs.
>   The pennate (comb-like) muscles are characterized by muscle fascicles that are disposed at an oblique angle to the line of contraction of the muscle. There are three types of pennate muscles.
>   1. In **unipennate muscle**, the tendon (or bone) lies on one side and muscle fibers run obliquely from it (extensor digitorum longus, flexor pollicis longus, lateral two lumbricals and palmar interossei).
>   2. In **bipennate muscle**, the tendon (or bone) lies in the center and muscle fibers reach it from either side obliquely (rectus femoris, soleus, medial two lumbricals and dorsal interossei).
>   3. In **multipennate muscle**, there are numerous tendinous septa that receive fibers from various directions as in acromial fibers of deltoid and in subscapularis.
> - Two types of muscle contraction (depending on movement of joint):
>   1. In **isometric contraction** there is no movement of a joint but there is increase in the tone of muscle. On lifting a heavy suitcase the flexor muscles contract without moving the elbow joint.
>   2. In **isotonic contraction** the same muscles shorten to hold a baby.
> - Depending on the actions of the muscles they are divided into following types:
>   - Prime mover is the main muscle that performs a particular action, for example, in flexed forearm the biceps brachii is the main supinator and in extended forearm the supinator muscle is the main supinator.
>   - Fixator is the muscle that contracts isometrically to stabilize the prime mover. The examples of fixator muscles are quadratus lumborum (which fixes the 12th rib during inspiration facilitating contraction of diaphragm) and rhomboid muscles fixing the scapula during overhead abduction of arm.
>   - Antagonist is the term used for a muscle that opposes the action of a prime mover as exemplified by contraction of triceps brachii (the extensor of elbow) during flexion movement of that joint.
>   - Synergist is the term used for a muscle, which helps other muscle (prime mover) in performing its stipulated action. The flexors and extensors of carpus (flexor carpi radialis and extensor carpi radialis) and extensor carpi radialis longus and brevis and extensor carpi ulnaris) contract simultaneously to stabilize the wrist joint when long flexor or extensor muscles of the digits contract.

Cardiac Muscle

The cardiac muscle is present in the heart, where it is called **myocardium**. It resembles skeletal muscle structurally in having cross striations. It resembles smooth muscle functionally in being involuntary. The contraction (beating of the heart) is initiated inherently by the pace maker located in the sinuatrial node. The contraction of cardiac muscle is not totally dependent on the nerve supply although the strength and rate of contraction are influenced by both sympathetic and parasympathetic nerves of autonomic nervous system.

Histology of Cardiac Muscle (Fig. 2.20)

The cardiac myocytes (muscle cells) are short uninucleated cells. The nuclei are centrally placed. The muscle cells are joined end-to-end at junctional specializations called **intercalated discs**, which are visible under light microscope as transverse dark lines arranged like steps in a staircase. In cardiac muscle, a muscle fiber is made up of a chain of myocytes (unlike in the skeletal muscle, where muscle fiber is a single cell). The cardiac muscle fibers are disposed parallel to each other. They branch and anastomose with myocytes of adjacent fibers. The branches are compactly arranged and have the same parallel orientation like the parent fiber. The cross striations of cardiac muscle are not very prominent. The cardiac muscle fibers show diads (combination of T tubule and terminal cistern of sarcoplasmic reticulum on one side only) at the level of Z discs (unlike the skeletal muscle fibers).

 ADDED INFORMATION

Electron Microscopy of Intercalated Disc (Fig. 2.21)

The intercalated discs are located between the ends of two contiguous myocytes. They have a transverse part (corresponding to the step of staircase) and a longitudinal part (corresponding to the connection between the two steps). At this site, the plasma membranes of the two myocytes are joined by macula adherens (desmosome) and gap junctions. The desmosomes are seen in the transverse part of the intercalated disc. They help to rapidly transmit force of contraction from one myocytes to another. The gap junctions are present in the longitudinal part of the disc. They provide electrical coupling of the cardiac myocytes to enable the cardiac muscle to function as physiological syncytium.

Smooth Muscle (Plain or Visceral Muscle)

The smooth muscle is non-striated and involuntary. It functions under the control of autonomic nerves. It is found in the walls of blood vessels, gastrointestinal tract, biliary tract, respiratory tract, urinary passages, genital ducts including uterus, muscles of eyeball, Muller's muscle in the upper eyelid, and dartos muscle in scrotum and arrector pili muscles of the skin.

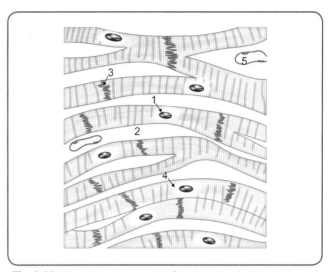

Fig. 2.20: Microscopic structure of cardiac muscle **Key: 1.** Central nucleus; **2.** Branching fibres; **3.** Intercalated disc; **4.** Perinuclear halo; **5.** Capillary

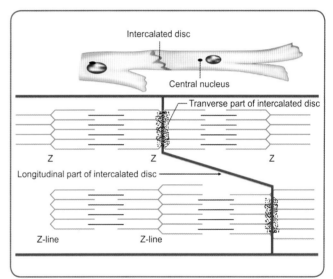

Fig. 2.21: Electron-microscopy appearance of intercalated disc in cardiac muscle fiber

Histology of Smooth Muscle (Fig. 2.22)

The smooth muscle fibers are elongated cells with broad central part and tapering ends. The muscle fibers show remarkable variation in length depending on the site. The oval or elongated nucleus is located in the central part of the cell. The acidophilic sarcoplasm contains myofibrils, which are responsible for the longitudinal striations seen under light microscope in addition to other cell organelles. There are no T tubules in smooth muscle fiber. A network of delicate reticular fibers envelops the muscle fibers to bind the cells to each other and the gap junctions join the neighboring cells to facilitate intercellular transmission of electric impulse (Fig. 2.10).

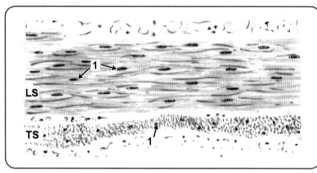

Fig. 2.22: Smooth muscle
Key: 1. Oval centrally placed nuclei

 ADDED INFORMATION

Regeneration of Muscular Tissue

The skeletal, cardiac and smooth muscles show difference in their capacity to regenerate after injury:
- The skeletal muscle fiber being multinucleate lacks capacity for mitosis. However the muscle fibers show limited capacity of regeneration due to presence of mesenchymal cells (satellite cells) in the their epimysium. The satellite cells act as reserve myoblasts.
- The cardiac muscle lacks both the satellite cells and the capacity for mitosis. Hence after myocardial infarction the damaged cardiac muscle is replaced by scar tissue.
- The smooth muscle cells are mononucleated and hence are capable of mitoses and active regeneration.

Basic differences between skeletal, cardiac and smooth muscle fibers are discussed in Table 2.3.

TABLE 2.3: Comparative features of skeletal, cardiac and smooth muscle fibers

Features	Skeletal	Cardiac	Smooth
Shape	Long cylindrical	Short cylindrical and branching	Spindle-shaped
Striations	Very prominent	Not so prominent	Absent
Nucleus	Multiple, flattened peripherally placed	Single, oval centrally placed	Single, oval, centrally placed
Intercalated disc	Absent	Present	Absent
T tubules and sarcoplasmic reticulum	Triads	Diads	Absent
Mitochondria	++	+++	+

NEURAL OR NERVOUS TISSUE

The neural tissue is composed of specialized cells called *neurons* which are supported by neuroglial cells. The neurons receive information from external and internal environment via the sensory fibers of the peripheral nerves. The information is processed and integrated in the central nervous system (CNS). The response or the command of the CNS is transmitted to the effector organs (muscle, glands, viscera, etc.) for desired effect. In this way the nervous tissue governs and coordinates the functions of all the organs of the body.

Subdivisions of Nervous System

- *Central nervous system (CNS)* includes brain and spinal cord.
- *Peripheral nervous system (PNS)* includes peripheral nerves (cranial and spinal nerves), sensory ganglia, autonomic ganglia and autonomic nerves.
- *Autonomic nervous system* (ANS) consists of sympathetic and parasympathetic parts which are further subdivided into central and peripheral. The ganglionated sympathetic chains (paravertebral in location) and the peripheral parasympathetic ganglia in the head and neck and in the viscera are part of peripheral autonomic nervous system.

Basic Components of Nervous Tissue

- Neuron or nerve cell consisting of cell body and neuronal processes (axons and dendrites).
- Neuroglia in CNS and Schwann and satellite cells in PNS.
- Synapses which are specialized junctions between two neurons.

The neurons are the structural and functional units of the nervous tissue. They are specialized for reception of stimuli, their integration and interpretation and lastly their transmission to other neurons, muscle cells and secretory cells. Neurons give off radiating processes from their cell bodies. These processes are of two types, dendrites and axons. The synapse is a site of close contact between two neurons for easy transmission of information from neuron to neuron. The neuroglia cells serve to support the neurons and their processes in CNS while Schwann cells and satellite cells serve similar function in PNS.

Classification of Neurons

According to the number of processes (Fig. 2.23):
- *Unipolar neurons:* It have a single process and are found only in early embryonic stage.

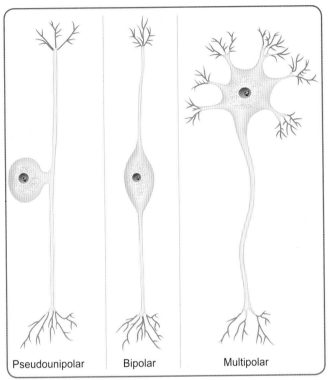

Fig. 2.23: Classification of neurons depending on the number of processes

- **Pseudounipolar neurons:** These neurons possess one very short process, which soon divides into a peripherally directed long process and a centrally directed short process. These neurons are found in sensory ganglia of dorsal roots of spinal nerves and cranial nerves. They are also known as dorsal root ganglia. The neurons of the mesencephalic nucleus of trigeminal nerve belong to this category.
- **Bipolar neurons:** These neurons have one dendrite and one axon. They are found in retina, olfactory epithelium and sensory ganglia of vestibular and cochlear nerves.
- **Multipolar neurons:** The neurons possess one long axon and multiple short dendrites. They are found in grey matter of central nervous system (spinal cord, cerebral and cerebellar cortex, intracerebral and intracerebellar nuclei in addition to cranial nerve nuclei in brainstem) and in autonomic ganglia.

According to the function of neurons:

- **Motor neurons** conduct impulses to skeletal muscles (neurons of ventral horn of spinal cord).
- **Sensory neurons** receive stimuli from external and internal environment.

According to the location of neuronal cell body:

- **Upper motor neurons (UMN):** These are the ones whose cell bodies are located in the motor area of cerebral cortex and their long axons become the corticospinal fibers. These fibers terminate on anterior horn cells of spinal cord at varying levels. The giant pyramidal cell of Betz is an example of UMN.
- **Lower motor neurons (LMN):** They belong to both CNS and PNS as their cell bodies are located in ventral horn of spinal cord and their axons leave the spinal cord as ventral roots, enter the spinal nerves and join the peripheral nerves to supply the skeletal muscles. Lower motor neurons are also present in brainstem in the motor nuclei of oculomotor, trochlear, trigeminal, abducent, facial, glossopharyngeal, accessory, vagus and hypoglossal nerves. The axons of these neurons leave the brainstem via the aforesaid cranial nerves, and supply the various skeletal muscles in head and neck.

According to the length of the axons:

- **Golgi type I:** These neurons have very long axons. They are called **projection neurons** as they carry impulse to distant sites. Examples are: pyramidal neurons of cerebral cortex and motor neurons of spinal cord.
- **Golgi type II:** These neurons have short axons. They are called **local circuit neurons** as they convey impulse to neighborhood neurons. Interneurons on spinal grey and cerebral gray are the examples.

Microscopic Structure of Neuron (Fig. 2.24)

The body of a neuron is called **perikaryon**. It contains a euchromatic (in which chromatin is uncoiled and active) and vesicular nucleus with prominent nucleolus. The area of cell body that gives origin to the axon is called **axon hillock.**

- The cytoplasm shows characteristic Nissl bodies (rough endoplasmic reticulum studded with ribosomes) (Fig. 2.18). The Nissl bodies are basophilic and are dispersed throughout the cytoplasm and in the dendrites but absent in axon hillock and axon. They are involved in protein synthesis. The absence of centriole is responsible for the inability of the neurons to divide. The neurons are arrested in G_0 phase of the cell cycle.
- Lysosomes are prominent feature of the cytoplasm. They contain hydrolytic enzymes necessary for phagocytosis. Aging neurons show cell inclusions, which are golden brown lipofuscin pigment (known as **wear and tear pigment**) derived from lysosomes.
- The cell bodies also contain microtubules and microfilaments (for internal support), neurofilaments, plenty of mitochondria and large Golgi complex.
- The dendrites are the cell processes that are close to cell body. They contain all the cytoplasmic contents of the cell body. They tend to branch and are capable of forming a dendritic tree for networking with processes of other neurons.

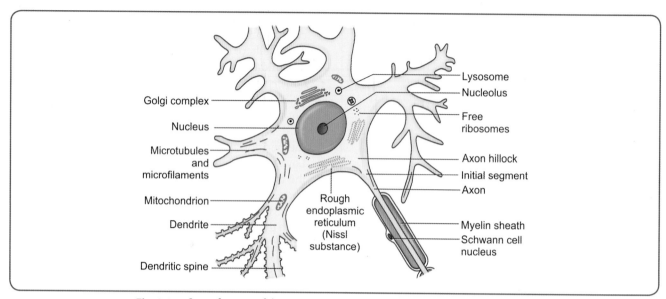

Fig. 2.24: Some features of the structure of a neuron as seen by electron microscope

- The axon arises from cell body at axon hillock and lacks Nissl bodies. The cytoplasm of axon is called *axoplasm* and its plasma membrane is called *axolemma*. Axons are either myelinated or nonmyelinated. The axons transmit action potential. They terminate by forming synapses with other neurons, muscle fibers and secretory units of exocrine glands.

Synapse

The interneuronal synapse is the specialized site of contact for cell-to-cell transmission of nerve impulse. It consists of three parts, the terminal bouton or presynaptic membrane of presynaptic neuron, synaptic cleft and postsynaptic membrane of postsynaptic neuron. The terminal bouton contains vesicles filled with neurotransmitter. The synaptic cleft is a narrow extracellular space between the two neurons. The synaptic vesicles release the neurotransmitter into the synaptic cleft. As soon as the neurotransmitter comes in contact with plasma membrane of postsynaptic neuron, action potential is generated by depolarization.

Neuroglia

The neuroglia cells are commonly called *glia* (*glia means glue*) cells. They are non-neuronal cells in CNS, where they outnumber the neuronal population. The glia cells are capable of mitotic cell division throughout life. The glia cells play a role equivalent to connective tissue in other organs of the body.

Neuroglia cells in CNS (Table 2.4)

- Oligodendrocytes (cells with few processes)
- Astrocytes (fibrous and protoplasmic types)
- Microglia
- Ependymal cells
- Retinoglial cells or Muller's cells

Neuroglia cells in PNS (Table 2.4)

- Schwann cells (neurolemmocytes or peripheral glia)
- Satellite cells (amphicytes or capsular gliocytes)

Myelination in PNS and CNS

The axons are either myelinated or nonmyelinated. The myelin sheath is formed outside the axolemma and is laid by Schwann cells in PNS (for example in the axons of sciatic nerve and of hypoglossal nerve) and by oligodendrocytes in CNS (for example in axons of optic nerve and of the white matter of brain and spinal cord). Unmyelinated axons are surrounded by Schwann cells(without deposition of myelin sheath) hence speed of impulse transmission is slow in them.

Myelination process by schwann cells (Fig. 2.25)

- The myelin sheath of a single long axon is provided by several Schwann cells lying along the length of an axon. The axon is engulfed along its length by several Schwann cells. The lipid rich plasma membranes of Schwann cells tightly wrap around the axon several times with

TABLE 2.4: Features of neuroglia cells in central nervous system (CNS) and peripheral nervous system (PNS)

Name	Origin	Location	Functions
Oligodendrocytes	Neural tube	CNS	Myelination of axons in CNS
Astrocytes	Neural tube	CNS	Regulation of ionic milieu of neurons in CNS
Ependymal cells	Neural tube	Lining ventricles and central canal of spinal cord	Production of cerebrospinal fluid (CSF) in ventricles
Microglia	Mesenchymal cells in bone marrow	CNS	Phagocytosis
Retinoglial cells (Muller's cells)	Optic vesicle from diencephalon	Retina	Support of retinal neurons
Schwann cells	Neural crest	Peripheral nerves in PNS	Myelination of peripheral nerves
Satellite cells	Neural crest	Around sensory and autonomic neurons in PNS	Insulation of neurons and maintaining their ionic milieu in PNS

the help of mesaxon (by which the axon is suspended from the plasma membrane surrounding it).

- Several concentric layers of plasma membrane and its lipid form the myelin sheath around the axon between the axolemma and the neurilemma or Schwann cell sheath. The myelin sheath shows areas of remnants of cytoplasm of Schwann cells called **Schmidt Lantermann clefts**.
- The myelin sheath is interrupted at regular intervals at nodes of Ranvier or nodal gaps that denote the limit of adjacent Schwann cells. The segment of myelin sheath between two nodes is called **internode** and this segment is myelinated by a single Schwann cell.
- The myelin sheath is necessary for insulation of nerve fibers so that nerve impulse can jump from node-to-node for faster conduction (saltatory conduction).

Myelination process by oligodendrocytes (Fig. 2.25)

The processes of oligodendrocytes wrap around parts of several axons to produce myelin sheath outside the axolemma. There is no neurilemma around the myelinated axons in CNS as the cell body of the oligodendrocytes is away from the axon unlike in the case of peripheral nerve which is wrapped by several Schwann cells.

Regeneration of Injured Axons

In PNS, for example in injury to ulnar nerve, axons regenerate due to close proximity of several Schwann cells. In CNS, for example in optic nerve, axons are incapable of regeneration.

 CLINICAL CORRELATION

Faulty Myelination
- **Guillain Barre-syndrome (GBS)** is a disorder in which the peripheral nerves lose their myelin sheath due to degeneration of Schwann cells. This results in slow transmission of nerve impulses causing muscle weakness and abnormal sensations starting in the legs and spreading towards arms and upper body.
- **Leprosy of Hensen's disease**: Schwann cells are attacked by lepra bacilli causing disruption of myelin sheath around the sensory nerves producing abnormal sensations initially and patches of sensory loss on the skin later.
- **Multiple sclerosis (MS)** is a disorder of brain and spinal cord caused due to degeneration of oligodendrocytes leading to demyelination of nerve fibers inside the white matter.

Tumors of Neuroglia
- Ependymoma is the tumor arising from ependymal cells.
- Astrocytoma is a tumor arising from astrocytes.
- Oligodendroglioma arises from oligodendrocytes.
- Schwannoma is the tumor arising from Schwann cells encircling nerve fibers in peripheral nerves.

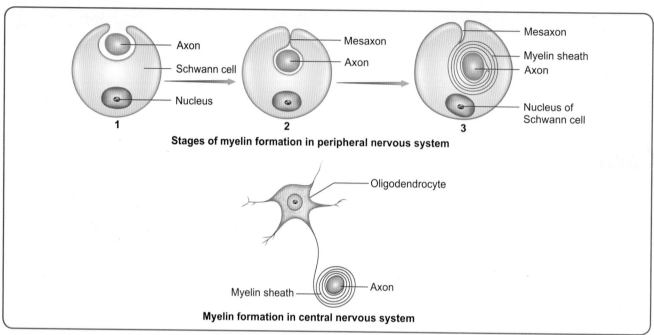

Fig. 2.25: Myelination of nerve fiber in peripheral nervous system by Schwann cells and myelination of nerve fiber in central nervous system by oligodendrocyte

STUDENT INTEREST

Neuron is a highly specialized cell, which is the structural and functional unit of the neural tissue. Types of neurons depending on the number of processes are pseudounipolar, bipolar and multipolar. Learn to draw these, and study the sites where they are located in the nervous system. Histological features of neurons must also be studied. Remember that nucleus of neuron presents '**an eye of an owl**' appearance (nucleus is large, spherical and vesicular with prominent nucleolus). Nissl bodies in the cytoplasm are basophilic clumps of rough endoplasmic reticulum. Axon conducts impulses away from the cell body but dendrites carry impulses towards the cell body. The axons are either short or long. Long axons form the nerve fibers of the peripheral nerves. The cytoplasm of axon is called **axoplasm** and its cell membrane is called **axolemma**. It contains all the organelles of neuronal cell body except Nissl bodies. Axons in central nervous system (CNS) are myelinated by oligodendrocytes and in peripheral nervous system (PNS) by Schwann cells.

Mature neurons are incapable of cell division. Axons in peripheral nerve like sciatic or ulnar nerve regenerate by activity of closely associated Schwann cells. Axons in CNS (like axons in optic nerve) are incapable of regeneration because there is no neurilemmal sheath around the axons.

3

Cartilage, Bones and Joints

Chapter Contents

CARTILAGE

The cartilage is a specialized or sclerous connective tissue in which the firm consistency of the extracellular matrix (fibers and ground substance) allows the cartilage to bear mechanical stresses without distorting its shape.

Components

Like the general connective tissue, the cartilage is composed of three basic elements:
1. *Cells:* Chondrocytes and chondroblasts
2. *Fibers:* Collagen or elastic
3. *Ground substance:* Sulfated glycosaminoglycans or chondroitin sulphate, proteoglycans and a large proportion of hyaluronic acid.

General Features

- *Perichondrium* is the outer covering of the cartilage. It is absent in articular cartilages covering the articular ends of the bones. The perichondrium is composed of two layers called *inner cellular* and *outer fibrous*. The inner cellular layer contains a row of undifferentiated perichondrial cells that have a potential to turn into chondroblasts if occasion demands. The outer fibrous layer contains dense irregular connective tissue and plenty of blood vessels and sensory nerves.
- The cartilage is avascular. The nourishment is provided by perichondrial blood vessels by a process of diffusion through the ground substance.
- The cartilage grows by interstitial and appositional processes. By appositional process new cartilage is added to the surface of old cartilage by the cells of perichondrium. By interstitial process new cartilage is added internally to the old cartilage by chondrocytes, which are inside the lacunae and which have retained their abilities to synthesize matrix and divide. Thus, appositional growth is called *surface growth* and interstitial growth is called *internal growth*.

Histological Types of Cartilage

- Hyaline cartilage
- Elastic cartilage
- Fibrocartilage

Hyaline Cartilage (Fig. 3.1)

The hyaline cartilage is the most commonly occurring cartilage in the body. It is found in the adults in nose, larynx (thyroid, cricoid and part of arytenoid cartilages), trachea, extrapulmonary bronchi, intrapulmonary

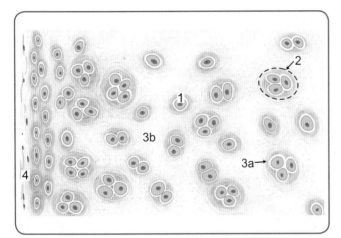

Fig. 3.1: Microscopic structure of hyaline cartilage
Key: 1. Chondrocyte; **2.** Cell nest; **3a.** Territorial matrix;
3b. Interterritorial matrix; **4.** Perichondrium

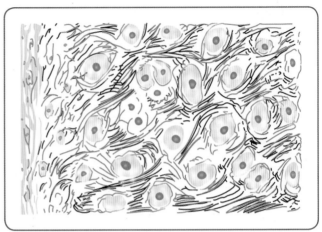

Fig. 3.2: Microscopic structure of elastic cartilage. Section stained by Verhoeff's method in which elastic fibers are stained bluish

bronchi, articular cartilages and costal cartilages. The hyaline cartilage has a tendency to calcify and ossify as age advances.

The hyaline cartilage appears transparent like a glass. It is covered with perichondrium. It contains homogeneous and highly basophilic matrix with collagen fibers (which are masked) and the chondrocytes.

Chondroblasts and chondrocytes

The inner cellular layer of perichondrium shows a layer of potential chondroblasts. These cells secrete the ground substance. Once the chondroblasts are surrounded by matrix they become mature chondrocytes. The unique feature of chondrocytes is that they retain the capacity to divide and continue to secrete the matrix. When chondrocytes divide they form groups of two or four chondrocytes which reside inside spaces called the *lacunae*.

Matrix of hyaline cartilage

The matrix of hyaline cartilage contains type II collagen fibers, which are masked by the ground substance. It is basophilic and exhibits metachromasia. The matrix is divisible into territorial and interterritorial parts according to the location and intensity of staining. The more basophilic territorial matrix surrounds the lacunae like a capsule. The less basophilic interterritorial matrix is found in between the lacunae.

Elastic Cartilage (Fig. 3.2)

The elastic cartilage occurs in the pinna of the ear, larynx (epiglottis, tips of arytenoid cartilages, corniculate and cuneiform cartilages) and cartilaginous part of the auditory tube. It appears yellow in color in fresh state due to the presence of abundant yellow elastic fibers in its matrix. The elastic fibers branch and anastomose to form a meshwork inside the matrix. The matrix also contains a few type II collagen fibers. The ground substance is basophilic and the chondrocytes are housed in lacunae either singly or in groups of two. The cells appear closely placed as intercellular ground substance is lesser than in the hyaline cartilage. Unlike the hyaline cartilage, elastic cartilage retains its histological characters throughout life because it does not undergo calcification and ossification with advancing age.

Fibrocartilage (Fig. 3.3)

The fibrocartilage is found in all secondary cartilaginous joints like symphysis pubis, manubriosternal joint

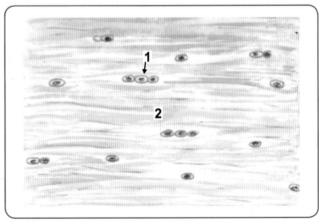

Fig. 3.3: Microscopic structure of fibrocartilage
Key: 1. Chondrocytes **2.** Ground tissue with collagen fibers

and intervertebral joints as an intraarticular plate of fibrocartilage joining the articulating bones. The intervertebral discs (joining the vertebral bodies) are composed of a ring shaped annulus fibrosus (which is a fibrocartilage) surrounding the inner nucleus pulposus (which is a gelatinous hygroscopic jelly). The fibrocartilages are also found inside some joints, for example as menisci of knee joint, articular disc of temporomandibular joint, joints of clavicle, inferior radioulnar joint and in labrum of hip and shoulder joints.

The fibrocartilage is called white fibrocartilage because of large proportion of collagen fibers and minimum ground substance in its matrix. The collagen fibers are type I and are arranged in large interlacing bundles. The chondrocytes are fewer in number and are seen as a single row between the adjacent bundles. The fibrocartilage lacks perichondrium.

🔬 CLINICAL CORRELATION

Osteoarthritis results when there is degeneration of articular cartilage (which lacks perichondrium and hence the capacity for regeneration). The degeneration of this cartilage causes difficulty in walking if weight bearing joints like hip and knee are affected. Incapacitation of joints of hand results in painful day to day activities (performed by hand).

BONE OR OSSEOUS TISSUE

The bone is the hardest and very strong connective tissue in the body. Paradoxically, it is a highly vascular and dynamic tissue in the body. The bone tissue undergoes a continuous turn over throughout life.

Components of Osseous Tissue

Like any other connective tissue, the bone consists of cells, matrix and fibers. However, the matrix of bone is mineralized so much so that bone is the body's storehouse of calcium and phosphorous.

Bone Cells (Figs 3.4A to C and Flowchart 3.1)

There are four types of cells in the bony tissue:
1. *Osteoprogenitor cells* are the least differentiated bone forming cells. They are present in the cellular layers of periosteum and endosteum. They are the stem cells of the bone since they turn into osteoblasts.
2. *Osteoblasts* are the bone forming cells. During bone development, they are seen on the periosteal surface and around interosseous blood vessels. Osteoblast is a round

Flowchart 3.1: Components of bone

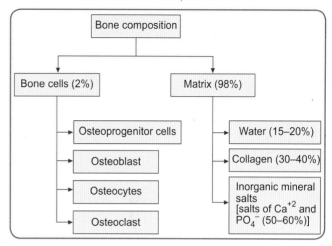

cell with single nucleus and highly basophilic cytoplasm. It is characterized by a well-developed rough endoplasmic reticulum, Golgi complex and mitochondria. It secretes type I collagen fibers and ground substance of bone matrix (osteoid). The osteoblast is rich in alkaline phosphatase, which is necessary during mineralization of the osteoid (Fig. 3.4A).

3. *Osteocytes* are mature form of osteoblasts. The cell bodies of these cells are trapped inside the lacunae within a bone and their protoplasmic processes extend into the canaliculi, which radiate from the lacunae. The processes of adjacent osteocytes meet each other inside canaliculi at gap junctions, which provide pathway for transport of nutrients (there are no blood vessels inside the lacunae and canaliculi). The osteocytes are metabolically active since they play a role in minimal secretion of bone matrix required for maintenance (Fig. 3.4B).

4. *Osteoclasts* are the macrophages of bone tissue and are derived from monocytes in blood circulation. They are largest in size among bone cells. They are multinucleated cells having lysosomes containing acid phosphatase. They are intensely eosinophilic due to plenty of lysosomes. A zone of peripheral cytoplasm and plasma membrane adjacent to their osseous surface is referred to as ruffled border. Multiple cytoplasmic processes and lysosomes are found along this border. This is to destroy the bone to create a depression in the bone, which is known as Howship's lacuna or resorption bay (in which the osteoclast resides). The activity of osteoclast is controlled by calcitonin (secreted by thyroid gland) and parathormone (secreted by parathyroid glands) (Fig. 3.4C).

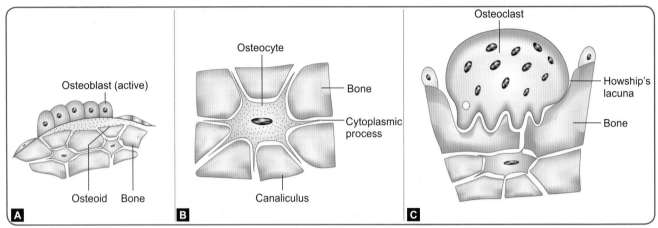

Figs 3.4A to C: Bone cells **A.** Osteoblast on bone surface; **B.** Osteocyte in lacuna; **C.** Osteoclast in Howship's lacuna

Bone Matrix

The matrix of the bone approximately consists of 15 to 20 percent water, 30 to 40 percent collagen, minimum proteoglycans and 50 to 60 percent inorganic mineral salts which are mainly the crystals of hydroxyapatite $Ca_{10}(PO4)_6 OH_2$. It is the calcium in the bone that makes it opaque in radiographs. The above proportions clearly indicate that bone is the largest store of body calcium.

Microscopic Structure of Bone

There are two types of bony tissue, spongy and compact depending on the bony architecture.

Structure of Spongy Bone (Cancellous Bone) (Fig. 3.5) Trabecular, cancellous

The bony lamellae are arranged as interconnecting rods and plates (bony trabeculae). There are spaces between the interconnecting bony tissues. These spaces are called **marrow cavities** as they are filled with red marrow. The bony lamellae contain collagen fibers. The osteocytes reside between lamellae in specialized lacunae. The processes of osteocytes pass through minute canals called

canaliculi, which originate from the lacunae and travel through the lamellae to connect with the cell processes of the neighboring lacunae. Spongy bone tissue is present in epiphyses of long bones. For example, in humerus it is present in head, greater and lesser tubercles at the upper end and in epicondyles, capitulum and trochlea at the lower end. Similarly spongy bone occurs in head, greater and lesser trochanters in upper end of femur and in the lower end of femur. All short, irregular bones (vertebrae), flat bones (sternum, scapulae) and skull bones contain spongy bone.

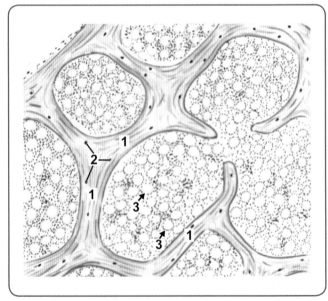

Fig. 3.5: Microscopic structure of cancellous bone
Key: 1. Trabeculae; **2.** Nuclei of osteocytes; **3.** Bone marrow

Structure of Compact Bone [Cortical/Dense]

The compact bone is found in the diaphysis of long bones. The pattern of lamellae in compact bone is quite unique. There are three different types of lamella in compact bone:
1. Haversian system or Osteon
2. Interstitial lamellae
3. Circumferential lamellae

Lamellae of haversian system or osteon (Fig. 3.6)

A single unit of Haversian system is called an *osteon*.

Composition of an osteon

- Haversian canal (containing capillaries, nerve fibers and areolar tissue) located in the center of osteon.
- Lamellae forming concentric rings of bony matrix around the Haversian canal.
- Lacunae containing cell bodies of osteocytes, in between the adjacent lamellae.
- Canaliculi containing processes of the cell bodies of osteocytes (radiating from the lacunae).

Note: Canaliculi connect the Haversian canal to all the lacunae in that osteon thus bringing the nourishment from the Haversian canal to all osteocytes via canalicular network. Volkmann's canals provide an additional source of blood supply and nerve supply to the compact bone. These canals carry blood vessels and nerves from periosteal and endosteal surfaces to the osteons. The Volkmann's canals are horizontally disposed and are not surrounded by concentric rings of lamellae.

Interstitial lamellae

These lamellae fill the gaps between the regular osteons of Haversian system.

Circumferential lamellae

The outer circumferential lamellae are arranged in parallel bundles deep to the periosteum, encircling the entire bone. The inner circumferential lamellae are likewise seen deep to endosteum surrounding the marrow cavity.

Periosteum (Fig. 3.7)

Periosteum is the outer covering of a bone. It is composed of two layers, outer fibrous and inner cellular. The fibrous layer is composed of dense irregular type of connective tissue. The cellular layer consists of osteoprogenitor cells. The periosteum has rich blood supply. A few of periosteal blood vessels enter the bone via Volkmann's canals. The outer layer of periosteum is very sensitive as it is richly innervated by somatic sensory nerves. The periosteum gives attachments to tendons and ligaments. The collagen fibers of the tendon occasionally enter the outer part of compact bone, where they are embedded in the matrix. Such extensions of collagen fibers from the tendons are called *Sharpey's fibers*. The periosteum performs several functions like nutrition and protection to the bony tissue. In the developing bone in both intramembranous and endochondral ossification, the osteoprogenitor cells in

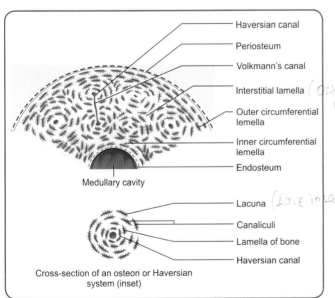

- Haversian canal
- Periosteum
- Volkmann's canal
- Interstitial lamella *(osteon old [fragment])*
- Outer circumferential lemella
- Inner circumferential lemella
- Endosteum

Medullary cavity

- Lacuna *(lace in [fragment])*
- Canaliculi
- Lamella of bone
- Haversian canal

Cross-section of an osteon or Haversian system (inset)

Fig. 3.6: Microscopic structure of compact bone in cross-section (Note the basic unit of Haversian system or osteon in the inset)

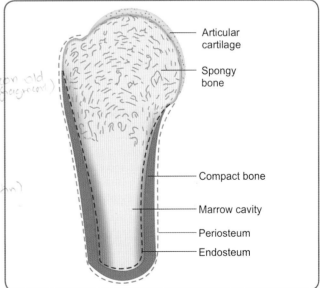

- Articular cartilage
- Spongy bone
- Compact bone
- Marrow cavity
- Periosteum
- Endosteum

Fig. 3.7: Longitudinal section of bone showing some features

the cellular layer of periosteum lay down subperiosteal bone. In well developed bone too these cells grow into osteoblasts (when bone is injured) to help in repair of bone by regeneration.

 CLINICAL CORRELATION

The cervical rib is an extra rib arising from seventh cervical vertebra. When present, it produces neurovascular symptoms by compressing brachial plexus and subclavian vessels. To relieve the symptoms a surgeon performs the surgical removal of cervical rib along with the periosteum. If the surgeon performs subperiosteal resection, the cervical rib will regenerate from the cellular layer of periosteum that is left behind and the patient will once again come back with the symptoms of cervical rib.

Endosteum

Endosteum is a highly vascular layer of loose connective tissue lining the medullary cavity in the long bones and marrow spaces in the spongy (cancellous) bones. It also lines the Haversian canals and Volkmann's canals. It is composed of a single very thin layer of flattened osteoprogenitor (osteogenic) cells. It plays a role in nutrition of osseous tissue and providing ready supply of new osteoblasts for repair and growth of bone. During bone surgeries like intramedullary nailing, care is taken not to injure the endosteum as its injury will not only jeopardize the reparative function of bone but also deprive the blood supply to the inner part of the cortex.

STUDENT INTEREST

Cross-section and longitudinal section of compact bone has to be studied to understand the microscopic structure of a bone. Basic unit of bone is Haversian system or osteon. At its center lies the Haversian canal containing vessels and nerves. Around the Haversian canal, there are concentric rings of bone tissue called *lamellae*. In between lamellae there are spaces called *lacunae* from which arise radiating canaliculi. The cell body of osteocyte lies in the lacuna and the cell processes of the osteocyte lie in the canaliculi. Through canaliculi cell processes of neighboring osteocytes communicate.

Development and Ossification of Bone

Embryologically, the bones develop from undifferentiated mesenchymal cells which have the ability to change into osteogenic cells either directly or indirectly via the cartilage cells.

- If a bone forms directly from osteogenic cells of the mesenchyme, the process of ossification is called *intramembranous*. The bones developed by intramembranous ossification are spongy bones. They are called *membrane bones*. Their examples are the bones of the face including mandible, the bones of the vault of the skull and clavicle.
- If a bone forms indirectly from osteogenic cells derived from the cartilage cells of the cartilage model of the developing bone, the process of ossification is called *endochondral* or *intracartilaginous* (for details of steps in ossification refer to histology texts). The bones developed by endochondral ossification are called *cartilage bones*. Their examples are ear ossicles, hyoid bone, long bones of limbs, vertebrae and bones of cranial base.

Growth in Diameter of a Bone

The bone grows in thickness by a process of appositional growth. In this process, the osteoblasts from cellular layer of periosteum deposit bone tissue under the periosteum. In the case of a long bone these is corresponding resorption of bone from endosteal side by the osteoclasts. The net result of these two diametrically opposite processes is increase in diameter without increase in width of compact bone. In this way bone can grow in thickness even after the growth in length stops (refer epiphyseal plate below).

 CLINICAL CORRELATION

Bone Diseases due to Nutritional Deficiency
- *Scurvy* (vitamin C deficiency) affects the synthesis of collagen in the bone as vitamin C is essential in this process. The osteoid is scanty and hence the bone tissue is thin.
- *Rickets* (vitamin D deficiency in children) affects the mineralization of osteoid. Vitamin D deficiency leads to poor absorption of calcium and in turn poor mineralization. There are widespread effects of poor mineralization on the skeleton.
- *Osteomalacia* is found in adults, who suffer from inadequate intake of vitamin D or of calcium.
- *Osteoporosis* is more common in postmenopausal women. When resorption of bone is more than formation of bone, the bone density is reduced and hence bones become fragile and prone to fracture due to slightest trauma.

Types of Bones

- *Long bones* are found in limbs. Their parts are similar to earlier mentioned parts of a developing long bone, except that they lack growth plate. They are composed of compact bone, are cartilage bones and contain medullary or marrow cavity. The only exception to this is the clavicle, which is the only long bone without marrow cavity, is a membrane bone and with two primary centers of ossification. In adults the yellow marrow fills medullary cavity and red marrow fills the epiphyses. The hemopoesis (production of erythrocytes, platelets, monocytes and granulocytes) takes place in red marrow. So hemopoesis takes place only in the ends of long bones in adults. There is one subtype of long bones called short long bones like metacarpals, metatarsals and phalanges. These bones have epiphysis at one end only unlike the long bones, which have epiphyses at both ends.

- **Short bones** are seen in hands and feet. The examples in the hand are the carpal bones (scaphoid, lunate, triquetral, pisiform in proximal row and trapezium, trapezoid, capitate and hamate in distal row). The examples in foot are the tarsal bones (talus, calcaneus, cuboid, navicular and three cuneiform bones). They are composed of spongy bone. So hemopoesis occurs throughout life in them. They are covered with periosteum like the long bones and their articular surfaces are covered with articular hyaline cartilages.
- **Flat bones** are seen in bones of the vault of skull, namely frontal bone, parietal bones and occipital bone. Scapula, sternum and ribs are the other examples. The peculiarity of flat bones of skull is that they show sandwich like arrangement of structure. There are two thin plates or tables of compact bone enclosing a space called diploe, which contains red hemopoetic marrow and diploic veins in spongy bone. The diploic veins open into adjacent dural venous sinuses.
- **Irregular bones** are the ones that have complex and atypical shapes. The examples are hip bones, vertebrae, temporal bone, sphenoid, ethmoid, maxilla, etc. The vertebrae and the hip bones are the sites of hemopoiesis.
- **Sesamoid bones** are like sesame seeds and develop in the tendons of some muscles. They are devoid of medullary cavity and periosteum. The largest sesamoid bone is the patella, which develops in tendon of quadriceps femoris muscle. A smaller sesamoid bone found in lateral head of gastrocnemius is called fabella. The pisiform bone develops in the tendon of flexor carpi ulnaris. Each of the two heads of flexor hallucis brevis contains a separate sesamoid bone.
- **Pneumatic bones** are flat or irregular bones containing a large cavity filled with atmospheric air. The bones containing paranasal air sinuses inside them are maxilla, ethmoid, frontal and sphenoid. The temporal bone houses air containing cavities like middle ear, mastoid antrum and mastoid air cells.

Structure of Long Bone

The long bone consists of three parts—diaphysis, metaphysis and epiphysis (Fig. 3.8). A tubular cavity called **marrow cavity** (containing red marrow) passes through the diaphysis. It is lined by a cellular layer called **endosteum**. It is covered by periosteum.

The developing long bone consists of four parts, diaphysis, metaphysis, epiphyseal plate or growth cartilage and epiphysis.

Diaphysis

The diaphysis is the shaft of a long bone. It is the first part to ossify. The primary center of ossification appears before birth in the cartilage model of the bone in the center of diaphysis (between sixth and eighth weeks of intrauterine life). The diaphysis is composed of compact bone.

Metaphysis

The metaphysis is the funnel-shaped region at either end of the diaphysis. It intervenes between the growth cartilage and the diaphysis. It is the most vascular part of the developing bone as newly formed spongy bone from ossification zone of growth cartilage is laid down here. There is an anastomotic arterial ring surrounding the metaphysis. Because of its high vascularity and stasis of blood at this site due to looping arterioles, the metaphysis is the common site of osteomyelitis in growing children.

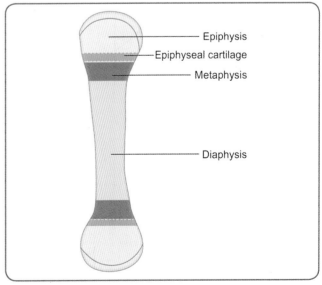

Fig. 3.8: Parts of long bone

Epiphyseal Plate or Growth Plate

The epiphyseal plate or growth cartilage is a thin plate of cartilage located between the metaphysis and epiphysis at either end. This is a region of great activity as it is responsible for linear growth in bone.

Five zones of epiphyseal plate (Fig. 3.9)

- Zone of resting cartilage closest to epiphysis
- Zone of proliferation
- Zone of hypertrophy
- Zone of calcification
- Zone of ossification

When full height is achieved the cartilaginous epiphyseal plate turns into bone. The time of closure of the epiphysis varies for different bones and for the two ends of the same bone. After closure the peripheral margin of the epiphyseal plate is indicated by epiphyseal line of the bone.

Epiphysis

The epiphysis is the upper and lower end of a long bone. However, in case of short-long bones (metacarpals, metatarsals, phalanges and in case of the ribs) there is epiphysis at one end only. The epiphyses are cartilaginous until secondary centers of ossification appear in them after birth (lower end of femur is the only exception where secondary center appears just before birth or at term). Thus, epiphysis is defined as part of bone that develops from secondary centre of ossification. It contains spongy bone and red marrow throughout life. The articular surface of the epiphysis is covered with articular cartilage (which is hyaline type but without perichondrium).

Types of epiphyses

- ***Pressure epiphysis*** develops at the articulating ends of long bones. The examples are head of femur, head of humerus and capitulum and trochlea at lower end of humerus.
- ***Traction epiphysis*** develops at the line of muscular pull. The examples are greater and lesser trochanters in femur, greater, lesser tubercles in humerus, medial and lateral epicondyles of humerus, etc.
- ***Atavistic epiphysis*** is present as a separate bone in lower animals but in human skeleton it fuses with other bone. The example in human is coracoid process of scapula and posterior tubercle of talus (called os trigonum).

Growing End of Long Bone and Rule of Ossification

The growing end of the long bone is determined by the rule of ossification in which the epiphysis where the center of ossification appears first unites with the shaft (diaphysis) first.

- In ***upper limb***, the upper end of humerus and lower ends of radius and ulna are the growing ends.
- In ***lower limb***, the lower end of femur and upper ends of tibia and fibula are the growing ends. However the fibula breaks the rule of ossification as the center of ossification appears first in lower end but fuses first.

Generally, the epiphyses of limb bones fuse with the shaft by the age of 18 to 20 years in males and two years earlier in females. Therefore, after the epiphyseal fusion in long bones persons do not grow in height.

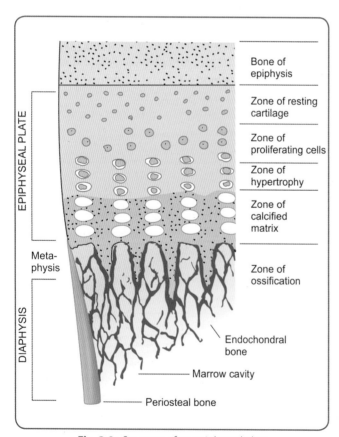

Fig. 3.9: Structure of an epiphyseal plate

EPIPHYSEAL PLATE

DIAPHYSIS

Bone of epiphysis

Zone of resting cartilage

Zone of proliferating cells

Zone of hypertrophy

Zone of calcified matrix

Zone of ossification

Meta-physis

Endochondral bone

Marrow cavity

Periosteal bone

CLINICAL CORRELATION

Disorders of Epiphyseal Plate

Since epiphyseal plates are present until the growth in length of long bones stops its disorders can occur only in pediatric age group and teenagers. Traumatic injury to epiphyseal plate can lead to shortening of the limb. There can be excessive length of the limb if the vascularity of the plate is increased due to inflammation.

You must know the definition of diaphysis, metaphysis and epiphysis in a long bone. You also must know the three basic types of epiphyses (traction, pressure and atavistic) with examples. In a developing long bone, there is growth cartilage or epiphyseal plate at both ends between the metaphysis and epiphysis. The epiphyseal plate or growth cartilage is temporary in existence as it is a place where growth in height takes place. After the specific height is achieved the growth cartilage turns into bone and individual no longer grows in height.

Blood Supply of Long Bone (Fig. 3.10)

The long bone is richly supplied with blood from four sources. These arteries anastomose with each other at the metaphysis. Hence, metaphysis is the most vascular part of a long bone.

1. *Nutrient artery* is the primary source. It enters the shaft via a nutrient foramen. Inside the bone it travels in nutrient canal to enter the medullary cavity where it terminates into the ascending and descending branches (which remain in contact with the endosteum). These branches supply medullary branches inwards and cortical branches outwards to the inner two-third of the shaft. In intramedullary nailing of long bones these arteries are vulnerable to injury. The ascending and descending branches run to the level of metaphysis, where they anastomose with epiphyseal and metaphyseal arteries. The nutrient foramen is located on the surface of the bone. Its direction indicates the direction of course of the nutrient artery inside the nutrient canal. The artery runs opposite to that of the growing end of a long bone. It is described by the following dictum in the case of limbs–"*Towards the elbow I run and away from the knee I flee*". The direction of nutrient foramen helps in identifying the growing end of a long bone.

2. *Numerous periosteal arteries* arise from the muscular arteries of the attached muscles. Therefore, bones like tibia and femur, which give attachments to large number of muscles, receive rich supply from the periosteal arteries. These arteries supply approximately the outer third of the bone.

3. *Metaphyseal arteries* (juxta-epiphyseal arteries) arise from the arterial anastomosis around the adjacent joint and enter through numerous vascular foramina located on the articular ends of the bones.

4. *Epiphyseal arteries* are the branches of arterial anastomosis around the adjacent joint.

Blood supply of long bone is a "Must Know" topic.

JOINS

The joints are known as *arthroses*. Broadly, the joints are grouped into two types—*synarthroses* and *diarthroses*.

1. *Synarthroses* or *immovable joints* are immovable as the articulating bones are united by solid bonds of special connective tissue.

2. *Diarthroses* or *synovial joints* are movable and have a cavity within them.

Synarthroses (Immovable Joints)

There are two types of synarthroses (immovable joints):

1. *Fibrous joints* in which the connecting bond is connective tissue.

2. *Cartilaginous joints* in which the connecting bond is a plate of cartilage.

Fibrous Joints (Figs 3.11A to C)

There are three types of fibrous joints—suture, syndesmosis and gomphosis.

1. The *suture* is the most common type. The flat cranial bones unite by sutural ligaments. The types of sutures are serrate, denticulate, plane, squamous and schindylesis (or wedge and groove). The only example of schindylesis is the joint between vomer and rostrum of sphenoid.

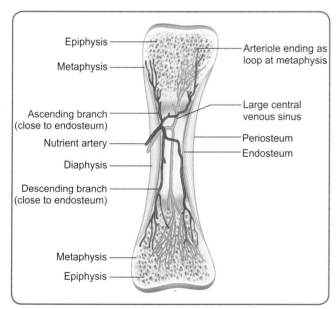

Epiphysis

Metaphysis

Ascending branch (close to endosteum)

Nutrient artery

Diaphysis

Descending branch (close to endosteum)

Metaphysis

Epiphysis

Arteriole ending as loop at metaphysis

Large central venous sinus

Periosteum

Endosteum

Fig. 3.10: Blood supply of a developing long bone

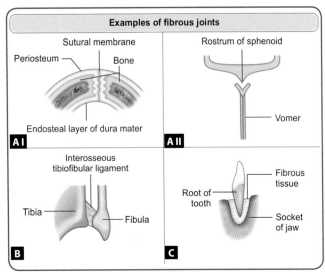

Figs 3.11A to C: Subtypes of fibrous joints **A.** Suture; **AI.** Serrate type of suture; **AII.** Wedge and groove suture or schindylesis; **B.** Syndesmosis; and **C.** Gomphosis

2. *Syndesmosis* is the fibrous joint in which the articulating bones are united by interosseous membrane or ligament, for example, inferior tibiofibular joint, middle radioulnar joint and middle tibiofibular joint (Fig. 3.11B).
3. *Gomphosis* is a peg and socket type of fibrous joint seen between the teeth and alveolar sockets (Fig. 3.11C).

Cartilaginous Joints (Figs 3.12A and B)

There are two types of cartilaginous joints—*synchondroses* and *symphyses*.

1. In *synchondroses* or *primary cartilaginous joints*, the articulating bones are joined by hyaline cartilage. The primary function of these joints is growth. Once

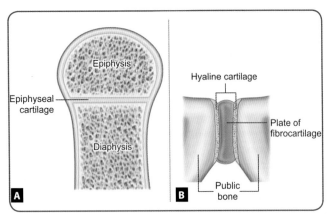

Figs 3.12A and B: Subtypes of cartilaginous joints **A**. Primary cartilaginous joint or synchondrosis; **B.** Secondary cartilaginous joint or symphysis

the growth is achieved the synchondroses turn into synostoses. Hence synchondroses are temporary joints. The best examples of this variety are, joint between diaphysis and epiphysis of long bones and the joint between basisphenoid and basiocciput at the base of the skull. The first costosternal or chondrosternal joint is also included in this category.

2. In *symphyses* or *secondary cartilaginous joints*, the articulating bones are united by fibrocartilaginous plate. These joints are midline in location in the body and are permanent. The joints between vertebral bodies (connected by intervertebral discs), symphysis pubis (joint between two pubic parts of hip bones joined by a plate fibrocartilage), manubriosternal joint, and lumbosacral joint and sacrococcygeal joint are the examples of secondary cartilaginous joints.

Diarthroses (Synovial Joints) (Figs 3.13A to F)

Types of synovial joints are described as below:

- *Plane joints* (Fig. 3.13A) are between the flat surfaces of articulating bones (examples—intercarpal joints, intertarsal joints, facet joints of vertebrae and sacroiliac joints).
- *Hinge joint* (Fig. 3.13B) allows movements around transverse axis (examples—elbow joint, ankle joint and interphalangeal joints).
- *Pivot joint* (Fig. 3.13C) allows rotation movements along a vertical axis (examples—superior radioulnar joint and median atlanto-axial joint).
- *Bicondylar* or *condylar joints* (Fig. 3.13D) allow conjunct and adjunct rotations (examples—temporomandibular joint and knee joint).
- *Ellipsoidal joints* are biaxial joints (examples—wrist joint and the metacarpophalangeal joints).
- *Saddle* or *sellar joint* (Fig. 3.13E) is biaxial. Its articulating surfaces are reciprocally concavo-convex (example—the first carpometacarpal joint or trapeziometacarpal joint of thumb).
- *Ball and socket type of joints* (Fig. 3.13F) are freely mobile as they are multiaxial (examples—hip joint, shoulder joint, talocalcaneonavicular joint and incudostapedial joint inside middle ear).

Basic Structure of Synovial Joints (Figs 3.14A and B)

- Articulating ends of the bones taking part in the synovial joints are enclosed in a fibrous capsule.
- The articular surfaces of the bones are lined by articular cartilage. Histologically the articular cartilage is a thin layer of hyaline cartilage covering the epiphysis where bone takes part in a joint. The articular cartilage is

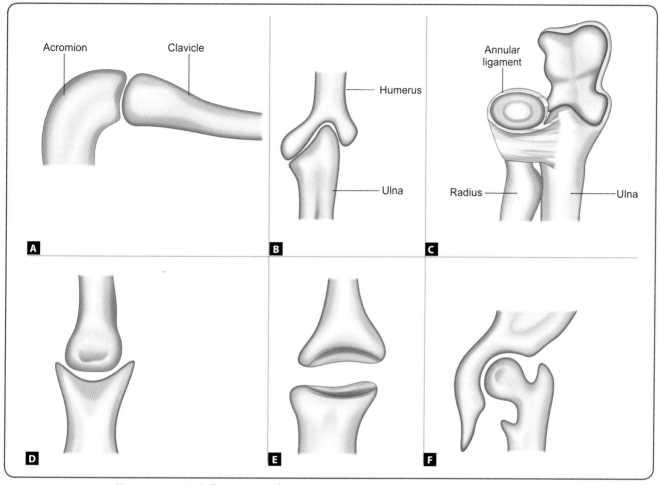

Figs 3.13A to F: Different types of synovial joints **A.** Plane joint; **B.** Hinge joint; **C.** Pivot joint; **D.** Condyloid joint; **E.** Saddle joint; **F.** Ball and socket joint

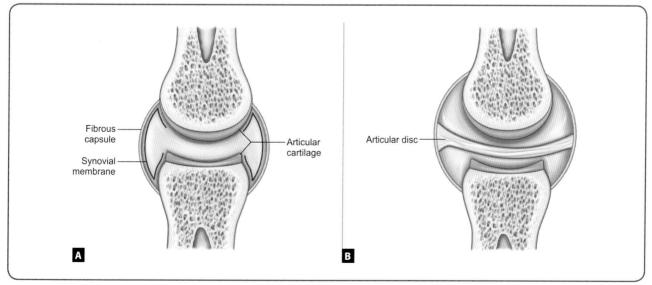

Figs 3.14A and B: Basic structure of synovial joints **A.** Features of synovial joint; **B.** Articular disc inside the synovial joint

devoid of perichondrium (because of which it lacks nerve supply and capacity to regenerate). Its only nutritional source is synovial fluid. Degeneration of the articular cartilage as age advances is the root cause of osteoarthritis.

- The internal surface of the fibrous capsule and the non-articular parts of articulating bones inside the capsule are lined by synovial membrane.
- The joint cavity is filled with synovial fluid, which is secreted by synovial membrane. The synovial fluid is of the consistency of egg white. It is a lubricant and provides nutrition to articular cartilages.
- In some joint, fibrocartilaginous articular discs may be present and the fibrous capsule of the joint is strengthened by ligaments.
- The synovial joints allow free movements.

Movements of Synovial Joints (Fig. 3.15)

The following movements take place in the various synovial joints of the body.

Flexion and extension

The flexion indicates bending or decreasing the angle between the two articulating bones of the joints. In flexion of elbow joint, ventral surfaces of arm and forearm approximate. On the contrary in case of knee joint, the dorsal surfaces of leg and thigh approximate during flexion.

The extension indicates straightening or increasing the angle between two articulating bones. In elbow extension forearm and arm align in straight line. Similarly, in knee extension the lower limb becomes a straight pillar.

Abduction and adduction (Fig. 3.15)

The abduction means a moving away from the median plane in a coronal plane. For example, moving upper limb away from the side of the body is abduction at shoulder joint.

The adduction means moving towards the median plane in a coronal plane. For example, moving the upper limb towards the side of the body is adduction at shoulder joint.

Lateral and medial rotation (Fig. 3.15)

In rotation movement the bone moves around itself along its longitudinal axis.

The medial rotation or internal rotation turns the anterior surface of the bone towards median lane.

The lateral rotation or external rotation turns the anterior surface of the bone away from median plane.

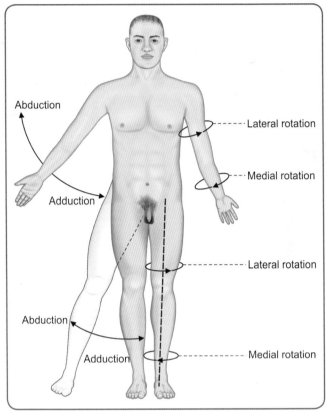

Fig. 3.15: Various movements of synovial joints

Supination and pronation (Fig. 3.16A)

The supination is the movement of forearm by rotating the radius along a longitudinal axis so that the hand faces anteriorly.

The pronation is the movement of forearm by rotating the radius along a longitudinal axis so that the dorsum of hand faces anteriorly.

Opposition and reposition (Fig. 3.16B)

In opposition the tip of thumb is brought in contact with the tip or base of the other finger.

In reposition the opposed thumb is brought back to resting position.

Dorsiflexion and plantarflexion (Fig. 3.16C)

In dorsiflexion, the ankle joint turns the dorsum upwards so that it faces the anterior surface of leg. In this movement one can walk on ones heel.

In plantarflexion, the ankle joint turns the dorsum of foot inferiorly so that the sole faces posteriorly. In this movement one can walk on ones toes.

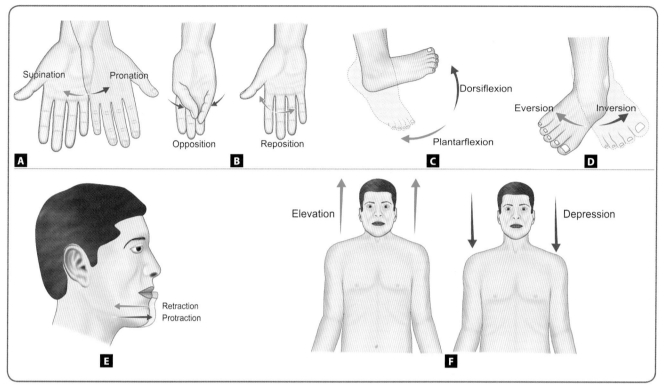

Figs 3.16A to F: Movements synonial joints **A.** Supination-pronation; **B.** Opposition-reposition; **C.** Dorsiflexion-plantarflexion; **D.** Eversion-inversion; **E.** Retraction-protraction; **F.** Elevation-depression

Inversion and eversion (Fig. 3.16D)

In inversion, the lateral margin of the foot is raised so that the sole faces medially. A fully inverted foot is automatically plantarflexed.

In eversion, the medial margin of foot is raised so that the sole faces laterally. A fully everted foot is automatically dorsiflexed.

Protraction and retraction (Fig. 3.16E)

In protraction, the bone moves anteriorly (as forward movement of mandible or scapula).

In retraction, the bone moves posteriorly (as backward movement of mandible or of scapula).

Elevation and depression (Fig. 3.16F)

In elevation, the part moves upwards as in elevating the scapula in shrugging of shoulders.

In depression, the part moves downwards as in depressing the scapula while standing at ease.

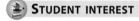 **STUDENT INTEREST**

Classification of joints is a "Must Know" topic.

4

Vascular Tissue and Lymphatic Tissue

Chapter Contents

VASCULAR TISSUE

The cardiovascular or circulatory system consists of heart, the arteries, capillary beds (surrounding the tissues) and the veins.

The heart is mainly composed of cardiac muscle (myocardium) and is lined internally by *endocardium* and covered externally by *epicardium* or visceral pericardium. The endocardium of heart is continuous with endothelium lining the blood vessels that arise from the heart and empty into the heart. As shown in Figure 4.1, the heart is the central pump though which oxygenated blood enters the systemic arterial tree down to the level of tissues and receives deoxygenated blood via the systemic veins.

The arterial system consists of large artery or aorta that begins from the left ventricle) followed by medium-sized arteries and then the arterioles which end in the capillary bed (that feeds the tissues).

The venous system consists of venules (that begin in the capillary bed and drain the tissues) followed by medium-sized veins and then large-sized veins (superior vena cava and inferior vena cava) which empty into the right atrium.

TISSUES OF THE WALL OF BLOOD VESSELS

All the blood vessels irrespective of sizes are lined internally by simple squamous epithelium which is called *endothelium*. Outer to the endothelium the vascular wall of both arteries and veins, consists of connective tissue (elastic and collagen fibers) and smooth muscle.

TUNICS OF THE WALL OF BLOOD VESSEL

- Tunica intima
- Tunica media
- Tunica externa or adventitia
  - The *tunica intima* consists of endothelium, subendothelial connective tissue and internal elastic lamina. The endothelial cells rest on the basement membrane and are linked by tight junctions and by gap junctions. The subendothelial tissue is made up of collagen and elastic fibers and a few smooth muscle cells.
  - The *tunica media* lies between the internal elastic and external elastic laminae.
  - The *tunica adventitia* is outer to external elastic lamina.

Some characteristics of the media and adventitia differentiate the large-sized and medium-sized arteries and veins in a histological section.

The endothelium is a very important layer of all blood vessels including capillaries. It acts as a semipermeable barrier between the blood inside the capillaries and the tissue fluid.

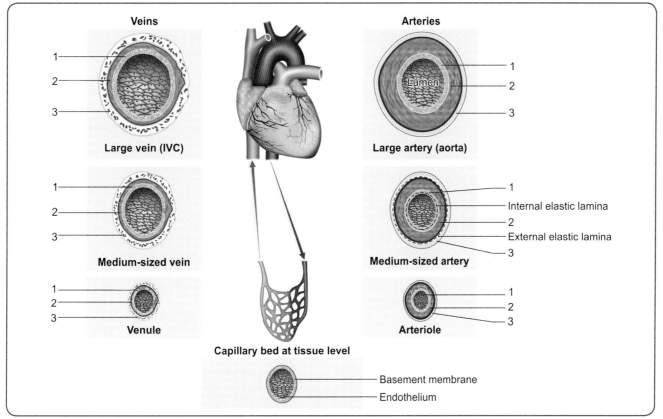

Fig. 4.1: Schematic representation of the structure of arteries, veins and capillaries in the cardiovascular system **Key: 1.** Tunica intima; **2.** Tunica media; **3.** Tunica adventitia

Functions of Endothelium

- Its main function is to monitor the bidirectional exchange of small molecules and restrict the transport of some macromolecules at tissue level.
- It maintains the tone of blood vessels by relaxing and contracting the smooth muscle in the vascular wall. This is controlled by secretion of nitrous oxide (vasodilator) and endothelin (vasoconstrictor).
- The angiotensin converting enzyme secreted by endothelial cells of lung capillaries converts circulating angiotensin I to angiotensin II which is a potent vasoconstrictor.
- The endothelial cells of arteries usually contain storage granules called Weibel–Palade bodies which contain von Willibrand factor involved in coagulation and hemostasis.
- An intact endothelium does not allow platelets to adhere to it due to its ability to produce prostacyclin (an inhibitor of platelet aggregation and clot formation).
- The endothelium of capillaries allows migration of leukocytes from blood to tissues. This migration is increased during injury to the endothelium.

ARTERIES

The arteries carry blood away from the heart under high pressure. They consist of following types:
- Large-sized or elastic or conducting arteries like aorta.
- Medium-sized or muscular or distributing arteries like brachial and femoral.
- Arterioles or resistance vessels.
- Capillaries (continuous, fenestrated and sinusoids).

Unique Types of Arteries

- The **anatomical end arteries** are the ones whose branches do not take part in anastomosis. The best example is central artery of retina.
- The **physiological end arteries take** part in anastomosis with other arteries but the anastomoses are not sufficient in the event of the sudden blockage of one of the main arteries. The best example is coronary arteries which are physiological end arteries though anatomical they are not end arteries.
- The **vasa vasora** are the tiny capillary like vessels (both veins and arteries) that supply large veins (superior and inferior vena cavae) and arteries (aorta and its

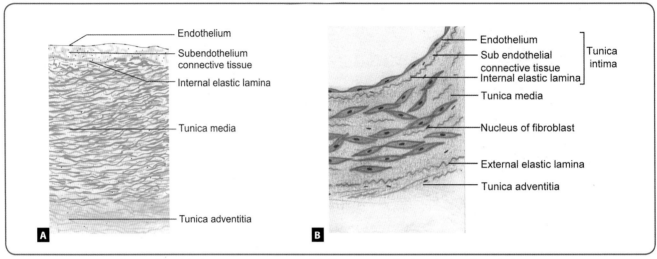

Figs 4.2A and B: Microscopic structure of **A.** Elastic artery; **B.** Muscular (medium size) artery

large branches like subclavian, common carotid, brachiocephalic, etc.). The vasa vasorum literally mean vessels of the vessel.

- They are of two types, vasa ***vasorum interna*** and ***vasa vasorum externa***. The former arise from the lumen of the parent vessel and the latter arises from the neighboring arteries which could be branches of the parent vessel or branches of other arteries. They are usually seen in the tunica externa in a histological section of the blood vessel. The outer wall of the large blood vessel (media and adventitia) is supplied by vasa vasorum. It is believed the abdominal aorta below the level of renal artery has no vasa vasorum hence the infrarenal part of aorta is more prone to aneurysm.

Histology of Arteries

- The ***large-sized or elastic arteries*** (Fig. 4.2A) are identified by the presence of large tunica media containing elastic fibers and a series of concentrically arranged perforated or fenestrated elastic laminae interspersed with smooth muscle fibers. The tunica adventitia shows collagen and elastic fibers for the support of vasa vasorum and nervi vascularis.
- The medium-sized or muscular arteries are (Fig. 4.2B) characterized by presence of circularly disposed smooth muscle fibers in tunica media and by a prominent internal elastic lamina (which is not prominent in the large-sized artery).

 CLINICAL CORRELATION

- ***Atherosclerosis is*** a degenerative disease of the tissues of the wall of arteries. The basic pathology is damage to the endothelial cells (due to hypertension, smoking, diabetes, etc.) leading to increased permeability, accumulation of lipoproteins and death of endothelial cells in patches.

Contd…

Contd…

 CLINICAL CORRELATION

There is exposure of subendothelial tissue in the areas of these patches. The smooth muscle fibers of tunica media migrate into the subendothelial layer where they imbibe lipoproteins along with macrophages. These changes lead to formation of atherosclerotic plaques which narrow the arteries eventually.
- ***Intravascular thrombus*** may form if the endothelium suffers damage. It may obstruct the artery.

Arterioles

The arterioles are less than 0.1 mm in diameter. Structurally they are similar to medium-sized arteries from which they begin except for the absence of internal elastic lamina. Near their termination they are made up of thin layer of intima surrounded by one or two layers of smooth muscle fibers. The arterioles offer resistance to blood flow by changing their diameter, hence the name resistance vessels. Constriction of arterioles raises the blood pressure and relaxation decreases the blood pressure.

Capillaries

The terminal arterioles break-up into capillaries which are thin-walled and endothelium-lined microscopic blood vessels connecting terminal arterioles and venules. The lumen of the typical capillary is equal to that of the diameter of the RBC. The capillaries form rich network or capillary bed surrounding the cells of the tissues since they are the main exchange vessels of nutrients, oxygen and metabolic byproducts between blood inside them and the cells.

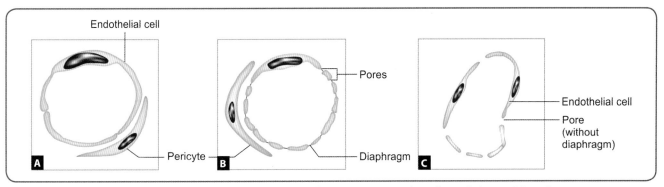

Figs 4.3A to C: Structure of **A.** Continuous capillaries; **B.** Fenestrated capillaries; **C.** Sinusoidal capillaries

The endothelial cells of the capillaries are elongated in the direction of blood flow. They are held together by tight junctions and gap junctions. The capillaries are normally associated with perivascular contractile cells called pericytes which have the capacity to transform in to smooth muscle fiber after tissue injury and repair.

Types of Capillaries (Figs 4.3A to C)

- **Continuous capillaries** (Fig. 4.3A) have continuous basement membrane with a distinct continuity of endothelial cells. There is transcytosis of macromolecules in both directions across the cytoplasm of endothelial cells. The continuous capillaries are seen in muscular tissue, skin, connective tissue, lungs and brain.
- **Fenestrated capillaries** (Fig. 4.3B) are characterized by presence of tiny pores in the endothelial layer. The pores are closed by a very thin diaphragm which allows dissolved substances and macromolecules to pass through easily. They are found in glomeruli of kidney, intestinal villi and endocrine glands.
- **Sinusoidal capillaries** (Fig. 4.3C) are wider and irregular in shape compared to typical capillaries. The lining endothelium is discontinuous as there are gaps between the endothelial cells as well as in the basal lamina. The flow of blood in the irregular sinusoids is rather sluggish. These sinusoids are found in red bone marrow, liver, suprarenal gland, pituitary gland and red pulp of the spleen.

VEINS

The basic structure of the vein is similar to that of the artery except that the lumen of the vein is large-sized and large veins.
- The post-capillary venules are the smallest veins which receive blood from the arterial capillaries at the tissue level. They are structurally similar to the large capillaries as they take part in exchanges between blood and the tissues. The post-capillary venules converge in to larger collecting venules.
- The collecting venules become the muscular venules when surrounded by smooth muscle fibers. The collecting veins join to form small veins with three distinct tunics.

- The histological section of a medium-sized vein is identified by its collapsed lumen. Its wall is composed of tunica intima which is made up of endothelial cells resting on a basement membrane and supported by subendothelial connective tissue. There is no internal elastic lamina. The tunica media is composed of a few circularly arranged smooth muscle fibers and scattered collagen fibers. The tunica adventitia consists of a thin layer of fibroelastic connective tissue containing vasa vasorum and Nervi vascularis (Fig. 4.4).
- The large-sized vein like vena cavae is composed of the same three layers as the medium-sized vein. The tunica intima is lined by endothelial cells resting on basement membrane supported by subendothelial connective tissue. The internal elastic lamina is indistinct. The tunica media is relatively thinner and contains collagen fibers and few smooth muscle fibers and elastic fibers. The tunica adventitia is characteristically the well developed layer as it contains longitudinally running bundles of smooth muscle fibers embedded in elastic and collagen fibers.

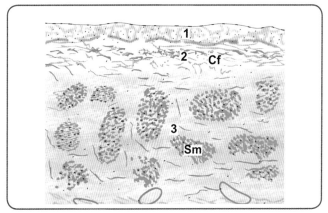

Fig. 4.4: Microscopic structure of vein **Key: 1.** Tunica intima; **2.** Tunica media; **3.** Tunica adventitia; **Cf.** Collagen fibers; **Sm.** Smooth muscles

LYMPHATIC TISSUE

The lymphatic tissue is functionally a part of the immune system of the body. It is distributed in the body as aggregations of lymphocytes in specific lymphatic organs (such as lymph nodes, spleen, tonsils and thymus) and as diffuse lymphoid tissue in MALT or GALT (mucosa or gut associated lymphatic tissue), BALT (bronchus associated lymphatic tissue) and SALT (skin associated lymphatic tissue).

Basically the lymphatic tissue is composed of lymphocytes [B-lymphocytes, T-lymphocytes, NK cells (natural killer), plasma cells and macrophages] supported by reticular fibers of connective tissue. The lymphatic tissue of the numerous lymph nodes found in the body filters the lymph, which is the tissue fluid or transudate of blood, containing particulate matter like cell debris, microbes and plasma proteins taken up by the lymphatic vessels and carried to regional lymph nodes. The filtered lymph from all regions of the body (except the right half of thorax, right upper limb and right half of head and neck) is collected in a big lymphatic duct called thoracic duct, to be poured into the blood circulation at the junction of left internal jugular and left subclavian vein (Fig. 4.5). The lymph from the areas mentioned in the bracket is collected by right lymphatic duct, to be poured into the corresponding venous junction on the right side.

FUNCTIONS OF LYMPHATIC TISSUE

- Production of cells like lymphocytes, plasma cells, etc. which have the ability to recognize and neutralize antigens (microbes, tumor cells and toxins).
- Phagocytosis of foreign cells such as microbes and cancer cells by macrophages, which are part of mononuclear phagocytic system (MPS) of the body.

TYPES OF LYMPHOCYTES

There are three types of lymphocytes namely, T-lymphocytes, B-lymphocytes and NK (natural killer)-lymphocytes.

1. ***T-lymphocytes*** originate in bone marrow but mature in thymus, from where they migrate to other lymphoid organs via blood circulation. Amongst the three types of lymphocytes the maximum population of T-lymphocytes is present in blood circulation. T lymphocytes are responsible for cell mediated immunity in which the microbes are killed by release of lymphokines which attach the T-lymphocytes to the

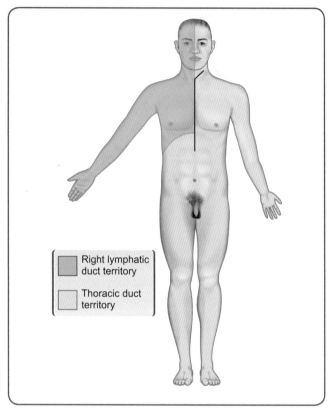

Fig. 4.5: Area of drainage of lymph of the body by thoracic duct and by right lymphatic duct into the venous circulation (of)

surface of the microbes. The example of cell mediated immunity is polio immunization.

2. ***B-lymphocytes*** originate in bone marrow but undergo maturation in either the bone marrow or in GALT. The plasma cells are modified B lymphocytes. They produce antibodies (immunoglobulin) to destroy the microbes and toxins. This type of immunity is called humoral immunity. Example of humoral immunity is tetanus toxoid. There are five types of immunoglobulins in the body (IgG that crosses placental barrier, IgA, IgM, IgE in allergic reactions and IgD).

3. ***NK cells*** originate in bone marrow. They are called natural killer cells because they attack virus infested cells and cancer cells without stimulation. They do not have surface receptors.

PRIMARY LYMPHOID ORGANS

The thymus and bone marrow are the primary lymphoid organs in human being. The thymus consists of 100% T-lymphocytes.

SECONDARY LYMPHOID ORGANS

The lymph nodes and spleen are secondary lymphoid organs in human being. They approximately consist of 60% T-lymphocytes and 40% B-lymphocytes.

LYMPHATIC TISSUE WITHIN OTHER ORGANS

- GALT (Gut Associated Lymphatic Tissue) includes Waldeyer's ring (composed of nasopharyngeal tonsil, bilateral palatine tonsils, bilateral tubal tonsils and lingual tonsils), Peyer's patches in small intestine and aggregations in vermiform appendix (abdominal tonsil).
- BALT (Bronchus Associated Lymphatic Tissue) is present in the wall of the bronchial tree.
- SALT (Skin Associated Lymphatic Tissue) is found in the skin (refer to Langerhans cells in the epidermis in chapter 5).

THYMUS (FIG. 4.6)

The thymus is composed of T-lymphocyte population only. It is unique in having a stroma of reticuloendothelial cells (referred to as epitheliocytes) inside its numerous lobules (Fig. 4.6).

Each **thymic lobule** consists of peripheral cortex of densely packed lymphocytes and central medulla of loosely packed lymphocytes. The epitheliocytes developmentally belong to endoderm of third pharyngeal pouches. These cells form an internal lining for the capsule and the septa of thymus. They also cover the surfaces of blood vessels inside the thymus. This arrangement indicates the role of epitheliocytes in forming a blood-thymus barrier, which prevents the contact between the lymphocytes of thymus and the antigens in the blood. The

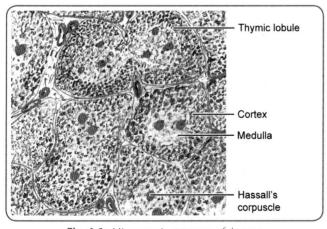

Fig. 4.6: Microscopic structure of thymus

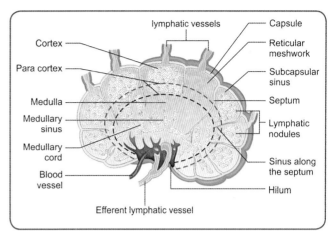

Fig. 4.7: Microscopic structure of lymph node

stem cells of bone marrow reach the cortex of each lobule via blood circulation and begin mitotic divisions to form T-lymphocytes. There are no lymphatic follicles in thymus and hence no germinal centers. T-lymphocytes enter the medulla to leave the thymus via venules or efferent lymph vessels. The characteristic **Hassall's corpuscles** of thymus are composed of degenerating epitheliocytes forming a homogeneous eosinophilic mass encircled by concentrically arranged epitheliocytes.

LYMPH NODE

The lymph nodes are small encapsulated structures seen along the path of lymphatic vessels that bring lymph to them for filtration. In keeping with this function, the lymph nodes have both afferent and efferent lymph vessels. The afferent vessels pierce the capsule to pour lymph in the subcapsular sinus.

The **interior of lymph node** (Fig. 4.7) is divided into **outer cortex** and **inner medulla**. The stroma consists of trabeculae and reticular connective tissue. The cortex is characterized by presence of well defined lymphatic nodules, which may show germinal centers. The cortex has densely packed lymphocytes while medulla shows cord like arrangement of lymphocytes. The inner part of cortex is called paracortex, which shows diffusely arranged T-lymphocytes. The lymph from subcapsular sinus percolates along cortical sinuses into the medullary sinuses, from where it leaves by efferent lymphatic vessels at hilum of lymph nodes.

SPLEEN (FIG. 4.8)

The spleen is the largest lymphoid organ in the body. It performs immunological functions, takes part in destruction of damaged and aged erythrocytes, filters

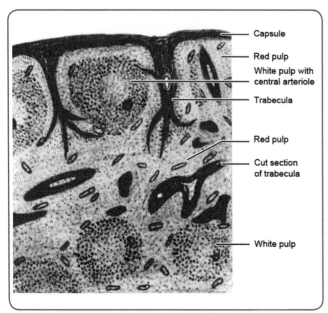

Capsule

Red pulp

White pulp with central arteriole

Trabecula

Red pulp

Cut section of trabecula

White pulp

Fig. 4.8: Microscopic structure of spleen

blood, produces B and T-lymphocytes and acts as reservoir of blood. A dense connective tissue capsule extends into the substance of spleen as characteristic trabeculae, which carry blood vessels inside. The splenic parenchyma is supported by delicate reticular fibers and cells. Being a highly vascular organ the spleen has plenty of venous sinusoids. Its parenchyma consists of white pulp and red pulp.

The white pulp is composed of periarterial lymphatic sheaths (PALS) and lymphatic follicles, scattered all over the interior. The lymphatic follicle surrounding an eccentrically placed central arteriole is actually a localized enlargement of PALS. It contains both T- and B-lymphocytes. The PALS contains only T-lymphocytes. The lymph from white follicle drains via efferent lymph vessels that leave the hilum of spleen and empty in to pancreatico splenic lymph nodes.

The red pulp is composed of splenic cords (cords of Billroth) separated by blood filled venous sinusoids. The splenic cords are composed of lymphocytes, macrophages, granulocytes, plasma cells, RBCs and reticular cells and the reticular fibers. The red pulp appears red because of the presence of innumerable venous sinusoids filled with blood. The blood flow in red pulp can take two routes to open into the venous sinusoids. In closed circulation, the arterial capillaries directly join the venous sinusoids. In open circulation, arterial capillaries open in to splenic cords and from there in to venous sinusoids. In compromise theory of circulation, there is closed circulation when the spleen is contracted and open circulation when the spleen is distended.

PALATINE TONSIL

The palatine tonsils (part of MALT) are the collections of lymphatic tissue subjacent to the stratified squamous non-keratinized epithelium of oropharynx. The epithelium dips into the substance of tonsils as 15 to 20 tonsillar crypts. The crypts branch once inside the tonsil. In this way, the lymphatic follicles with germinal centers are brought in intimate contact with the epithelium (at the so-called lymphoepithelial symbiosis). This facilitates direct contact between the antigen (microbes ingested through the oral cavity) and the lymphocytes inside the tonsils. Thus, the tonsil offers first line of defense to the body against antigens (bacteria, viruses, etc.) as soon as they are swallowed in the food or the drink.

5

Skin, Hypodermis and Deep Fascia

SKIN

The skin covers the external surface of the body. The skin is considered the widest organ of human body as it performs a variety of functions.

Functions of Skin

- The keratin of skin serves as an effective barrier against invasion by microorganisms and against chemicals, heat and abrasions. It prevents excessive evaporation of water from skin surface thus guarding against dehydration.
- Body temperature is regulated by dilatation (cooling) and constriction (warming) of blood vessels.
- The skin serves as a sensory organ because it perceives external sensations via sensory receptors located in it. The touch sensations are carried by Meissner's corpuscles located in dermal papillae close to dermoepidermal junction and Merkel's discs associated with cells in stratum basale in epidermis of thick skin, Krause's end bulbs and by Ruffini endings in the dermis. The pain and temperature sensations are carried by free nerve endings. The pressure and vibration is subserved by lamellated Pacinian corpuscles (located deep in the dermis).
- Synthesis of vitamin D in keratinocytes of epidermis with the help of ultraviolet rays in sunlight is a major metabolic activity of the skin.

- The cutaneous blood vessels store around 5% of the body's blood volume. The skin therefore is a blood reservoir.
- The skin acts like an excretory organ by eliminating limited amounts of nitrogenous wastes from the body in the sweat.
- Intradermal injections are given in the dermis. The best example is intradermal injection of tuberculin in (Mantoux test) the skin of ventral surface of forearm for diagnosis of tuberculosis. Other common example of intradermal injection is testing for penicillin sensitivity before giving intramuscular penicillin injection to avoid anaphylactic reaction due to penicillin.
- The skin is an active immune organ of the body as it contains immunocompetent cells in epidermis and dermis. The skin-associated lymphatic tissue (SALT) is involved in induction and regulation of the primary immune response.

Layers of Skin

Histology of Skin

Basically, the skin consists of two layers, namely outer epidermis and inner dermis.
- *Epidermis* is derived from ectoderm, is an avascular layer and lacks lymphatics.
- *Dermis* is derived from mesoderm, is a vascular layer, and contains lymphatics, nerve endings and pilosebaceous units in thin skin.

Contd...

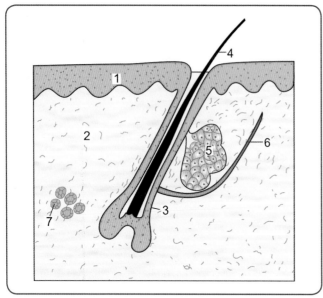

Fig. 5.1: Thin skin (Schematic representation)
Key: 1. Epidermis; 2. Dermis; 3. Hair follicle; 4. Hair; 5. Sebaceous gland; 6. Arrector pili muscle; 7. Swat glands

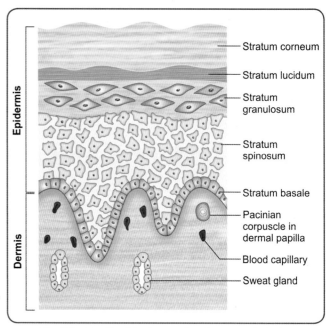

Fig. 5.2: Details of the layers of epidermis in thick skin

Contd…

> Depending on the thickness of epidermis, there are two types of skin, thick skin and thin skin.
> - The **thin skin** (Fig. 5.1) is characterized by thin epidermis with marked reduction in keratinized layer and absence of stratum lucidum. It is hairy skin hence the dermis contains abundant pilosebaceous units in addition to sweat glands. It covers the entire body except the palms and soles.
> - The **thick skin** (Fig. 5.2) is characterized by broad epidermis, is hairless and glabrous. It covers the palms and flexor surfaces of digits as well as soles. Its dermis presents plenty of sweat glands but no pilosebaceous units (hair follicles, sebaceous glands and erector pili muscles).

Epidermis

Layers of epidermis in thick skin from deep to superficial (Fig. 5.2)

- The **stratum basale** is the deepest layer consisting of a single row of low columnar keratinocytes resting on a well-defined basement membrane. These cells are attached to the basement membrane by hemidesmosomes. They undergo rapid and repeated mitotic divisions. Hence, this layer is also known as stratum germinativum. As the new cells are formed they move towards stratum spinosum. The basal layer also contains Merkel cells, Langerhans cells and melanocytes (and occasional lymphocytes).
- The **stratum spinosum** or prickly layer is composed of several layers of keratinocytes. These polygonal cells are attached to one another by desmosomes. On staining

with H and E, the desmosomes appear as small spines or thorns on the cells (hence the name stratum spinosum for this layer and the name prickle cells for keratinocytes). The cytoplasm of these cells contains keratin filaments.
- The **stratum granulosum** consists of rows of flattened and degenerating keratinocytes. The presence of darkly staining keratohyalin granules is the distinctive feature of these cells.
- The **stratum lucidum** appears a clear transparent band. It consists of a few rows of flat, dead keratinocytes and is present only in thick skin of sole and palm.
- The **stratum corneum** is fairly thick outermost layer of dead keratinized cells devoid of nuclei and cell organelles. These cells are gradually sloughed off by a process called **desquamation**.

Epidermal cells (Fig. 5.3)

Apart from the keratinocytes the epidermis has a population of non-keratinocytes (melanocytes, Langerhans cells, Merkel cells and a few lymphocytes).

The epidermis is composed of following four major cell types:
1. **Keratinocytes** are the most abundant cells. They are derived from surface ectoderm.
2. **Melanocytes** are pigment producing cells that are derived from neural crest. They are scattered in stratum basale and thier processes enter the stratum spinosum. They protect the stratum basale or germinativum cells and the dermis from ultraviolet rays of sunlight (Fig. 5.4).

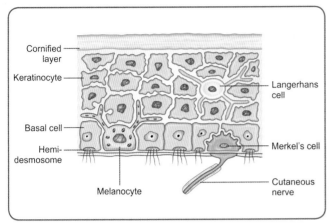

Fig. 5.3: Schematic diagram to show location of different cells of epidermis

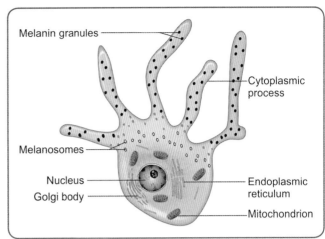

Fig. 5.4: Melanocyte showing dendritic processes

3. ***Langerhans cells*** originate from stem cells in bone marrow and migrate into the skin to perform immune function. They are located in stratum spinosum. They are dendritic antigen presenting cells. It forms an important part of skin-associated lymphatic tissue (SALT) along with T lymphocytes, dermal dendritic cells (DDC), keratinocytes and local lymphatics and associated lymph nodes. SALT is responsible for induction and regulation of the primary immune response. The Langerhans cell that is sensitized by the antigen moves via the lymphatics in the dermis to the local lymph node where it activates the proliferation of antigen specific and cytotoxic T lymphocytes.

4. ***Merkel's cells*** are seen the stratum basal of thick skin. They are intimately associated with expanded terminal discs of sensory nerves forming receptors concerned with touch. Hence, they fall in the category of mechanoreceptors. Markel's cells are seen in stratum basale.

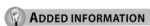 **ADDED INFORMATION**

Surface Epidermal Ridges
The following sites in the body (palm, sole, finger pads and toe pads) present surface elevations due to epidermal thickenings (somewhat similar to epidermal ridges projecting in dermis). These epidermal irregularities are variously described as papillary ridges or friction ridges or surface ectodermal ridges. They form intricate patterns, which are unique for every individual. This is the basis of personal identification from finger prints. The study of these patterns is known as dermatoglyphics.

Dermal-Epidermal Junction

The basement membrane of epidermis is the demarcation line between epidermis and dermis. The anchoring fibers between the two layers are composed of both collagen and elastic fibers. This junction is wavy as it is characterized by dermal papillae and epidermal ridges (peg-like extensions of epidermis into dermis), which increase the area of adhesion between the two layers. It is this junctional tissue that is defective in a disease called ***epidermolysis bullosa*** (EB). This is an inherited disorder characterized by recurrent blister formation on skin in response to trivial trauma like rubbing or pressure.

Dermis

It is the second major skin region containing strong, flexible connective tissue. It is composed of two layers, ***papillary*** and ***reticular***.

Papillary layer

This layer is characterized by areolar connective tissue with collagen and elastic fibers along with fibroblasts. The upward projections on dermis indenting the basement membrane of epidermis are called ***dermal papillae***. The papillae contain capillary loops, Meissner's corpuscles and free nerve endings.

Reticular layer

This layer is composed of dense irregular connective tissue along with blood vessels and Pacinian corpuscles for vibration and pressure sense. The collagen fibers add to its strength and resiliency. The elastic fibers provide stretch-recoil properties. These fibers tend to atrophy as age advances resulting in wrinkling of skin. The bundles of collagen fibers are arranged parallel to one another. They are oriented along the long axis of limbs but along the perpendicular axis in the trunk. The cleavage lines of Langer (tension lines) on the skin are produced along the direction of the collagen bundles. The cleavage lines have surgical importance. The skin incision placed along these lines heals with a fine scar compared to the incision placed across them, which heals with a thick irregular scar.

Cells of dermis

- Fixed cells of organized structures like Schwann cells of sensory nerves, endothelial cells of cutaneous vessels, smooth muscle cells of hair follicles.
- Free cells performing different functions like connective tissue cells, T and B lymphocytes and dermal dendritic cells (DDC).

Glands of Skin

- The **sweat glands** (Fig. 5.5) are coiled tubular glands which are located deep in the reticular layer of dermis. Their long ducts pass through the dermis and then the epidermis to open at skin pores. The part of ducts in dermis is lined by stratified cuboidal epithelium while the part in the epidermis is lined by stratified squamous epithelium. The main function of sweat glands is to prevent overheating of the body. There are two types of sweat glands in the body. The **eccrine sweat glands** are the most common and are widely distributed in the body. They are supplied by postganglionic cholinergic sympathetic nerve fibers. The **apocrine sweat glands** are localized to the skin of axilla, ano-genital region and

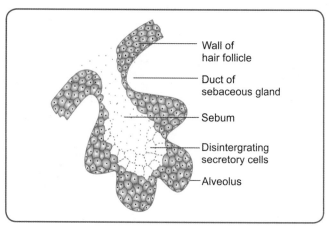

Fig. 5.6: Microscopic structure of sebaceous gland

areola. They are supplied by postganglionic adrenergic sympathetic nerve fibers.

- The **sebaceous glands** (Fig. 5.6) are part of a complex called **pilo-sebaceous unit**, which consists of sebaceous gland, arrector pilorum muscle, hair shaft and hair follicle. The gland is located in the triangle formed by epidermis, slanting side of hair shaft and arrector pilorum muscle (Fig. 5.1).
- It opens by a short duct into the shaft of adjacent hair follicle. The gland secretes an oily secretion called sebum (lipid and cell debris), which softens the skin and the hair. Its mode of secretion is holocrine (associated with death of secreting cell, also known as **programmed death** or **apoptosis**). Sebaceous glands are under the control of secondary hormones.
- The arrector pilorum muscle is a smooth muscle that connects the undersurface of the hair follicle to dermal papilla. It is supplied by postganglionic sympathetic fibers. Contraction of these muscles compresses the secretory units of the glands thereby helping in expelling the secretion out into the ducts and into the hair shaft. The contraction of muscles straightens the shafts of the hair follicles and exerts a pull on the skin surface causing dimpling known as **gooseflesh**. The arrector pili muscles develop from mesenchyme.

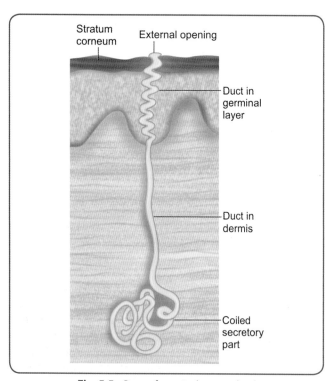

Fig. 5.5: Parts of a typical sweat gland

🔖 CLINICAL CORRELATION

- The **basal cell carcinoma** arises from cells of basal layer. The squamous cell carcinoma begins in keratinocytes of stratum spinosum. The melanoma is the cancer of melanocytes. It is a highly metastatic cancer.
- **Albinism** is an autosomal recessive disorder in which an individual lacks the ability to synthesize melanin. The melanin pigment is absent in hair, iris and skin.

Contd...

Contd…

CLINICAL CORRELATION

- **Vitiligo** is a common skin condition in which the melanocytes are destroyed due an autoimmune reaction resulting in bilateral depigmentation of the skin.
- In **psoriasis** the cells of basal layer proliferate at a rapid rate so that keratinization process completes much before its usual time frame and the poorly keratinized cells shed prematurely producing thick and scaly skin.
- **Acne** or **pimples** are small elevations on facial skin due to swelling of sebaceous glands. Under the influence of sex hormones the sebaceous glands secrete more sebum and if the ducts are blocked sebum accumulates. The swollen gland may be infected. Another condition affecting sebaceous glands is sebaceous cyst, which needs surgical removal. The scalp is the most favorite site for sebaceous cysts.
- The **leprosy bacilli**, which enter the skin from intimate contact with a patient of infective type of leprosy travel proximally in the perineurium of the cutaneous nerves. They destroy the Schwann cells causing demyelination. This blocks impulse conduction causing cutaneous patches of sensory loss in the area of distribution of the affected nerve.

HYPODERMIS OR SUPERFICIAL FASCIA

This layer lies subjacent to the dermis and is composed of variable amount of subcutaneous adipose tissue (panniculus adiposus), areolar connective tissue, cutaneous vessels, cutaneous lymphatics and sensory nerves. It is visible after placing an incision in the skin with a surgical knife and reflecting skin flaps in living as well as in dead. The panniculus carnosus is the subcutaneous muscle in quadrupeds. It is inserted into the skin. This muscle is represented in human beings by palmaris brevis, muscles of facial expression, platysma, dartos, subcutaneous part of sphincter ani externus and corrugator cutis ani. Of the above muscles dartos and corrugator cutis ani are smooth muscles.

CLINICAL CORRELATION

Subcutaneous Injections

Some drugs are administered in subcutaneous tissue, especially where slow absorption is desirable. The most common example is subcutaneous injection of insulin. The local anesthetics are injected subcutaneously. Similarly, low

Contd…

Contd…

CLINICAL CORRELATION

molecular weight heparin is given by this route (usually in anterior abdominal wall) in post-angioplasty patients and after coronary bypass surgeries.

DEEP FASCIA

This is a tough fibrous membrane deep to the superficial fascia. In the limbs and neck its arrangement is such that there are fascial compartments enclosing some structures. The purpose of such compartmentalization is to prevent spread of infection from one to the other. In the limbs it forms partitions (intermuscular septa) which separate the compartments comprising muscles, nerves and vessels. In the leg, the tightly enclosed fascial compartments assume functional significance in facilitating venous return against gravity. In palm, it forms fascial spaces of surgical importance. The deep fascia does not have uniform appearance. So, depending on functional requirements its appearance and terminology change. There are a few sites in the body devoid of deep fascia (face, scalp and anterior abdominal wall).

Modifications of Deep Fascia

- The **retinacula** around wrist and ankle are the thickened bands of deep fascia. They serve the purpose of strapping down the tendons of long flexor and extensor muscles.
- The **palmar** and **plantar aponeuroses** are the thickened and flattened parts of deep fascia in palm and sole respectively. Their function is to protect the underlying nerves and vessels.
- The **fascial sheaths** around neurovascular bundles are seen in neck as carotid sheath and as axillary sheath, which is extension of prevertebral fascia of neck surrounding the axillary vessels.
- The **interosseous membranes** of forearm and leg are modified deep fascia.
- The **fibrous sheaths around** tendons are found around flexor tendons of fingers.
- The **fascial sheaths** are formed around muscles in certain locations. The psoas major muscle on posterior abdominal wall is covered with psoas sheath.

6

Descriptive Anatomical Terms

Chapter Contents

ANATOMICAL POSITION

The position of a person standing erect, looking directly forwards, with arms resting by the side of the body, feet together and palms facing forwards is described as *anatomical position*.

The relationship of anatomical structures to each other are described with the assumption that person is in anatomical position. To illustrate this concept let us take a simple example of direction of forearm in supine position of body and anatomical position of body. The forearm faces upwards in former and towards front in the latter position. Therefore, to have uniformity in describing anatomical interrelations anatomical position of the body is the gold standard.

VARIOUS ANATOMICAL TERMS

Different descriptive anatomical terms are enlisted in Table 6.1 and Fig. 6.1.

DIRECTIONAL TERMS OF HUMAN BODY

Additional Descriptive Terms for Position of Body

- **Supine position** is the one in which subject is lying on the back with face looking upwards (Fig. 6.2).
- **Prone position** is the one in which subject is lying on the belly with face looking downwards (Fig. 6.3).

TABLE 6.1: Descriptive anatomical terms (Fig. 6.1)		
Term	**Definition**	**Example**
Superior/cranial	Towards head	Nose is superior to mouth
Inferior/caudal	Towards feet	Knee joint is inferior to hip joint
Anterior/ ventral	Towards the front	The toes are anterior to heel
Posterior /dorsal	Towards the back	The heel is posterior to the toes
Medial	Towards the midline of body	The eye is medial to ear of same side
Lateral	Away from the midline of body	The ear is lateral to the eye of same side
Proximal	Nearer the attachment of limb to the trunk	Shoulder is proximal to elbow
Distal	Away from the attachment of limb to the trunk	The palm is distal to forearm
Superficial	Near the surface of body	The skin is superficial to muscles and bones
Deep	Away from the surface of body in inward direction	The lungs are deeper to rib cage
Superolateral	Nearer the head but away from median plane	The ears are superolateral to chin
Superomedial	Nearer the head and median plane	The nose is superomedial to angle of mouth of both sides

Contd...

Contd…

Term	Definition	Example
Inferolateral	Nearer the feet but away from median plane	The shoulder is inferolateral to the point of chin
Inferomedial	Nearer the feet and median plane	The anterior ends of floating ribs run inferomedially
Ipsilateral	Occurring on the same side of body	Right upper limb is ipsilateral to right lower limb
Contralateral	Occurring on opposite sides of body	Right upper limb is contralateral to left lower limb

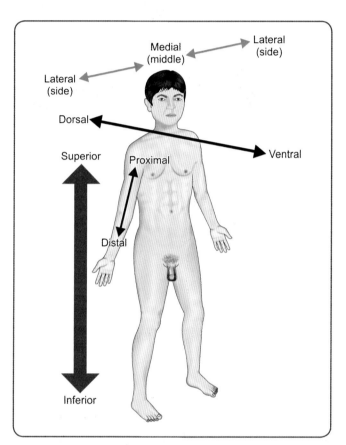

Fig. 6.1: Commonly used terms of relationship and comparison

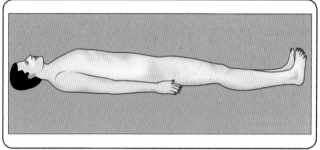

Fig. 6.2: Supine position

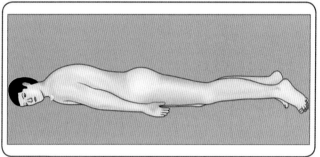

Fig. 6.3: Prone position

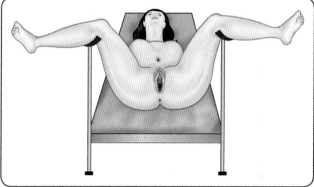

Fig. 6.4: Lithotomy position

- ***Lateral position*** is either right lateral or left lateral in which subject lies on one side of the body.
- ***Lithotomy position*** (Fig. 6.4) is the one in which subject lies in supine position with hip joints in flexed and abducted positions and knee joints in partially flexed positions. This position is adopted for performing cadaveric or surgical dissection of perineum and also during per vaginum (PV) examinations, vaginal deliveries and procedures like dilatation and curettage (D and C) in gynecological practice.

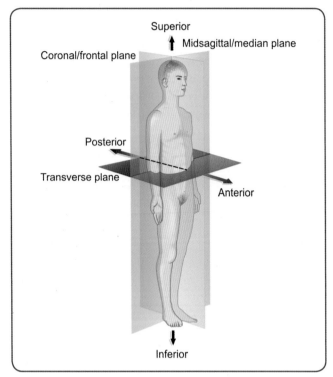

Fig. 6.5: Anatomical position of the body and anatomical planes

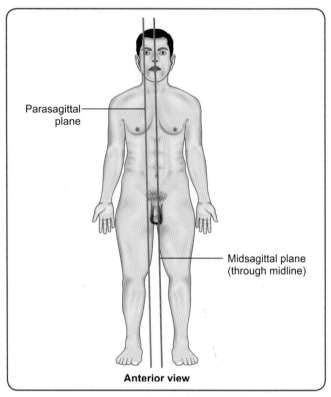

Fig. 6.6: Sagittal planes

DIRECTIONAL PLANES OF HUMAN BODY (FIG. 6.5)

In order to understand relations of internal structures (organs inside the body) the body is conventionally cut in the following planes. Individual organs can also be studied by using similar planes of sectioning.

- *The midsagittal plane or median plane* is a vertical plane that divides the body lengthwise into two equal halves. It is called midsagittal because it passes along the length of sagittal suture of the skull.
- *The sagittal plane* or *parasagittal* is any plane passing parallel to the median plane for dividing the body into unequal longitudinal halves (Fig. 6.6).

- *The coronal or frontal plane* divides the body into anterior and posterior halves. It is so called because it is passes through or parallel to the coronal suture of the skull. The coronal plane is at right angles to the midsagittal plane.
- *The transverse or horizontal plane* divides the body or organs into superior and inferior sections. It is at right angles to both midsagittal and coronal planes.

The aforementioned anatomical terms are universally used by clinicians all over the world. In fact these terms are the integral part of the international vocabulary of health care professionals.

7

Clinicoanatomical Problems and Solutions

CASE 1

A six feet tall 14-year-old school student, an aspirant for school basket ball team, undergoes physical fitness examination. The examination revealed that the boy had long limbs (the tips of his fingers reached just below his knees), the sternum showed incurving (pes cavum), the joints were very loose and flexible. He was sent for cardiac and ophthalmic check up because of the family history of Marfan's syndrome and the findings of physical examination.

Questions and Solutions

1. Enumerate the four basic tissues of the body.

Ans. Epithelium, connective tissue, muscular tissue and neural tissue

2. Which basic tissue is affected in Marfan's syndrome?

Ans. Connective tissue

3. Name the three histological components of this tissue.

Ans. Connective tissue cells, connective tissue fibers and matrix (ground substance)

4. Name the three types of fibers in this tissue.

Ans. Collagen, reticular and elastic

5. Which connective tissue fiber is defectively formed in this syndrome?

Ans. Synthesis of elastic fibers is defective in Marfan's syndrome

6. Describe the physical and chemical properties of the above fibers and enumerate their distribution in the body.

Ans. The elastic fibers impart elasticity to the tissues. They are composed of a protein called elastin. They run singly and individual fibers branch and anastomose. They are highly refractile. They stain poorly with ordinary hematoxylin and eosin stains. Special stains like orcein, resorcin-fuchsin and Verhoeff's are used to visualize them. The elastic fibers are produced by fibroblasts and smooth muscle cells. They are widely distributed in the body. They occur in loose areolar tissue, ligaments of joints, dermis of skin, lung, large arteries (tunica media of aorta is mainly composed of elastic fibers), ligamentum nuchae, ligamenta flava (connecting the laminae of adjacent vertebrae), suspensory ligament of lens, elastic cartilage, etc.

7. Why is the student referred to cardiologist and ophthalmologist?

Ans. The cardiac check up in a suspected case of Marfan's syndrome is necessary to find out the presence of aortic aneurysm (dilatation of aortic wall due to defective elastic fibers in its wall). The ophthalmic check up is to rule out visual problems due to dislocation of lens (lens is held in position by the suspensory ligament, which is composed of elastic fibers).

SINGLE BEST RESPONSE TYPE MULTIPLE CHOICE QUESTIONS

1. The luminal cells belonging to the following type of epithelium are provided with extra reserve of plasma membrane:
   a. Stratified squamous
   b. Transitional
   c. Stratified cuboidal
   d. Stratified columnar

2. The secondary center of ossification appears in following part of the developing bone:
   a. Diaphysis
   b. Metaphysis
   c. Epiphyseal plate
   d. Epiphysis

3. Which of the following connective tissue cells is active in tissue healing:
   a. Plasma cell
   b. Myofibroblast
   c. Mast cell
   d. Leukocyte

4. The prickles that characterize the keratinocytes in stratum spinosum represent:
   a. Ribosomes
   b. Tight junctions
   c. Desmosomes
   d. Hemidesmosomes

5. The following cell migrates into epidermis during embryonic life and may turn into skin cancer:
   a. Keratinocyte
   b. Langerhans
   c. Fibroblast
   d. Melanocyte

6. The reticular layer of dermis consists of following type of connective tissue:
   a. Loose areolar
   b. Dense irregular
   c. Dense regular
   d. Adipose tissue

7. Which of the following are pressure receptors in skin:
   a. Merkel's discs
   b. Meissner's corpuscles
   c. Pacinian corpuscles
   d. Ruffini's endings

8. Which of the following is the frontal plane:
   a. Sagittal
   b. Midsagittal
   c. Coronal
   d. Horizontal

9. Which of the following is found inside Volkmann's canal:
   a. Blood vessel
   b. Process of osteocytes
   c. Sharpey's fiber
   d. Lymphatic vessel

10. The linear growth of a long bone is disrupted by a fracture passing through:
    a. Diaphysis
    b. Epiphysis
    c. Epiphyseal plate
    d. Metaphysis

11. Laminin is a structural protein mainly found in:
    a. Plasma membrane
    b. Nuclear membrane
    c. Basal lamina of basement membrane
    d. Reticular lamina of basement membrane

12. What is the surface modification seen in epithelial cells of epididymis:
    a. Microvilli
    b. Ruffles
    c. Stereocilia
    d. Cilia

13. Which of the following is not a fibrous joint:
    a. Schindylesis
    b. Symphysis
    c. Gomphosis
    d. Syndesmosis

14. Which of the following is a pressure epiphysis:
    a. Os trigonum
    b. Radial tuberosity
    c. Head of radius
    d. Fabella

15. Which of the following cells is a histiocyte:
    a. Plasma cell
    b. Fibroblast
    c. Macrophage
    d. Monocyte

16. Metachromasia is characteristic of following cell:
    a. Plasma cell
    b. Melanocyte
    c. Macrophage
    d. Mast cell

17. T-tubule in a skeletal muscle is part of:
    a. Smooth endoplasmic reticulum
    b. Rough endoplasmic reticulum
    c. Sarcolemma
    d. Myofilaments

18. Myelination of axons of optic nerve and of sciatic nerve is the function of which of the following pair (cells are arranged in the order of the nerves):
    a. Satellite cells and oligodendroglia
    b. Protoplasmic astrocytes and Schwann cells
    c. Fibrous astrocytes and ependymal cells
    d. Oligodendroglia and Schwann cells

19. Which of the following is a resistance vessel:
    a. Medium-sized artery
    b. Medium-sized vein
    c. Arteriole
    d. Venule

20. The neurons of following site are example of upper motor neuron:
    a. Motor cortex of cerebrum
    b. Cerebellar cortex
    c. Ventral horn of spinal cord
    d. Motor nuclei of cranial nerves

21. Structural component of bone responsible for tensile strength is:
    a. Calcium
    b. Phosphorus
    c. Collagen
    d. Hydroxyapatite

22. Where does the conversion of procollagen to tropocollagen occur:
    a. Rough endoplasmic reticulum
    b. Smooth endoplasmic reticulum

c. Extracellular compartment

d. Golgi complex

23. The osteoclast is formed by undergoing the following processes:

a. Apoptosis

b. Cytokinesis and karyokinesis

c. Cytokinesis but no karyokinesis

d. Karyokinesis but no cytokinesis

24. Which of the following is the outer covering of the peripheral nerve:

a. Perineurium

b. Neurilemma

c. Epineurium

d. Endoneurium

25. Lipofuscin pigment in aging neurons is derived from which of the following:

a. Nissl granules

b. Neurofibrils

c. Golgi bodies

d. Lysosomes

KEY TO MCQs

1. b	2. d	3. b	4. c	5. d	6. b	7. c	8. c
9. a	10. c	11. c	12. c	13. b	14. c	15. c	16. d
17. c	18. d	19. c	20. a	21. c	22. c	23. d	24. c
25. d							

Section 2

GENERAL EMBRYOLOGY

8

General Embryology including Basic Genetics and Genetic Causes of Birth Defects

Chapter Contents

INTRODUCTION

General embryology includes the prenatal development of the embryo and fetus. The prenatal development takes place inside the uterus of the mother. The prenatal period (gestation period) is divisible into germinal or pre-embryonic (first three weeks), embryonic (four to eight weeks) and fetal (from nine weeks until birth). The embryonic period is the critical period of organogenesis. The embryonic tissues are highly susceptible to teratogenic agents like viruses, drugs, radiation, etc. during organogenesis.

The new life begins as a zygote, which is a unicellular organism. A new human being is created by the complex processes of multiplication and differentiation from this unique cell. The zygote is formed by the union of sperm (a male gamete) and a secondary oocyte (a female gamete). The gametes are haploid cells (23 chromosomes) unlike the somatic cells of the body, which are diploid (46 chromosomes). They are formed in gonads. The oocytes develop in ovaries and sperms develop in testes.

GAMETOGENESIS

The formation of gametes by conversion of primordial germ cells into gametes is known as gametogenesis.

Oogenesis

The formation of mature ovum from the oogonium is called **oogenesis**. It takes place in the ovaries.

Spermatogenesis

The formation of sperm from the spermatogonium is called **spermatogenesis**. It takes place in the testes.

Significance of Meiosis or Reduction Divisions during Gametogenesis

The germ cell is the only cell in the body that has the capacity to undergo meiotic divisions. During prophase of meiosis I, homologous maternal and paternal chromosomes exchange chromatid segments during crossover (Fig. 8.29) to ensure genetic variation in daughter cells and then move from each other during anaphase I to go to new daughter cells ensuring the haploid status of the daughter cells. During meiosis II there in no replication of DNA in the haploid cells but there is splitting of chromosomes during anaphase II (Fig. 8.25) like in mitosis so that each gamete retains the haploid status and half the amount of DNA.

Stages in Oogenesis (Fig. 8.1)

The process of oogenesis is quite lengthy as it begins in the ovaries of the female fetus (before birth) and continues up to the end of reproductive life of the female.

- *Oogonia* are the primordial germ cells which divide by mitosis to increase their number during embryonic and fetal life. Their number is highest during 4th to 5th month of intrauterine life.
- *Primary oocytes* differentiate from some oogonia that enlarge. The primary oocytes enter the prophase of first meiotic division in female fetus and remain arrested in this stage until the onset of puberty. From puberty onwards during each ovarian cycle one primary oocyte begins to mature and completes its first meiotic division just before ovulation. The products of first meiotic division are unequal. The larger cell is called secondary oocyte and the much smaller cell is called the first polar body.
- *Secondary oocyte* immediately enters the second meiotic division which is completed only if it is penetrated by the sperm after ovulation. The products

of second meiotic division are unequal. The larger cell is called the ovum and the smaller cell is called second polar body. If not fertilized the secondary oocyte does not complete the meiosis and is thrown out of the uterus with the next menstrual flow. The polar bodies degenerate.

Ovarian Cycle (Fig. 8.2)

The ovarian cycle begins at the age of puberty. The ovary undergoes cyclic changes which are repeated every 4 weeks starting at puberty and ending at menopause. The ovarian cycle is regulated by gonadotrophic hormones secreted by anterior pituitary. It consists of following three stages:

1. Preovulatory or follicular stage
2. Ovulation
3. Postovulatory or luteal stage

Preovulatory or Follicular Stage

Under the influence of follicle stimulating hormone (FSH) the ovarian follicles undergo maturation changes.

- Primordial follicles which consist of primary oocyte surrounded by a single row of spindle-shaped follicular cells begin to grow.
- Primary follicles are formed when the spindle-shaped follicular cells become columnar in shape and become multilayered. The primary oocyte enlarges and a thick and pale covering called zona pellucida appears between the follicular cells and the oocyte.

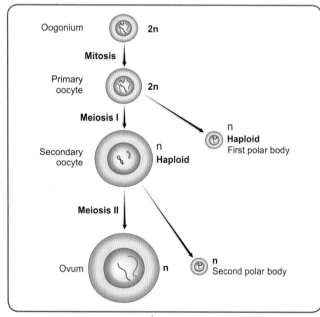

Fig. 8.1: Stages in oogenesis

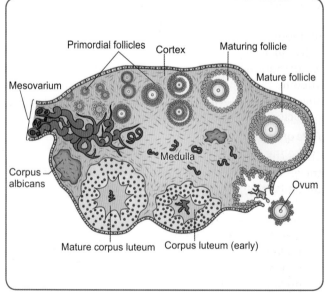

Fig. 8.2: Section of ovary showing stages in ovarian cycle including ovulation

- Secondary follicles are formed when the follicular cells proliferate to form membrana granulosa and the primary oocyte further increases in size and its nucleus becomes larger and vesicular.

  Theca interna (secretory cells) and theca externa (thickly packed fibers and spindle-shaped cells) are discernible around the secondary follicle. They are derived from the spindle-shaped cells of the stroma of ovarian cortex.
- Tertiary follicle is characterized by formation of a fluid filled antrum inside the membrana granulosa.
- Graafian follicle is the mature follicle, which is very large in size (2 to 5 mm). It bulges out of the surface of the ovary in to the peritoneal cavity, as the time of ovulation nears. The theca interna becomes more prominent and its estrogen secreting cells constitute thecal gland. The primary oocyte is surrounded by cumulus oophorus. Just before ovulation, the primary oocyte completes first meiotic division and gives rise to secondary oocyte with a haploid nucleus and the first polar body.

Ovulation (Fig. 8.2)

Ovulation means release of secondary oocyte (surrounded by zona pellucida and cells of corona radiata derived from cumulus oophorus) from the surface of the ovary in to the peritoneal cavity, after the rupture of Graafian follicle under the influence of LH (luteinizing hormone) surge in the plasma. The ovulation takes place 14th day prior to the onset of the next menstrual period.

Secondary Oocyte

The liberated secondary oocyte is picked up by the fimbriated end of the uterine tube. It is in the process of undergoing second meiotic division. It is a very large cell and measures about 140 microns in diameter. It is surrounded by corona radiata, zona pellucida and vitelline membrane (cell membrane). The perivitelline space is present between the vitelline membrane and zona pellucida. The nucleus contains 23 chromosomes.

Fate of Secondary Oocyte

The secondary oocyte surrounded by various coverings travels through the uterine tube assisted by cilia and gentle muscular contractions.

- If during this journey through the uterine tube the secondary oocyte is penetrated by the sperm the fertilized secondary oocyte completes its second meiotic division. This is also an unequal division in which an ovum and second polar body are formed. The polar body occupies the perivitelline space.

- If the secondary oocyte is not fertilized, it dies within one day and is discharged from the uterus.

Postovulatory Stage

This stage of ovarian cycle is also called luteal stage. Its duration is always fourteen days. This is useful in calculating the time of ovulation. For example if a woman's menstrual cycle is of 35 days her ovulation time is (35–14 = 21), i.e. on 21st day of the menstrual cycle.

Corpus luteum

The ruptured Graafian follicle is converted into corpus luteum under the influence of luteinizing hormone. Corpus luteum is a temporary endocrine gland.
- At first the outer wall of the Graafian follicle collapses and the cavity is filled with blood.
- The granulosa cells and theca interna cells begin to proliferate and are filled with yellowish lipochrome pigment and change in to lutein cells which secrete progesterone and estrogen.

Fate of corpus luteum

- Corpus luteum of pregnancy develops if the liberated secondary oocyte is fertilized. It functions for 3 to 4 months under the influence of human chorionic gonadotropin. After fourth month of pregnancy the corpus luteum of pregnancy undergoes slow regression.
- Corpus luteum of menstruation develops if fertilization does not take place. Its functional life is 14 days after which it degenerates to form corpus albicans or white body.

Endometrial or menstrual cycle (Fig. 8.3)

The wall of endometrium consists of three layers:
1. Endometrium or mucosa lining the uterus
2. Myometrium or muscular wall
3. Perimetrium or peritoneal covering

From puberty until menopause, the endometrium undergoes changes in a cycle of 28 days under the influence of the hormones secreted by the ovary.

Stages of menstrual cycle

- Follicular or proliferative stage (under control of estrogen)
- Secretory or progestational stage (under control of progesterone)
- Menstrual

Figure 8.3 shows the correlation between endometrial changes and ovarian changes during normal menstrual cycle and during pregnancy. After implantation of blastocyst, the endometrium changes in to the decidua.

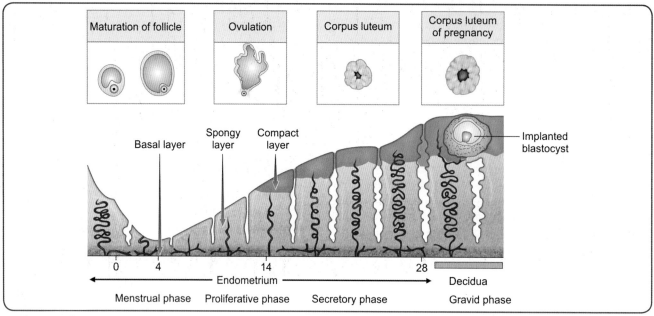

Fig. 8.3: Changes in uterine mucosa (endometrial cycle) in relation to ovarian cycle. (Note the implantation of blastocyst in secretory endometrium and formation of corpus luteum of pregnancy in the ovary)

🔖 **STUDENT INTEREST**

Oogenesis begins before birth in the ovaries of female fetus. The primordial germ cells form oogonia which undergo repeated mitotic divisions. Some of the oogonia are arrested in prophase of meiosis I and are surrounded by follicular cells to form primordial follicles. At puberty the primordial follicle grows in to secondary follicle or Graafian follicle. Just before ovulation due to surge in luteinizing hormone the primary oocyte completes its first meiotic division to form secondary oocyte (haploid cell) and first polar body. The secondary oocyte cannot complete the second meiotic division unless fertilized by sperm. If not fertilized the secondary oocyte is thrown out of uterus through next menstrual flow. The estrogen is secreted by theca interna cells of Graffian follicle and progesterone is secreted by lutein cells of corpus luteum during each ovarian cycle to prepare the endometrium of uterus for implantation.

Note: Corpus luteum and Graafian follicle are short-note questions.

Stages in Spermatogenesis (Fig. 8.4)

The process of formation of sperms begins by the age of puberty in the seminiferous tubules in male. The spermatogonia begin to divide mitotically. Some spermatogonia enlarge into primary spermatocytes, which first meiotic division to give rise to two equal haploid cells known as secondary spermatocytes. Following the second meiotic division of the two secondary spermatocytes four spermatids are formed.

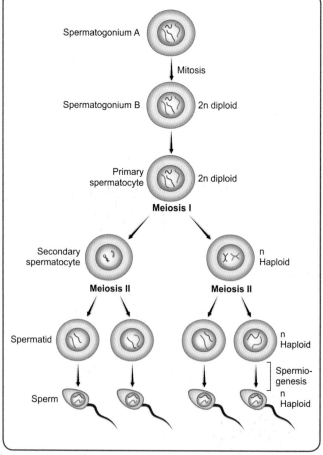

Fig. 8.4: Stages in spermatogenesis

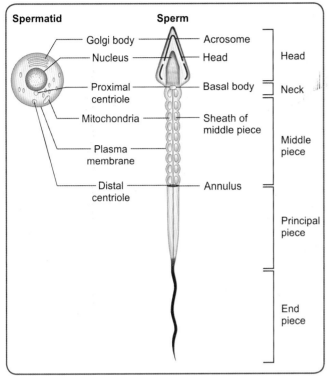

Fig. 8.5: Process of spermiogenesis in which different cell organelles of spermatid give rise to different parts of a sperm

Spermiogenesis (Figs 8.4 and 8.5)

The rounded spermatids change into motile elongated sperms by a process called *spermiogenesis*. The nucleus of spermatid becomes the head of sperm. The acrosomal granules in Golgi body become the acrosomal cap covering a large area of the nucleus. One centriole occupies the neck and the middle piece contains axial filament that is surrounded by mitochondrial sheath. The caudal end of middle piece is limited by ring-like second centriole. The principal piece consists of axial filament surrounded by fibrous sheath. The last segment is the long tail piece consisting of axial filament. The entire sperm thus formed is covered with plasma membrane.

🛈 STUDENT INTEREST

Spermatogenesis begins at puberty in male, when the primordial germ cells differentiate in to spermatogonia, which in turn give rise to primary spermatocytes. The primary spermatocytes undergo meiosis I to form two haploid secondary spermatocytes. The secondary spermatocytes undergo second meiotic division to form two haploid spermatids. Lastly the round spermatid undergoes spermiogenesis to change in to highly motile elongated sperm. The time taken by the spermatogonium to change into sperm is around 64 days.

FERTILIZATION

The union of secondary oocyte and sperm takes place normally in the ampulla of uterine tube or fallopian tube. The following events occur in the gametes preparatory to the fertilization:

- At the time of fertilization, the ovulated secondary oocyte is surrounded by a glycoprotein layer called zona pellucida, which is covered by cells of corona radiata (derived from cumulus oophorus). The perivitelline space is located between the zona and the vitelline membrane (which is the plasma membrane of the secondary oocyte).
- After entering the female genital tract, the sperms undergo capacitation (functional changes) and acrosomal reaction in the uterine tube.
- The capacitation means the removal of glycoproteins, cholesterol and seminal proteins from plasma membrane around the acrosomal cap of the sperm. Only the capacitated sperms are able to penetrate the corona radiata.
- The head of the sperm binds with the zona pellucida and triggers the acrosomal reaction and release of acrosomal enzymes, which create a path in zona pellucida.
- Once the sperm reaches the perivitelline space zona reaction is induced by secondary oocyte to prevent the entry of other sperms.
- The secondary oocyte completes its second meiotic division as soon as the head of the sperm enters its cytoplasm. The nucleus in the head of sperm develops into male pronucleus and nucleus of fertilized ovum develops into female pronucleus. After losing their nuclear envelopes the pronuclei fuse and chromosomes intermingle to form a new diploid cell called *zygote*.

Effects of Fertilization

- Restoration of the species specific chromosome number (46 in the case of human).
- Determination of the chromosomal sex of the zygote (if a Y bearing sperm fertilizes the ovum it results in male zygote and if X bearing sperm fertilizes the ovum it results in female zygote).
- Initiation of the process of cleavage in which the zygote undergoes rapid mitotic divisions to form smaller cells called *blastomeres*.

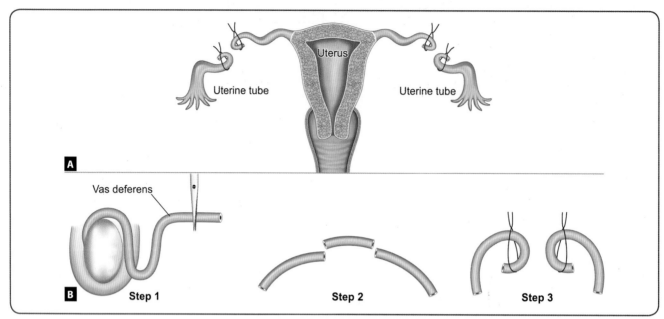

Figs 8.6A and B: A. Tubectomy (Family planning operation in female); **B.** Vasectomy (family planning operation in male)

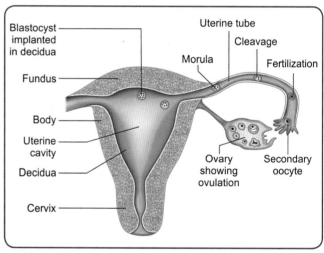

Fig. 8.7: Cleavage and morula formation (events in early embryogenesis) in the uterine tube

Cleavage of Zygote and Formation of Morula (Fig. 8.7)

The cleavage is a process, in which, there are rapid repeated mitotic divisions of zygote immediately after fertilization. The smaller and smaller cells thus formed are called **blastomeres**. The morula (resembling mulberry) is formed at 16-cell stage. It is covered by zona pellucida. Gradually,

the morula adds to its cell population as it travels from the uterine tube to the uterine cavity.

Blastocyst Formation

The morula changes into the blastocyst (Fig. 8.8) inside the uterine cavity as follows:
- There is accumulation of fluid inside the morula through zona pellucida followed by segregation of cells of morula into inner cell mass and outer cell mass enclosing a cavity.

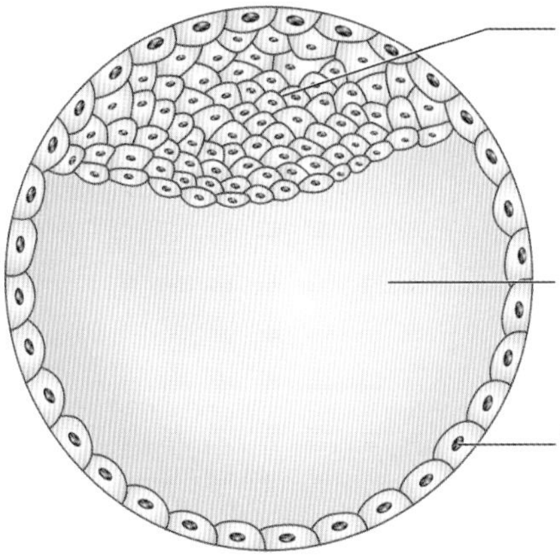

Fig. 8.8: Conversion of morula in to blastocyst in the uterine cavity

- Soon the cavity of blastocyst enlarges and the flattened cells of outer cell mass around it are called the trophoblast.
- The inner cell mass is attached to trophoblast at the embryonic pole of the blastocyst.
- The zona pellucida disappears by fifth day after fertilization.
- The blastocyst begins implantation in endometrium by sixth or seventh day after fertilization.
- The inner cell mass develops into the embryo and the trophoblast develops into chorion, which later takes part in the formation of placenta (the nutritive organ).
- The trophoblast subdivides into inner cytotrophoblast and outer syncytiotrophoblast. The latter begins to secrete human chorionic gonadotropin (hCG) hormone and by the end of second week (after missed period) the hormone can be detected in the urine sample of pregnant woman by radioimmunoassay. This is the basis of pregnancy test.

Implantation of Blastocyst (Fig. 8.3)

It is a process by which blastocyst is embedded in to the secretory endometrium. The syncytiotrophoblast erodes the endometrial tissue creating a passage for the blastocyst to enter and embed inside the endometrium. This is the characteristic interstitial implantation in human being.

Normal site of implantation (Fig. 8.9A)

The implantation of the blastocyst usually occurs in the endometrium lining the posterior wall of the body of the uterus (nearer the fundus).

STUDENT INTEREST

Remember that zygote changes in to morula in the uterine tube by a process of cleavage. At 16-cell stage inner cells of morula form inner cell mass and surrounding cells form the trophoblast. The inner cell mass is the forerunner of embryo and trophoblast gives rise to protective and nutritive fetal membranes. The morula changes in to blastocyst inside the uterine cavity. It is the blastocyst that implants in the secretory endometrium on the posterior wall of uterus nearer the fundus in normal cases. After implantation in to the endometrium, the endometrium changes in to decidua. Learn the three subdivisions of decidua.

Decidua

The decidua is the name given to the endometrium after the implantation is completed. The human chorionic gonadotrophin (hCG) secreted by syncytiotrophoblast is responsible for the decidual reaction in which stromal cells of endometrium are converted into enlarged decidual cells as they are filled with abundant glycogen and lipids. Histologically the decidua is very much thicker, edematous, vascular, glandular and cellular than the endometrium.

Subdivisions and Fate of Decidua

After complete implantation of blastocyst the decidua is divisible into three parts.

1. ***Decidua basalis*** covers the blastocyst on the side facing the uterine wall. It takes part in the maternal component of the placenta.
2. ***Decidua capsularis*** covers the blastocyst on the side facing the uterine cavity.
3. ***Decidua parietalis*** is the most extensive, does not cover the blastocyst but lines the rest of uterine cavity.

The decidua capsularis fuses with the amnion and chorion laeve to form chorioamniotic membrane. As the amniotic cavity expands further, there is complete obliteration of uterine cavity when chorioamniotic membrane fuses with decidua parietalis.

CLINICAL CORRELATION

Abnormal Sites of Implantation

- The blastocyst may be implanted nearer the cervix of uterus. This results in formation of placenta which may cover the internal os (upper opening of cervical canal). This condition is called ***placenta previa.***

Contd...

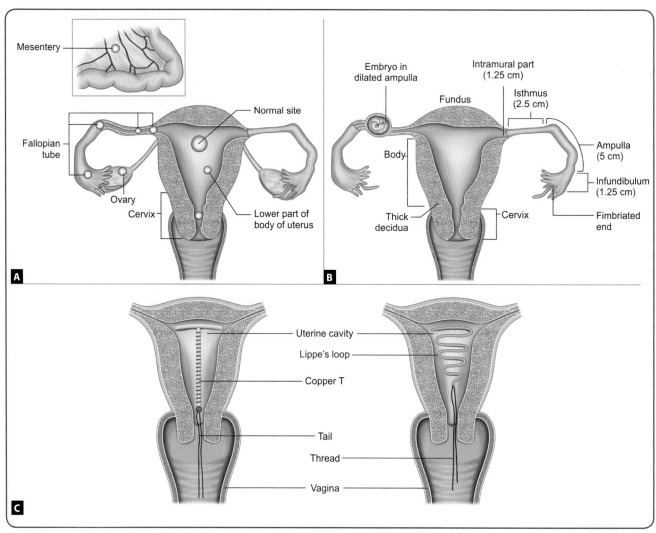

Figs 8.9A to C: A. Showing normal site of implantation on posterior wall of uterus nearer the fundus (also note the abnormal sites of implantation); **B.** Tubal pregnancy in which implantation takes place in the ampulla of uterine tube (Note the four parts of uterine tube with the length of each part); **C.** Copper T and Lippe's loop in uterine cavity (temporary contraceptive measures)

Contd…

⚕ CLINICAL CORRELATION

- Implantation in uterine tube is called tubal pregnancy (Fig. 8.9B). When the products of conceptus grow inside the tube it produces symptoms like pain in lower abdomen. The natural fate of tubal pregnancy is rupture of the tube leading to severe hemorrhage in the peritoneal cavity. It is a surgical emergency.
- The rare sites of implantation are ovarian surface, peritoneum, surface of intestine and rectouterine pouch.

Contraceptive Device to Prevent Implantation

IUCD (intrauterine contraceptive device) like copper–T is inserted in to the uterine cavity to prevent implantation (Fig. 8.9C).

Formation of Bilaminar Embryonic Disc (Figs 8.10A and B)

At the beginning of second week the cells of inner cell mass differentiate into two layers called ***ectoderm*** and ***endoderm***. Subsequent to this amniotic cavity and yolk sac cavity are formed.

Endoderm

The cells closer to the cavity of blastocyst arrange in a single layer to form endoderm.

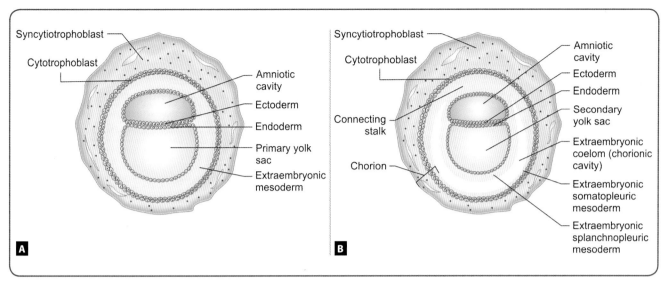

Figs 8.10A and B: A. Formation of bilaminar embryonic disc from inner cell mass of blastocyst (also note the amniotic cavity above the ectoderm and primary yolk sac below the endoderm); **B.** Bilaminar embryonic disc surrounded by extraembryonic coelom (note the development of secondary yolk sac and chorion at this stage)

Ectoderm

The ectoderm is formed from the rest of the cells of the inner cell mass which become columnar cells and lie above the endoderm.

Amniotic Cavity (Figs 8.10A and B)

The amniotic cavity appears between ectoderm and adjacent trophoblast. The roof of this cavity is formed by amniogenic cells which are delaminated from the trophoblast. They produce amniotic fluid.

Primary Yolk Sac (Fig. 8.10A) and Secondary Yolk Sac (Fig. 8.10B)

Soon the endodermal cells grow to line the cavity of the blastocyst, which is now called ***primary yolk sac***. Concurrently, the cells of primary yolk sac proliferate to form the extraembryonic mesoderm between the trophoblast externally and the amniotic cavity and yolk sac cavity internally. The extraembryonic mesoderm splits to form extraembryonic coelom except adjacent to the roof of amniotic cavity. Here the mesoderm forms connecting stalk (the forerunner of umbilical cord). The extraembryonic coelom compresses the primary yolk sac reducing its size. The reduced primary yolk sac is converted in to secondary yolk sac.

Chorion (Fig. 8.10B)

The formation of extraembryonic coelom subdivides the extraembryonic mesoderm into outer somatopleuric layer and inner splanchnopleuric layer. The somatopleuric layer of extraembryonic mesoderm lies subjacent to the trophoblast. The combination of the aforesaid two layers is known as chorion. The chorion is divisible into chorion frondosum and chorion laeve. The chorion frondosum contributes to the fetal part of placenta and the chorion laeve fuses with amnion and decidua capsularis to form chorioamniotic membrane.

Prochordal Plate (Fig. 8.11A)

- At the end the second week, the prochordal plate appears at the cranial end of the bilaminar embryonic disc as some endodermal cells become columnar. It appears as a rounded thickened area.
- At this site the columnar endodermal cells are firmly adherent to the ectoderm.
- The prochordal plate confers the central craniocaudal axis to the embryonic disc.
- The intraembryonic mesoderm does not enter the prochordal plate.
- After the folding the embryonic disc, in the fourth week, the prochordal plate moves ventral to the notochord intervening between the endodermal foregut and the ectodermal stomodeum.

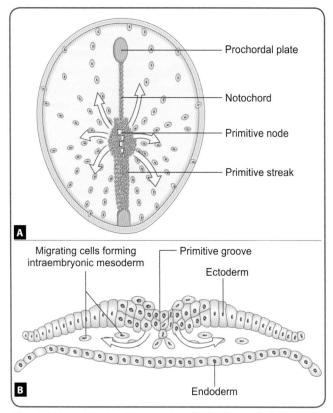

Figs 8.11A and B: Primitive streak and primitive node showing the process of gastrulation

- It ruptures at the end of fourth week to establish communication between the foregut and the oral cavity.

Primitive Streak and Gastrulation (Figs 8.11A and B)

The third week after fertilization is characterized by gastrulation, which is crucial in converting the bilaminar embryonic disc into trilaminar embryonic disc (gastrula). This process establishes the three germ layers, (1) endoderm, (2) mesoderm and (3) ectoderm.

Formation of primitive streak

The primitive streak is the primary organizer of the embryo. It makes its first appearance in the midline at the caudal end of the disc by proliferation of the ectodermal cells. Then it elongates in cranial direction and ends in a rounded area called ***primitive node*** or ***primitive knot*** or ***Hensen's node***.

Gastrulation

The ectodermal cells begin to proliferate and migrate towards the groove in the primitive streak to invaginate

between the ectoderm and endoderm. These invaginated cells give rise to the intraembryonic mesoderm or secondary mesoderm. After this the circular bilaminar disc is converted into pear-shaped trilaminar disc.

The intraembryonic mesoderm fails to invaginate into the prochordal plate at the cranial end and cloacal membrane at the caudal end. These two bigerminal sites are destined to breakdown in due course of development.

Fate of primitive streak

Normally by fourth week of embryonic life the primitive streak regresses and disappears.

> **⚕ CLINICAL CORRELATION**
>
> **Remnants of Primitive Streak Cells**
>
> Occasionally pluripotent cells (stem cells) of primitive streak do not perish in sacrococcygeal region and proliferate to give rise to sacrococcygeal teratoma. Such tumors contain tissues derived from the ectoderm, mesoderm and endoderm.
>
> **Teratogenic Effects on Primitive Streak**
>
> The gastrulation process is highly sensitive to teratogenic effects.
> - High doses of alcohol intake by mothers during this sensitive or critical period of development can affect cells in cranial midline of embryo producing holoprosencephaly (small forebrain, fusion of lateral ventricles of brain, and hypertelorism in which eyes are very close to each other).
> - Gastrulation process is susceptible to teratogenic insult leading to formation of insufficient intraembryonic mesoderm at the caudal end of the embryonic disc. Since this mesoderm contributes to development of lower limbs, urogenital organs and lumbosacral vertebrae, there is fusion of lower limb (mermaid like appearance), vertebral abnormalities, renal agenesis and abnormalities of genital organs. These combined defects are known as ***caudal dysgenesis*** or ***sirenomelia*** (Fig. 8.12).

Formation of Notochord

- The primitive node and primitive pit (a depression in the center of primitive node) play a key role in the formation of notochord. The cells of primitive node divide and invaginate the primitive pit (also called blastopore) to move in cranial direction in the midline until they reach the prochordal plate. This cellular plate extending from primitive node to the prochordal plate is called the ***notochordal process*** (Fig. 8.11A)
- The notochordal process elongates in caudal direction as a result of gradual regression of primitive streak and primitive node

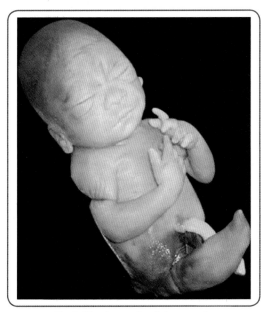

Fig 8.12: Anomaly of sirenomelia

- The canalization of notochordal process results in formation of notochordal canal, which opens into amniotic cavity by blastopore.
- The cells in the floor of the notochordal canal are intercalated (merged) with underlying endodermal cells. Soon after this, the process of breaking down of

notochordal and endodermal cells of the floor begins at the caudal end. This creates a temporary curved passage called neurenteric canal, which communicates the yolk sac cavity with the amniotic cavity blastopore.
- As the process of breakdown of the floor is completed, the notochordal canal is converted into the notochordal plate (which is between the endoderm and the ectoderm).
- The notochordal plate changes into definitive notochord (resembling a solid cellular rod) by a process of fusion of its margins.

Significance of Notochord

- The notochord provides the central axis to the embryonic disc. The vertebral canal is laid down around the notochord
- The notochord induces the overlying ectodermal cells to become neuroectodermal cells and form the neural tube (the forerunner of brain and spinal cord).

Fate of Notochord

The notochord regresses after the development of vertebrae around it. Its remnants are:
- Nucleus pulposus of intervertebral discs.
- Apical ligament attached to the dens of axis vertebra.

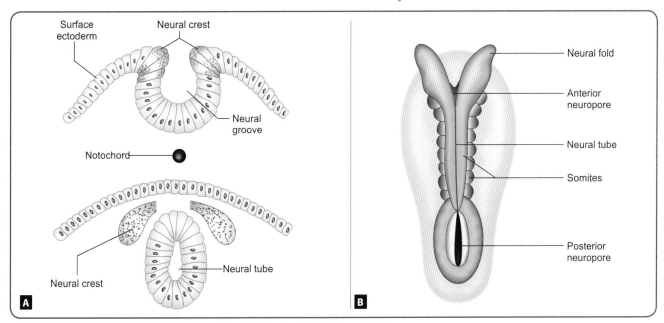

Figs 8.13A and B: A. Formation of neural tube from surface ectoderm; **B.** Dorsal surface of embryonic disc showing anterior and posterior neuropores at the ends of developing neural tube

The chordoma is the tumor arising from cells of at the cranial end of the notochord seen at the base of the cranium. It has a tendency to spread to the nasopharynx.

Prochordal plate, primitive streak and notochord are short note questions. Study the topic with the help of simple diagrams.

Formation of Neural Tube or Neurulation (Fig. 8.13A)

- The neuroectodermal cells of the neural tube are differentiated from the ectoderm overlying the notochord under the inductive influence of the notochord.
- The neuroectodermal cells gather to form a neural plate in the midline dorsally. The neural plate has broad cranial end and narrow caudal end.
- It develops a neural groove centrally and raised edges (neural folds) on either side. As the neural groove deepens the folds come closer until they fuse
- The neural tube is formed by fusion of the neural folds of the neural plate.
- The closure of neural groove is a gradual process. It begins in the cervical region and extends in cranial and caudal directions. Therefore, for some time, the neural tube is in communication with amniotic cavity by a cranial opening (anterior neuropore) and a caudal opening (posterior neuropore) as shown in figure 8.13B.
- The time of closure of anterior neuropore is around day twenty-fifth and that of posterior neuropore is around day twenty-seventh.

Neural Tube Defects (NTD)

The failure of closure of neuropores gives rise to neural tube defects (NTD) which are of two types.
- Anencephaly (Figs 8.14A and B) results due to failure of closure of anterior neuropore.
- Spina bifida defects of different severities occur due to failure of closure of posterior neuropore. In meningocele, there is protrusion of spinal pia-arachnoid producing a CSF filled sac. In meningomyelocele, there is protrusion of pia-arachnoid and spinal cord tissue in the CSF filled sac while in rachischisis; there is exposure of neural tissue through the defect in the back.

The NTDs can be prevented by peri-conceptional intake of folic acid by the prospective mothers.

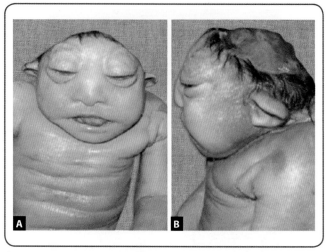

Figs 8.14A and B: A and B. Frontal view and lateral profile of a newborn with the anomaly of Anencephaly (Note the degenerated brain tissue exposed through deficient cranial vault)

Neural Crest (Fig. 8.13A)

During the process of fusion of neural folds a few junctional cells at the crest or summit of the neural folds separate and give rise to a cluster of cells called neural crest on either side.

Derivatives of Neural Crest Cells (Fig. 8.15)

- Autonomic ganglia (sympathetic and parasympathetic)
- Sensory or dorsal root ganglia of spinal and cranial nerves
- Adrenal medulla
- Schwann cells
- Melanocytes
- Pia-arachnoid

Subdivisions of Intraembryonic Mesoderm (Fig. 8.16A)

From medial to lateral side the intraembryonic mesoderm is subdivided into three parts as follows:
1. Paraxial mesoderm
2. Intermediate mesoderm
3. Lateral plate mesoderm

Paraxial Mesoderm

The paraxial mesoderm is located dorsally on either side of the midline. It is a thickened column of mesoderm, which breaks up into segments called *somites* in the craniocaudal direction. The somite period of embryonic life extends from day 20 to day 35.

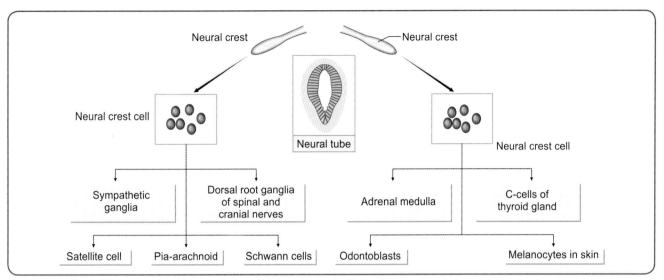

Fig. 8.15: Derivatives of neural crest cells

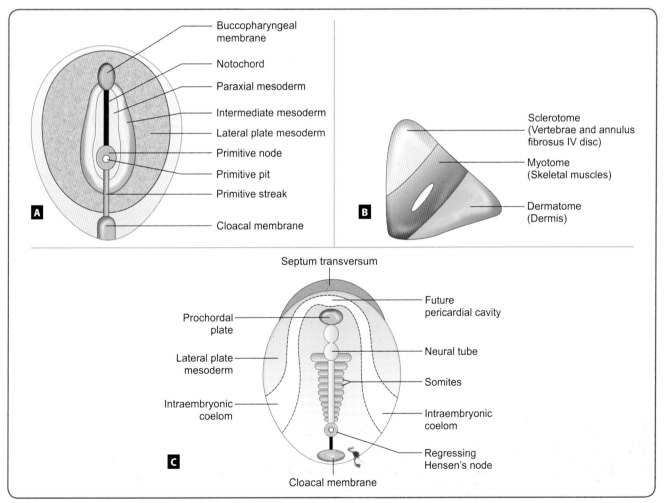

Figs 8.16A to C: A. Trilaminar embryonic disc showing three subdivisions of intraembryonic mesoderm into paraxial mesoderm, intermediate mesoderm and lateral plate mesoderm; **B.** Subdivisions of somite into sclerotome (medially), myotome (in the middle); and **C.** Splitting of lateral plate mesoderm to form intraembryonic coelom (Note the septum transversum at the cranial end of embryonic disc)

Number of pairs of somites is about 42 to 44 (4 occipital, 8 cervical, 12 thoracic, 5 lumbar, 5 sacral and 8–10 coccygeal). Of these, the first occipital somite and 5 to 7 coccygeal somites degenerate.

Each somite is subdivided into three parts as follows (Fig. 8.16B):
1. Laterally placed dermatome (forming dermis of skin)
2. Centrally placed myotome (forming skeletal muscles)
3. Medially placed sclerotome (forming vertebrae and annulus fibrosus of intervertebral discs).

Intermediate Mesoderm

The intermediate mesoderm is located between the paraxial mesoderm medially and lateral plate mesoderm laterally. It develops in to organs of excretion (kidneys, ureters and part of urinary bladder) and organs of reproduction (gonads, genital ducts, etc.).

Lateral Plate Mesoderm (Fig. 8.16C)

The lateral plate mesoderm is organized in the shape of inverted U. The right and left halves of the lateral plate mesoderm are continuous cranial to the prochordal plate.
- It splits into two layers—(1) the somatopleuric intraembryonic mesoderm and (2) the splanchnopleuric intraembryonic mesoderm.
- These layers enclose a cavity called *intraembryonic coelom*. This cavity is the forerunner of pericardial cavity, pleural cavities and the peritoneal cavity.
- A small part of lateral plate mesoderm cranial to pericardial coelom fails to split. This un-split part is known as septum transversum, which is the most cranial landmark of the trilaminar germ disc.

✤ CLINICAL CORRELATION

Neural tube develops in to central nervous system (CNS) (brain and spinal cord). Time of closure of anterior and posterior neuropores must be studied. Failure of closure of anterior neuropore leads to anencephaly. Neural crest is important because it is a source of diverse structures. It gives rise to sensory ganglia, Schwann cells, satellite cells or amphicytes, sympathetic ganglia, parasympathetic ganglia, adrenal medulla, melanocytes, pia-arachnoid, etc. Intraembryonic mesoderm is a very important topic. The derivatives of its three subdivisions are to be understood. Paraxial mesoderm divides in to somites and each somite divides in to sclerotome, myotome and dermatome.

Folding of Embryonic Disc

The pear-shaped two-dimensional embryonic disc is converted into a three-dimensional cylindrical human like form by a process of embryonic folding.

- The folding in the median plane produces ventrally directed cranial fold and a caudal fold. Folding in transverse plane produces ventrally directed two lateral folds. As a result of cranial folding the septum transversum (the most cranial landmark of trilaminar disc) is shifted caudal to the pericardium, which itself is brought ventral to the foregut.
- The ectodermal depression called *stomodeum* is located between the pericardial bulge and the head bulge.
- The buccopharyngeal membrane (derived from prochordal plate) separates the foregut and the stomodeum. The buccopharyngeal membrane breaks down at end of fourth week.
- The caudal end of hindgut is closed by the cloacal membrane, which breaks down at seventh week.
- The ectoderm lines the external surface of embryo and the amniotic cavity completely surrounds the embryo. The amnio-ectodermal junction is shifted around the umbilicus.
- The yolk sac is partly taken inside the embryo to form primitive gut consisting of foregut, midgut and hindgut.
- The body stalk (the forerunner of umbilical cord) is now attached to the ventral surface of the embryo and contains inside it extraembryonic mesoderm, extraembryonic part of the yolk sac, allantois and the left umbilical vein and umbilical arteries.

FETAL MEMBRANES (FIGS 8.17A AND B)

The fetal membranes develop simultaneously with embryo and the fetus to take care of the protection and nourishment of the embryo and the fetus. The fetal membranes being extraembryonic structures are discarded after the baby is delivered. The fetal membranes are:
- Yolk sac
- Allantois
- Amnion
- Chorion
- Umbilical cord

Yolk Sac

The yolk sac is divisible into three sacs—(1) primary yolk sac, (2) secondary yolk sac and (3) definitive yolk sac.
- The primary yolk sac (Fig. 8.10A) is formed from the cavity of the blastocyst after it is lined by endodermal cells in the second week.
- With formation of extraembryonic coelom the primary yolk sac decreases in size and is now called secondary yolk sac (Fig. 8.10B). The main functions of the secondary yolk sac during third week are angiogenesis and formation of primordial germ cells, which migrate

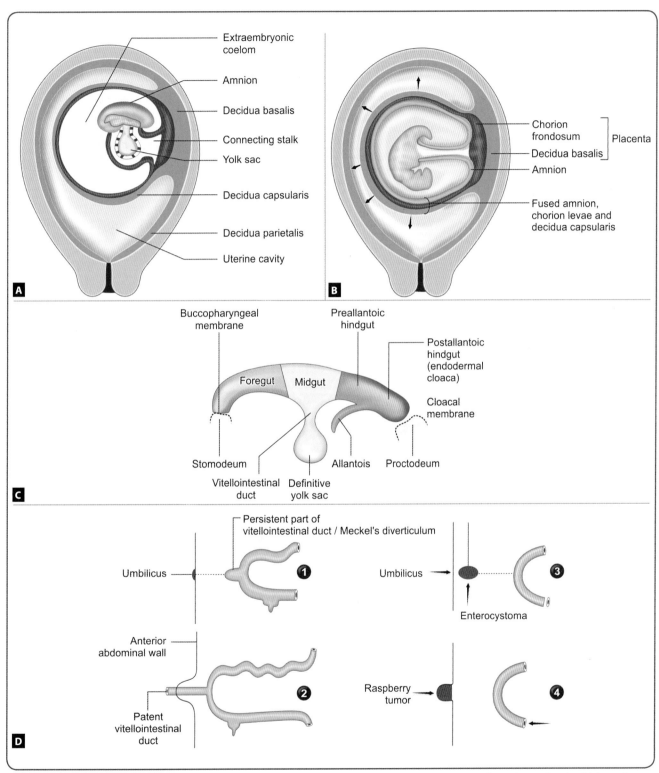

Figs 8.17A to D: A and B. Position of various fetal membranes (amnion, yolk sac, connecting stalk, etc.) just after the folding of embryo and in the growing fetus (Note that the amniotic cavity expands at the expense of extraembryonic coelom and uterine cavity); **C.** Fate of yolk sac after folding of embryo; **D.** Anomalies of vitellointestinal duct
Key: 1. Meckel's diverticulum; **2.** Umbilical fecal fistula; **3.** Enterocystoma; **4.** Raspberry tumor at umbilicus

to the developing gonads and give rise to oogonia or spermatogonia.

- After folding of the embryo, secondary yolk sac is subdivided into three parts (Fig. 8.17C) as follows:
    1. Midgut of the primitive gut (intraembryonic).
    2. Vitellointestinal duct (partly intraembryonic and partly in the umbilical cord).
    3. Definitive yolk sac (inside the umbilical cord).

Fate of definitive yolk sac and vitellointestinal duct

- Definitive yolk sac atrophies.
- Vitellointestinal duct atrophies in its entire extent. Occasionally it persists in its proximal part as Meckel's diverticulum or ileal diverticulum. The anomalies of vitellointestinal duct are shown in Figure 8.17D.

Allantois

The allantois is a small diverticulum from the yolk sac into the connecting stalk before the folding of embryo. It performs the function of hemopoeisis.

After the embryonic folding, the allantois appears as a diverticulum from the hindgut.

The allantois divides the hindgut in to pre-allantoic part and post-allantoic part (also known as *endodermal cloaca*). The endodermal cloaca is subdivided into anterior part called *urogenital sinus* and posterior part called rectum by *urorectal septum*.

Now the allantois is shifted to urogenital part of cloaca. Its intraembryonic part is called urachus, which extends from the urogenital sinus up to the umbilicus. Its extraembryonic part enters the umbilical cord. After birth the urachus changes into median umbilical ligament extending from the apex of urinary bladder to the umbilicus and it raises a peritoneal fold called median umbilical fold.

If the urachus remains patent at birth the urine leaks out at umbilicus (weeping umbilicus) as illustrated in a photograph of an infant (Fig. 48.13).

Amnion

The amnion is a transparent membrane that forms the amniotic sac containing amniotic fluid.

The amnion consists of amniogenic cells (which arise from the trophoblast) and the extraembryonic mesoderm in the second week of gestation. The amnio-ectodermal junction is evident at each end of the ectodermal layer and the amniotic cavity is located above the ectodermal layer (Fig. 8.10A).

After folding of the embryonic disc, the amniotic cavity surrounds the embryo as the bilateral amnio-ectodermal junctions come together and fuse around the umbilical opening on the embryonic ventral surface (Fig. 8.17B).

The initial expansion of the amniotic cavity takes place at the expense of extraembryonic coelom. With the disappearance of extraembryonic coelom, the amnion fuses with chorion laeve and decidua capsularis to form chorioamniotic or amnio-chorio-decidual membrane. Further expansion of the amniotic cavity takes place at the expense of uterine cavity, which is obliterated with the fusion of chorioamniotic membrane with the decidua parietalis (Figs 8.17A and B).

The fluid-filled amniotic cavity provides shock proof environment for the fetus. At the time of childbirth the amnio-chorio-decidual or chorioamniotic membrane forms a hydrostatic bag, which helps in dilatation of the cervical canal during childbirth.

The amount of amniotic fluid at full term is around 800 to 1000 mL. The amniotic fluid is formed from various sources like secretion of amniogenic cells, diffusion from maternal tissues across the chorioamniotic membranes, diffusion from maternal blood in intervillous space and urine secreted by fetal kidneys. The amniotic fluid is drained across the chorioamniotic membranes. In addition to this, the fetus regularly swallows the amniotic fluid. The swallowed amniotic fluid is absorbed from respiratory and gastrointestinal tract into the fetal blood from which it reaches the placenta via umbilical arteries.

🔖 CLINICAL CORRELATION

- *Hydramnios* or *polyhydramnios* is a condition in which volume of amniotic fluid is abnormally high.
- *Oligohydramnios* is a condition in which volume of amniotic fluid is less than normal.
- *Amniocentesis* (Fig. 8.34A) is a procedure for removing amniotic fluid for prenatal diagnosis of certain diseases like Down syndrome, neural tube defects and inborn errors of metabolism. For further details refer to "Prenatal Diagnosis under Genetics".

Chorion

The chorion consists of trophoblast (syncytiotrophoblast and cytotrophoblast) lined internally by somatopleuric layer of extraembryonic mesoderm or primary mesoderm (Fig. 8.10B). It is formed during the second week of gestation and it surrounds the embryonic disc uniformly initially.

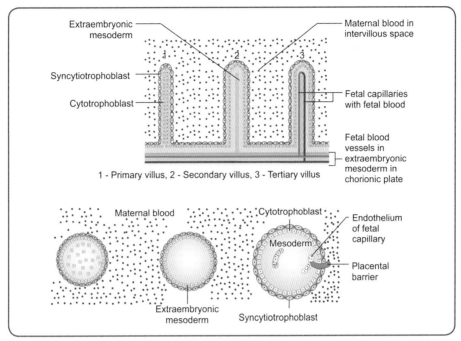

Fig. 8.18: Stages in the formation of Chorionic Villi (Primary, Secondary and Tertiary) [Note the tissue layers (placental barrier) between blood in fetal capillaries in the tertiary villi and maternal blood in the intervillous space]

Establishment of Uteroplacental Circulation

After implantation, the syncytiotrophoblast erodes the decidua so that lacunar spaces are created in it. Erosion of uterine blood vessels fills the lacunar spaces with maternal blood. This is the beginning of uteroplacental circulation. Soon the finger-like columns of syncytiotrophoblast extend between the lacunae all around.

Three stages in formation of chorionic villi (Fig. 8.18)
1. ***Primary chorionic villi*** are formed when columns of syncytiotrophoblast are invaded by a single layer of cytotrophoblast.
2. ***Secondary villi*** are formed when the underlying extraembryonic mesoderm or primary mesoderm invades the core of primary villi.
3. ***Tertiary villi*** are formed when fetal capillaries develop in the mesodermal core of secondary villi. The tertiary villi are the functional units of the placenta.

Chorion Frondosum and Chorion Laeve

- Chorionic villi in contact with decidua basalis grow vigorously like a bush hence, are called ***chorion frondosum***.
- Chorionic villi in contact with decidua capsularis degenerate and become smooth hence are called ***chorion laeve***.

PLACENTA

The placenta is a vital organ of temporary existence essential for intrauterine growth and development of the fetus. It attaches the fetus to the uterus of mother. It is called ***composite organ*** as both maternal and fetal tissues (which are genetically different) contribute to its development. Fully formed placenta is composed mainly of fetal tissue and of maternal tissue. The placenta starts developing soon after implantation and is fully functional around third to fourth month of pregnancy. The placenta is shed after the childbirth. A normal full term placenta is disc shaped with a diameter of 15 to 20 cm and weight of 500 to 600 g. It presents a smooth fetal surface and a rough maternal surface. The fetal surface is transparent as it is covered with amnion. The umbilical cord is attached to this surface usually at the center. The maternal surface is rough due to presence of cotyledons, which are aggregations of chorionic villi separated by grooves occupied by placental septa. About fifteen to twenty cotyledons are seen on the maternal surface.

Structure of Mature Placenta (Fig. 8.19)

The placental tissues are arranged in following order from fetal to maternal surface:

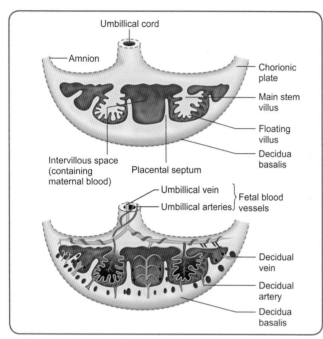

Fig. 8.19: Structure of mature placenta and the position of fetal (umbilical arteries and umbilical vein) and maternal blood vessels (decidual arteries and veins) in the placenta

- Chorionic plate is covered on fetal surface by amnion and gives attachment to umbilical cord. In the stroma deep to amnion is found the connective tissue supporting the main branches of umbilical vein and arteries. Still deeper are the layers of cytotrophoblast and syncytiotrophoblast.
- Intervillous space containing stem villi, anchoring villi and free or floating villi in addition to maternal blood
- Basal plate consists of outer wall of intervillous space comprising cytotrophoblastic shell having pores for spiral arteries and corresponding veins, fibrinoid deposits and maternal decidua.

Developmental Sources of Placenta

Placenta develops from two sources:
1. Fetal component—from chorion frondsum
2. Maternal component—from decidua basalis

Development of Cytotrophoblastic Shell in Placenta

As the chorionic villi of chorion frondosum grow into decidua basalis, a cytotrophoblastic shell is formed on the fetal surface of the decidua basalis by the cytotrophoblastic

cells that come out through the tips of syncytiotrophoblast and spread to form a wall on the adjacent decidual surface.

Types of Chorionic Villi inside Placenta

- The *stem villi* or *anchoring villi* are the first to grow. They extend from the chorion (on the fetal side) to the cytotrophoblastic shell (on the maternal side) to which they are fixed.
- The *free villi* or *floating villi* or *branch villi* arise from the stem villi. They extend into the intervillous space which is filled with maternal blood. The spiral arteries in the decidua basalis pierce the cytotrophoblastic shell and the high pressure arterial blood is sprayed like a garden hose on the floating chorionic villi in the intervillous space. The venous blood is collected by spiral veins passing through the cytotrophoblastic shell. The floating chorionic villi are the real sites of gaseous exchange between the maternal blood in the intervillous space and the fetal blood in the fetal capillaries inside the floating villi. As the maternal blood comes in direct contact with the chorionic villi in the human species, the placenta is described as hemochorial.

Placental Barrier

The tissues between the fetal blood in the fetal capillaries inside the floating chorionic villi and the maternal blood inside the intervillous space constitute the placental barrier.

Starting from fetal side towards intervillous space the placental barrier consists of following tissues:
- Endothelium of fetal capillaries
- Primary mesoderm or extraembryonic mesoderm
- Cytotrophoblast
- Syncytiotrophoblast

Towards the end of the pregnancy (towards term) the placental barrier thins out to such an extent that it consists of endothelium of fetal capillaries and syncytiotrophoblast only.

Functions of Placenta

- Exchange of blood gases.
- Passage of nutrients and immunoglobulin G (IgG) type antibodies from maternal to fetal side.
- Passage of metabolic waste from fetal to maternal side.
- Production of hormones like human chorionic gonadotropin, human placental lactogen, estrogen, progesterone and relaxin.

CLINICAL CORRELATION

Placenta Previa

- First degree placenta previa means the site of attachment of placenta is in the lower uterine segment. In this case the placenta completely or partially covers the internal os of cervix.
- Second degree placenta previa
- Third degree placenta previa
- Fourth degree placenta previa

Vesicular Mole

The vesicular mole is a condition in which chorionic villi degenerate producing grape-like cystic swellings.

Gestational Carcinoma

The choriocarcinoma or gestational carcinoma is a highly malignant pathology of chorionic villi.

STUDENT INTEREST

Placenta is a "Must know" topic. Placenta is composed of maternal tissues and fetal tissues. Maternal tissue is decidua basalis and fetal tissue is chorion frondosum. Read about decidua basalis and chorion frondosum. The chorionic villi pass through three stages during development, primary, secondary and tertiary. The tertiary villi are the functional units of placenta. They float in the intervillous space which contains maternal blood. The tertiary chorionic villus is covered with outer layer of syncytiotrophoblast and inner layer of cytotrophoblast. The core of the villus contains primary mesoderm supporting the fetal capillaries. The syncytiotrophoblast is in direct contact with the maternal blood. The fetal blood inside the capillaries and the maternal blood in the intervillous space are separated by placental barrier, which is composed of syncytiotrophoblast, cytotrophoblast, primary mesenchyme and endothelium of fetal capillaries. Towards the term of gestation, the placental barrier thins out and consists of only two layers (syncytiotrophoblast and endothelium of fetal capillaries).

Umbilical Cord

At birth, the umbilical cord is attached to the center of the fetal surface of placenta to the center of the anterior abdominal wall of fetus (location of future umbilicus). It is approximately 50 to 60 cm long and 2 cm in diameter. It is highly twisted due to which it presents false knots. The cord is covered with a shining membrane called amnion.

The umbilical cord develops from the connecting stalk of the embryonic disc. The extraembryonic mesoderm inside the connecting stalk becomes Wharton's jelly of the umbilical cord. Wharton's jelly supports the vessels and

some remnants inside the umbilical cord, namely a single umbilical vein (carrying oxygenated blood to the fetus), two umbilical arteries (carrying deoxygenated blood from the fetus) and remnants of vitellointestinal duct, definitive yolk sac and of allantois.

 CLINICAL CORRELATION

- A very long umbilical cord may prolapse into cervical canal during childbirth. The prolapsed cord and the umbilical vessels inside it may be compressed by fetal head resulting in hypoxia to the fetus.
- Occasionally the cord encircles the neck of the fetus in utero causing fetal distress.
- Nowadays, cord blood is stored in cord blood banks in a frozen state to provide a future source of pluripotent stem cells (which can be used for stem cell therapy in case the donor develops blood cancer). The cord blood cells can be injected into bone marrow, where they carry on the function of hemopoesis.

ADDED INFORMATION

The organogenetic period (4th to 8th weeks) is regarded as the critical period of human embryonic development as during this period there is maximum cell division and cell differentiation and highest susceptibility to teratogenic agents (viruses, drugs, chemicals, ionizing radiation, etc.). Congenital anomalies (birth defects) in various organs are the feared complication if pregnant mother is exposed to teratogens during organogenetic period. For example, the developing limbs are most susceptible to tranquilizers like thalidomide during 24 to 36 days after fertilization (critical period for developing limbs). Such exposure leads to anomalies like amelia (absence of limbs) and phocomelia (absence of a part of limb as shown in Fig. 8.20). A pregnant mother suffering from German measles due to exposure to rubella virus during critical period of development of the eyes, heart and ears (4 to 5 weeks after fertilization) is in danger of having the baby born with congenital cataract, cardiac defects and deafness (rubella syndrome).

Twinning and Multiple Births

Multiple births result from simultaneous intrauterine development of two or more embryos. The most common form of multiple births is twinning in which two embryos grow together.

Classification of Twins

- Monozygotic or identical or uniovular twins
- Dizygotic or fraternal or non-identical or binovular twins
- Conjoined twins (Siamese twins)

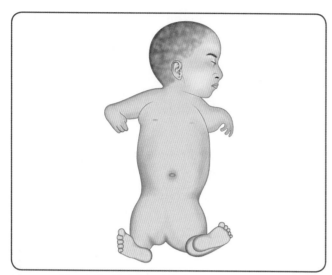

Fig. 8.20: Thalidomide baby with phocomelia

Monozygotic Twins

They are genetically identical, have same blood groups, identical fingerprints and are of same sex. They are formed by splitting of the zygote at different stages. Sometimes splitting can occur at 2-cell stage of zygote. But usually, splitting of inner cell mass of blastocyst occurs. Each part of the inner cells mass proceeds to become an independent embryo (within the common blastocele. Each embryo has a separate amniotic sac but a common placenta.

Dizygotic Twins or Fraternal Twins

This type of twinning is more common than monozygotic twinning. In dizygotic twinning two embryos are formed from two separate zygotes (which result by simultaneous fertilization of two secondary oocytes by two sperms). They are genetically different; their sex may be same or different and appearance is like siblings born to same parents. Since blastocyst implant separately, each has its own amniotic sac and placenta.

Conjoint Twins

These are a type of twins which are fused to each other physically. They arise due to incomplete splitting of primitive node or primitive streak. According to the site of fusion they are named as follows:
- Craniopagus (back to back fusion of heads)
- Pyropagus (fusion by lower back)
- Thoracopagus (fusion by ventral walls of thorax so that twins face each other).

Conjoint twins can survive and live a full life as illustrated by the lives of Chang and Eng Bunker born on 11th May 1811 in Thailand and lived in United States.

Multiple Births

A unique case of multiple births (of surviving octuplets) in California became international news in January 2009.

BASIC GENETICS AND GENETIC FACTORS IN CAUSATION OF CONGENITAL ANOMALIES

The magnitude of the problem of congenital anomalies due to genetic causes can be appreciated taking a look at the prevalence of genetic diseases in the developing countries (1 out of 50 newborns with major congenital anomaly (like anencephaly), 1 out of 100 newborns with monogenic disease (e.g. hemophilia) and 1 out of 200 newborns with major anomaly of chromosome 21 (Down syndrome). It is estimated that 50% of mental retardation is due to genetic causes of which 30% is due to Down syndrome.

The genetic diseases are caused by and large either by gene mutation or by chromosomal defects.

Monogenic Diseases

The monogenic diseases occur due to mutation of DNA sequence of a single gene. The genes are the specific units of the chromosomal DNA. The normal function of the gene is to produce the proteins, which carry out most of life functions. When the gene is altered or mutated, its protein product can no longer carry out its normal functions and the consequence of this is a genetic disease.

Modes of Inheritance of Monogenic Diseases

Autosomal dominant inheritance

Autosomal dominant disorders arise due to a defective dominant gene on the autosome that expresses in a single dose (heterozygous state).

The distinguishing features are:
- The dominant gene and the disease appear in every generation hence described as vertically transmitted disorders.
- Sons and daughters are equally affected.
- If one parent is affected half the children (50%) are at risk of inheriting the gene and are affected. If both parents are affected all the children (100%) are affected.

Examples of the diseases transmitted by autosomal dominant mode are:
- Achondroplasia (circus dwarf)
- Huntington's chorea
- Marfan's syndrome
- Osteogenesis imperfecta
- Neurofibromatosis
- Familial hypercholesterolemia

Autosomal recessive inheritance

Autosomal recessive disorders occur when both the genes on a pair of autosome are affected and it is well known that recessive gene expresses as disease only in double dose (homozygous state). This means both the parents must carry this gene to pass on to the offspring to express as disease.

The distinguishing features of autosomal recessive mode are:

- These diseases are more common in consanguineous marriages (cousin marriages or maternal uncle-niece marriages).
- When both the parents carry the affected gene there is chance of 25% children affected by the disease. If one parent carries the gene there is probability of 50% children being normal and 50% being the carriers of the disease (carrier means carrying the affected gene but showing no signs of disease).
- The disease may skip a few generations (unlike the autosomal dominant inheritance).
- The affected child may not have the affected through an affected parent.

Examples of diseases transmitted by autosomal recessive mode are:

- Albinism
- Cystic fibrosis
- Hemoglobinopathies (sickle cell anemia, B- thalassemia, etc)
- Inborn errors of metabolism including phenylketoneuria and hemocystineuria.

X-linked disorders

X-linked diseases arise due to defective gene on X-chromosome. The male receives maternal X-chromosome (hemizygous state) which means whether the mutant gene on it is recessive or dominant it will express. The female has two X-chromosomes. She may be heterozygous (when a gene on one X-chromosome is affected) or homozygous (if genes on both X-chromosomes are affected). The noteworthy feature of all X-linked inheritance is that father does not transmit the defective gene on X-chromosome to the sons but transmits it to the daughters.

X-linked recessive inheritance

Distinguishing features of this mode are:

- There is no father to son transmission of the gene (because fathers do not pass on X-chromosome to the sons) but sons are affected more by the disease compared to daughters.

- Affected fathers transmit the defective gene only to the daughters that become carriers.
- An affected mother equally transmits the gene to sons and daughters.
- The marriage between affected man and carrier woman will produce 25% affected sons, 25% carrier daughters and 50% normal children. If both parents are affected all children will be affected. A marriage between affected man and normal woman will produce 50% normal sons and 50% carrier daughters.

The examples of X-linked recessive inheritance are:

- Red-green color blindness
- Hemophilia or bleeder's disease
- Glucose-6-phosphatase dehydrogenase deficiency (G6PD deficiency)
- Duchenne muscular dystrophy (DMD)

X-linked dominant inheritance

X-linked dominant disorders arise from an affected heterozygote female if one dominant gene is affected on the X-chromosome.

Distinguishing features of this mode are:

- The disease manifests in heterozygous female and hemizygous male.
- Affected heterozygous female transmits the gene equally to daughters and sons.
- The marriage between the affected woman (heterozygous affected) and normal man is likely to produce 25% affected daughters, 25% affected sons, 25% normal daughters and 25% normal sons.
- The marriage between affected man and normal woman is likely to produce affected daughters and normal sons.

One example of this mode of inheritance is vitamin D resistant rickets.

Holandric inheritance

Holandric or Y-linked inheritance is from father to son. There are very few genes on Y chromosome hence diseases by this mode of inheritance are not seen. The hairy pinna is the only example of this inheritance.

Polygenic or Multifactorial Diseases

The polygenic or multifactorial diseases are caused by a combination of environmental factors and mutation of multiple genes. Some examples of multifactorial diseases are cancers, atherosclerosis, hypertension, Alzheimer's disease, schezophrenia, epiliepsy, diabetes and obesity.

ADDED INFORMATION

Mitochondrial Inheritance

Mitochondrial inheritance is a mode by which mutant genes inherited from mother's mitochondria cause some rare genetic diseases. The non chromosomal DNA is located in the mitochondria DNA (mtDNA). It is to be noted that mitochondria of the zygote are derived only from the ovum (from mother) and the sperm (from father) does not contribute any cell organelles to the zygote. Therefore a mutant mitochondrial gene in the mother will be inherited by all her offspring irrespective of sex. The affected sons do not transmit the mutant gene but affected daughters do. Leber's hereditary optic neuropathy (LHON), Leigh's syndrome and Kearns-Sayre syndrome are the examples of mitochondrial inheritance.

GENETIC DISEASES DUE TO CHROMOSOMAL DEFECTS

To understand the chromosomal defects it is essential to have prior knowledge of normal chromosomes and method of studying them (karyotyping) in the laboratory.

General Features of Normal Chromosomes

- The chromosomes are located inside the nucleus of the cell.
- They carry the genes which contain DNA-protein packages on specific positions called loci and pass them on from one generation to the next through reproductive process.
- The number of chromosomes is species specific. In human it is 46 in somatic cells. The 46 chromosomes are arranged in 23 pairs of homologous chromosomes (one member of the pair being derived from mother and the other from the father).
- The somatic cells are known as diploid (symbolically designated by 2n) and the gametes containing 23 chromosomes are known as haploid (symbolically designated by n).
- The 46 chromosomes are divided into 44 autosomes and 2 sex chromosomes (normal female has XX sex chromosomes and normal male has XY sex chromosomes).
- The chromosomes are best visible during cell division (mitosis and meiosis) under a light microscope.

Parts of a Chromosome (Fig. 8.21A)

Each chromosome presents two chromatids held together by a primary constriction called centromere which is a non-staining gap. The centromere divides the chromosome in to an upper short or (p) arm and a lower long or (q) arm. The free ends or tips of chromatids are called telomeres. They close the ends of chromatids and make them insensitive to the proximity of neighboring chromatids.

Morphological Types of Chromosomes (Fig. 8.21B to E)

Depending upon the position of centromere, the chromosomes are classified into four types.

1. **Metacentric chromosome** presents the centromere near its central point so that (p) arm equals to (q) arm (p = q).
2. **Sub-metacentric chromosome** presents the centromere near the intermediate point so that (q) arm is longer than (p) arm (p < q).
3. **Acrocentric chromosome** presents a centromere near the end of short arm. It is characterized by long (q) arms and very short (p) arms. The (p) arms bear satellites. Such chromosomes are known as **SAT-chromosomes**.
4. **Telocentric chromosomes** present centromere at one end where the long arms meet. They lack short arms and satellites. They are not seen in human being.

Karyotyping and Karyotype

The karyotyping is a method of chromosome preparation and staining used for identification of individual chromosome under the microscope in the metaphase of cell division (Fig. 8.22). The enlarged photomicrograph of the stained metaphase spread is taken. Then individual chromosomes are cut out and arranged in homologous pairs in descending order of their heights. This photographic representation of the entire chromosome complement is called **karyotype**. The karyotyping is indicated to detect chromosomal anomalies (both structural and numerical).

Common Techniques for Studying Chromosomes

- Blood culture, Giemsa banding and karyotyping.
- FISH (fluorescent *in situ* hybridization) is a rapid method as no culture is necessary.

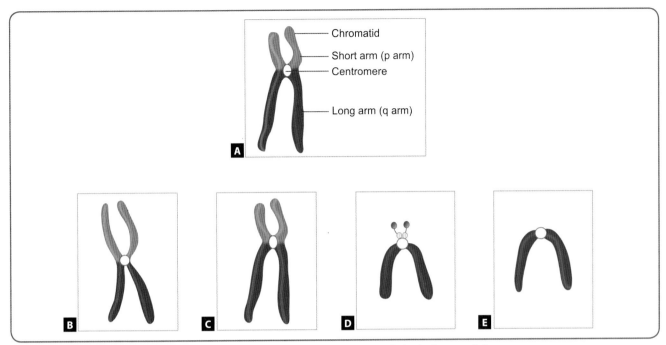

Figs 8.21A to E: A. Parts of chromosome; **B to E.** Morphological types of chromosomes
(**B.** Metacentric; **C.** Submetacentric; **D.** Acrocentric, telocentric)

Blood Culture, Giemsa Banding and Karyotyping

- 5 mL venous blood is collected in heparinized syringe and red cells are separated off by centrifugation.
- The white cell suspension is transferred to culture vials containing culture medium, fetal calf serum, phytohemagglutinin (mitogenic agent extracted from French beans) and antibiotics.
- Culture vials are kept in incubator at 37° centigrade (body temperature) for 3 days.
- After about 70 hours colchicine is added to the culture to arrest the mitoses at metaphase by preventing spindle formation.
- After centrifugation for 5 minutes, supernatant is discarded and cell pellet at the bottom of the test tube is treated with hypotonic solution.
- The cells swell on treatment with hypotonic solution there by separating the chromosomes from each other.
- The cells are fixed in a solution of acetic acid and methanol in the ratio of 1:3.
- The cells are dropped on a chilled slide from a height to release the chromosomes out of the cells. The chromosomes are stained with Giemsa.
- The chromosomes are identified by their banding patterns and their photographic representation in descending order of height (karyotype) is prepared (Fig. 8.22).

Denver Classification of Chromosomes

From their banding patterns and lengths of the arms, the chromosomes are classified into 7 groups.

1. *Group A* consists of pairs of following chromosome numbers 1, 2 and 3 (total chromosome number being 6). The chromosomes of this group are metacentric and the longest.
2. *Group B* consists of pairs of chromosome numbers 4 and 5 (total chromosome number is 4). They are submetacentric and long.
3. *Group C* consists of pairs of chromosome numbers from 6 to 12 and X chromosome (total number in female is 16 and in male is 15). They are of medium height and submetacentric.
4. *Group D* consist of pairs of chromosome numbers 13, 14, and 15 (total number is 6). They are medium-sized and acrocentric chromosomes bearing satellites on short arms (SAT chromosomes).
5. *Group E* consists of pairs of chromosomes numbers 16, 17 and 18 (total number is 6). They are shorter than group D chromosomes but submetacentric.
6. *Group F* consists of pairs of chromosome numbers 19 and 20 (total number is 4). They are short metacentric.
7. *Group G* consists of pairs of chromosome numbers 21 and 22 and Y chromosome (total number is 4 in female and 5 in male). They are shortest acrocentric SAT chromosomes.

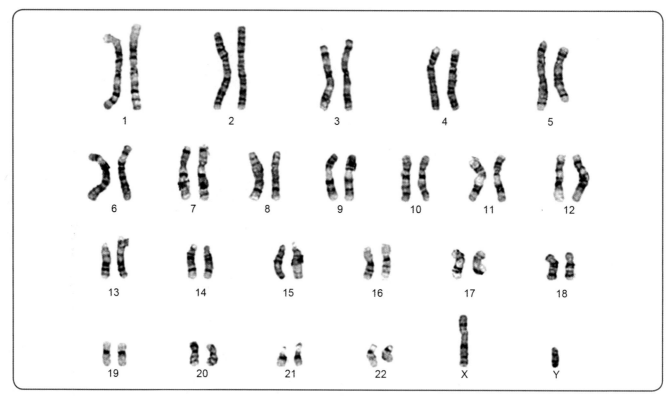

Fig. 8.22: Karyotype of a normal male (46, XY)

Sex Chromosome (Figs 8.23A and B)

X and Y chromosomes are called sex chromosomes because they determine the sex of zygote at the time of fertilization (Table 8.1). If Y-bearing sperm fertilizes the secondary oocyte the resultant zygote develops into male. If X-bearing sperm fertilizes the secondary oocyte the resultant zygote develops into female.

Role of Y Chromosome in Sex Differentiation

- Until 6 weeks of development, the genital organs are undifferentiated. Hence, it is known as indifferent stage (neither male nor female external genitalia are distinctly identifiable). The reproductive organs consist of gonads and genital ducts of both sexes, Wolffian and Mullerian.
- In the presence of SRY gene (that produces testis determining factor) the indifferent gonad develops in to testis.
- Sertoli cells in fetal testis secrete Mullerian inhibiting factor (MIF), which suppresses the Mullerian ducts

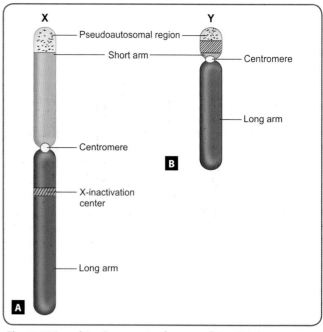

Figs 8.23A and B: Comparative features of X and Y chromosomes

TABLE 8.1: Comparative features of X and Y chromosomes

Features	X chromosome	Y chromosome
Length	Long	Very short
Group	C-medium-sized, submetacentric	G-short acrocentric with satellites
Staining with Quinacrine dye	—	Vivid fluorescence in interphase and metaphase
Pseudoautosomal region	Xpter (at terminal part of p arm)	Ypter (at terminal part of p arm)
Number of genes	Several X-linked genes on both arms	SRY gene on (p) arm
X-inactivation	On band Xq13 on either paternal or maternal	No X-inactivation
Center	X chromosomes	

and stimulates the growth of Wolffian ducts to form male genital ducts (epididymis, vas deferens, seminal vesicles and ejaculatory ducts).

- Leydig cells of fetal testis secrete testosterone to stimulate the development of indifferent external genitalia on male line.
- In the female, due to absence of SRY gene, the indifferent gonad develops in to ovary. In the absence of MIF, the Mullerian ducts differentiate in to female genital ducts (fallopian tubes, uterus and vagina) and the indifferent external genitalia develop on female line. The Wolffian ducts regress.

Sex Chromatin or Barr Body (Figs 8.24A to C)

It is the heterochromatic and inactive X-chromosome found inside the nuclei of somatic cells of the female in the interphase of cell cycle. It is usually found in cells of buccal mucosa (adjacent to nuclear membrane), in neurons (attached to nucleolus) and in neutrophils (drum stick from nucleus). This condensed clump of chromatin is intensely basophilic. It is named Barr body after its discoverer Murray L Barr who along with Bertram discovered it in neurons of the female cats in the year 1949. It is in the year 1962 that Mary Lyon explained the reason and time of X-inactivation. According to Lyon hypothesis, the inactivation of one sex chromosome (either maternal X or paternal X) takes place from around 16th week of embryonic life. The condensed X chromosome lags in replication of DNA as it is out of sync with the rest of chromosomes. There is X-inactivation gene on the long arm of X chromosome.

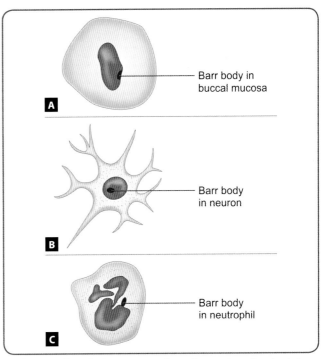

Figs 8.24A to C: Appearance of sex chromatin or Barr body in various somatic cells of normal female

Significance of barr bodies

The number of Barr bodies is one less than the number of X chromosomes. Therefore, by counting the number of Barr bodies by a simple buccal smear test one can find out the numerical anomalies of sex chromosomes (Table 8.2).

Structural Anomalies of Chromosomes

These include change in the structure of chromosome by breakage of chromosome and subsequent reunion of broken piece. This may result in abnormal genotype and consequently the altered phenotype (genetic disease). There are different types of structural anomalies.

TABLE 8.2: Number of Barr bodies in normal and abnormal number of sex chromosomes

Normal female	XX	1 Barr body
Normal male	XY	0 Barr body
Turner syndrome in female	XO	0 Barr body
Isochromosome X	46 Xi (Xq)	1 Barr body
Klinefelter syndrome in male	47 XXY	1 Barr body
Superfemale	47 XXX	2 Barr bodies

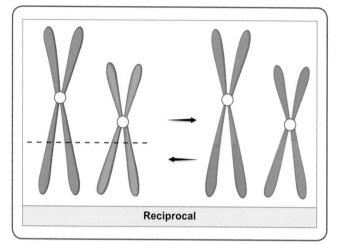

Fig. 8.25: Reciprocal translocation in which there is reciprocal transfer of broken segments of two non-homologous chromosomes

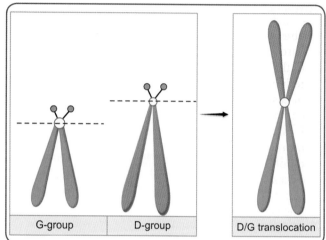

Fig. 8.26: Robertsonian translocation or D/G translocation in which acrocentric chromosomes break at their centromeres and there is fusion of long arms of D and G group chromosomes

Deletion

- There may be a loss of a piece of one arm or loss of piece of both arms of a chromosome. Cri du chat (or cat's cry) syndrome is due to deletion of short arm of chromosome 5 (designated by the symbol 5p-).
- A ring chromosome is formed if there is deletion at both ends and the broken arms unite to form a ring-shaped chromosome.

Translocation

The translocation is the defect in which there is break in two different chromosomes and later exchange of the broken parts. So the genetic material is transferred from one chromosome to another.

Reciprocal translocation (Fig. 8.25)

This involves breakage of two non-homologous chromosomes with exchange of fragments. This type of translocation with no loss of genetic material and no change in chromosome number may be problematic during segregation in meiosis. This may lead to early abortion.

Robertsonian translocation (Fig. 8.26)

This translocation, e.g. D/G translocation results when two acrocentric chromosomes (belonging to groups D and G) break at their centromeres and there is subsequent fusion of their long arms. Interestingly the short arms of these chromosomes are lost. Thus the total chromosomal number is reduced by one (45 chromosomes). The chromosome formula of a male with Robertsonian translocation is 45, XY, t (14q, 21q). Such an individual is called ***carrier of translocation***. The carrier is a normal person. However, at the time of meiotic segregation a few gametes with translocated chromosome (14/21) and normal chromosome number 21 may be formed. Union of a sperm with Robertsonian translocation and a normal ovum results in translocation Down syndrome which is indicated by the formula 46 XX or XY, t (14q, 21q).

Isochromosome

The isochromosome is an abnormal chromosome, which is produced due to transverse division at centromere. There is separation of short and long arms. Thus, the isochromosome is composed of two long arms only. This anomaly common in X chromosome and is the cause of Turner's syndrome in some patients. The isochromosome is nonfunctional chromosome. Hence, this type of Turner's syndrome is characterized by 46 chromosomes but is Barr body negative. The chromosome formula of isochromosome X Turner's syndrome is 46 X, I (Xq).

Philadelphia Chromosome (Ph[1] Chromosome)

This is an acquired abnormality of chromosomes in white blood cells in peripheral blood and bone marrow of patients with chronic myeloid leukemia (CML). Philadelphia chromosome is a shortened chromosome 22 due to replacement of a segment of its long arm by a small fragment of long arm of chromosome 9 (which is elongated). During the exchange of genetic material, BCR gene on chromosome 22 and ABL gene on chromosome 9 fuse on Philadelphia chromosome to form a hybrid gene, which produces a fusion protein. This anomaly is designated symbolically as t (22q, 9q).

Numerical Anomalies of Chromosomes

- The basic cause of numerical anomalies of chromosomes (both autosomal and sex chromosomal) is the nondisjunction of chromosomes during the reduction division of gametogenesis in the majority of cases. The gametes formed due to nondisjunction contain abnormal number of chromosomes. So after fertilization with normal gamete the zygote has either more chromosomes than normal number or fewer chromosomes than normal number.
- Occasionally, after union of both normal gametes and formation of normal zygote, there is nondisjunction in one cell line during rapid mitotic divisions or cleavage of the embryo. This is the basis of mosaicism (having two cell lines in body tissues with differing numbers of chromosomes).

To understand the basis of numerical chromosomal anomalies like nondisjunction it is essential to revise the basics of cell cycle, mitosis and meiosis.

Cell Cycle in Somatic Cells (Fig. 8.27)

The interphase of cell cycle is a between two mitotic divisions. It is divisible into G_1 (gap 1), S (synthesis) and G_2

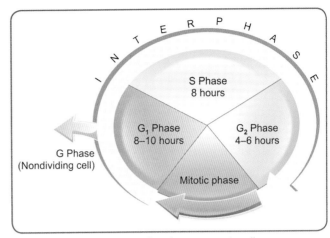

Fig. 8.27: Cell cycle in a somatic cell

(gap 2) phases. The cell that does not divide exits the cell cycle to enter G_0 phase.

During G_1 phase, there is duplication of cell organelles. During S phase, there is replication of DNA. During G_2 phase, enzymes and other proteins are formed.

The stages in mitosis are depicted in Figure 8.28 and stages of meiosis are depicted in Figs 8.29A and B.

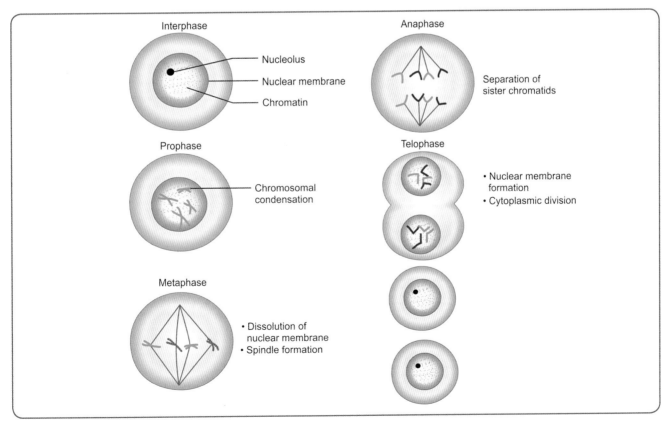

Fig. 8.28: Stages in mitosis

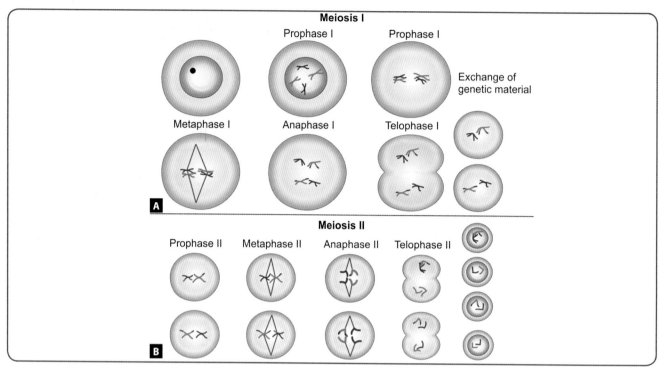

Figs 8.29A and B: Stages in meiosis I and meiosis II

Nondisjunction during Gametogenesis (Fig. 8.30)

Nondisjunction means failure of separation of one member of the homologous pair of chromosomes during anaphase of oogenesis or spermatogenesis. Nondisjunction may occur during meiosis I or meiosis II. Sometimes it may occur during rapid mitotic divisions of cleavage producing two cell lines with varying numbers of chromosomes (mosaicism). However, nondisjunction is more common during reduction division of the process of oogenesis. The reason for this is that the primary oocytes remain arrested in metaphase I for protracted period (from before birth until the time of ovulation). The homologous chromosomes fail to separate and both copies of the same chromosome move into one daughter cell and while the other daughter cell receives no copy of the same chromosome. This explains why there is increase in the incidence of numerical chromosomal anomalies like Down syndrome with advanced maternal age.

Types of Numerical Chromosomal Anomalies

There are two categories as follows:
1. Aneuploidy
2. Polyploidy

Aneuploidy

Aneuploidy is an abnormality in which the chromosome number is not an exact multiple of the haploid number (23 = n). The gamete may show one chromosome less (22 = n-1) or one chromosome more (24 = n+1). After fertilization with normal gamete the zygote is formed either with monosomy (22 + 23 = 45 chromosomes, i.e. 2n–1) or with trisomy (24 + 23 = 47 chromosomes, i.e. 2n+1).

- *Monosomy* is characterized by a single copy of the paired chromosome. Monosomy of X chromosome (45X) is compatible with life but monosomy of autosomes is not compatible with life. Such embryos are aborted very early.
- *Trisomy* is characterized by three copies of the same chromosome. Trisomy of chromosome 21 resulting in Down syndrome is very common in population.

Polyploidy

It is a numerical anomaly in which the chromosome number is an exact multiple of haploid number but more than diploid (69, 92, etc).

- In *triploidy*, the chromosome number is 69. This occurs during second meiotic division when chromosome number is doubled but cell division fails to take place. In this way one gamete will have 46 chromosomes and if this gamete is fertilized by normal gamete the result will be (46 + 23 = 69 chromosomes) triploidy.
- In *tetraploidy*, the cells have 92 chromosomes. This anomaly is produced due to failure of separation of cells during first mitotic division of the zygote.

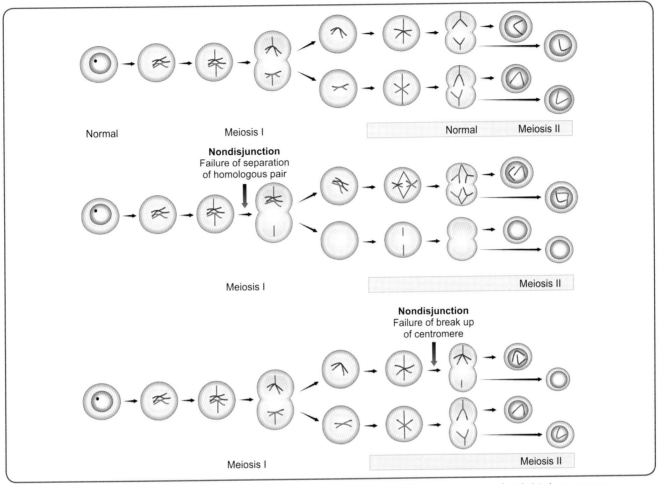

Fig. 8.30: Nondisjunction during gametogenesis producing gametes with 22 chromosomes and with 24 chromosomes

---

⊘ **CLINICAL CORRELATION**

Down Syndrome (Trisomy 21)

Down syndrome is an autosomal numerical anomaly in which there are three copies of chromosome 21 instead of normal two copies. It is the most important single cause of mental retardation in children. There is a strong association between advanced maternal age and Down syndrome.

Cytogenetic Types of Down Syndrome

- Free trisomy with three copies of chromosome 21 (47, XX or XY + 21) occurs in 95% of Down patients. The cause of free trisomy is nondisjunction during oogenesis.
- Translocation Down syndrome is seen in 4% of Down patients. Its cytogenetic formula is 46, XX or XY, t (14q, 21q). One of the parents carries the structural anomaly D/G translocation which is transmitted during gametogenesis to a few gametes and if the gamete carrying D/G translocation takes part in fertilization the anomaly is transmitted to the zygote will have 46 chromosomes and D/G chromosome and extra copy of chromosome 21 (attached to D).
- Mosaic Down syndrome is seen in 1% patients of Down patients. It is due to non-disjunction during cleavage in one cell line in the embryo. This results in some cells with 46 chromosomes and some cells with 47 chromosomes. The cytogenetic notation of a boy with mosaic Down syndrome is 46, XY/47, XY + 21.

Clinical Features (Fig. 8.31)

Phenotype of Down syndrome is typical. The short statured patient has Mongoloid facies, low bridge of nose, upward and laterally slanting eyes, low set ears and protruding furrowed tongue. The palms show characteristic Simian crease (single palmar crease). There is clinodactyly which means incurving fifth digit. In the feet, there is wide gap between first and second digits.

Contd...

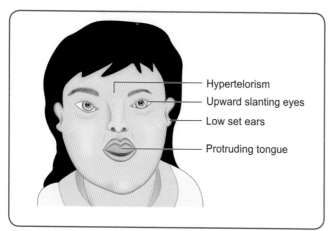

Fig. 8.31: Mongoloid facies in Down syndrome (Trisomy 21)

Contd...

🔬 CLINICAL CORRELATION

Klinefelter's Syndrome

This is the trisomy involving sex chromosomes as a result of nondisjunction of X chromosomes during oogenesis. When a gamete with two X chromosomes is fertilized by Y-bearing sperm the result is a zygote with three sex chromosomes (XXY). This is called **Klinefelter's syndrome** with 47, XXY karyotype. This patient is phenotypically male but he is Barr body positive.

Clinical Features (Fig. 8.32)

The grown-up patients present thin and tall stature with poorly developed male secondary sexual characters. There is hypogonadism with azoospermia (sterility) and gynecomastia.

Turner's Syndrome (Fig. 8.33)

This is a monosomy of X chromosome. There are three ways by which Turner's syndrome results:

1. As a result of nondisjunction of a pair of X chromosomes during oogenesis, if a gamete without X chromosome is fertilized by a normal X bearing sperm the result will be monosomy of X (45 X) which is phenotypically female but without Barr body.
2. Presence of a structural anomaly called **isochromosome X** in one of the gametes produces isochromosome X Down syndrome. The karyotype of isochromosome X Turner is 46X, i(Xq). This patient has normal number of chromosomes but is Barr body positive.
3. The mosaic Turner syndrome (46 XX/45 X) is produced if there is nondisjunction in X-chromosome pair during mitosis one cell lines of the zygote.

Clinical Features

The affected female has short stature, low hair line, webbed neck, decreased carrying angles and lymphedema over feet. They have poorly developed secondary sexual characters with streak gonads. Often patients come to doctors with the complaint of amenorrhea.

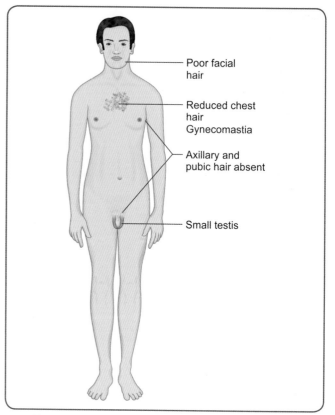

Fig. 8.32: Phenotype of Klinefelter's syndrome (47, XXY)

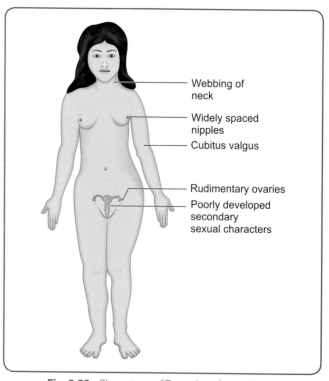

Fig. 8.33: Phenotype of Turner' syndrome (45, X)

Contd...

Contd...

Contd...

CLINICAL CORRELATION

Prenatal Diagnosis of Genetic Diseases

Prenatal diagnosis (PND) is an important part of clinical genetics. The primary purpose of PND is to detect all types of abnormalities of embryo or fetus like neural tube defects (NTD), syndromes associated with chromosomal anomalies, cleft lip, cleft palate, cystic fibrosis, thalassemia, sickle cell anemia, and hemophilia to name a few genetic diseases, before birth. This is to make the parents aware about the impending traumatic event in their life and give them a chance to be prepared psychologically, socially and financially to accept a disabled baby. It can also give parents time to think about another option called MTP (medical termination of pregnancy) if a serious abnormality is detected very early in embryonic period. So the foremost concern under the delicate situation is to advise the parents to seek genetic counseling from experts in the field.

Methods of Prenatal Diagnosis

Prenatal diagnosis are described under two methods: (1) noninvasive methods; (2) invasive methods.

Noninvasive Methods

- Fetal visualization by ultrasound scan to determine fetal age in cases where date of conception is not clear and to evaluate progress in fetal growth. It is used specifically for detecting thickness of nuchal translucency at 11 to 13 weeks in pregnancies at risk for Down syndrome.
- Screening test in mother for NTD in fetus is done to find out level of maternal serum alpha fetoprotein. The alpha fetoprotein is produced in the embryo by yolk sac and later in fetus by liver. It enters the amniotic fluid and into the maternal blood. MS AFP level reflects the AFP level in fetus. Rise in MSAFP after 16 week indicates possibility of NTD such as spina bifida or anencephaly.
- Screening (triple test) for Down syndrome in maternal serum is done by measuring three parameters (triple test for beta-HCG, uE3 (unconjugated estriol) and MS AFP). Increase in HCG, decrease in alpha fetoprotein and decrease in estriol indicate probability of Down. If inhibin-A is measured along with above three parameters it is called quadruple test (quad test for Down syndrome screening).

Invasive Methods

- ***Amniocentesis*** (Fig. 8.34A) is done during 16–20 weeks of gestation. The amniotic fluid sample is drawn by passing a needle in to the amniotic cavity under the guidance of ultrasound. Rise in alpha fetoproteins is indicative of neural tube defects. The amniotic fluid can be used for biochemical analysis and the fetal cells (amniocytes shed from fetal skin) can be cultured for chromosome analysis (Fig. 8.34B).
- ***Chorionic villus sampling*** (Fig. 8.35) is done during 9–12 weeks of gestation. A catheter is passed either through the vagina or through abdomen under ultrasound guidance to suction out a small amount of tissue from chorionic villi. The chorion cells are dividing cells hence the results of chromosome analysis are available much quicker than culture method by amniocentesis.

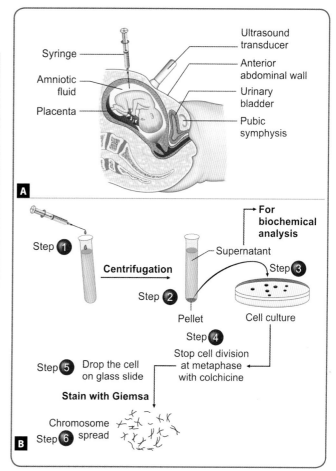

Figs 8.34A and B: A. Amniocentesis via anterior abdominal wall and; **B.** Biochemical analysis of amniotic fluid and culture of amniotic cells for karyotyping (both for prenatal diagnosis of genetic diseases)

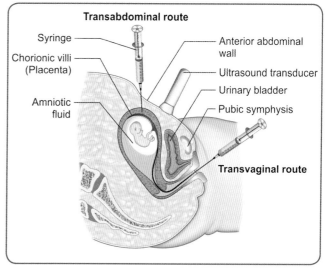

Fig. 8.35: Chorionic villus sampling (CVS) for prenatal diagnosis of genetic diseases

9

Clinicoanatomical Problems and Solutions

CASE 1

A 25-year-old woman with a history of two missed menstrual periods was rushed to the hospital because she had intense lower abdominal pain. Vaginal examination revealed early pregnancy and ultrasound of pelvic cavity revealed empty uterus and fluid in the pouch of Douglas. This is a case of ectopic pregnancy.

Questions and Solutions

1. Name the common site of ectopic pregnancy.

Ans. Uterine tube

2. Which embryological event normally takes place at this site?

Ans. Fertilization

3. Which embryological event takes place at this site to cause ectopic or tubal pregnancy?

Ans. Implantation of blastocyst in the uterine tube

4. What is the natural fate of tubal pregnancy?

Ans. Rupture of the uterine tube with bleeding in the peritoneal cavity and accumulation of blood in the pouch of Douglas is the natural fate of tubal pregnancy.

5. Describe the embryological process of transformation of zygote into blastocyst.

Ans. The zygote undergoes a series of rapid mitotic divisions called cleavage, as a result of which there is increase in the number of cells and gradual decrease in the size of cells (now called blastomeres). Around third day after fertilization the 16-cell stage is reached. This stage of the embryo is called morula (mulberry like). The blastomeres of morula are held together tightly inside the zona pellucida. When the morula reaches the uterine cavity it changes into blastocyst as follows. It begins to absorb fluid through zona pellucida. The fluid enters the intercellular spaces, which coalesce to form a cavity called blastocele. The blastomeres segregate to form embryo blast and trophoblast. The embryo blast consists of a clump of cells called inner cell mass at the embryonic pole. The trophoblast consists of flattened cells forming the outer limit of blastocele. The trophoblast divides into outer syncytiotrophoblast and inner cytotrophoblast. The syncytiotrophoblast secretes human chorionic gonadotrophic (hCG) hormone. Only when on day five the blastocyst loses its zona pellucida, is it ready for implantation in the endometrium of uterus.

6. What is the normal site of implantation?

Ans. The body of uterus near fundus (either on anterior wall or posterior wall) is the site of implantation since this site has maximum blood supply.

7. Which is the surgical contraceptive measure in women that prevents fertilization?

Ans. Tubectomy

8. Write briefly on decidua.

Ans. After implantation of blastocyst inside the endometrium, the endometrium is called decidua. The decidua is histologically recognized by decidual reaction, which shows characteristic changes in the stromal cells and the stroma of endometrium under the influence of hCG hormone. The stromal cells enlarge by accumulating glycogen and lipids. The stroma becomes edematous by accumulation of fluid. The decidua is divisible into three parts—(1) decidua basalis, (2) decidua capsularis and (3) decidua parietalis. At the site of implantation the decidua is divided into decidua basalis and decidua capsularis. The decidua basalis is in contact with the embryonic pole of the blastocyst and the decidua capsularis covers the abembryonic pole. The decidua parietalis is most extensive layer as it lines the rest of the uterine cavity. As pregnancy progresses the decidua basalis forms the maternal component of placenta. The decidua capsularis and the decidua parietalis fuse with each other to obliterate the uterine cavity. Ultimately, they fuse with the amnion.

CASE 2

A congenitally malformed baby shows fusion of lower limbs, vertebral anomalies, imperforate anus, renal agenesis and genital anomalies. This is known as caudal dysgenesis or sirenomelia. This anomaly is believed to result from teratogenic effects during third week of embryogenesis.

Questions and Solutions

1. Which is the major event during third week of prenatal development?

Ans. The gastrulation is the process that establishes all three germ layers (ectoderm, mesoderm and endoderm) and changes the bilaminar embryonic disc into trilaminar embryonic disc during third week by formation of intraembryonic mesoderm.

2. Which structure is responsible for gastrulation?

Ans. The primitive streak (which develops as midline linear thickening of ectoderm) is instrumental for the process of gastrulation. It is composed of pluripotent cells. Its cranial end is called primitive node. The cells originating from the node insinuate cranially in the midline and form notochord. From the rest of the primitive streak there is continuous migration of cells in all directions between the ectoderm and endoderm giving rise to intraembryonic mesoderm. The primitive streak rapidly shrinks in size and disappears during the fourth week.

3. What is the unique feature of the primary organizer?

Ans. The primitive streak is the primary organizer. It is composed of pluripotent cells and hence highly susceptible to teratogenic effects.

4. Give the subdivisions of intraembryonic mesoderm.

Ans. The subdivisions of the intraembryonic mesoderm on each side from medial to lateral are paraxial mesoderm, intermediate mesoderm and lateral plate mesoderm. The paraxial mesoderm undergoes segmentation into somites (about 42 to 44 pairs). Each somite divides into sclerotome, myotome and dermatome. The

intermediate mesoderm is the forerunner of urinary and genital organs. The lateral plate mesoderm splits into somatopleuric and splanchnopleuric layers enclosing a cavity called intraembryonic coelom (forerunner of serous cavities of body, which are pleural, pericardial and peritoneal).

5. What is the basic defect in caudal dysgenesis or sirenomelia?

Ans. There is insufficient formation of intraembryonic mesoderm in caudal region of the embryo. This is responsible for fusion of lower limbs and genitourinary and vertebral anomalies.

CASE 3

A 44-year-old woman consults her obstetrician when she misses two periods. The obstetrician confirms the pregnancy and advices her to undergo triple test, amniocentesis and chorionic villus sampling (CVS).

Questions and Solutions

1. Considering the age of the mother, which chromosomal anomaly (in the unborn) is suspected by the obstetrician?

Ans. Down syndrome or trisomy 21 is the most common chromosomal anomaly found in elderly women who are above 35 years of age.

2. Describe the clinical features of condition.

Ans. Down syndrome babies present typical phenotype. The short statured children have Mongoloid facies, low bridge of nose, upward and laterally slanting palpebral fissures (Mongoloid eyes), low set ears and protruding furrowed tongue. The palms show characteristic Simian crease (single palmar crease) and clinodactyly (incurving 5th digit). In the feet, there is wide gap between first and second digits. Down syndrome babies are born with mental retardation (the most agonizing factor to the parents).

3. What is triple test?

Ans. It is a noninvasive screening test for Down syndrome in which three biochemical parameters are tested in maternal serum—hCG, AFP and unconjugated estriol (uE3). There is increase in hCG and decrease in the level of other two parameters in this syndrome.

4. How is amniocentesis performed?

Ans. Amniocentesis is a procedure by which a sample of amniotic fluid is withdrawn from the amniotic cavity surrounding the fetus by 16 weeks of gestation. This procedure is done under ultrasound guidance so that placenta is protected. The amniotic fluid contains fetal cells that are shed from the skin. These cells are cultured to obtain a karyotype of fetus to confirm prenatal diagnosis of trisomy 21.

5. What is chorionic villus sampling?

Ans. Chorionic villus sampling is done during 9 to 12 weeks of gestation. A catheter is passed either through vagina or through abdomen under ultrasound guidance to suction out a small amount of tissue from the chorionic villi (chorionic villi belong to fetal component of placenta). At this stage the cells of cytotrophoblast are mitotically active hence the cell culture is not needed and results of chromosome analysis are available much quicker compared to amniocentesis.

6. Give reason for high risk of free trisomy 21 or Down syndrome baby in mothers over 40 years.

Ans. There is extra copy of chromosome 21 in free trisomy 21 (chromosome formula: 47 + 21 in male and 47 + 21 in female). This is a numerical chromosomal anomaly of autosome. Therefore the basic cause is nondisjunction of chromosome pair 21 during gametogenesis. Nondisjunction means failure of separation of one of the homologous chromosome pair during anaphase of meiosis. The nondisjunction occurs more commonly during oogenesis because the primary oocyte remains arrested in metaphase for protracted period (from before birth until the time of ovulation). This implies that with increase in the maternal age there is proportionate increase in duration of the arrested metaphase of primary oocyte. This is likely to cause failure of the homologous chromosomes 21 to separate with the consequence two copies of chromosome 21

enter into the secondary oocyte while the first polar body receives no copy. If the secondary oocyte bearing 2 copies of chromosome 21 is fertilized by normal sperm bearing one copy of chromosome 21 the net result is a zygote with 3 copies of chromosome 21 (trisomy 21).

7. What is translocation Down syndrome?

Ans. The translocation is the structural anomaly of chromosomes in which there is break in two different chromosomes and later fusion of the broken parts. So the genetic material is transferred from one chromosome to another. The Robertsonian translocation or (D/G translocation) results when two acrocentric chromosomes (belonging to groups D and G) break at their centromeres and subsequently there is fusion of their long arms (the short arms of the chromosomes are lost). Thus the total chromosomal number is reduced by one (45 chromosomes).

The chromosome formula of a male with Robertsonian translocation is 45, XY, t(14q, 21q) and of female is 45, XX, t(14q, 21q). Such an individual is called carrier of D/G translocation. The carrier is a normal person. However, at the time of meiotic segregation (gametogenesis) a few gametes may show a homologus pair of translocated chromosome (14/21) and a normal 21 chromosome. Union of such a gamete carrying two copies of 21 (one free copy and another as part of translocated chromosome) with a normal gamete at the time of fertilization will result in translocation Down syndrome. The chromosome formula of translocation Down syndrome will be 46 XX, t(14q, 21q) in female and 46, XY, t(14q, 21q) in female.

SINGLE BEST RESPONSE TYPE MULTIPLE CHOICE QUESTIONS

1. A couple with a history of first born with mental retardation came for genetic counseling. The karyotype of the couple revealed Robertsonian translocation in father. Which of the following configurations correctly indicates the above translocation:
   a. A/C
   b. D/G
   c. C/F
   d. A/E

2. Which of the following is the feature of Y chromosome:
   a. Telocentric
   b. Metacentric
   c. Acrocentric
   d. Submetacentric

3. Which is the critical period of organogenesis in an embryo:
   a. 1 to 3 weeks
   b. 2 to 3 months
   c. 4 to 8 weeks
   d. 12th week

4. Which of the following in an embryo represents oral cavity:
   a. Stomodeum
   b. Prochordal plate
   c. Primitive knot
   d. Primitive pit

5. A cell that does not divide is arrested in following phase:
   a. Metaphase
   b. G_1
   c. G_2
   d. G_0

6. Which of the following is distinguishing feature of autosomal dominant inheritance:
   a. Expresses in homozygous state
   b. The disease appears to skip a generation
   c. If one parent is affected 25% offspring are affected
   d. Offspring of both sexes are equally affected

7. All the following cells contain 23 chromosomes except:
   a. First polar body
   b. Second polar body
   c. Primary oocyte
   d. Secondary oocyte

8. The failure of closure of anterior neuropore results in:
   a. Rachischisis
   b. Meningocele
   c. Anencephaly
   d. Spina bifida occulta

9. After ovulation the secondary oocyte is arrested in:
   a. Prophase of meiosis I
   b. Prophase of metaphase II
   c. Metaphase of meiosis II
   d. Metaphase of meiosis II

10. Chorion consists of following layers:
    a. Trophoblast and extraembryonic mesoderm
    b. Amnion and extraembryonic mesoderm
    c. Syncytiotrophoblast and cytotrophoblast
    d. Ectoderm and endoderm

11. Which of the following cells undergoes first meiotic division:
    a. Primordial germ cell
    b. Primary spermatocyte
    c. Secondary spermatocyte
    d. Spermatid

12. At which time in the life of a female the germ cells are highest in the ovaries:
    a. Birth
    b. Menarche
    c. 5 months of intrauterine life
    d. 25 years

13. The time of completion of first division of meiosis by primary oocyte is:
    a. After fertilization
    b. Just after ovulation
    c. Just before ovulation
    d. At ovulation

14. Mullerian inhibiting factor is produced by:
    a. Cytotrophoblast
    b. Syncytiotrophoblast
    c. Leydig cells of fetal testis
    d. Sertoli cells of fetal testis

15. Sex determining region is located on the following chromosome:
    a. Short arm of Y
    b. Short arm of X
    c. Long arm of Y
    d. Long arm of X

16. Which of the following possibilities is true if a woman carrying an autosomal recessive gene is married to a normal man:
    a. All children affected
    b. 25% children carrier
    c. All children carrier
    d. 50% normal and 50% carrier

17. On staining with quinacrine, the cells of buccal mucosa show two fluorescent spots. This is indicative of which of the following:
    a. Two Y chromosomes
    b. Two Barr bodies
    c. Two nuclei
    d. Two foreign bodies

18. A man affected with X-linked recessive disorder marries a normal woman. What is the probability of having normal sons:
    a. 25%
    b. 50%
    c. 0%
    d. 100%

19. The following trait expresses only in homozygous state:
    a. Sex linked recessive
    b. Autosomal recessive
    c. Sex linked dominant
    d. Autosomal dominant

20. Which of the following is the final fate of prochordal plate:
a. Nucleus pulposus
b. Atlas
c. Buccopharyngeal membrane
d. Degeneration

21. Ideal time for performing chorionic villus sampling is:
a. 20 weeks
b. 5–6 weeks
c. 10–12 weeks
d. 16 weeks

22. The dermis of the skin develops from the following embryonic source:
a. Ectoderm
b. Intermediate mesoderm
c. Septum transversum
d. Somites

23. The corona radiata is formed from following source:
a. Theca interna cells
b. Cumulus oophorus
c. Follicular cells
d. Ovarian stroma

24. Amniotic cavity obliterates the uterine cavity by fusion of chorioamniotic membrane with:
a. Decidua basalis
b. Decidua capsularis
c. Decidua parietalis
d. Chorion levae

25. What is not true about human placenta:
a. Placental barrier is formed by endothelium of fetal and maternal capillaries
b. Full term normal placenta weighs around 500–600 g
c. Chorionic vessels are seen through amnion on fetal surface of placenta
d. Maternal part develops from decidua basalis

26. The human placenta belongs to the following type:
a. Hemoendothelial
b. Endotheliochorial
c. Epitheliochorial
d. Hemochorial

27. High level of alpha fetoprotein in maternal serum after 16 weeks is indicative of which of the following conditions in the fetus:
a. Trisomy 21
b. Marfan's syndrome
c. Anencephaly
d. Monosomy X

28. The neural tube develops under the inductive effect of:
a. Primitive streak
b. Primitive node
c. Notochord
d. Prochordal plate

29. Thalidomide baby is characterized by:
a. Agenesis of all limb
b. Phocomelia
c. Sirenomelia
d. Syndactyly

30. The extraembryonic mesoderm develops from:
a. Amnion
b. Trophoblast
c. Primitive node
d. Yolk sac

KEY TO MCQs

1. b	**2.** c	**3.** c	**4.** a	**5.** d	**6.** d	**7.** c	**8.** c
9. d	**10.** a	**11.** b	**12.** c	**13.** c	**14.** d	**15.** a	**16.** d
17. a	**18.** c	**19.** b	**20.** c	**21.** c	**22.** d	**23.** b	**24.** c
25. a	**26.** d	**27.** c	**28.** c	**29.** b	**30.** b		

Section 3

UPPER LIMB

10

Bones of Upper Extremity

Chapter Contents

CLAVICLE

The clavicle or collar bone is the long bone that is placed horizontally at the junction of the pectoral region and posterior triangle of the neck. It transmits weight of upper limb to its lateral one-third via coracoclavicular ligament and transmits it to the axial skeleton (sternum) through its medial two-third.

Unique Features

- It is a long bone that is S shaped.
- It is the only subcutaneous long bone that is placed horizontally in the body.
- It is the only long bone without medullary cavity.
- It is the first long bone to ossify.
- There are two primary centers, which appear during fifth to sixth weeks of intrauterine life.
- It is the only long bone to ossify in membrane.

- Supraclavicular nerves (cutaneous branches of cervical plexus) cross in front of the clavicle. Sometimes they pierce the clavicle.

Parts

The clavicle presents a shaft and two ends, sternal (or medial) and acromial (or lateral). The shaft is divisible into lateral one-third and medial two-third.

Lateral One-third (Figs 10.1 and 10.2)

The lateral one-third is flat. It presents two surfaces and two margins.

Surfaces

- Superior surface is subcutaneous.
- Inferior surface bears a conoid tubercle and a trapezoid line. The conoid tubercle provides attachment to conoid part and trapezoid line gives attachment to trapezoid part of coracoclavicular ligament.

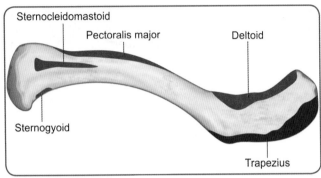

Fig. 10.1: Muscles attached to superior and anterior aspects of clavicle

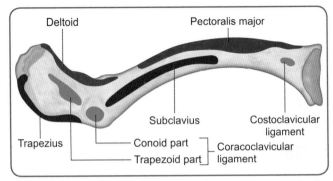

Fig. 10.2: Muscles and ligaments attached to inferior aspect of clavicle

Margins

- Concave anterior margin gives origin to deltoid muscle.
- Convex posterior margin gives insertion to trapezius muscle.

Medial Two-third (Figs 10.1 and 10.2)

Surfaces

The medial two-third of the shaft is roughly cylindrical with four surfaces as follows:

- ***Anterior surface*** is convex forwards. It gives origin to clavicular head of pectoralis major.
- ***Posterior surface*** is concave backwards. It has important vascular relations. At its medial end, it is related to three veins (internal jugular vein, subclavian vein and the beginning of brachiocephalic vein).

  The rest of the posterior surface forming the boundary of the cervico-axillary canal or apex of axilla (Fig. 12.3) is related to anterior and posterior divisions of the three trunks of the brachial plexus and the third part of subclavian artery with accompanying vein.

  The origin of sternohyoid muscle encroaches on the medial end of this surface from the posterior surface of the manubrium sterni.
- ***Superior surface*** provides origin to clavicular head of sternomastoid muscle in its medial half.
- ***Inferior surface*** bears a subclavian groove in its long axis. The subclavian groove gives insertion to subclavius muscle and its margins give attachment to clavipectoral fascia. The nutrient foramen is located at the lateral end of the subclavian groove.

Sternal or Medial End

The sternal end is larger and quadrangular and articulates with the clavicular notch of manubrium sterni and first costal cartilage to form sternoclavicular joint (Fig. 15.1).

Acromial or Lateral End

The acromial end is flattened from above downwards. It is articulated with acromion of scapula to form acromioclavicular joint (Fig. 15.1).

Ligaments (Fig. 10.2)

- The coracoclavicular ligament is composed of conoid and trapezoid parts. It is located below the clavicle as it extends from the coracoid process to the conoid tubercle and trapezoid line. This ligament is important in weight transmission from the upper limb to the lateral one-third of clavicle.
- The costoclavicular ligament is attached to the rough impression on the inferior surface of the sternal end of the clavicle and to the first costal cartilage and adjacent first rib.
- The interclavicular ligament passes between the medial ends of the right and left clavicles via suprasternal space.

Growing End

The sternal end is the growing end.

Blood Supply

The nutrient artery of the clavicle arises from clavicular branch of acromiothoracic artery.

 STUDENT INTEREST

Every student is adviced to remember the unique features of clavicle. Holding it in anatomical position is possible only if you know its medial and lateral ends and superior and inferior surfaces. The attachments of muscles and ligaments and ossification fall under MUST KNOW category. Remember its joints are unique in that they take part in movements of scapula.

Ossification

The clavicle is ossified by intramembranous process of ossification. It has two primary centers and one secondary center. The primary centers appear in the shaft at 5th or 6th week of intrauterine life and fuse on day 45. The secondary center appears in sternal end at puberty or a little later and fuses with the shaft by 20 to 25 years.

⚕ CLINICAL CORRELATION

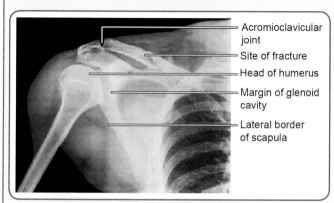

Acromioclavicular joint
Site of fracture
Head of humerus
Margin of glenoid cavity
Lateral border of scapula

Fig. 10.3: Radiograph showing fracture of right clavicle

- **Fracture of Clavicle:** The junction of medial two-third and lateral one-third of the clavicle is the weakest site since it is located at the differently shaped and differently curved parts of the bone. Therefore, the junctional site is liable to fracture. The clavicle is the most commonly fractured bone (Fig. 10.3). When the clavicle fractures medial to the attachment of the coracoclavicular ligament, its two fragments are displaced in the directions, corresponding to the muscle pull (Fig. 10.4). The medial fragment is shifted upwards due to sternomastoid whereas the lateral fragment is drawn downwards by the weight of the upper limb. The contraction of pectoralis major pulls the lateral fragment medially (by adduction of the arm). This results in overriding of the two fragments and shortening of the clavicle. The time honored method of treating the fracture of clavicle by figure of eight sling is still in practice (Fig. 10.5).
- If clavicles are congenitally absent due to defective intramembranous ossification **(cleidocranial dysostosis)**, the shoulders droop anteriorly and are thus approximated in front of the chest. This is because of absence of the function of clavicles to brace back the shoulders.

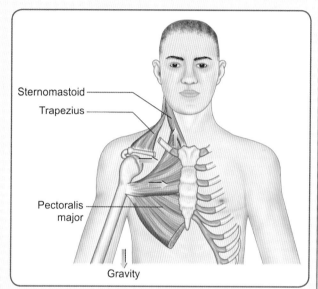

Sternomastoid
Trapezius
Pectoralis major
Gravity

Fig. 10.4: Overlap of fragments of broken clavicle due to pull of the muscles attached to clavicle

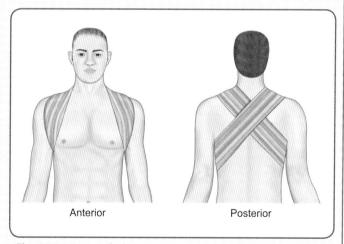

Anterior

Posterior

Fig. 10.5: 'Figure of 8' bandage to immobilize the fractured clavicle

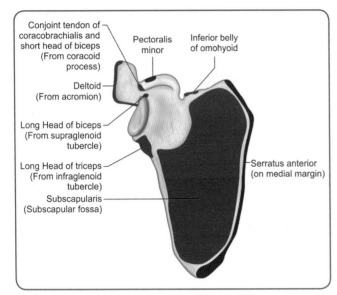

Fig. 10.6: Muscles attached to ventral or costal surface of scapula including those attached to coracoid process

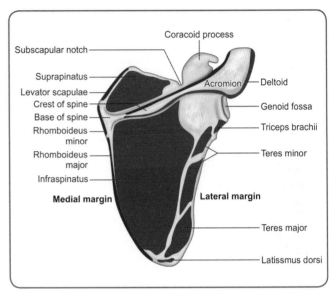

Fig. 10.7: Muscles attached to dorsal surface of scapula including to those attached to crest of the spine and the acromion process

SCAPULA

The scapula is a large flat triangular bone. It is located on the posterolateral aspect of thoracic cage. It articulates with the humerus at the shoulder joint and with the clavicle at the acromioclavicular joint. The scapula is suspended from the cranium by trapezius and held close to the thoracic cage by serratus anterior muscle.

General Features (Figs 10.6 and 10.7)

The scapula presents two surfaces, three margins, three angles and three processes.

Surfaces

- **Ventral or costal or subscapular surface** is concave and faces anteromedially. It is characterized by three radiating ridges which provide attachments to intramuscular tendons of subscapularis muscle. The subscapularis muscle takes origin from the medial two-third of the costal surface.
- **Dorsal surface** is convex and faces posteriorly. It is characterized by a shelf-like projection called the spine which divides this surface into smaller supraspinous and larger infraspinous fossae. The supraspinous fossa gives origin to supraspinatus and infraspinous fossa to infraspinatus muscles. Free lateral margin of the spine of scapula bounds the spinoglenoid notch through which suprascapular nerve and accompanying vessels pass from supra spinous fossa to the infraspinous fossa.

Margins

- **Superior margin** is thin and sharp. It is characterized by suprascapular notch near the base of coracoid process. This notch is converted into foramen by transverse scapular ligament. The suprascapular artery passes above the ligament and the suprascapular nerve passes through the foramen. The inferior belly of omohyoid arises from this margin just medial to the suprascapular notch.
- **Lateral margin** is the thickest. Its upper extent is up to the infraglenoid tubercle (from which long head of triceps brachii originates). Its dorsal surface gives origin to teres minor above and teres major below. Its costal surface is marked by a rod-like ridge which provides a lever for the serratus anterior when the muscle pulls the inferior angle of scapula upwards against gravity while abducting the arm above 90°.
- **Medial or vertebral** margin extends from superior to inferior angle. Its costal aspect provides insertion to serratus anterior. Its dorsal aspect provides insertion to levator scapulae above the root of the spine, to rhomboideus minor opposite the root of the spine and the rhomboideus major below the root of the spine.

Angles

- **Superior angle** is at the junction of superior and medial margins. It lies deep to the muscles.
- **Lateral or glenoid** angle is broad and bears a pear-shaped glenoid cavity or glenoid fossa for articulating with the head of humerus at shoulder joint. The

supraglenoid tubercle lies just above it. It gives origin to long head of biceps brachii.

- **Inferior angle** is covered by latissimus dorsi. Its costal surface gives insertion to lower four (5th to 8th) digitations of serratus anterior.

Processes

- **Spine of the scapula** is a shelf-like projection from the dorsal surface. The spine has two surfaces and three margins. Its superior surface contributes to supraspinous fossa and its inferior surface corresponds to infraspinous fossa. The spine is attached to dorsal surface of scapula by its anterior margin. Its lateral free margin bounds the spinoglenoid notch (Fig. 10.8). The crest of the spine is the posterior margin of the spine. The trapezius is inserted into the upper lip of the crest and the deltoid takes origin from the lower lip of the crest.
- **Coracoid process** (crow's beak) is shaped like a bent finger. It is an example of atavistic epiphysis. It gives attachment to three muscles (short head of biceps and coracobrachialis arise from its tip and pectoralis minor is inserted into its medial margin) and three ligaments (coraco-acromial ligament, coracoclavicular ligament and coraco-humeral ligament).
- **Acromion** projects forward from the lateral end of the spine (almost at right angles) and overhangs the glenoid cavity. It has two margins (medial and lateral), two surfaces (superior and inferior) and a tip. Its inferior surface is related to subacromial bursa. The acromial angle is the junction of lower lip of the crest of spine and the lateral margin of acromion. The medial margin provides insertion to trapezius and lateral margin provides origin to acromial fibers of deltoid.

Refer to figures 10.6 and 10.7 for the parts and muscular attachments of scapula.

Palpable Parts

- Tip of coracoid process (felt through the infraclavicular fossa)
- Superior margin of scapula and angle of acromion
- Crest of the spine of scapula
- Medial margin of scapula
- Inferior angle of scapula

Vertebral Levels

- Superior angle—second thoracic vertebra.
- Base of spine—third thoracic spine.
- Inferior angle—seventh thoracic vertebra (a useful landmark on the back).

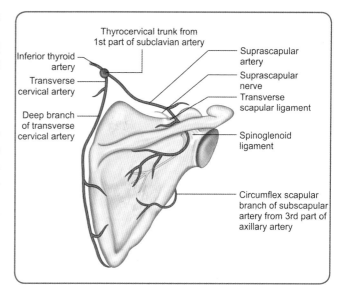

Fig. 10.8: Neurovascular relations of scapula (Note the suprascapular nerve passing under the transverse scapular ligament and suprascapular artery above the same ligament. Also note the same structures passing through the spinoglenoid foramen under the spinoglenoid ligament)

Neurovascular Relations (Fig. 10.8)

The suprascapular notch is converted into suprascapular foramen by superior transverse ligament.

- The suprascapular artery passes above the ligament to enter the supraspinous fossa and suprascapular nerve passes through the foramen.
- The suprascapular nerve and artery enter the infraspinous fossa via spinoglenoid notch which frequently is converted into a foramen by spinoglenoid ligament.

  The suprascapular nerve is liable for entrapment at two sites, suprascapular notch and spinoglenoid notch.
- The lateral margin is related to circumflex scapular artery (a branch of subscapular) that turns round this margin between two sets of fibers of teres minor muscle.
- The medial margin is related to the deep branch of the transverse cervical artery or the dorsal scapular artery.

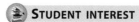 **STUDENT INTEREST**

> Suprascapular artery passes above the transverse scapular ligament and suprascapular nerve below it (through the suprascapular foramen). Mnemonic: ARMY above NAVY relation. Remember that suprascapular nerve is a branch from the upper trunk of brachial plexus and suprascapular artery is a branch of thyrocervical trunk of the first part of subclavian artery.

Ossification

The scapula is ossified by the process of endochondral ossification. **One primary center** appears near the glenoid cavity at 8th week of intrauterine life. There are **seven secondary centers**. They appear in the following sequence – in the middle of coracoid process during first year, remaining six centers appear during puberty at the root of coracoid process (subcoracoid center), two appear in acromion, one for medial border of scapula, one for inferior angle and one for the lower two-third of the rim of glenoid cavity. The secondary center that appears first in the coracoid process fuses with the rest of bone by 15th year. The other secondary centers fuse by 25th year.

🎵 CLINICAL CORRELATION

Pulsating Scapula

The arteries related to the scapula form anastomoses on the dorsal and costal aspects of scapula. The anastomoses enlarge in obstruction to blood flow either in the first part of the subclavian artery or the third part of the axillary artery causing pulsating scapula.

Winged Scapula or Winging of Scapula (Fig. 10.9)

Winged scapula is the deformity in which the vertebral border and inferior angle of scapula protrude posteriorly due to paralysis of serratus anterior muscle in injury to long thoracic nerve.

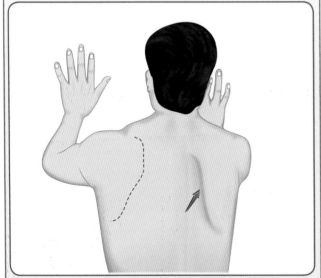

Fig. 10.9: Winging of right scapula due to injury to long thoracic nerve or nerve of Bell

HUMERUS

It is the long bone of the arm articulating with glenoid cavity of scapula at the shoulder joint and with bones of forearm, the radius and ulna at the elbow joint.

General Features

The humerus presents upper end, shaft and lower end.

Upper End

The upper end presents a head, three necks (anatomical, surgical and morphological), greater tubercle, lesser tubercle and intertubercular sulcus or bicipital sulcus (groove).

Head

The hemispherical head bears articular surface for articulating with glenoid cavity of scapula. It is directed medially and backwards.

Neck

- The anatomical neck is a slight constriction that demarcates the head from the rest of the upper end of humerus. It gives attachment to the capsule of the shoulder joint except at its inferomedial part.
- The surgical neck encircles the junction of upper end and the shaft. It is vulnerable to fracture, in which case the axillary nerve and posterior circumflex humeral vessels are liable to injury (as these structures are closely related to medial part of surgical neck).
- The morphological neck corresponds to the epiphyseal line between the upper end and the shaft. In the adult, its position is about half cm above the surgical neck.

Tubercles

- The **greater tubercle** projects from the lateral part of the upper end. Its posterior surface shows three facets for insertion of supraspinatus, infraspinatus and teres minor (from above downwards).
- The **lesser tubercle** projects anteriorly from the upper end. It provides insertion to subscapularis.
- The **intertubercular sulcus** or bicipital groove is between the greater and lesser tubercles. Its main content is the tendon of long head of biceps brachii covered with synovial sheath. Its lateral and medial lips provide insertion respectively to the pectoralis major and to the teres major. Its floor provides insertion to the latissimus dorsi.

Shaft

The shaft of humerus is cylindrical in upper half and triangular in the lower half. It presents three margins (medial, lateral and anterior) and three surfaces (anterolateral, anteromedial and posterior).

Margins

- The *medial margin* begins in the medial lip of bicipital groove and runs downwards to continue as medial supracondylar ridge in the distal shaft. The coracobrachialis is inserted into the middle of medial margin.
- The *lateral margin* is prominent only in lower part where it is known as lateral supracondylar ridge. Its proximal part is barely discernible. The brachioradialis muscle arises from the upper 2/3rd of the lateral supracondylar ridge while the extensor carpi radialis longus arises from its lower third.
- The *anterior margin* begins in the lateral lip of intertubercular sulcus in its upper one-third and then it forms the anterior margin of the deltoid tuberosity. Distally this margin is smooth.

Surfaces

- The *anterolateral surface* is bounded by anterior and lateral margins. A little above its middle it is marked by a V-shaped deltoid tuberosity which provides insertion to the deltoid muscle. Its lower half provides origin to brachialis muscle.
- The *anteromedial surface* is bounded by anterior and medial margins. Its upper part forms the floor of intertubercular sulcus. A nutrient foramen is seen on this surface somewhere near its middle. It is directed downwards indicating that the upper end of humerus is its growing end. The lower half of the anteromedial surface provides origin to brachialis.

- The *posterior surface* is bounded by medial and lateral margins. The middle one-third of the posterior surface presents a radial or spiral groove, which houses the radial nerve and profunda brachii vessels. The upper part presents an oblique ridge from which the lateral head of triceps brachii takes origin (above the level of radial groove). The medial head of triceps takes origin from the posterior surface below the level of radial groove.

Lower End

The lower end presents articular and nonarticular parts.

Articular parts

- The rounded *capitulum articulates* with the disc-shaped head of radius at the humeroradial articulation.
- The pulley-like *trochlea* (lying medial to capitulum) has longer and larger medial flange. It articulates with trochlear notch of the upper end of ulna at humeroulnar articulation. The humeroradial and humeroulnar articulations together form the elbow joint.

Nonarticular parts

- There are three fat-filled depressions at the lower end of the shaft. There are two fossae on the anterior aspect. The radial fossa lodges head of radius and coronoid fossa lodges coronoid process of ulna in flexed elbow. The olecranon fossa is present on posterior aspect and it receives olecranon process of ulna in extended elbow.
- The *medial epicondyle* is a prominent bony projection on the medial side of lower end. It can be easily felt on the medial side of the elbow. The relations of medial epicondyle are important. The ulnar nerve can be palpated against its posterior surface. The medial epicondyle is called funny bone because a hit on it by a hard object evokes painful and tingling sensations along the medial side of forearm and the hand. The anterior aspect of medial epicondyle presents area for common flexor origin for five muscles (pronator teres, flexor carpi radialis, palmaris longus, flexor carpi ulnaris and humeral head of flexor digitorum superficialis).

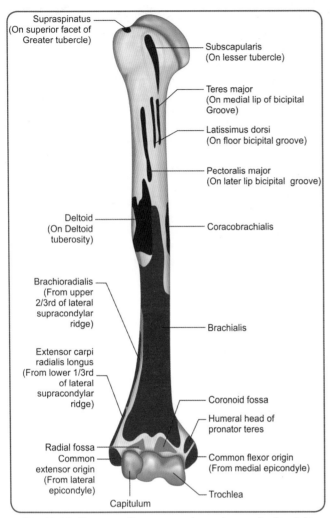

Fig. 10.10: Features of humerus and muscles attached to right humerus on anterior aspect

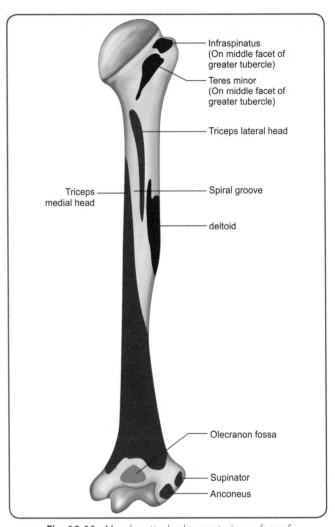

Fig. 10.11: Muscles attached to posterior surface of right humerus

- The *lateral epicondyle* is smaller than the medial epicondyle. Its anterior surface presents area for common extensor origin for four muscles (extensor digitorum, extensor carpi radialis brevis, extensor carpi ulnaris and extensor digiti minimi), below which it gives origin to supinator. The posterior surface of lateral epicondyle gives origin to anconeus.

Note: For muscular attachments of humerus, refer to figures 10.10 and 10.11.

STUDENT INTEREST

Medial epicondyle is referred to as funny bone. The ulnar nerve can be rolled against its posterior surface.

ADDED INFORMATION

Supracondylar spur is a small hook-like process that may be occasionally present on the shaft of humerus. It arises from anteromedial surface about 5 cm above the medial epicondyle. If it is attached to the medial epicondyle by *ligament of Struthers*, a foramen is created through which median nerve and brachial artery pass.

Growing End

The upper end of humerus is its growing end (the nutrient foramen is directed towards the elbow). The nutrient artery takes origin from profunda brachii artery.

🕉 **CLINICAL CORRELATION**

Nerves Related to Humerus (Fig. 10.12)

• Axillary nerve is related to surgical neck; hence, it is injured in fracture of surgical neck and in anterior dislocation of humeral head.

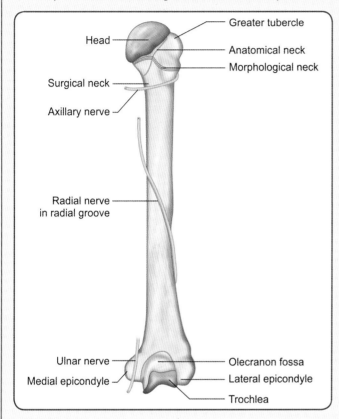

Head
Greater tubercle
Anatomical neck
Morphological neck
Surgical neck
Axillary nerve
Radial nerve
in radial groove
Ulnar nerve
Medial epicondyle
Olecranon fossa
Lateral epicondyle
Trochlea

Figs 10.12: Axillary, Radial and Ulnar Nerves in direct relation to humerus (viewed from posterior aspect);

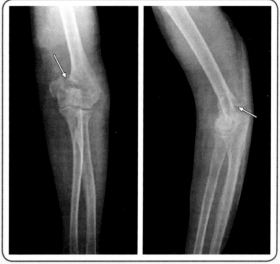

Fig. 10.13: Radiographs showing supracondylar fracture of the shaft of humerus in AP and lateral views (arrows showing)

• Radial nerve is related to posterior surface of shaft at radial or spiral groove; hence, it is injured in fractures of mid-shaft and due to careless intramuscular injection into triceps muscle.
• Ulnar nerve is related to posterior aspect of medial epicondyle, where it can be palpated when thickened (as in leprosy) and is injured in fracture of medial epicondyle.

Supracondylar Fracture of Humerus

The fracture of distal end of humerus just above the epicondyles is called supracondylar fracture (Fig. 10.13). It occurs most often in children as a result of a fall on the outstretched hand. The distal fragment of humerus moves backward and upward. The proximal fragment moves forwards causing compression of the brachial artery (Fig. 18.7C) which may result in necrosis and contracture of flexor muscles of forearm (known as ***Volkmann's ischemic contracture***).

Ossification

• The primary center for shaft appears in 8th week of intrauterine life.
• The upper end has three epiphyses ossified form three secondary centers, which appear in first year (head), second year (greater tuberosity) and fifth year (lesser tuberosity). All the three epiphyses join together at sixth year and form a cup-shaped common epiphysis, which fuses with the shaft by eighteenth year.

• The lower end ossifies by four secondary centers. The center for medial epicondyle appears at fifth year and fuses with the shaft by eighteenth to twentieth year. The other centers appear at first year (for capitulum), at tenth year (trochlea) and at eleventh to twelfth year (for lateral epicondyle). The epiphyses of lateral epicondyle, trochlea and capitulum fuse together and then join the shaft by sixteen years.

RADIUS

The radius is the lateral bone of the forearm. It is the weight-bearing bone; hence, more prone to fractures compared to the ulna.

Articulations

- Elbow joint
- Proximal (superior) radioulnar joint
- Middle radioulnar joint
- Inferior (distal) radioulnar joint
- Wrist joint.

General Features

The parts of the radius are upper end, shaft and lower end.

Upper End

The upper end consists of disc-shaped head, neck and radial or bicipital tuberosity.

- A shallow depression (covered with articular cartilage) on the upper surface of the head articulates with capitulum of humerus at elbow joint.
- The head moves inside the annular ligament during pronation and supination of forearm at the superior radioulnar joint. The circumference of the head articulates with radial notch of ulna medially. The annular ligament encircles the head and is attached to the anterior and posterior margins of the radial notch (Fig. 20.2).

> ### 📖 STUDENT INTEREST
>
> ***Annular ligament*** is not attached to the radial head but is attached to the margins of radial notch of ulna. The annular ligament and the radial notch of ulna together form an osseofibrous ring for the head of radius to rotate during pronation and supination.

- The neck of radius is a slight constriction below the head. The head and neck rotate freely within the annular ligament because capsule is not attached to them.
- The radial tuberosity lies below the medial part of the neck. The rough posterior part of the tuberosity gives insertion to biceps brachii muscle. Its smooth anterior part is covered by a synovial bursa.

Shaft (Fig. 10.14)

The shaft presents three margins and three surfaces.

Margins

- The ***anterior margin*** extends from anterior margin of radial tuberosity to the styloid process at lower end. The upper oblique part of the anterior margin is referred to as anterior oblique line (which gives origin to radial head of flexor digitorum superficialis).
- The ***interosseous*** or ***medial margin*** is the sharpest. The interosseous membrane is attached to its lower three-fourth. Through the interosseous membrane radius is connected to ulna
- The ***posterior margin*** is well marked only in the middle third. Its upper third is called posterior oblique line.

Surfaces

- The ***anterior surface*** lies between the anterior and interosseous margins. An upwardly directed nutrient foramen is located on the upper part of this surface. The flexor pollicis longus arises from its upper three-fourth and pronator quadratus is inserted in its lower fourth.
- The ***posterior surface*** lies between posterior and interosseous margins. The abductor pollicis longus arises from its middle third and extensor pollicis brevis arises just distal to the previous muscle.
- The ***lateral surface*** lies between anterior and posterior margins. Supinator is inserted into its upper one-third. The pronator teres is inserted into the middle part (area of maximum convexity) of lateral surface.

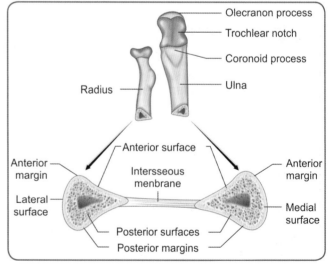

Fig. 10.14: Schematic diagram to depict margins and surfaces of both radius and ulna

It is noteworthy that the muscles of pronation (pronator teres and pronator quadratus) and of supination (biceps brachii and supinator) are inserted into the radius (Fig. 20.4).

Note: The muscular attachments of radius, are shown in figures 10.15 and 10.16

Lower End

The lower or distal end of the radius is expanded and is characterized by five surfaces and a styloid process.

- The ***anterior surface*** of lower end is in the form of a thick prominent ridge which is palpable even through the overlying tendons. The radial pulse is felt on the lateral end of the anterior surface (lateral to the tendon of flexor carpi radialis) (Fig. 19.6).
- The ***posterior surface*** of the lower end presents four grooves and prominent Lister's tubercle or dorsal tubercle. The tendon of extensor pollicis longus produces an oblique groove on the medial aspect

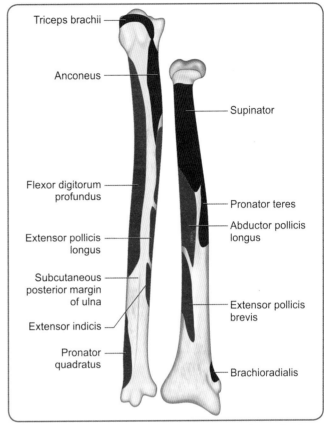

Fig. 10.16: Muscular attachments to posterior surfaces of radius and ulna

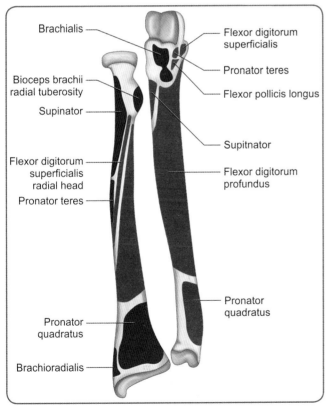

Fig. 10.15: Muscular attachments to anterior surfaces of radius and ulna

of Lister's tubercle and the shallow groove lateral to the tubercle is faintly divided to lodge the tendons of extensor carpi radialis brevis medially and extensor carpi radialis longus laterally (Fig. 10.17). The groove medial to the tendon of extensor pollicis longus is for tendons of extensor digitorum and extensor indicis.

- The ***medial surface*** of lower end presents ulnar notch for articulation with ulnar head at inferior radioulnar joint.
- The ***lateral surface*** of lower end is crossed by abductor pollicis longus and extensor pollicis brevis tendons. The brachioradialis is inserted into the lowest part of this surface just above the base of styloid process.
- The styloid process of radius extends from the lateral surface and is longer than the ulnar styloid process. It can be felt in the floor of anatomical snuff-box.
- The articular area on the inferior surface of lower end articulates with scaphoid, lunate and triquetral bones to form the wrist joint.

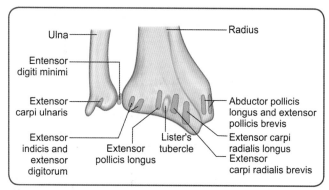

Fig. 10.17: Showing the tendons related to dorsal aspect of lower ends of radius and ulna

Growing End

The lower end of the radius is the growing end.

Ossification

The shaft ossifies from primary center, which appears at 8th week of intrauterine life. The upper end ossifies by secondary center which appears at 4th year and fuses with the shaft by 16 years. The lower end ossifies by secondary center which appears by first year and fuses with shaft by 18th year.

✄ CLINICAL CORRELATION

Colles' Fracture

This is the fracture of the lower end of the radius (Fig. 10.18). It commonly occurs in elderly women due to a fall on outstretched hand. The wrist and hand show a dinner fork deformity (Fig. 10.19A), which occurs due to the displacement of the lower fragment of radius in the posterior and upward direction. As a result, the radial styloid process moves upward until it is at the same level or at a higher level than that of ulnar styloid process (Fig. 10.19B).

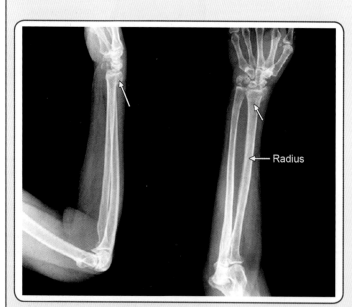

Fig. 10.18: Radiograph showing Colle's fracture of lower end of right radius (arrows showing)

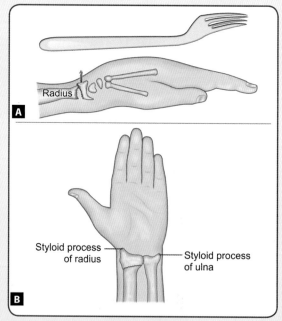

Figs 10.19A and B: A. Dinner fork deformity in Colle's fracture due to dorsal displacement of distal fragment of radius; **B.** Same levels of styloid processes of radius and ulna due to proximal displacement of distal fragment of radius in Colle's fracture

Pulled Elbow or Subluxation of Head of Radius

In this condition, the head of radius escapes out from the grip of the annular ligament. This is more common in children below 5 years of age.

Smith's Fracture

In this fracture distal fragment of fractured lower end of radius is displaced in anterior direction (reverse to what is seen in Colles' fracture).

ULNA

The ulna is the medial bone of the forearm.

Articulations

- Elbow joint
- Superior (proximal) radioulnar joint
- Middle radioulnar joint
- Inferior (distal) radioulnar joint

Note: The ulna is excluded from taking part in the wrist joint by an articular disc.

General Features

The ulna consists of proximal or upper end, shaft and distal or lower end.

Upper End

The upper end has two processes (olecranon and coronoid) and two notches (radial and trochlear).

Olecranon process

It is hook-shaped and projects upward. It has five surfaces as follows:

1. The **anterior surface** is articular as it forms the upper part of the trochlear notch
2. The **posterior surface** is subcutaneous. It is separated from the skin by a subcutaneous bursa. The inflammation of this bursa is the cause of a student's elbow
3. The **superior surface** in its posterior part provides insertion to the triceps brachii. Violent contraction of triceps brachii may fracture the olecranon process.
4. The **lateral surface** provides insertion to anconeus.
5. The medial surface is continuous with the medial surface of the shaft.

Coronoid process

It projects forward from the shaft just below the olecranon process. It presents four surfaces:

1. The **superior surface** is articular as it forms the lower part of the **trochlear notch**.
2. The **anterior surface** is rough and gives insertion to brachialis muscle and continues down as ulnar tuberosity. The sharp medial margin of this surface provides attachments to ulnar head of pronator teres besides the anterior thick part (or band) of the triangular ulnar collateral ligament.

3. The **lateral surface** bears a radial notch for articulation with the circumference of the head of radius. The annular ligament is attached to the anterior and posterior margins of the radial notch. A small depressed area called **supinator fossa** (below the radial notch) presents sharp posterior margin called supinator crest. The supinator fossa and crest give origin to supinator muscle.
4. The **medial surface** of coronoid process is continuous with the medial surface of the shaft. It gives origin to fibers of flexor digitorum profundus.

Trochlear notch

The trochlear notch is formed by articular surfaces of olecranon and coronoid processes. It articulates with the trochlea of humerus in the formation of elbow joint.

Radial notch

This notch is also articular. It is present on the lateral surface of the coronoid process for articulation with the circumference of head of radius in the formation of superior radioulnar joint.

Shaft (Fig. 10.14)

The shaft of ulna has three margins (anterior, posterior and interosseous) and three surfaces (anterior, medial and posterior).

Margins

- The **anterior margin** is thick and rounded. It intervenes between the medial and anterior surfaces. It gives origin to fibers of flexor digitorum profundus.
- The **posterior margin** is subcutaneous. The deep fascia of forearm is attached to it. Through the deep fascia the posterior margin provides origin to flexor digitorum profundus, flexor carpi ulnaris and extensor carpi ulnaris.
- The **lateral or interosseous margin** provides attachment to interosseous membrane.

Surfaces

- The **anterior surface** is bounded by anterior and lateral margins. It provides origin to flexor digitorum profundus in upper three-fourth and to pronator quadratus from the oblique ridge in its lower fourth. The nutrient foramen (directed towards elbow) is located in its upper part.

- The *medial surface* is bounded by anterior and posterior margins. It gives origin to flexor digitorum profundus in its upper three-fourth. Its lower fourth is subcutaneous.
- The *posterior surface* is bounded by posterior and lateral margins. It is divided by an oblique line into smaller upper and larger lower areas. The anconeus is inserted into the smaller upper part. The lower larger area is further divided into medial and lateral parts by a vertical line. The lateral part provides origin from above downward to abductor pollicis longus, extensor pollicis longus and extensor indicis.

Note: The muscular attachments of ulna are shown in figures 10.15 and 10.16.

Lower End

The lower tapering end of ulna shows the head and styloid process.

- The *head of ulna* articulates with the ulnar notch of the radius at the inferior radioulnar joint. The articular disc of this joint is placed below the ulnar head, because of which the ulnar head is excluded from the wrist joint.
- The *ulnar styloid process* projects downwards from the posteromedial aspect of the lower end. It is palpable in supinated position of forearm about one cm proximal to the plane of radial styloid process. The groove between the ulnar head and styloid process (on the dorsal aspect) is occupied by tendon of extensor carpi ulnaris (Fig. 10.17).

Growing End

The lower end of ulna is its growing end.

Ossification

- The shaft ossifies from primary center, which appears at 8th week of intrauterine life.
- The upper surface of olecranon process ossifies by secondary center which appears at 9th to 10th year and fuses with the shaft by 17 years.
- The lower end ossifies by secondary center which appears by fifth year and fuses with shaft by 19th year.

Pediatric Elbow

The epiphyses at the lower end of humerus and upper end of radius and ulna are depicted in the radiograph of pediatric elbow (Fig. 10.20) of a twelve-year-old child. The order of appearance of secondary centers in these epiphyses is remembered by the mnemonic CRITOE (Fig. 10.21) which

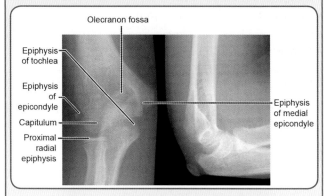

Fig. 10.20: Radiograph showing various epiphyses at the elbow in a child between 11 and 12 years

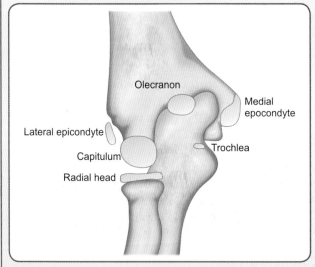

Figs 10.21: Pediatric elbow showing CRITOE which gives the order of appearance of ossification centers in the bony parts around elbow joint:– **C**apitulum–first year, **R**adial head–3-4 years, **I**nternal or medial epicondyle–5-6 years, **T**rochlea–7-8 years, **O**lecranon process–9 years, **E**xternal or lateral epicondyle–11 years

Contd…

Contd...

 CLINICAL CORRELATION

stands for capitulum (first year), radial head (3–4 years), internal (media) epicondyle (5–6 years), trochlea (7–8 years), olecranon (9 years) and external (lateral) epicondyle (11 years). If a twelve-year-old boy suffers avulsion fracture of medial epicondyle and the radiograph of his elbow shows no medial epicondyle but a well-marked lateral epicondyle, trochlea and olecranon, it means the avulsed piece of medial epicondyle must be searched in the radiograph.

Point of Elbow (tip of olecranon process)

At the back of the elbow, there are three palpable bony points, namely medial epicondyle of humerus, lateral epicondyle of humerus and the tip of olecranon process of ulna. In the extended elbow, these points lie in a straight horizontal line (Fig. 18.7A). In flexed elbow, they form an equilateral triangle (Fig. 18.7B). These bony points are examined to differentiate posterior dislocation of the elbow joint and the supracondylar fracture of humerus. In posterior dislocation (Figs 18.7C and 18.8), the olecranon process moves backward from the lower end of humerus resulting in loss of the normal shape of the triangle. In supracondylar fracture, the normal bony relation is retained (since the olecranon shifts backward along with lower end of humerus). The brachial artery is in danger of compression by the anteriorly displaced proximal fragment as shown in figure 18.7C.

Ulnar Fractures

The shaft of ulna may be fractured along with radius or singly. The olecranon may fracture in the fall on the point of elbow.

BONES OF HAND (FIG. 10.22)

The bones of hand consist of eight carpal bones, five metacarpal bones and fourteen phalanges (total of twenty-seven bones).

Carpal Bones

The carpal bones are arranged in two rows.

Proximal Row

The bones in the proximal row are (from lateral to medial) scaphoid, lunate, triquetral and pisiform. The proximal row is convex proximally and concave distally.

Distal Row

The bones in the distal row are (from lateral to medial) trapezium, trapezoid, capitate and hamate. The distal row is convex proximally and flat distally.

Characteristic Features of Individual Carpal Bones

- Scaphoid is boat shaped. Its neck or waist subdivides the scaphoid into proximal and distal segments. A tubercle projects from its lateral side. It lies in the floor of anatomical snuff-box, where it can be palpated. Tubercle gives attachment to flexor retinaculum.
- Lunate is shaped like a lunar crescent (shape of half moon).
- Triquetral is pyramidal in shape.
- Pisiform is pea shaped. It is a sesamoid bone in the tendon of flexor carpi ulnaris. It presents only one articular facet and that is for palmar surface of triquetral. The insertion of flexor carpi ulnaris into the pisiform is extended by pisohamate and pisometacarpal ligaments. Both flexor retinaculum and extensor retinaculum are attached to the pisiform.
- Trapezium is quadrilateral in shape and bears a crest and a groove. The crest provides origin to the three thenar muscles. The groove is converted in to osseofibrous tunnel as its margins give attachments to two slips of flexor retinaculum. This small tunnel lodges the tendon of flexor carpi radialis. Distally the trapezium articulates with the base of first metacarpal bone to form the first carpometacarpal joint, which imparts unique mobility to the human thumb.
- Trapezoid is irregular like a baby's shoe. Distally it articulates with base of second metacarpal bone.
- Capitate is the central carpal bone and also the largest carpal bone bearing a big head. Distally it articulates with base of third metacarpal bone.
- Hamate has a hook-shaped process at its base projecting laterally. The flexor retinaculum is attached medially and distally to the hook of hamate. The base of the hook is in contact with the deep branch of the ulnar nerve. Distally, the hamate articulates with bases of fourth and fifth metacarpal bones.

 STUDENT INTEREST

Mnemonic

For sequence of carpal bones from lateral to medial side:
Proximal row—***Sona Looks Too Pretty***.
Distal row—***Try To Captivate Her***.
Point to remember: Lateral bones of both rows (scaphoid and trapezium) and medial bones of both rows (pisiform and hamate) give attachment to the flexor retinaculum.

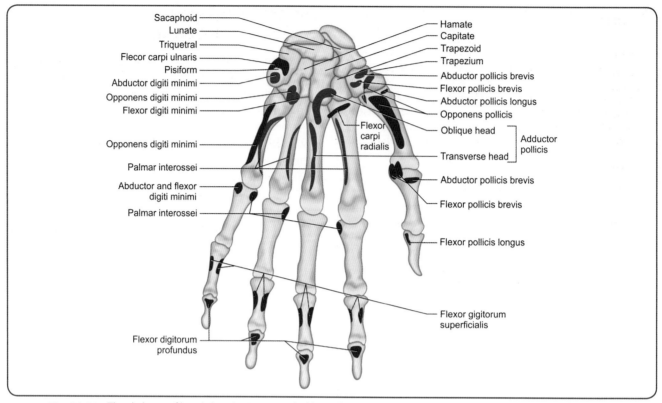

Fig. 10.22: The skeleton of hand showing insertion (in blue color) and origin (in red color) of the intrinsic muscles of hand

⚕ **CLINICAL CORRELATION**

The *carpal tunnel* is an osseofibrous tunnel formed by anterior concavity of carpus (carpal bone as one unit) and flexor retinaculum, which is attached to the four pillars of the carpus. On lateral side, the proximal pillar is the tubercle of scaphoid and distal pillar is the crest of trapezium. On the medial side, the proximal pillar is the pisiform and distal pillar is the hook of hamate.

The carpal tunnel contains following tendons—
- Flexor digitorum superficialis (FDS)–4
- Flexor digitorum profundus (FDP)–4
- Flexor pollicis longus (FPL)–1

Thus a total of nine tendons and median nerve are packed inside the carpel tunnel.

Compression of median nerve in carpal tunnel gives rise to symptoms and signs which collectively are called carpal tunnel syndrome.

Ossification

The ossification of carpal bones helps in determining the bone age. Each carpal bone ossifies from a single center, which appears after birth.

Capitate is the first bone to ossify and pisiform is the last to ossify. The carpal bones are cartilaginous at birth.

Time of Appearance of Ossification Centers (Fig. 10.23)

Capitate—second month
Hamate—end of third month
Triquetral—third year
Lunate—fourth year
Scaphoid, trapezium and trapezoid—fifth year
Pisiform—tenth to twelfth year

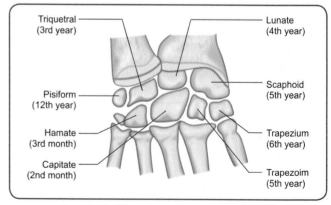

Fig. 10.23: Time of appearance of ossification centers of carpal bones

Fracture of Scaphoid

- Of all the carpal bones, the scaphoid is the most commonly fractured. The distal half of scaphoid lies close to the distal row of carpal bones and proximal half lies in the proximal row of carpal bones. The waist or narrow part, which is between the two halves, lies in the intercarpal line. Hence it is subjected to maximum stresses. This is the reason why waist of scaphoid is the common site of fracture. The artery supplying the scaphoid enters through its distal half (Fig. 10.24A). In case of fracture of the waist the blood supply to the proximal half is affected leading to nonunion of the fracture or avascular necrosis of the proximal half.
- In fracture of scaphoid, pain and tenderness are felt in the anatomical snuff-box.

Dislocation of Lunate

The lunate is commonly dislocated in the anterior direction, which may cause compression of the median nerve inside the carpal tunnel (Fig. 10.24B).

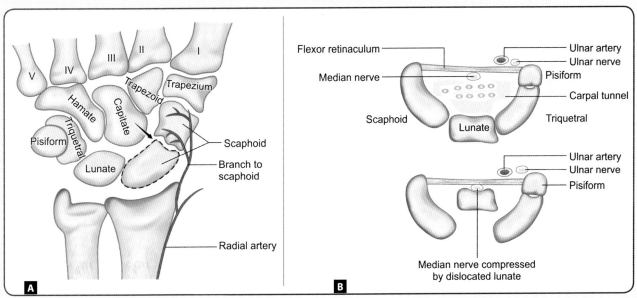

Figs 10.24A and B: A. Fracture of scaphoid bone through waist (arrow) and avascular necrosis of proximal half of scaphoid;
B. Showing normal anatomy of carpal tunnel and anterior dislocation of lunate bone inside the carpal tunnel causing compression of median nerve in a schematic diagram

🏛 **STUDENT INTEREST**

Scaphoid is the most common carpal bone to fracture and lunate is the most common to dislocate anteriorly and injure the medial nerve inside the carpal tunnel. Appearance of centers of ossification in carpal bones is a MUST KNOW topic.

Metacarpal Bones

The five metacarpal bones are numbered from lateral to medial. They are miniature long bones.

Parts

Each metacarpal bone consists of head distally, shaft and base proximally.

- The **heads** of the metacarpals are prominently visible on the dorsum of hand on making a fist. They are called knuckles in common language. The heads articulate with bases of corresponding proximal phalanges to form metacarpophalangeal joints.
- The **shafts** are concave on palmar aspect.
- The **base of each** metacarpal bone articulates with carpal bone/bones of distal row. The first metacarpal articulates with trapezium, the second with trapezoid, third with capitate and fourth and fifth with hamate.

Unique Features of First Metacarpal Bone

- It is the shortest and strongest.
- It is the modified first phalanx of thumb.
- It is not in line with the other four metacarpals as it is more anteriorly placed.

- It gives great mobility to the thumb by its saddle type of articulation with the trapezium.
- Its base does not articulate with adjacent metacarpal bone (to maintain its independence) unlike the other metacarpals, which articulate with each other at their bases.
- Its mode of ossification is like that of phalanx. Phalanges ossify by one primary centre and one secondary center at the bases (the second to fifth metacarpals ossify by one primary center in the shaft and one secondary center in the head).

 CLINICAL CORRELATION

Bennett's Fracture

It is the fracture of the base of the first metacarpal bone involving the first carpometacarpal joint. This is often caused by direct blow with a closed fist, as in boxing.

Boxer's Fracture

The most common site of boxer's fracture is neck of fifth metacarpal bone.

Phalanges

The phalanges of each hand are 14 in number, thumb has 2 and the remaining four fingers have 3 each. Each phalanx presents a base, shaft and head. The head of distal phalanx is nonarticular and is marked anteriorly by tuberosity.

JOINTS OF HAND

Metacarpophalangeal (MCP) Joints

The metacarpophalangeal (MCP) joints (which are five in number) are the articulations between the base of proximal phalanx and the head of metacarpal bone. The movements of flexion, extension, adduction and abduction take place at the medial four MCP joints. The first MCP joint permits only flexion and extension.

Interphalangeal Joints of Medial Four Digits

- The proximal interphalangeal (PIP) joints are between the heads of proximal phalanges and bases of middle phalanges.
- The distal interphalangeal (DIP) joints are between the heads of middle phalanges and bases of distal phalanges.

The interphalangeal joints permit only flexion and extension.

Interphalangeal Joint of Thumb

The thumb has only one interphalangeal joint because there are only two phalanges in the thumb.

Note: For origin (red color) and insertions (blue color) of the muscles in the anterior aspect of carpal bones, metacarpal bones and phalanges, refer to figures 10.22.

11

Pectoral Region and Breast

Chapter Contents

The pectoral region is the name given to the front of the chest or thorax. This region contains the breast or mammary glands, pectoral muscles, clavipectoral fascia, origin of platysma and pectoral nerves.

SURFACE MARKING (FIG. 11.1)

- The clavicle lies horizontally in the upper part of pectoral region on either side. It articulates with manubrium sterni medially and with acromion laterally. Since it is subcutaneous, it is felt through the skin in its entire extent.
- The coracoid process of scapula is palpable in the infraclavicular fossa (deltopectoral groove).
- The sternum (breastbone) is located in the midline. The manubrium sterni, body and xiphoid process are the three parts of sternum from above downward. All parts of sternum are palpable.
- The sternal angle or angle of Louis is the palpable transverse ridge indicating the manubriosternal joint. The second costal cartilage articulates with the sternum at the sternal angle. Therefore, sternal angle is an important landmark during examination of the chest of the patient as it indicates the position of the second rib from which the other ribs are counted downwards.

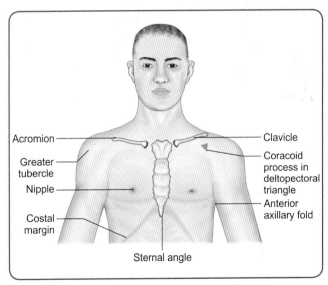

Fig. 11.1: Surface marking in pectoral region

- The epigastric fossa is a depression in the infrasternal angle. The epigastric fossa overlies the xiphoid process.
- The nipple is variable in position in females. In males and in prepubertal females, the nipple lies in fourth intercostal space just medial to the midclavicular line.

- The anterior axillary fold produced by pectoralis major muscle is a visible landmark when the muscle contracts against resistance.

> **STUDENT INTEREST**
>
> The sternal angle or angle of Louis is an important landmark for the clinician. It is palpable as a transverse ridge and indicates the position of second costal cartilage and second rib on either side. Platysma is an interesting muscle. Learn it in pectoral region and then revise it in head and neck region. In clinical training, you will be testing contraction of platysma muscle in a patient for assessing function of facial nerve.

SUPERFICIAL FASCIA

- The main feature of the superficial fascia is the presence of breasts or mammary glands.
- The *platysma* (Fig. 11.2) seen in the upper part of the pectoral region is a thin subcutaneous muscle. It takes origin from the deep fascia covering the upper part of pectoralis major and adjacent deltoid muscle. It crosses the clavicle to enter the neck and is inserted into the lower margin of the body of mandible partly and into the facial muscles around the mouth. In its course through the neck, the platysma lies in the superficial fascia of the neck. The platysma is supplied by the facial nerve (seventh cranial nerve) in the neck (for the actions and clinical testing of platysma, refer to muscles of facial expression in chapter 62).

Cutaneous Nerves (Fig. 11.3)

- The skin above the sternal angle is supplied by the medial, intermediate and lateral supraclavicular nerves

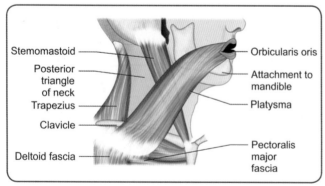

Fig. 11.2: Origin of platysma from fascia covering deltoid and pectoralis major muscles in the pectoral region (Note the platysma crossing the clavicle to pass through neck and reach the mouth by crossing the mandible)

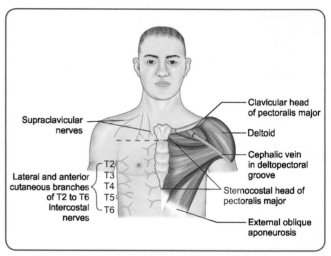

Fig. 11.3: Cutaneous innervation of pectoral region on right side (supraclavicular nerves from cervical plexus and intercostal nerves) and line of discontinuous dermatomes at the level of sternal angle. Note the origin of pectoralis major muscle on the left side

(C3, C4), which arise in the neck from the cervical plexus. These nerves descend to the pectoral region by crossing in front of the clavicle or frequently by piercing it. The medial supraclavicular nerve supplies the skin overlying the manubrium. The intermediate nerve supplies the skin over the upper part of pectoralis major muscle and the lateral nerve supplies the skin over the shoulder.

- The anterior cutaneous branches of the second to the sixth intercostal nerves enter the pectoral region along the lateral margin of sternum after piercing the sternocostal head of pectoralis major and the deep fascia. These branches are accompanied by corresponding arteries (which are the branches of internal thoracic artery). The area of supply of these cutaneous nerves extends from the anterior median plane to the midclavicular line.
- The lateral cutaneous branches of the intercostal nerves appear along a vertical line just behind the anterior axillary fold. They supply the skin beyond the midclavicular plane.

Line of Discontinuous Dermatomes

Since the first intercostal nerve does not give cutaneous branches to the pectoral region C4 and T2 dermatomes approximate each other (Fig. 11.3) at the level of sternal angle. This interruption in the sequential order of dermatomes occurs due to the fact that C5 to T1 dermatomes are dragged into the upper limb bud during embryonic life.

 STUDENT INTEREST

Cutaneous nerves on the anterior chest wall above the level of sternal angle are derived from cervical plexus and below that level are derived from intercostal nerves. At the junctional line (level of sternal angle) C4 dermatome meets T2 dermatome (Fig. 11.3).

DEEP FASCIA

The deep fascia of the pectoral region is called ***pectoral fascia*** because it covers the pectoralis major muscle. It is continuous with the periosteum of the clavicle and of the sternum. It passes over the deltopectoral groove to become continuous with the fascia covering the deltoid. The upper portion of the pectoral fascia gives origin to fibers of platysma. At the lower margin of pectoralis major, the pectoral fascia and the fascia covering the latissimus dorsi are connected by the axillary fascia, which lies in the floor of the axilla. The suspensory ligament of axilla connects the axillary fascia to the clavipectoral fascia at the lower margin of pectoralis minor.

Deltopectoral Triangle (Figs 11.1 and 11.3)

The boundaries of this triangle are the upper margin of pectoralis major medially, anterior margin of deltoid laterally and the clavicle superiorly. The triangle contains cephalic vein, deltoid branch of thoracoacromial artery and the deltopectoral lymph nodes. The coracoid process of scapula projects in its upper part.

MUSCLES

Pectoralis Major (Fig. 11.3)

This is the largest muscle of the pectoral region. It forms the anterior axillary fold.

Origin

- The ***clavicular head*** takes origin from the anterior surface of the medial half of the clavicle.
- The ***sternocostal head*** arises from the front of the manubrium, body of the sternum and from second to sixth costal cartilages.
- The aponeurotic fibers arise from the aponeurosis of the external oblique muscle of the anterior abdominal wall.

Insertion

The pectoralis major is inserted into the lateral lip of the intertubercular sulcus of humerus by a U-shaped bilaminar tendon (the two limbs of the U being called anterior and posterior laminae). The anterior lamina is formed by clavicular fibers. It is inserted into the lower part of the lateral lip. The posterior lamina is formed by aponeurotic fibers. It is inserted into the upper part of the lateral lip. The base of the U is formed by sternocostal fibers.

Nerve Supply

By medial pectoral (C8, T1) and lateral pectoral (C5, C6, C7) nerves.

Actions

- The contraction of entire muscle produces medial rotation and adduction of arm as, for example, while putting the hand on one's hip and pushing inward forcibly.
- The contraction of clavicular part alone produces flexion of arm. This part becomes prominent, when the arm is flexed against resistance, e.g. in pushing the edge of a heavy table.
- The contraction of sternocostal part produces extension of the flexed arm against resistance, for example, while pulling a heavy table by holding on the edge of the table.
- In climbing on a rope or a tree, the sternocostal part of pectoralis major along with latissimus dorsi (Fig. 14.3) produces a very powerful movement of extension of the arms from fully flexed position.

CLINICAL CORRELATION

- ***To test the function of pectoralis major,*** the subject abducts the arms to about 60° and then flexes the elbows. Now the subject attempts to bring the arms together. The examiner watches for the prominence of the anterior axillary folds. (Another method of testing the muscle function is by asking the subject to place hands on the hips and press firmly inward and observe for the prominence of anterior axillary folds).
- ***Poland anomaly*** is congenital absence of pectoralis major muscle, as a result of which the anterior axillary fold is absent.

Pectoralis Minor (Fig. 11.4)

This is a triangular muscle in the anterior wall of axilla, placed posterior to the pectoralis major. It has anterior and posterior surfaces and upper (medial) and lower (lateral) margins.

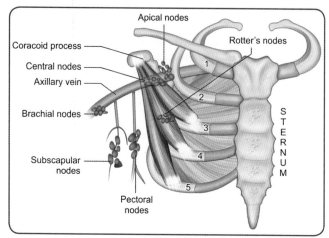

Fig. 11.4: Origin and insertion of pectoralis minor muscle and its relations to the various groups of axillary lymph nodes

Origin

From the outer surfaces of third, fourth and fifth ribs near the costal cartilages

Insertion

Into the medial margin and upper surface of the coracoid process of scapula

Relations

The pectoralis minor muscle is completely enclosed in the *clavipectoral fascia*.

- *Anterior:* Interpectoral lymph nodes (Rotter's nodes) and the pectoralis major muscle.
- *Posterior:* Second part of axillary artery, axillary vein and cords of brachial plexus.
- *Lower (lateral) margin:* Lateral thoracic vessels and anterior group of axillary lymph nodes.

Nerve Supply

Medial pectoral nerve and (lateral pectoral nerve through communication with medial pectoral nerve).

Actions

- Protraction of scapula along with serratus anterior muscle.
- Depression of scapula along with lower fibers of trapezius.

 CLINICAL CORRELATION

The pectoralis minor muscle is a key surgical landmark for identifying axillary lymph nodes during surgical dissection of axilla. These nodes are grouped into three levels, depending on their relation to pectoralis minor muscle. Level-I nodes (anterior, posterior and lateral groups) are located below and lateral to the lower margin of the muscle. Level-II nodes (central group) are located behind and the interpectoral or Rotter's nodes in front of the muscle. The level-III nodes (apical group) lie above the upper margin of the muscle.

STUDENT INTEREST

Both pectoralis major and pectoralis minor muscles are clinically very important, especially in diagnosis and surgical treatment of breast cancer. Hence, their origin, insertion, nerve supply, actions and relations to breast, anterior axillary wall and to axillary vessels must be thoroughly revised.

Subclavius

This is a very small muscle in the upper end of anterior wall of axilla deep to the pectoralis major.

Origin

By a narrow tendon from the first costochondral junction
Insertion: Into the subclavian groove on the lower surface of the clavicle

Nerve Supply

From nerve to subclavius (a branch of upper trunk of brachial plexus).

Action

The subclavius steadies the clavicle during movements of the scapula.

Clavipectoral Fascia (Figs 11.5A and B)

The clavipectoral fascia is located in the anterior wall of axilla deep to the pectoralis major.

Vertical Extent

The clavipectoral fascia splits twice to enclose two muscles (subclavius and pectoralis minor) and it forms

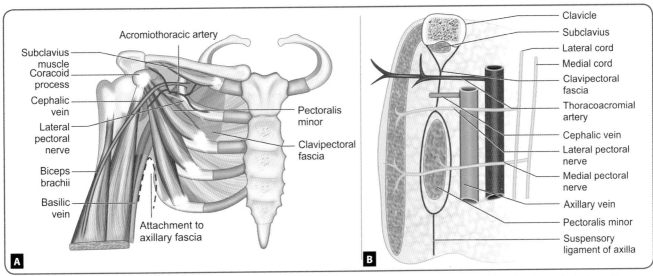

Subclavius muscle
Coracoid process
Cephalic vein
Lateral pectoral nerve
Biceps brachii
Basilic vein
Acromiothoracic artery
Pectoralis minor
Clavipectoral fascia
Attachment to axillary fascia

Clavicle
Subclavius
Lateral cord
Medial cord
Clavipectoral fascia
Thoracoacromial artery
Cephalic vein
Lateral pectoral nerve
Medial pectoral nerve
Axillary vein
Pectoralis minor
Suspensory ligament of axilla

Figs 11.5A and B: A. Schematic diagram to depict the vertical extent of clavipectoral fascia and the structures that pierce it; **B.** Simplified diagram depicting clavipectoral fascia

two ligaments (costocoracoid ligament and suspensory ligament of axilla).

- Superiorly, it splits to enclose the subclavius muscle and its two layers are attached to inferior surface of clavicle at the lips of subclavian groove. At the lower margin of subclavius, the two layers unite to form a single sheet of strong clavipectoral fascia, which bridges the gap between the subclavius muscle and the upper margin of pectoralis minor muscle.
- The fascia splits to enclose the pectoralis minor muscle. At the lower margin of the pectoralis minor the two layers unite to form the suspensory ligament of axilla, which becomes continuous with the axillary fascia.

Horizontal Extent

- Medially, the strong part of clavipectoral fascia is attached to the first rib medial to subclavius and blends with the fascia covering the first two intercostal spaces.
- Laterally, it is attached to the coracoid process of scapula and to the fascia covering the short head of biceps brachii.

Costocoracoid Ligament

The part of clavipectoral fascia between the first rib and the coracoid process is known as costocoracoid ligament.

Structures Piercing Clavipectoral Fascia

- Cephalic vein
- Acromiothoracic (thoracoacromial) artery
- Lateral pectoral nerve
- Lymphatics (from superficial structures in pectoral region).

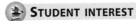 **Student Interest**

Mnemonic
***Structures piercing clavipectoral fascia:* CALL** – **C**ephalic vein, **A**cromiothoracic artery, **L**ateral pectoral nerve, **L**ymphatics
Note: Clavipectoral fascia is a short note question in theory.

Pectoral Nerves

- The ***medial pectoral nerve (C8, T1)*** arises from the medial cord of the brachial plexus. It lies behind the first part of axillary artery initially but soon curves forward to give a communicating ramus to the lateral pectoral nerve in front of the axillary artery. The medial pectoral nerve supplies both pectoralis minor and major muscles.
- The ***lateral pectoral nerve (C5, C6, C7)*** arises from the lateral cord of the brachial plexus. It travels forward on the lateral side of axillary artery and pierces the clavipectoral fascia and clavicular fibers of pectoralis major muscle, which it supplies.

BREAST OR MAMMARY GLANDS

The breasts or mammary glands are a pair of modified sweat glands, located in the superficial fascia of the pectoral region. Each breast is composed of glandular tissue and fibrofatty stroma. The breast is covered with the skin, areola and nipple. In male, the breasts are rudimentary. In female, after the onset of puberty, the breasts grow in size.

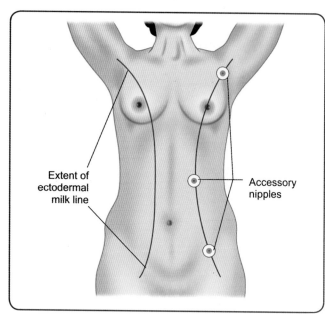

Fig. 11.6: Development of breast in pectoral region from ectodermal milk line (also note the sites of accessory nipples on left side)

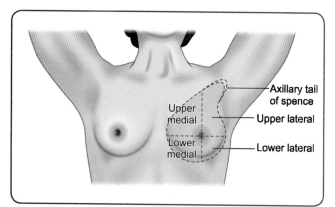

Fig. 11.7: Quadrants of breast and axillary tail of Spence

🧬 EMBRYOLOGIC INSIGHT

In the seven-week embryo, ectodermal milk line appears on the ventral body wall on each side, extending from the limb bud of the upper limb to that of the lower limb. The milk lines in the pectoral region give rise to a pair of glands and the remaining milk lines disintegrate (Fig. 11.6).

⚕ CLINICAL CORRELATION

Congenital Anomalies
- Accessory nipples (polythelia) may be found anywhere along the milk line
- A complete accessory breast (polymastia) may develop along the milk line
- Amastia or amazia is bilateral agenesis of breast and athelia is absence of nipple
- In Poland anomaly, there is complete or partial absence of glandular tissue but the nipple is normal. The pectoralis major muscle is partly or fully absent in this anomaly.

Extent

The breast extends vertically from the second to the sixth ribs and in the transverse plane, from the sternal margin to the midaxillary line.

Parts

The breast consists of a broad base in contact with the chest wall and a pointed apex, which bears the nipple. A projection of the glandular tissue from the upper and outer quadrant of the breast, into the axilla, is called *axillary tail of Spence* (Fig. 11.7). This deep part of the breast passes through an opening (foramen of Langer) in the axillary fascia. It is in direct contact with the anterior group of axillary lymph nodes. Due to this proximity, cancer of the axillary tail may be mistaken for an enlarged anterior lymph node.

📖 STUDENT INTEREST

Breast lies in superficial fascia except the axillary tail of Spence which projects into the axilla by passing through foramen of Langer in the axillary fascia.

Relations of Base of Breast (Fig. 11.8)

The base of the breast is in contact with the pectoral fascia, deep to which it rests on three muscles. The pectoralis major muscle is in contact with the greater part of the base. The serratus anterior is related superolaterally and the aponeurosis of external oblique muscle of the abdomen inferiorly. These three muscles form the bed of the mammary gland. Between the base and the pectoral fascia, there is a retromammary space filled with loose connective tissue and fat. This space allows some degree of mobility to the breast. When the pus collects in this space it is called retromammary abscess.

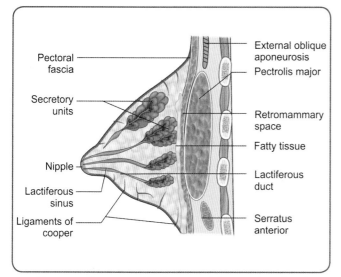

Fig. 11.8: Structure of the breast and the muscles related to its base

Nipple and Areola

The nipple lies approximately in the fourth intercostal space unless the breast is pendulous. It is covered with thick hairless skin, which contains involuntary muscle and is rich in sensory receptors needed for the sucking reflex. About 15–20 lactiferous ducts open by 15–20 minute apertures at the summit of the nipple. The areola is the rounded area of pigmented skin that encircles the nipple. Permanent darkening of the areola and nipple occurs during first pregnancy. The areola contains involuntary muscles, sebaceous glands and sweat glands. The sebaceous glands enlarge during pregnancy as subcutaneous tubercles (Montgomery tubercles). The oily secretion of these glands is a protective lubricant to nipple during lactation.

Gross Structure (Fig. 11.8)

The breast parenchyma is arranged in 15–20 lobes. Each lobe has one main *lactiferous duct*, which converges toward the nipple. The number of lactiferous ducts is equal to that of the lobes. Each lactiferous duct receives numerous smaller ducts and as it approaches the nipple,

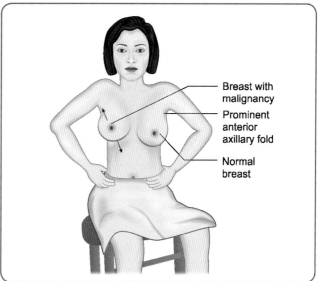

Fig. 11.9: Testing mobility of breast on contracted pectoralis major muscle (Note that normal breast is freely mobile but a breast with malignancy loses mobility due to fixation of breast to underlying pectoral fascia)

it dilates beneath the areola to form the lactiferous sinus, and then narrows again to reach its opening at the summit of the nipple. The lactiferous ducts converge towards the nipple in a radiating manner. Therefore, while draining a breast abscess a radial incision is placed to avoid injury to these ducts. *The ligaments of Cooper* are the special thickened parts of stromal tissue, which serve to anchor the gland to the overlying skin at certain points. They also connect the base of the gland to the pectoral fascia, without hampering the mobility of the normal gland on the contracted pectoralis major muscle (Fig. 11.9).

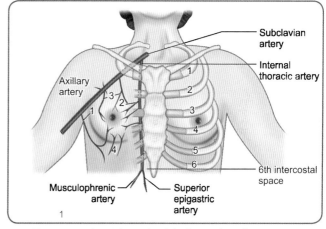

Fig. 11.10: Arterial supply of the breast from four sources

Histology

The breast consists of parenchyma (secretory acini and ducts), connective tissue stroma, adipose tissue, blood vessels and lymphatics and is covered with skin.
- **Nonlactating breast** is composed of abundant fatty tissue and stromal tissue. The ill-defined lobules contain ducts only (secretory acini are lacking)
- **Lactating breast** has a markedly different structure. The lobules are well developed and contain dilated acini and ducts. Acini may be distended with milk. There are plenty of blood vessels. The stroma and fatty tissue are markedly reduced.

Mode of Secretion

The breast is a compound tubuloalveolar gland. According to its mode of secretion, it is classified as both **merocrine** and **apocrine gland**. The release of protein molecules without loss of plasma membrane falls under merocrine mode, whereas release of fat globules by loss of apical plasma membrane falls under apocrine mode.

Arterial Supply

The breast receives arteries mainly from four sources (Fig. 11.10).
1. **Lateral part** of breast by branches of lateral thoracic artery .

2. **Medial part** of breast by perforating cutaneous branches of internal mammary artery in the second, third and fourth intercostal spaces.
3. **Upper part** of breast by pectoral branches of acromiothoracic and superior thoracic arteries
4. **Base of breast** by posterior intercostal arteries in the second, third and fourth spaces.

Venous Drainage

The veins radiate from the circular venous plexus subjacent to the areola. They drain into the surrounding veins, namely axillary, internal thoracic and intercostal veins. The communication of posterior intercostal veins with the internal vertebral venous plexus (via intervertebral veins) is the basis of spread of cancer of breast to the vertebrae and skull bones (Fig. 11.15).

Lymphatic Drainage

The lymph vessels of breast are grouped into the superficial and deep sets.

Superficial Set

Superficial lymph vessels (Fig. 11.11A) drain the skin overlying the breast except that of nipple and areola.
- A few lymph vessels from the skin of the upper part of the breast directly reach the supraclavicular nodes by crossing the clavicle, whereas a few terminate into the deltopectoral nodes.

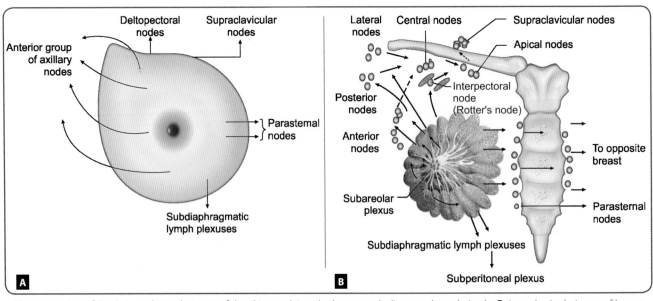

Figs 11.11A and B: A. Lymphatic drainage of the skin overlying the breast excluding areola and nipple; **B.** Lymphatic drainage of breast parenchyma (glandular tissue and lactiferous ducts) including areola and nipple

- The skin of the medial part drains into the internal mammary (parasternal) nodes of the same side. A few lymphatics cross over to communicate with the lymphatics of the opposite breast.
- The skin of the rest of the breast drains into the anterior group of axillary nodes.

Deep Set

The deep lymph vessels (Fig. 11.11B) drain the gland parenchyma and the skin of the nipple and areola. The lymph plexuses in the parenchyma around the lactiferous ducts and in the stroma communicate with the subareolar plexus of Sappey.

- The lymph vessels from the parenchymal plexuses and the subareolar plexus mainly drain into pectoral (anterior) group of axillary nodes. A few drain into the interpectoral or Rotter's nodes and others to the subscapular (posterior) and brachial (lateral) groups of axillary nodes. From these axillary nodes, the lymph passes to the central nodes and finally to the apical nodes. Some vessels from the peripheral part of superior quadrants pass directly into the apical group.
- About 75% of lymph from the breast drains into the axillary nodes.
- Rest of the parenchyma drains into the internal mammary or parasternal nodes.
- The lymph vessels that leave the deep surface of the breast reach the posterior intercostal nodes.
- A few lymph vessels from the base communicate via the rectus sheath on the anterior abdominal wall with the subperitoneal lymph plexuses.

🍵 STUDENT INTEREST

Lymphatic drainage of breast is very important because cancer of breast spreads mainly by lymphatic route and cancer of breast is a very common disease. About 75% of lymph from breast drains into the axillary lymph nodes, 20% drains into the internal mammary nodes and 5% drains into the posterior intercostal nodes. Mastectomy or surgical removal of the breast for cancer is accompanied by surgical dissection of the axilla for removing axillary lymph nodes.

👌 CLINICAL CORRELATION

Malignancy of Breast

The breast cancer in women is a global problem. The cancer usually arises from the epithelium of the ducts. The upper outer quadrant of the breast is the most common site of cancer. The early symptom of cancer is the presence of a painless hard lump in the breast. However, the patient may seek help of the surgeon at various stages of the cancer (Figs 11.12A to C).

Spread or Metastasis of Breast Cancer

The spread of cancer cells from the primary lesion in the breast is by three routes, lymphatic, local infiltration and blood borne.

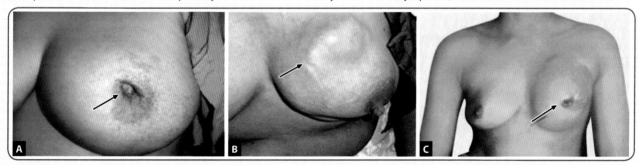

Figs 11.12A to C: Different presentations of breast cancer (indicated by arrows) in patients

Contd...

Contd…

Spread to Axillary Lymph Nodes

The axillary lymph nodes usually are involved in a very early stage of cancer. Therefore, clinical examination of breast is incomplete without the palpation of axillary lymph nodes (Fig. 11.13). The biopsy of lymph nodes is taken for histopathological confirmation of the diagnosis.

Local Spread

- Involvement of the ligaments of Cooper results in dimpling or puckering of skin. The fibrosed ligaments of Cooper, at the base of the breast cause fixation of the breast to the underlying pectoral fascia leading to loss of mobility of the breast.
- The blockage of cutaneous lymph vessels causes edema of the overlying skin. The points of openings of sweat ducts (sweat pores) do not show edema and hence remain depressed. As a result, the skin over the breast presents an appearance of an orange peel (peau d' orange appearance seen in figure 11.14).
- Retraction of the nipple may occur if the cancer cells invade the lactiferous ducts.

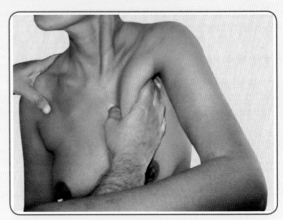

Fig. 11.13: Examination of anterior axillary (pectoral) lymph nodes in a patient

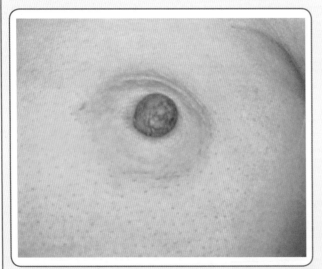

Fig. 11.14: Peau d'orange appearance of the skin of breast blockage of cutaneous lymph vessels by cancer cells causing elevation of skin surrounding the depressed pores of the ducts of sweat glands

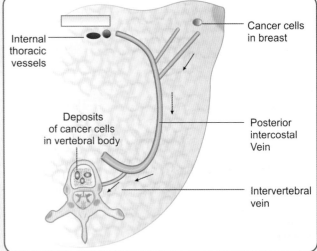

Fig. 11.15: Venous route of spread of cancer cells from the breast to the vertebral column

Distant Spread

- The cancer cells spread to subdiaphragmatic and hepatic nodes via the subperitoneal lymph plexuses. A few cells may drop in the peritoneal cavity to deposit on any organ, usually the ovary. The secondary deposits via peritoneal or transcoelomic route are called Krukenberg's tumors.
- The cancer cells spread to vertebral column, cranial bones, ribs and femur by entering the venous circulation. During rise in intrathoracic pressure (in acts like coughing, straining, etc.), there is reversal of blood flow in the intervertebral veins, which facilitates the spread into the internal vertebral venous plexus and into the vertebral bodies (Fig. 11.15) and cranial bones. For this reason, radiological examination of the skeleton is mandatory in breast cancer patients.

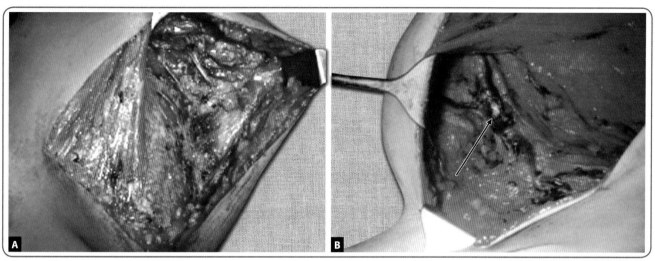

Figs 11.16A and B: A. Exposure of axilla during mastectomy operation; **B.** Dissection of axillary lymph nodes during mastectomy

---

💡 ADDED INFORMATION

Mastectomy (Figs 11.16A and B)

The breast cancer is surgically treated in the majority of cases. The surgical removal of breast is called mastectomy. To perform this operation the knowledge of anatomy of the breast, pectoral region and axilla is essential. Nowadays radical mastectomy (in which the breast, pectoral muscles, clavipectoral fascia, deltopectoral lymph nodes and axillary fat along with all the axillary lymph nodes are removed) is rarely performed. In its place the standard modified radical mastectomy is preferred. This procedure includes simple mastectomy with removal of axillary lymph nodes (level I and II) and the preservation of pectoral muscles. While dissecting the axillary lymph nodes the surgeon identifies the nerve to serratus anterior, nerve to latissimus dorsi and the intercostobrachial nerve in order to safeguard them. The surgeon also identifies axillary blood vessels and their major branches and tributaries.

Early Detection of Breast Cancer

The mammography is a soft tissue X-ray of the breast, with minimum radiation risk. It is taken by placing the breast in direct contact with ultra sensitive film and exposing it to low voltage X-rays. The presence of macrocacification is an indication of malignancy. This method is useful in locating clinically undetected lesion hence mammogram (Figs 11.17A and B) is a part of prevention or early detection of breast cancer in women.

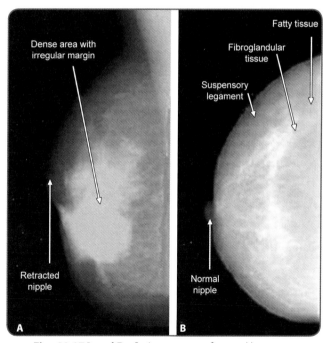

Figs 11.17A and B: A. Appearance of normal breast on Mammography; **B.** Retraction of nipple and a dense area with irregular margin (showing cancer mass) as seen on mammography

Contd...

Contd...

 ADDED INFORMATION

Gynecomastia (Fig. 11.18)

The gynecomastia is the abnormal enlargement of male breast. In some individuals, it may be idiopathic (without any cause). The pathological causes of gynecomastia are liver disease, hormone-secreting tumors, side effects of drugs and leprosy. Gynecomastia is one of the characteristic features in XXY sex chromosomal anomaly (Klinefelter's syndrome).

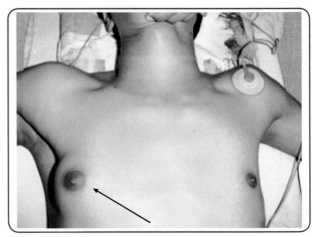

Fig. 11.18: Gynecomastia (enlarged breast in male) indicated by an arrow

Axilla and Axillary Lymph Nodes

AXILLA

The axilla is a roughly pyramidal space situated between the lateral surface of chest wall and the medial aspect of the upper part of the arm. The anatomy of axilla is important not only because it gives passage to the neurovascular structures of the upper limb but also because it is examined clinically for enlargement of axillary lymph nodes and dissected during mastectomy for removing lymph nodes in cancer of the breast.

Contents (Fig. 12.1)

- Axillary artery and its six branches
- Axillary vein and its tributaries
- Axillary lymph nodes
- Adipose tissue (axillary pad of fat)
- Infraclavicular part of brachial plexus (which includes three cords and their branches).
- Long thoracic nerve
- Intercostobrachial nerve
- Axillary tail of Spence.

Walls (Fig. 12.2)

When the arm is abducted, the narrow space of axilla increases in size forming a recognizable armpit bounded by anterior and posterior axillary folds.

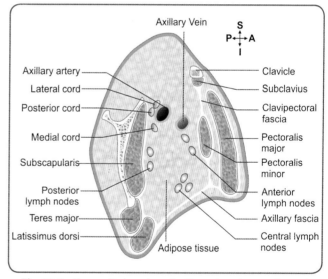

Fig. 12.1: Parasagittal section of axilla to show its anterior and posterior boundaries, some contents and extent of clavipectoral fascia

The axilla has anterior, posterior, medial and lateral walls, and a base and an apex.

- **The anterior wall** consists of the pectoralis major and deeper to it, pectoralis minor, clavipectoral fascia and subclavius muscle in that order from below upward. The lateral thoracic vessels and anterior or pectoral

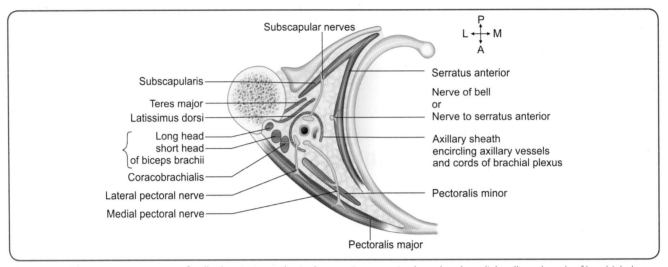

Fig. 12.2: Schematic cross-section of axilla showing muscles in the anterior, posterior, lateral and medial walls and cords of brachial plexus around the second part of axillary artery (Note that the cords of brachial plexus and axillary artery are inside the axillary sheath)

group of lymph nodes are present inside this wall. The anterior axillary fold formed by lower margin of pectoralis major muscle becomes prominent, when the arm is adducted against resistance.

- **The posterior wall** of axilla consists of (from above downward) the subscapularis, teres major and latissimus dorsi muscles. However, as the teres major and latissimus dorsi twist around each other, they come to lie in the same plane.

  The important relations of the posterior wall are the subscapular vessels, subscapular and thoracodorsal nerves and the posterior or subscapular lymph nodes. The posterior axillary fold is formed by the teres major and latissimus dorsi muscles and it becomes prominent when the arm is adducted against resistance.

- **The medial wall** of axilla consists of first four ribs with intervening intercostal muscles and the upper four digitations of serratus anterior muscle. The long thoracic nerve descends on the surface of serratus anterior muscle. The intercostobrachial nerve (lateral cutaneous branch of second intercostal nerve) pierces the serratus anterior to enter the axilla. As the nerve crosses from medial to lateral side of axilla it passes through the central group of axillary lymph nodes to join the medial cutaneous nerve of arm. Compression of intercostobrachial nerve due to enlarged central lymph nodes gives rise to pain in its area of supply (upper medial side of arm including the floor of axilla).

- **The lateral wall** of axilla is the narrowest as it is formed by the bicipital groove of the humerus with the tendon long head of biceps brachii. The conjoint tendon of coracobrachialis and short head of biceps brachii is closely related to this wall.

- **The base or the floor** of axilla is composed of (from below upward) the skin, superficial fascia and the dome-shaped axillary fascia. The axillary tail of Spence passes through the foramen of Langer in the medial part of axillary fascia to enter into the axilla.

- **The apex or cervicoaxillary canal** is the communicating passage between the axilla and the posterior triangle of the neck. The boundaries of the apex (Fig. 12.3) are the middle third of clavicle anteriorly, the superior margin of scapula posteriorly and the outer margin of the first rib medially. The structures that pass through the apex are axillary vessels, cords of brachial plexus, long thoracic nerve and the subclavian lymph trunk.

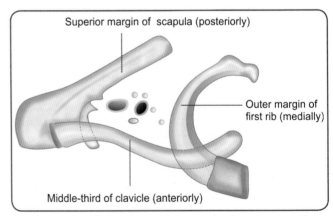

Fig. 12.3: Bony boundaries of the apex of axilla or cervicoaxillary canal

Serratus Anterior Muscle (Fig. 12.4)

This is a broad and flat muscle of the trunk in the medial wall of the axilla.

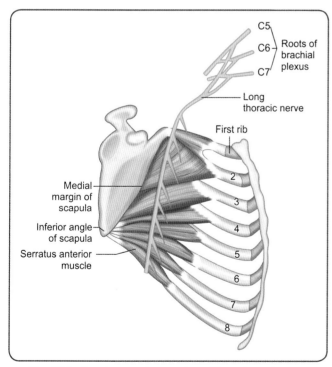

Fig. 12.4: Serratus anterior muscle and long thoracic nerve (nerve of Bell)

Origin

From anterior aspect of outer surfaces of upper eight ribs by eight fleshy digitations

Insertion

Into medial border of ventral (costal) surface of scapula as follows:
- First digitation into superior angle of scapula.
- Second, third and fourth digitations into the entire medial border of scapula.
- Lower four digitations into the inferior angle of scapula.

Nerve Supply

Long thoracic nerve (nerve of Bell)

Note: The long thoracic nerve descends on the superficial surface of serratus anterior and gives separate twig to each of its eight digitations.

Actions

- The serratus anterior muscle protracts the scapula with the help of pectoralis minor. Protraction of scapula is required during punching and pushing movements; hence, serratus anterior is called the boxer's muscle.
- The lateral rotation of scapula is brought about by lower five digitations of serratus anterior with the help of trapezius.

Testing Function of Serratus Anterior

The subject is asked to place the stretched hands on the wall and push forward. Normally the scapulae will remain fixed to the thoracic cage. If the medial border of the scapula is raised during this act it is indicative of weakness or paralysis of serratus anterior muscle.

Long Thoracic Nerve (Fig. 12.4)

This is also known as the nerve of Bell. It is a branch of the root stage of the brachial plexus. It is a purely motor nerve. The long thoracic nerve begins from C5, C6 and C7 nerve roots in the neck.

Cervical Course

The three roots pass downward behind the supraclavicular part of the brachial plexus. The C5 and C6 roots separately pierce the scalenus medius muscle and then unite with each other. This common trunk and the C7 root enter the axilla through its apex and unite with each other to form the long thoracic nerve

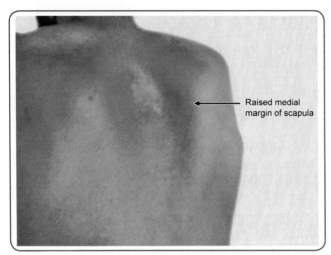

Fig. 12.5: Photograph showing winging of right scapula in a patient

Axillary Course

The long thoracic nerve is closely plastered to the lateral surface of serratus anterior muscle (the medial wall of the axilla). It gives separate twigs to each of the eight digitations of the muscle.

 CLINICAL CORRELATION

Winging of Scapula or Winged Scapula (Fig. 12.5)

The long thoracic nerve may be injured during surgical removal of axillary lymph nodes, leading to paralysis of serratus anterior muscle. Non-functioning of serratus anterior results in a deformity called winged scapula. In this, the medial border and inferior angle of scapula stand out from the chest wall and the patient experiences difficulty in abduction above 90°.

AXILLARY LYMPH NODES

The axillary lymph nodes are arranged into five groups. The area of their drainage includes the entire upper extremity and the thoracoabdominal walls up to the level of umbilicus on the front and up to the level of iliac crest on the back. The axillary nodes drain nearly 75% of the breast tissue.

Groups of Axillary Lymph Nodes

- The **anterior or pectoral group** of lymph nodes is located in the anterior wall of the axilla along the course of lateral thoracic vessels. These nodes receive lymph from major portion of breast tissue, anterior chest wall and anterior abdominal wall up to the level of umbilicus. Its efferent vessels mainly go to the central nodes. The axillary tail of Spence (deep part of mammary gland) lies in close contact with these nodes.

- The **posterior or subscapular group** is located in the posterior wall of axilla along the subscapular vessels. These nodes receive lymph from the posterior chest wall and posterior abdominal wall up to the level of iliac crest.

- The **lateral or brachial group** is located on the lateral wall of axilla along the axillary vein. The lymph nodes of lateral group receive lymph from the entire upper limb. A few vessels accompanying the cephalic vein drain in the deltopectoral nodes and others from lateral aspect of proximal arm terminate directly into the apical nodes. Some lymph vessels accompanying the basilic vein terminate in the epitrochlear (supratrochlear or cubital) nodes, the efferent vessels from which drain into the lateral group. Inflammatory lesion anywhere in the upper limb causes enlarged and painful lateral group of lymph nodes.

- The **central group** is composed of three or four large lymph nodes embedded in the fatty tissue along the axillary vein. These nodes receive lymph from anterior, posterior and lateral groups and drain in to the apical nodes. The intercostobrachial nerve passes through the central nodes. Therefore, when the central nodes are swollen, there is pain along the medial side of upper part of arm and the base of axilla due to compression of intercostobrachial nerve.

- The apical group consists of six to eight lymph nodes lying partly in the apex of the axilla and along the axillary vein in the triangular space between the axillary vein, outer margin of first rib and the upper margin of pectoralis minor muscle. These nodes receive lymph from the central group, deltopectoral or infraclavicular nodes and interpectoral nodes. They receive a few lymphatics directly from the superior peripheral region of the breast and a few from the proximal arm. The apical lymph nodes are the terminal nodes of the upper extremity. Their efferent vessels unite to form the subclavian lymph trunk, which terminates in the jugulovenous junction or the subclavian vein, or the jugular lymph trunk or the right lymph trunk, on the right side and the thoracic duct on the left side.

💡 **ADDED INFORMATION**

The surgeons include the interpectoral or **Rotter's nodes** as a sixth group of axillary lymph nodes. The interpectoral nodes are situated between the pectoralis major and minor muscles, closer to the anterior wall of axilla. They receive deep lymphatics from the breast and drain directly into the apical group or into the central group. (For levels of axillary lymph nodes refer to lymphatic drainage of breast in chapter 11).

STUDENT INTEREST

- The areas of drainage of each group of axillary lymph nodes must be studied in depth. For example, one must know the lower limit of drainage of anterior axillary nodes anteriorly and of posterior group of axillary lymph nodes posteriorly.
- The lymph drainage of the upper limb is also important.
- Keep in mind that intercostobrachial nerve is the lateral cutaneous branch of second intercostal nerve and it pierces the central lymph nodes during its course from medial to lateral side across the axilla.

CLINICAL CORRELATION

Axillary Lymphadenopathy

The enlargement of lymph nodes is called *lymphadenopathy*. The cancer of the breast causes painless enlargement of the axillary lymph nodes. The painful enlargement is due to any infective focus in the area of drainage of the axillary lymph nodes. The nodes are enlarged in generalized lymphadenopathy due to other causes like Hodgkin's lymphoma, lymphatic leukemia and AIDS.

Palpation of Axillary Lymph Nodes

While palpating the axillary lymph nodes in a patient, the examiner uses his or her right hand for the left axilla and left hand for the right axilla. The examiner supports the arm of the patient in a slightly abducted position so as to relax the axillary floor and walls. Standing in front of the patient, the semiflexed fingers are gently but firmly pushed into the floor of the axilla to palpate the nodes of pectoral group (Fig. 12.6), then central, apical and lateral nodes. Standing behind the patient, the examiner feels the subscapular nodes (Fig. 12.7).

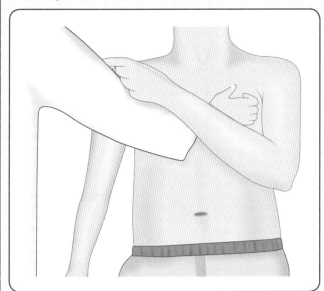

Fig. 12.6: Examination of pectoral or anterior group of lymph nodes standing in front of the patient

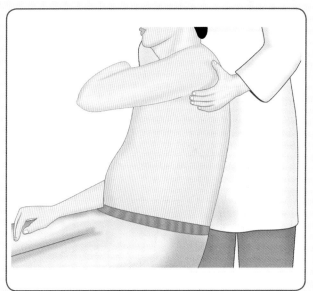

Fig. 12.7: Examination of subscapular or posterior group of axillary lymph nodes standing behind the patient

13

Brachial Plexus and Axillary Vessels

Chapter Contents

BRACHIAL PLEXUS

The brachial plexus is a nerve plexus which is responsible for the motor and sensory nerve supply of the upper limb including a few muscles of the trunk. Through its connections with the sympathetic ganglia, the branches of the brachial plexus provide pilomotor supply (to the arrector pili muscles of skin), sudomotor supply (to sweat glands) and vasomotor supply (to the smooth muscle of blood vessels) of the skin of the upper limb.

Location (Fig. 13.1)

The brachial plexus lies partly in the posterior triangle of the neck and partly in the axilla.

Parts

It is divisible into the supraclavicular and infraclavicular parts.
- **Supraclavicular** part consists of roots, trunks and divisions (located in the neck).
- **Infraclavicular** part consists of cords and their branches (located in axilla).

Note: The supraclavicular part of brachial plexus in the posterior triangle of neck and infraclavicular part in the axilla

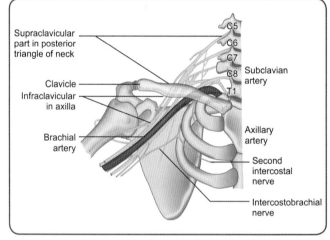

Fig. 13.1: Showing the location of entire brachial plexus in the body

Formation (Fig. 13.2)

The ventral rami of C5, C6, C7, C8 and T1 spinal nerves take part in the formation of the brachial plexus. Usually C4 ventral ramus contributes a small twig to C5 and T2 ventral ramus to T1.

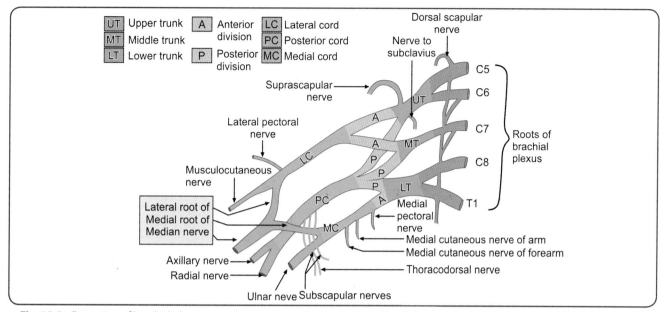

Fig. 13.2: Formation of brachial plexus: stage I – roots, stage II – trunks, stage III – divisions, stage IV – cords, stage V – branches of cords

Stages

Usually, five stages (roots, trunks, divisions, cords and branches) are described in the formation of brachial plexus.

Root stage

The roots of brachial plexus consist of C5, C6, C7, C8 and T1 ventral rami, which are located behind the scalenus medius and scalenus anterior muscles of the neck. The roots unite to form the trunks.

Branches from root stage

• Dorsal scapular nerve or nerve to rhomboids (C5).
• Long thoracic nerve or nerve of Bell (C5, C6, C7).

Trunk stage

There are three trunks (upper, middle and lower) in the brachial plexus.

1. The *upper trunk* is formed by union of C5 and C6 roots at the lateral margin of the scalenus medius.
2. The *middle trunk* is the continuation of C7 root (hence its root value is C7).
3. The *lower trunk* is formed by the union of C8 and T1 roots behind the scalenus anterior muscle.

The trunks of brachial plexus emerge through interscalene space (between scalenus anterior and scalenus medius muscles) to enter the lower part of posterior triangle, where they are superficially located above the clavicle. The upper and middle trunks lie above the subclavian artery and the lower trunk lies directly on the superior surface of the first rib along with the subclavian artery.

Note to students: You will understand the location and relations of trunks of brachial plexus when you study posterior triangle in head and neck region.

Branches of upper trunk

• Suprascapular nerve (C5, C6)
• Nerve to subclavius (C5, C6)

Division stage

As each trunk slants obliquely downward toward the middle third of the clavicle, it terminates into anterior and posterior divisions just behind the clavicle.

Cord stage (Table 13.1)

• The *lateral cord* is formed by the union of anterior divisions of upper and middle trunks (root value—C5, C6, and C7).
• The *medial cord* is the continuation of the anterior division of the lower trunk. Hence, its root value is C8, T1.
• The *posterior cord* is formed by the union of all the three posterior divisions. Its root value is C5, C6, C7, C8 and (T1).

Note: T1 fibers are usually absent because the slender posterior division of the lower trunk carries C8 fibers only.

Relations of Cords to Axillary Artery (Figs 13.9 and 13.10)

The cords are related to the first and second parts of the axillary artery.

TABLE 13.1: Branches of Cords	
Cords	**Branches**
Lateral cord	Lateral root of median—C5, C6, C7
	Lateral pectoral—C5, C6, C7
	Musculocutaneous—C5, C6, C7
Medial cord	Medial root of median—C8, T1
	Medial pectoral—C8, T1
	Medial cutaneous nerve of arm—C8, T1); after the intercostobrachial nerve joins it, the root value is C8, T1, T2)
	Medial cutaneous nerve of forearm—C8, T1
	Ulnar nerve—C8, T1
Posterior cord	Upper subscapular—C5, C6
	Lower subscapular—C5, C6
	Thoracodorsal—C6, C7, C8
	Axillary nerve—C5, C6
	Radial nerve—C5, C6, C7, C8, (T1)

1. Around the first part of the artery, the medial cord is in posterior position, whereas the lateral and posterior cords are in lateral position.
2. Around the second part of the artery, cords take up the positions as indicated by their names.

 ADDED INFORMATION

Prefixation of Brachial Plexus

A prefixed brachial plexus moves one segment higher than usual. In this type, the contribution from C4 is larger, that from T1 is reduced and that from T2 is absent.

Postfixation of Brachial Plexus

A postfixed brachial plexus moves one segment lower than usual. In this type, the contribution from T2 is larger, that from C5 is reduced and that from C4 is absent. Postfixed brachial plexus has mechanical disadvantage since the lower trunk is more angulated and hence, stretched on the upper surface of the first rib. This may, give rise to symptoms of compression of the lower trunk leading to Klumpke's palsy.

Connections with Sympathetic Chain

The ventral rami of the C5 to C8 and T1 spinal nerves receive postganglionic sympathetic fibers from the middle cervical and stellate ganglia of the sympathetic chain via the grey rami communicants (GRC). In this way, the branches of the plexus carry postganglionic sympathetic fibers to the upper limb. The ventral ramus of T1 presents

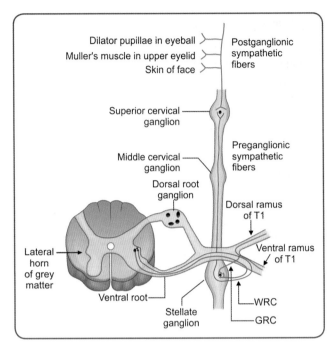

Fig. 13.3: Sympathetic connections of T1 root of brachial plexus showing grey ramus communicans (GRC) and white ramus communicans. The figure also depicts the long preganglionic sympathetic fibers (for head and face) terminating into superior cervical sympathetic ganglion and long postganglionic sympathetic fibers supplying the dilator pupillae muscle of eyeball, Muller's muscle in upper eyelid and skin of face. Injury to T1 root of brachial plexus or T1 ventral ramus (involving preganglionic sympathetic fibers for head and face) results in complete claw hand accompanied by Horner's syndrome

additional connection to stellate ganglion via the first white ramus communicans (WRC) (Fig. 13.3). The preganglionic sympathetic fibers in the first WRC supply the head and face. They synapse in the superior cervical ganglion, from where the postganglionic fibers supply the dilator muscle of the pupil, smooth muscle of the upper eyelid (Muller's muscle) and vasomotor, sudomotor and pilomotor supply to the skin of the head and face. The T1 ventral ramus may be avulsed in traumatic injury to the brachial plexus, which results in avulsion of preganglionic fibers for head and face. The symptoms and signs due to loss of sympathetic supply to the face and eye produce Horner's syndrome (refer to total brachial plexus avulsion in brachial plexus injuries given in clinical correlation box below).

Note: Preganglionic fibers are red and postganglionic fibers are green.

Brachial Plexus Injuries

The brachial plexus may be damaged due to trauma, compression and malignancy of breast and lung. The traumatic causes of the brachial plexus injury are forceps delivery, gunshot or stab injuries, fall from a height, post-fixation of plexus and automobile accidents. The plexus may be compressed due to aneurysm (dilatation) of the axillary artery.

Total Brachial Plexus Paralysis

This is a serious injury. The roots of the plexus are avulsed so the upper limb is paralyzed with total loss of sensation. There is paralysis of serratus anterior and rhomboid muscles. The damage to T1 ventral ramus (involving preganglionic sympathetic fibers) for head and face (Fig. 13.3) results in Horner's syndrome on the affected side. This syndrome consists of partial ptosis (due to paralysis of Muller's muscle of upper eyelid), constriction of pupil (due to paralysis of dilator pupillae muscle of eyeball), ipsilateral loss of sweating on face (due to loss of sudomotor supply) and flushing of ipsilateral face (due to loss of vasomotor supply).

Upper Trunk Palsy or Erb's Palsy

Erb's palsy in new born usually occurs due to forceps delivery, during which, there may be forceful separation of neck and shoulder with resultant stretching of the upper trunk (Erb's point). Hence, it is also known as obstetrical palsy.

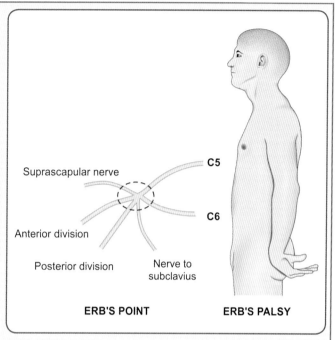

Figs 13.4A and B: A. The formation of Erb's point on upper trunk of brachial plexus and **B.** Typical waiter's tip position' of upper limb due to lesion at Erb's point

The Erb's point is described as the meeting point of six nerves (Fig. 13.4), which include ventral rami of C5 and C6, two branches (suprascapular and nerve to subclavius) of upper trunk and two divisions of upper trunk. In Erb's palsy, upper limb is held in porter's tip or policeman's tip or waiter's tip position, in which the arm is adducted and medially rotated and the forearm is extended and pronated. This characteristic position is due to paralysis of certain muscles and overaction of antagonistic muscles as shown in Table 13.2.

Lower Trunk Paralysis or Klumpke's Paralysis

The lesion of lower trunk is usually produced by traction on the lower trunk by a cervical rib (Fig. 13.5A) or forcible hyper-abduction of arm in a fall from a height or malignant infiltration of the lower trunk (as in Pancoast tumor of lung or carcinoma breast). This lesion results in complete claw hand (Fig. 13.5B), in which there is weakness in interossei and lumbricals supplied by T1 root via branches of ulnar and median nerves. In claw hand deformity, the fingers are hyper extended at metacarpophalangeal joints and hyper flexed at interphalangeal joints. The wrist joint is hyperextended due to paralysis of flexors of wrist and overaction of extensors. There is pain and numbness along the medial side of the arm, forearm and medial one-and -half fingers. Horner's syndrome may be produced due to injury to the ventral ramus of T1 spinal nerve or the first WRC.

Contd…

Contd…

TABLE 13.2: Paralysis of abductors and lateral rotators of arm and flexors and supinators of forearm and overaction of antagonistic muscles in Porter's tip position of upper limb

Position of limb	Muscles paralyzed	Muscles showing overaction
Adducted arm	Supraspinatus and deltoid	Adductors of arm
Medially rotated arm	Teres minor and infraspinatus	Medial rotators of arm
Extended forearm	Biceps brachii, brachialis and brachioradialis	Extensors of forearm
Pronated forearm	Biceps brachii and supinator	Pronators of forearm

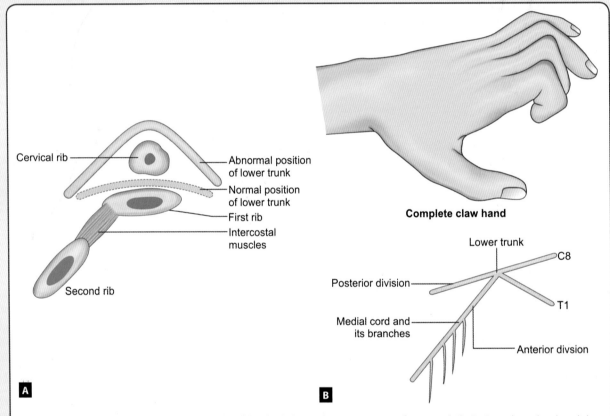

Complete claw hand

Figs 13.5A and B: A. Traction on lower trunk of brachial plexus due to presence of a cervical rib; **B.** Complete claw hand due to lesion of lower trunk of brachial plexus (Note that anterior division of lower trunk continues as medial cord of brachial plexus)

STUDENT INTEREST

- The brachial plexus is nerve plexus supplying the muscles and skin of upper limb and muscles of the trunk. If it is injured or the nerves arising from it are injured, the result is paralysis of muscle or muscles and loss of sensation on the skin. This causes hindrance in day-to-day simple activities. This is a MUST KNOW TOPIC.
- The location of brachial plexus is partly in neck and partly in axilla.
- By practicing the simple line diagram showing the stages of brachial plexus, one can imprint it in one's memory and then memorization is less troublesome.

Stage I— Roots C5 to C8 and T1 (total 5)

Stage II—Trunks (total 3) (upper trunk is formed by union of C5 and C6 roots, middle trunk is the continuation of C7 root and lower trunk is formed by union of C8 and T1 roots)

Stage III—Divisions (total 6—anterior and posterior from each trunk)

Stage IV—Cords (total 3—anterior divisions of upper and middle trunks unite to form lateral cord, anterior division of lower trunk continues as medial cord and all posterior divisions unite to form posterior cord)

Stage V—Branches arising from cords in axilla (3 from lateral cord, 5 from medial cord and 5 from posterior cord)

Remember: The branches arising from root stage (dorsal scapular nerve and long thoracic nerve) and the branches arising from upper trunk at Erb's point (suprascapular nerve and nerve to subclavius) arise in the neck.

ADDED INFORMATION

Brachial Plexus Block

The *brachial plexus block* is a preferred method of anesthesia for surgery on upper limb for complicated wounds of hand, fracture of forearm bones, reduction of shoulder joint, etc. The second stage of brachial plexus in the subclavian triangle at the root of the neck is accessible usually via supraclavicular approach (Figs 13.6A and B). Some anesthetists approach the second stage of brachial plexus via infraclavicular route.

AXILLARY ARTERY

The axillary artery is the main artery of the upper extremity. It begins as a continuation of the subclavian artery at the outer border of the first rib and continues as the brachial artery at the lower border of teres major muscle. The axillary artery and the cords of brachial plexus are wrapped in a fascial sheath(axillary sheath) derived from the prevertebral fascia of the neck.

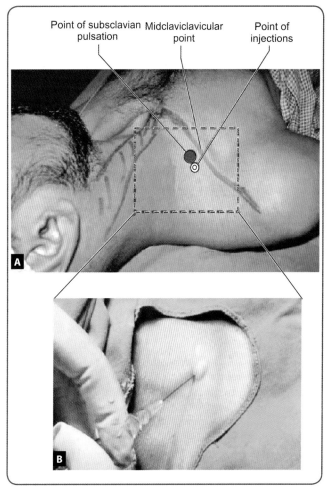

Figs 13.6A and B: Anesthetic block in supraclavicular part of brachial plexus in a patient (Note that the landmarks for the point of insertion of the needle are midclavicular point and site of pulsation of subclavian artery)

Variation

The axillary artery may divide into ulnar and radial arteries at the distal border of teres major. In such cases the brachial artery is absent.

Surface Marking (Fig. 13.7)

There are two methods of marking the axillary artery on the surface of the body.

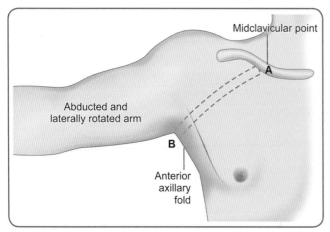

Fig. 13.7: Surface marking of axillary artery (as shown by dotted lines connecting points A and B)

1. With the arm abducted to 90° and the palm facing up, the first point is marked at midpoint of the clavicle. The second point is marked at the junction of the anterior two-third and posterior one-third of the line joining the lower ends of the anterior and posterior axillary folds. A line connecting these two points represents the axillary artery. The point of demarcation of axillary and brachial arteries is roughly at the level of the lower end of the posterior axillary fold, where pulsation of artery can be felt against the humerus.

2. With the arm abducted to 90° and the palm facing upwards, a mid clavicular point is marked. Another point is marked one cm below the midpoint of the line joining two epicondyles of humerus (just medial to the tendon of biceps brachii). The upper one third of the line joining the above two points represents the axillary artery.

    The second point is marked one cm below the midpoint of the line joining the two epicondyles of the humerus (just medial to the tendon of biceps brachii). The upper one third of the line joining the two points represents the axillary artery.

Course

As the axillary artery enters the axilla through the apex, it is in intimate relation to the medial wall of axilla, which is formed by the first two digitations of serratus anterior muscle. As it courses downwards with a lateral convexity, it comes in very intimate relation to the lateral wall of the axilla.

Parts or Subdivisions (Fig. 13.8)

The axillary artery is subdivided into three parts by the pectoralis minor muscle, which crosses it anteriorly.

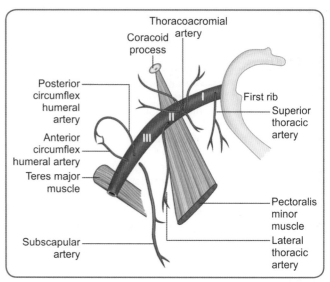

Fig. 13.8: Extent, parts and branches of axillary artery

1. The first part extends from the outer margin of the first rib to the upper margin of pectoralis minor.
2. The second part lies deep or posterior to the pectoralis minor.
3. The third part extends from the lower margin of the pectoralis minor to the lower margin of teres major.

Relations of First Part (Fig. 13.9)

Anterior: From superficial to deep, it related to the skin, superficial fascia along with platysma, deep fascia and the clavicular head of the pectoralis major muscle, the clavipectoral fascia and the structures that pierce it and the communication between medial and lateral pectoral nerves.

Posterior: From posterior to anterior to the first two digitations of the serratus anterior muscle and nerve to

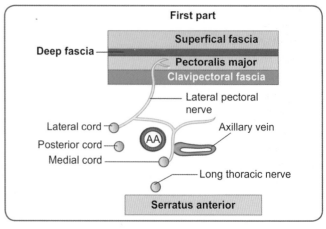

Fig. 13.9: Relations of the first part of axillary artery

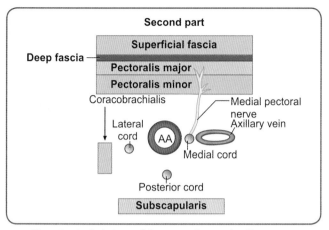

Fig. 13.10: Relations of the second part of axillary artery

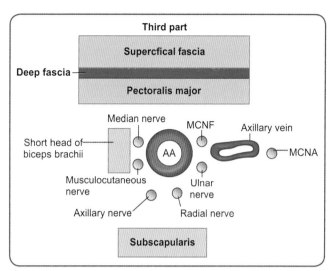

Fig. 13.11: Relations of the third part of axillary artery
Key: MCNA–Medial cutaneous nerve of arm,
MCNF–Medial cutaneous nerve of forearm

serratus anterior and to the medial cord of brachial plexus (giving origin to medial pectoral nerve).

Lateral: Lateral and posterior cords of brachial plexus.

Medial: to axillary vein closely as both vessels are enclosed in a fascial sheath.

Relations of Second Part (Fig. 13.10)

Anterior: From superficial to deep, it is related to the skin, superficial fascia, deep fascia and the clavicular head of pectoralis major and the pectoralis minor muscle (covered with clavipectoral fascia)

Posterior: Posterior cord and subscapularis muscle

Lateral: Lateral cord, coracobrachialis and short head of biceps brachii

Medial: Medial cord, medial pectoral nerve and axillary vein.

Relations of Third Part (Fig. 13.11)

Anterior: proximal relations are skin, superficial fascia, deep fascia and pectoralis major muscle including medial root of the median nerve.

Anterior: distal relations are skin and fasciae only.

Posterior: axillary nerve and radial nerve and muscles of posterior axillary wall (subscapularis muscle and tendons of teres major and latissimus dorsi).

Lateral: median nerve, musculocutaneous nerve and coracobrachialis and short head of biceps brachii.

Medial: medial cutaneous nerve of forearm, ulnar nerve and axillary vein.

🎓 STUDENT INTEREST

First and second parts of the axillary artery are related to the cords of the brachial plexus and the third part to the branches of the cords. You must practice the diagrams of relations of axillary artery as shown in figures 13.9, 13.10 and 13.11.

Branches (Fig. 13.6)

The axillary artery gives origin to six branches.

Single Branch of First Part

Superior thoracic artery.

Two Branches of Second Part

- *Acromiothoracic* or thoracoacromial artery pierces the clavipectoral fascia and then divides into clavicular, deltoid, pectoral and acromial branches.
- *Lateral thoracic artery*.

Three Branches of Third Part

- *Subscapular artery (Fig. 13.12)*, the largest branch, courses downwards along the posterior wall of the axilla lying on subscapularis muscle. It gives off a large circumflex scapular artery which passes through the triangular intermuscular space at the lateral margin of scapula (Fig. 13.5). The terminal part of the subscapular artery, which accompanies the thoracodorsal nerve, is called thoracodorsal artery.

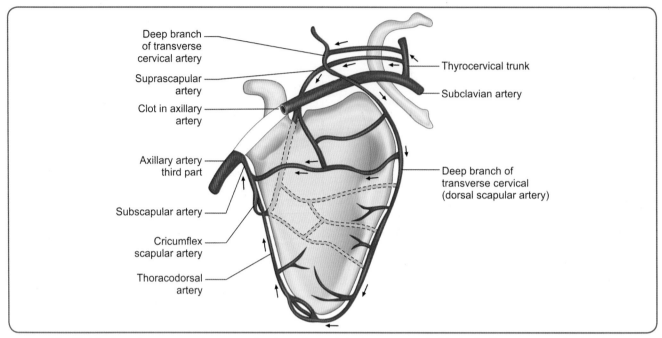

Fig. 13.12: Scapular anastomosis on ventral surface of scapula in the presence of a block of axillary artery proximal to the origin of its subscapular branch

- *Anterior circumflex humeral artery* travels on the anterior aspect of the surgical neck of the humerus and supplies mainly the shoulder joint and the deltoid muscle.
- *Posterior circumflex humeral artery* and the axillary nerve pass behind the surgical neck of humerus after passing through the quadrangular space. It ends by anastomosing with anterior circumflex humeral artery.

STUDENT INTEREST

Mnemonic
For branches of axillary artery— *Students Always Love Solving Algebra Problems*.

Scapular Anastomosis (Fig. 13.12)

The scapular anastomosis brings in to communication the first part of subclavian artery with the third part of the axillary artery through the anastomosis between the following branches from the first part of subclavian artery and of the third part of axillary artery.
1. Suprascapular artery, a branch of thyrocervical trunk of the first part of the subclavian artery.
2. Either the deep transverse cervical artery (a branch of the thyrocervical trunk of the first part of the subclavian artery) or the dorsal scapular artery (a branch of third part of subclavian artery).

3. Circumflex scapular branch of subscapular artery (from the third part of the axillary artery).

In case of a block in the subclavian or the axillary artery, the anastomosis around scapula enlarges to a considerable extent to provide adequate blood supply to the upper limb. The enlarged anastomosis may give rise to 'pulsating scapula'.

CLINICAL CORRELATION

Axillary Artery Pulse

The axillary artery pulse can be felt against the humerus in the lateral wall of axilla. In this location, the artery can be compressed to stop bleeding from it in case of stab injury or bullet injury in the axilla.

Aneurysm of Axillary Artery

The aneurysm (localized dilatation of the artery) of axillary artery presents as a soft pulsating swelling often palpable through the base of the axilla. It gives rise to symptoms and signs due to compression of the nerves of brachial plexus and of the axillary vein.

AXILLARY VESSELS

The axillary vein extends from the lower margin of teres major to outer margin of the first rib (where it continues as the subclavian vein).

Formation

The axillary vein may be formed in one of the two ways:

1. It is formed by the union of basilic vein and the venae comitantes accompanying the brachial artery (brachial veins) at the lower margin of teres major muscle.
2. It is the continuation of basilic vein at the lower margin of teres major and the brachial veins open into the axillary vein at the lower margin of the subscapularis.

Relations

The axillary vein lies medial to the axillary artery throughout its course. It is not inside the fascial sheath like the axillary artery. This is to allow free expansion of the vein. The axillary vein is related on the medial side to medial cutaneous nerve of arm and on lateral side to the medial cutaneous nerve of forearm and ulnar nerve.

Tributaries

- The **cephalic vein** from the upper limb is its largest tributary.
- The veins accompanying the branches of axillary artery are its other tributaries.

 CLINICAL CORRELATION

Axillary Vein Thrombosis

- Thrombosis in the terminal segment of the axillary vein at the apex of axilla may occur due to traction, as seen in people who have to keep the arm hyperabducted for long stretches of time (for example, during plastering or painting the ceiling).
- The apical, central and lateral (brachial) groups of axillary lymph nodes are very closely related to the axillary vein (Fig. 11.4). These nodes are removed during mastectomy by axillary dissection. If the axillary vein is injured during removal of the nodes post-operative thrombosis may occur. This leads to venous stasis causing edema of the upper limb and dilatation of the superficial veins of the pectoral region and of the upper limb.

14

Superficial Muscles of Back and Scapular Region

Chapter Contents

SUPERFICIAL MUSCLES OF BACK

The superficial muscles on the back of the chest are disposed in two layers. The outer layer is composed of two flat muscles, trapezius and latissimus dorsi (Fig. 14.1A) which connect the vertebral column to the bones of upper limb. They are also called superficial posterior thoraco-appendicular muscles. The inner layer consists of muscles under cover of the trapezius. They include deep thoraco-appendicular muscles (levator scapulae, and rhomboids) and scapulo-humeral muscles (deltoid, teres major, and teres minor, supraspinatus, infraspinatus and subscapularis).

Trapezius

This large triangular muscle covers the posterior aspect of the neck and the upper half of the trunk. The muscles of the two sides lie side by side in the midline along their linear attachment to the vertebral column and together form an outline of a trapezium. The trapezius is the only muscle that suspends the pectoral girdle from the cranium.

Origin (Fig. 14.1)

The trapezius has a wide origin from:
- Medial third of superior nuchal line
- External occipital protuberance
- Ligamentum nuchae
- Spine of seventh cervical vertebra
- Spines of all thoracic vertebrae and corresponding supraspinous ligaments.

Insertion

- **Upper fibers:** Into the posterior margin of lateral third of clavicle.
- **Middle fibers:** Into the medial margin of acromion and upper lip of crest of the spine of scapula.
- **Lower fibers:** Into a well-marked tubercle at the medial end of the spine of scapula.

Actions

- The upper fibers elevate the scapula along with levator scapulae (as in shrugging implying 'I don't know').
- The middle fibers cause retraction of scapula along with rhomboids (thus moving it towards the median plane, when a person clasps the hands behind the lower back as in 'stand at ease position').
- The upper and lower fibers of trapezius along with lower five digitations of serratus anterior bring about lateral or forward rotation of scapula.
- The cervical fibers of trapezius of both sides act together to extend the neck.

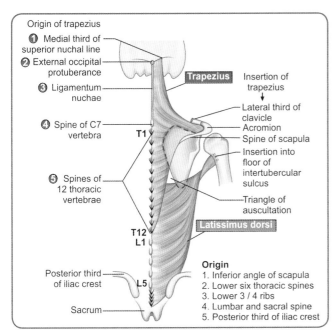

Origin of trapezius
❶ Medial third of superior nuchal line
❷ External occipital protuberance
❸ Ligamentum nuchae
❹ Spine of C7 vertebra
❺ Spines of 12 thoracic vertebrae
Posterior third of iliac crest
Sacrum

Trapezius Insertion of trapezius
↓
Lateral third of clavicle
Acromion
Spine of scapula
Insertion into floor of intertubercular sulcus
Triangle of auscultation

Latissimus dorsi

Origin
1. Inferior angle of scapula
2. Lower six thoracic spines
3. Lower 3 / 4 ribs
4. Lumbar and sacral spine
5. Posterior third of iliac crest

Fig. 14.1: Showing origin and insertion of trapezius and latissimus dorsi muscles

Nerve Supply

Is by spinal accessory nerve and branches from C3 and C4 ventral rami.

Testing Function of Trapezius

The subject is asked to raise shoulders towards the ears and simultaneously the examiner depresses the shoulders forcibly.

Muscles, Nerves and Vessels Under Cover of Trapezius (Figs 14.2A and B)

Muscles of the neck: Semispinalis capitis and splenius capitis

Muscles Attached to the Scapula
• Levator scapulae
• Rhomboid major
• Rhomboid minor
• Inferior belly of omohyoid
• Supraspinatus
• Infraspinatus
• Latissimus dorsi

Nerves
• Spinal part of accessory nerve or eleventh cranial nerve
• Dorsal scapular nerve.
• Third and fourth ventral rami of cervical spinal nerves.

Vessels
• Suprascapular vessels
• Superficial branch of transverse cervical artery and accompanying vein.
• Deep branch of transverse cervical artery and accompanying vein.

Levator Scapulae

Origin

From transverse processes of upper four cervical vertebrae

Insertion

Into medial margin of scapula opposite the supraspinous fossa

Rhomboideus Minor

Origin

From lower part of ligamentum nuchae and spines of seventh cervical and the first thoracic vertebrae

Insertion

Into medial margin of scapula opposite the root of the spine

Rhomboideus Major

Origin

From spines of second to fifth thoracic vertebrae and intervening supraspinous ligaments

Insertion

Into medial margin of scapula opposite the infraspinous fossa

Nerve Supply

Above three muscles receive branches from dorsal scapular nerve (C5). Levator scapulae muscle also receives twigs from C3 and C4 ventral rami in the posterior triangle of neck.

Actions

• The levator scapulae and rhomboid muscles stabilize the scapula during shoulder movements and transmit the body weight to the vertebral column, especially during lifting heavy weight.
• The levator scapulae muscle along with upper fibers of trapezius elevates the scapula.
• The rhomboid muscles along with middle fibers of trapezius retract the scapula.
• All the three muscles help in reverse or medial rotation of scapula.

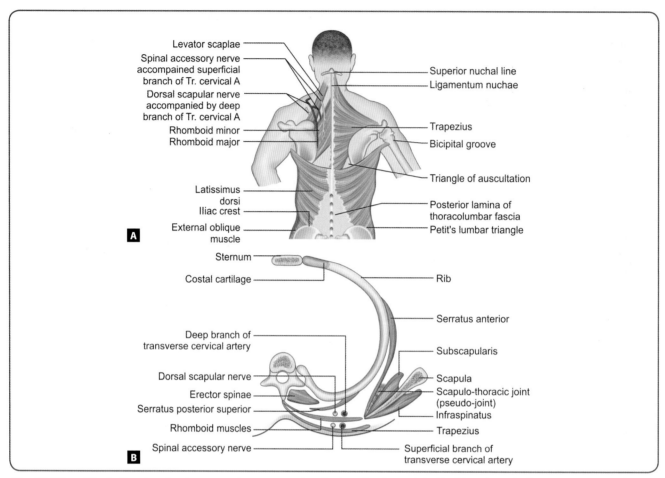

Figs 14.2A and B: A. Showing structures seen deep to trapezius after its reflection on left side (Note that spinal accessory nerve is deep to trapezius and dorsal scapular nerve is deep to rhomboids); **B.** Schematic diagram of the transverse section of the back showing arrangement of muscles, nerves and vessels from superficial to deep

Dorsal Scapular Nerve (Nerve to Rhomboideus)

This nerve takes origin from the C5 nerve root (first stage of brachial plexus) in the neck. It is a purely motor nerve. In its cervical course, the nerve passes through the scalenus medius muscle and comes to lie on the anterior aspect of the levator scapulae muscle in the posterior triangle. Here the deep branch of the transverse cervical artery (or the dorsal scapular artery) joins it. The neurovascular bundle thus formed descends in the back along the anterior surface of the levator scapulae muscle and the rhomboids. It supplies levator scapulae, rhomboid major and minor muscles.

🦴 STUDENT INTEREST

The dorsal scapular nerve or nerve to rhomboids takes origin from C5 root of brachial plexus in the neck. It travels all the way down on the anterior surface of levator scapulae, rhomboid minor and rhomboid major (muscles inserted into vertebral border of scapula) in company with dorsal scapular artery. It supplies the same three muscles.

Latissimus Dorsi (Figs 14.1 and 14.2A)

This is a large and flat muscle and is the only muscle that connects the pelvic girdle and the vertebral column to the upper limb. This muscle is part of the posterior axillary fold.

Origin

The latissimus dorsi has a wide origin from the following:
- Lower six thoracic spines and the intervening supraspinous ligaments.
- Spines of lumbar and sacral vertebrae (through the posterior lamina of thoracolumbar fascia).
- Outer lip of the posterior part of iliac crest.
- Lower three or four ribs.
- A few slips from the inferior angle of scapula.

Insertion

The muscle winds round the teres major muscle in the posterior wall of axilla, where it gives rise to a narrow flat tendon. The tendon of latissimus dorsi is inserted into the floor of the intertubercular sulcus (bicipital groove) of humerus.

Nerve Supply

The latissimus dorsi is supplied by thoracodorsal nerve, which accompanies the thoracodorsal artery (continuation of subscapular artery beyond the origin of circumflex scapular artery) to enter the muscle at the neurovascular hilum. This is of importance in reconstructive surgery.

Actions

- The latissimus dorsi brings about adduction and medial rotation of the arm.
- It brings about extension of arm along with teres major and posterior fibers of deltoid.
- It elevates the trunk as in climbing (Fig 14.3) by extending the flexed arms to the side against resistance. This action is performed along with pectoralis major muscle.
- Latissimus dorsi is active in coughing and sneezing, which are the expiratory processes.

Note: Latissimus dorsi is called 'swimmer's muscle' as it is used in back-stroke swimming. It is active in persons who use crutches

Testing Function of Latissimus Dorsi

When the subject is asked to adduct the arm abducted to 90^0 against resistance, the muscle can be felt in the posterior axillary fold. An alternative method is to ask the subject to cough and then feel the contraction of latissimus dorsi.

Triangles Related to Latissimus Dorsi (Figs 14.1 and 14.2A)

- **The triangle of auscultation** is located near the inferior angle of scapula. It is bounded inferiorly by the upper transverse margin of latissimus dorsi, medially by lateral margin of trapezius and laterally by medial

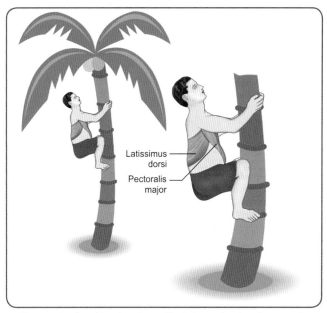

Fig. 14.3: Combined actions of latissimus dorsi and pectoralis major muscles in climbing on a tree

margin of scapula. The sixth and seventh ribs and the sixth intercostal space are in the floor of the triangle. The apical segment of the lower lobe of the lung is auscultated here after the patient folds the arms in front of the chest and flexes the trunk in order to expand the triangle.
- **The triangle of Petit or lumbar triangle** is located near the lower part of latissimus dorsi. It is bounded inferiorly by the iliac crest, laterally (anteriorly) by the free posterior margin of external oblique muscle and medially (posteriorly) by the lateral margin of latissimus dorsi muscle. The internal oblique muscle is in its floor. A rare hernia occurring through this triangle is called **lumbar hernia**.

MUSCLES OF SCAPULAR REGION

Deltoid (Fig. 14.4)

The deltoid muscle is triangular in shape. It surrounds the shoulder joint on all sides except inferomedially and is responsible for the rounded contour of the shoulder.

Origin

The deltoid muscle has V-shaped origin.
- **Anterior fibers:** from anterior margin of lateral third of clavicle.
- **Middle or acromial fibers:** from lateral margin of acromion. Only the acromial fibers are multipennate.
- **Posterior fibers:** from lower lip of the crest of scapular spine.

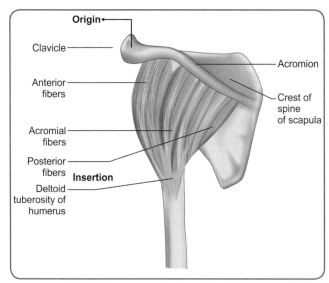

Fig. 14.4: Showing origin and insertion of deltoid muscle

Insertion

Into a V-shaped deltoid tuberosity on the lateral surface of humeral shaft.

Nerve Supply

Axillary nerve (C5, C6).

Actions

- **Anterior fibers:** Flexion and medial rotation of arm
- **Acromial (middle) fibers:** Abduction of arm from 15° to 90°.
- **Posterior fibers:** Extension and lateral rotation of arm.

Testing Function of Deltoid

The subject is asked to hold the arm in abducted position against resistance. Contracted deltoid muscle can be seen and felt.

 CLINICAL CORRELATION

Effects of Paralysis
- Loss of rounded contour of shoulder due to wasting of deltoid.
- Loss of ability to abduct the arm beyond 15–20°.

Intramuscular Injection
Deltoid is used for this purpose. The site of injection is the lower half of deltoid.

Structures under Cover of Deltoid

The structures are shoulder joint, subacromial bursa, axillary nerve, anterior and posterior circumflex humeral vessels, insertion of supraspinatus, infraspinatus and teres minor on greater tubercle, insertion of subscapularis on lesser tubercle, the rotator cuff, intertubercular sulcus and the insertion of muscles into it, coracoid process and structures attached to it, triangular and quadrangular intermuscular spaces, supraglenoid and infraglenoid tubercles.

Supraspinatus

Origin

From supraspinous fossa of scapula

Insertion

In to upper facet of greater tubercle of humerus

Nerve supply

Suprascapular nerve

Action

To initiate the abduction of the shoulder joint

Testing Function of Supraspinatus

The subject is asked to initiate abduction of the arm from the side, against resistance.

Special Features of Supraspinatus

- It is fused with the tendons of infraspinatus, teres minor and subscapularis muscles (SITS muscles) to form **rotator cuff** around the shoulder joint.
- The supraspinatus tendon is separated from the coracoacromial arch by the **subacromial bursa**. At the end of abduction, the greater tuberosity of humerus and the attached supraspinatus tendon (along with subacromial bursa) slide under the acromion.

 CLINICAL CORRELATION

- The tendon of **supraspinatus** shows degenerative changes from the age of forty and above. Hence, rupture, inflammation and calcium deposits in the tendon are very common. Supraspinatus tendonitis (with or without subacromial bursitis), calcification and rupture are some of the causes of supraspinatus syndrome. This presents with

Contd…

Contd...

 CLINICAL CORRELATION

> painful arc of abduction, which is characterized by painless abduction up to 60°, painful abduction from 60° to 120° and painless beyond this. The mid-abduction pain is due to impingement of inflamed and thickened tendon against the lateral edge of acromion.
> - Patients with **ruptured supraspinatus tendon or paralyzed supraspinatus** are not able to initiate abduction. But soon the patient learns to overcome this deficiency by tilting the shoulder of affected side away from the body to cover initial abduction, after which deltoid takes over.

Infraspinatus

Origin

From infraspinous fossa of scapula

Insertion

Into the middle facet on the greater tubercle of humerus

Nerve Supply

Suprascapular nerve

Action

Lateral rotator of arm.

Testing Function of Infraspinatus

The subject keeps the flexed elbow by the side of the trunk. Then the forearm is turned backwards against resistance (this is to test the lateral rotation of arm).

Teres Minor

Origin

From upper two-thirds of dorsal surface lateral margin of scapula by two sets of fibers. The circumflex scapular artery enters the infraspinous fossa through the two sets of fibers (Fig. 14.5).

Insertion

Into the lower facet on the greater tubercle of humerus.

Nerve Supply

Axillary nerve supplies via a branch that has pseudoganglion on it.

Action

Lateral rotator of arm.

Subscapularis

The subscapularis (Fig. 17.3) is a bulky multipennate muscle that fills the subscapular fossa. It forms the posterior wall of axilla.

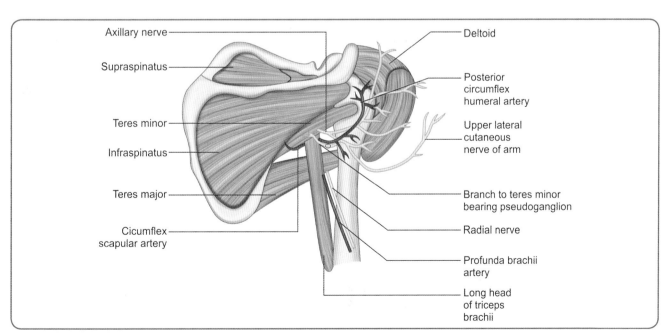

Fig. 14.5: Boundaries and contents of quadrangular and triangular intermuscular spaces

Origin

From medial two-thirds of subscapular fossa (anterior or costal surface of scapula)

Insertion

Into lesser tubercle of humerus by a wide tendon that lies immediately anterior to the capsule of shoulder joint. A subscapular bursa is in communication with the cavity of the shoulder joint.

Nerve Supply

By upper and lower subscapular nerves.

Actions

- Along with supraspinatus, infraspinatus and teres minor muscles, the subscapularis forms the rotator cuff around the shoulder joint to reinforce the capsule.
- The subscapularis is a medial rotator of the arm (when it is at the side of body).

Teres Major

Origin

From dorsal surface of lateral margin of scapula below teres minor.

Insertion

Into medial lip of intertubercular sulcus of humerus, just below the insertion of subscapularis muscle.

Nerve supply

Lower subscapular nerve

Actions

Adduction, medial rotation and extension of the arm

 STUDENT INTEREST

Note that teres minor is lateral rotator of arm and teres major is adductor, medial rotator and extensor of arm. Teres minor is supplied by axillary nerve and teres major by lower subscapular nerve. Also note that supraspinatus initiates abduction of arm and infraspinatus is lateral rotator of arm. Both supraspinatus and infraspinatus are supplied by suprascapular nerve.

INTERMUSCULAR SPACES (FIG. 14.5)

Three intermuscular spaces (one quadrangular and two triangular) are located under cover of the deltoid muscle in the shoulder region.

Qudrangular Space

Boundaries of quadrangular space (From anterior aspect)

- Superiorly by subscapularis
- Inferiorly by teres major
- Laterally by surgical neck of humerus
- Medially by long head of triceps brachii.

Boundaries of quadrangular space (From posterior aspect)

- Superiorly by teres minor
- Inferiorly by teres major
- Laterally by surgical neck of humerus
- Medially by long head of triceps brachii.

Contents of quadrangular space

- Axillary nerve
- Posterior circumflex humeral vessels
- Sagging part of capsule of shoulder joint.

Upper Triangular Space

Boundaries of upper triangular space

- Superiorly by inferior margin of teres minor
- Inferiorly by superior margin of teres major
- Apex (on lateral margin of scapula) by a point where teres major and minor meet
- Base by long head of triceps brachii.

Contents

The circumflex scapular artery, a branch of subscapular artery, winds round the lateral margin of scapula (Fig. 14.5).

Lower Triangular Space

Boundaries of lower triangular space

- Superiorly by inferior margin of teres major muscle
- Medially by the long head of triceps
- Laterally by shaft of the humerus.

Contents

The radial nerve and profunda brachii vessels pass through this space to reach the spiral groove.

AXILLARY NERVE

The axillary nerve (C5, C6) is also known as *circumflex nerve*. It is a mixed nerve containing both sensory and motor fibers. It is a branch of the posterior cord of brachial plexus.

Relations in axilla

The axillary nerve is located posterior to the axillary artery and anterior to the subscapularis muscle. The radial nerve lies on its medial side. On reaching the lower border of subscapularis, the nerve passes backwards into the quadrangular space along with posterior circumflex humeral vessels.

Relations in quadrangular space

The axillary nerve is related to the boundaries of the quadrangular space as follows:
Above: Teres minor (posteriorly) and subscapularis (anteriorly)
Below: Teres major
Medially: Long head of triceps brachii
Laterally: Surgical neck of humerus laterally
It is closely related to the inferomedial part of the fibrous capsule of the shoulder joint.

Distribution (Fig. 14.6)

- The trunk of axillary nerve gives off an articular twig to the shoulder joint and divides into anterior and posterior branches.
- The ***anterior branch of axillary nerve*** and the posterior circumflex humeral vessels wind round the posterior aspect of surgical neck of humerus to reach the anterior margin of the deltoid muscle. Along its course, the anterior branch gives motor branches to deltoid and a few cutaneous branches through the deltoid to the skin over the lower part of the deltoid.
- The ***posterior branch of axillary nerve*** gives a twig to teres minor, which bears a connective tissue swelling

called ***pseudoganglion***. After supplying the posterior part of deltoid, the posterior branch continues as the upper lateral cutaneous nerve of the arm, which supplies a patch of skin over the insertion of the deltoid extending up to its lower half.

Since the axillary nerve gives articular branch to the shoulder joint, supplies the muscles, which act on the joint and supplies the skin in the vicinity of the joint, it is said to obey Hilton's law.

✀ CLINICAL CORRELATION

Lesion of Axillary Nerve

The axillary nerve is liable to injury in fracture of the surgical neck of humerus or in anterior dislocation of humeral head.

Motor Loss

The weakness of deltoid causes inability to abduct the arm. The wasting of deltoid causes loss of rounded contour of the shoulder. The paralysis of teres minor results in weak lateral rotation of arm.

Sensory Loss (Fig 14.7)

There is sensory loss on outer aspect of lower half of deltoid, which is known as ***regimental badge anesthesia*** (Fig 14.7).
Note: A patient with dislocation of shoulder joint, experiences pain on movements of the joint. In order to test the integrity of the axillary nerve in a patient with dislocated shoulder, abduction cannot be tested. Therefore, sensory loss on the lower half of deltoid is the sign to observe.

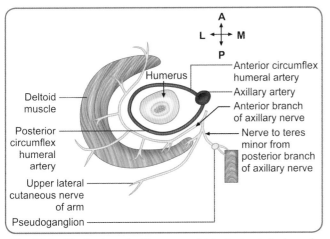

Fig. 14.6: Distribution of axillary nerve (Note that anterior branch of axillary nerve is accompanied by posterior circumflex humeral artery)

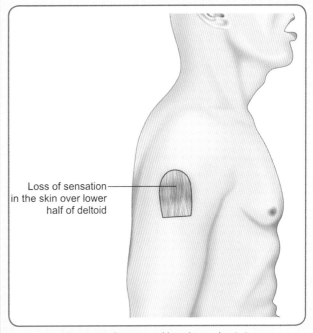

Fig. 14.7: Regimental band anesthesia in injury to axillary nerve

Axillary nerve (C5, C6) arises from posterior cord of brachial plexus in the axilla. Its course through quadrangular intermuscular space is very important. Here it is related to the dependent part of capsule of shoulder joint, hence liable to injury in dislocation of humeral head. Injury to axillary nerve results in loss of abduction from 20° to 90° due to paralysis of deltoid and regimental badge anesthesia (Fig. 14.7).

SUPRASCAPULAR NERVE

This nerve arises from the upper trunk of the brachial plexus in the posterior triangle of the neck. Its root value is C5, C6.

Cervical Course

The suprascapular nerve runs downwards and laterally posterior and parallel to inferior belly of omohyoid muscle. It leaves the posterior triangle by passing deep to the trapezius. The suprascapular artery, a branch of thyrocervical trunk from the first part of subclavian artery, accompanies the nerve to the scapular region.

Course in Scapular Region (Fig. 14.8)

The suprascapular nerve and vessels reach suprascapular notch of the superior margin of scapula. The suprascapular nerve enters the supraspinous fossa by passing through the foramen formed by the suprascapular notch and the transverse scapular ligament. However, the suprascapular artery passes over the ligament. After supplying the supraspinatus the nerve passes through the spinoglenoid notch to enter the infraspinous fossa. The spinoglenoid ligament (inferior transverse scapular ligament) bridges the spinoglenoid notch creating a tunnel for the nerve and the artery.

Distribution

- Just proximal to suprascapular notch articular branches are given off to the acromioclavicular joint
- Muscular branches to supraspinatus arise in supraspinous fossa
- Articular branches for shoulder joint arise in spinoglenoid notch
- The suprascapular nerve terminates in a few motor branches in the infraspinous fossa for the supply of infraspinatus muscle.

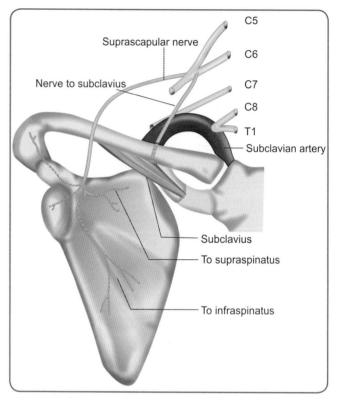

Fig. 14.8: Scheme to show the course of the suprascapular nerve and the nerve to the subclavius

- If the suprascapular nerve is injured proximal to the spinoglenoid notch both supraspinatus and infraspinatus muscles are paralyzed with resultant loss of initiation of abduction at the shoulder joint and weakness of lateral rotation of arm respectively.
- *Suprascapular nerve entrapment* occurs usually due to repetitive overuse of arm in overhead abduction as in the case of baseball, volleyball and tennis players besides weight-lifters and newsreel cameramen. The suprascapular nerve is liable for entrapment at suprascapular notch and at spinoglenoid notch. If compressed at suprascapular notch, both supraspinatus and infraspinatus are weakened. If compressed at spinoglenoid notch, only infraspinatus is affected (described as infraspinatus syndrome). The signs of infraspinatus syndrome are atrophy of infraspinatus muscle and difficulty in lateral rotation of arm. The symptom is dull aching pain in shoulder. The infraspinatus syndrome is so common in volleyball players that it is called 'volleyball shoulder'.

15

Pectoral Girdle and Shoulder Joint

Chapter Contents

PECTORAL GIRDLE

The pectoral or shoulder girdle consists of two bones—(1) clavicle; and (2) scapula. The clavicle articulates with the axial skeleton by the sternoclavicular joint, which is the only link between the upper limb and the trunk. It articulates with the scapula at the acromio-clavicular joint. The pectoral girdle is suspended from the cranium and cervical vertebrae by the trapezius muscle.

SPECIAL FEATURES

The subscapularis and serratus anterior muscles occupy the interval between the costal surface of scapula and the thoracic wall. There is a loose packing of areolar tissue between serratus anterior and thoracic wall as well as between the serratus anterior and subscapularis. This unit between the scapula and thoracic wall can be conceptualized as a scapulo-thoracic joint (Fig. 14.2B). In fact this pseudo-joint confers high mobility to the scapula, which is responsible for the high mobility of the shoulder joint.

GIRDLE JOINTS (FIG. 15.1)

There are two joints in the pectoral girdle—(1) sternoclavicular; and (2) acromioclavicular joints, where movements of scapula take place.

Sternoclavicular Joint

This is a saddle type of synovial joint. The articular disc completely divides the joint cavity (Fig. 15.1).

Articulating Ends

The sternal end of the clavicle and the clavicular notch on the manubrium sterni and the first costal cartilage are the articulating ends.

Ligaments

- The anterior and posterior ***sternoclavicular ligaments*** reinforce the fibrous capsule.
- The ***interclavicular ligament*** passing through the suprasternal space connects the medial ends of the two clavicles.
- The ***costoclavicular ligament*** is a powerful ligament that passes from first costochondral junction to the inferior surface of medial end of clavicle. It acts as a fulcrum during the movements of the scapula and prevents dislocation of the joint.

Posterior Relations

The joint is posteriorly related to brachiocephalic veins and trachea on both sides and the brachiocephalic artery (on the right side). These structures are in danger of injury if the joint is dislocated posteriorly.

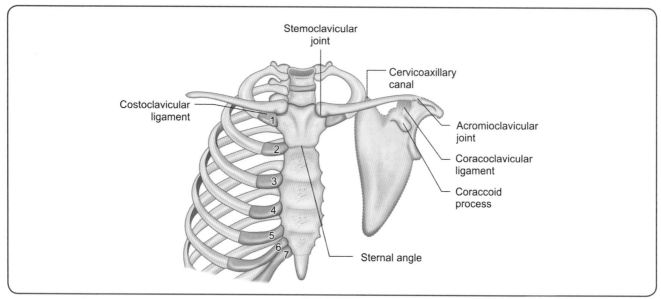

Fig. 15.1: Osseocartilaginous skeleton of thorax showing girdle joints (sternoclavicular and acromioclavicular)

Acromioclavicular Joint

This is a plane synovial joint. The joint is divided by incomplete articular disc projecting inside from the upper part of the capsule (Fig. 15.1).

Articulating Ends

The acromial end of the clavicle and the medial border of the acromion are the articulating ends.

Ligaments

- The *fibrous capsule* covers the joint and is strengthened superiorly by the acromioclavicular ligament.
- The *coracoclavicular ligament* is the main bond between clavicle and scapula. It is a very powerful ligament as it transmits the weight of the upper limb to the medial two-third of the clavicle. Its two parts are conoid and trapezoid. The *conoid part* is attached above to conoid tubercle of clavicle and below to the root of coracoid process. The *trapezoid part* is attached above to the trapezoid line of clavicle and below to the upper surface of coracoid process.

> ### ⊘ CLINICAL CORRELATION
>
> The acromioclavicular joint is prone to dislocation or shoulder separation, in which the fibrous capsule and the coracoclavicular ligament are torn. The scapula falls away from the clavicle and weight transmission to the axial skeleton becomes impossible.

Movements of Scapula (Figs 15.2A to F)

The girdle joints allow free sliding of the scapula on the thoracic wall.

- *Elevation and depression of scapula* take place around an anteroposterior axis passing through costoclavicular ligament (Figs 15.2A and B).
- *Protraction and retraction of scapula* take place around a vertical axis passing through costoclavicular ligament (Figs 15.2 C and D).
- *Lateral or forward* and *medial or return rotation of scapula* take place around an axis passing through acromioclavicular joint (Figs 15.2 E and F).

Elevation and Depression

When the lateral end of the clavicle is elevated, the scapula is also elevated along with it and the medial end of the clavicle is depressed. When the lateral end of the clavicle is depressed, the scapula is also depressed.

- *Muscles producing elevation:* The elevation of scapula (shrugging movement) is caused by contraction of the upper fibers of trapezius and the levator scapulae (Fig. 15.2A).
- *Muscles producing depression:* The depression of the scapula is produced by contraction of pectoralis minor along with lower fibers of trapezius (Fig. 15.2B).

Protraction and Retraction

During the protraction and retraction the lateral end of clavicle moves forwards or backwards respectively, along

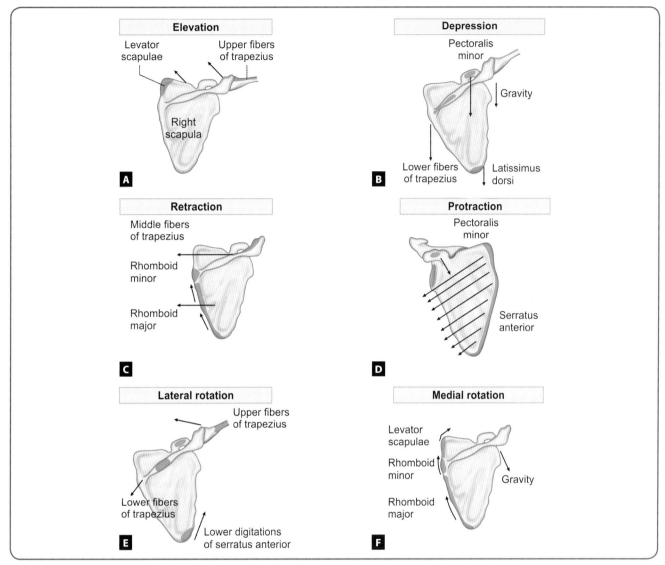

Figs 15.2A to F: Movements of scapula at girdle joints

with the scapula. Protraction is the movement used in punching, pushing and reaching forwards.
- **Muscles producing protraction:** Protraction of scapula is produced due to combined action of serratus anterior and pectoralis minor muscles (Fig. 15.2C).
- **Muscles producing retraction:** Retraction of scapula is produced due to combined action of middle fibers of trapezius and rhomboids (Fig. 15.2D).

Rotation of Scapula

The scapula shows forward or lateral rotation and medial or return rotation (Figs 15.2E and F). In lateral rotation, as the clavicle rotates upwards along its longitudinal axis, the scapula also rotates so that its acromion is lifted upwards and medially and the inferior angle is turned forwards and laterally. The net effect is on the glenoid cavity, which faces upwards. The forward or lateral rotation of the scapula is an integral part of abduction of shoulder joint above 90°.
- **Muscles producing forward rotation:** Forward rotation of scapula is produced by the lower five digitations of the serratus anterior along with upper and lower fibers of trapezius.
- **Muscles producing return rotation:** The medial or return rotation of scapula is due to the action of the muscles attached to the medial border of scapula assisted by gravity.

SHOULDER JOINT

The shoulder joint or the glenohumeral joint is a multiaxial synovial joint of ball and socket type, between the head of humerus and the glenoid cavity of scapula. The arm can be moved freely in all directions at the shoulder joint.

Articular Surfaces (Fig. 15.3)

The large hemispherical head of the humerus articulates with the smaller and shallower glenoid cavity of scapula. Both articular surfaces are covered with articular cartilage. The scapular articular surface is slightly deepened by glenoid labrum, which is a fibrocartilaginous rim attached to the margins of the glenoid cavity. Due to marked disproportion in the sizes of the two articular surfaces only a small part of the head of the humerus comes in contact with the glenoid cavity in any one position of the joint.

Fibrous Capsule (Fig. 15.3)

The fibrous capsule envelops the joint on all sides. The capsule is very lax.

- **Laterally**, the capsule is attached to the anatomical neck of the humerus except inferomedially, where the capsular attachment shifts one cm or more on the humeral shaft. This is the dependent part of the capsule.
- **Medially**, the capsule is attached to the margin of glenoid cavity outside the glenoid labrum. Since the capsule is attached to the root of the coracoid process the supraglenoid tubercle of the scapula becomes intracapsular.

- **Superiorly**, the capsule is deficient (between the tubercles of the upper end) for the passage of long head of the biceps brachii along with its synovial sheath.

The incongruity of the articulating surfaces of the shoulder joint and the laxity of its capsule confer great mobility to it but at the expense of stability. Therefore, the capsule is reinforced with the help of ligaments and tendons of the rotator cuff muscles.

Glenohumeral Ligaments (Fig. 15.4)

The superior, middle and inferior glenohumeral ligaments are the localized thickenings of the anterior aspect of the capsule.

💡 **ADDED INFORMATION**

- The **superior glenohumeral ligament** passes from the base of the coracoid process and adjacent glenoid labrum to the upper part of the anatomical neck.
- The **middle glenohumeral ligament** extends from the anterior margin of the glenoid cavity to the lesser tubercle deep to the insertion of subscapularis.
- The **inferior glenohumeral ligament** extends from the anterior and posterior margins of the glenoid cavity to the inferomedial part of the anatomical neck. In traumatic anterior dislocation, the inferior glenohumeral ligament is stretched or its attachment to glenoid labrum is torn. This is known as **Bankart lesion**, which predisposes to recurrent dislocation of shoulder joint.

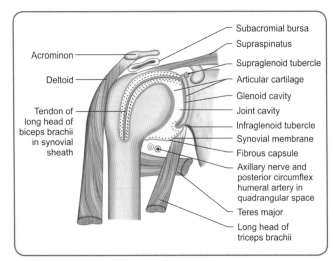

Fig. 15.3: Coronal section of shoulder joint to depict fibrous capsule and synovial membrane

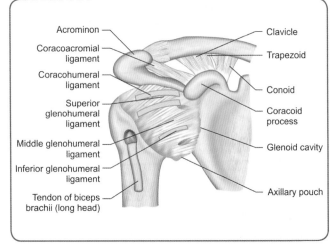

Fig. 15. 4: Glenohumeral ligaments of shoulder joint seen from the anterior aspect

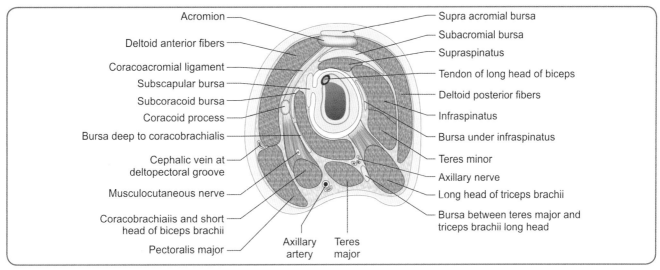

Acromion
Deltoid anterior fibers
Coracoacromial ligament
Subscapular bursa
Subcoracoid bursa
Coracoid process
Bursa deep to coracobrachialis
Cephalic vein at deltopectoral groove
Musculocutaneous nerve
Coracobrachiaiis and short head of biceps brachii
Pectoralis major

Supra acromial bursa
Subacromial bursa
Supraspinatus
Tendon of long head of biceps
Deltoid posterior fibers
Infraspinatus
Bursa under infraspinatus
Teres minor
Axillary nerve
Long head of triceps brachii
Bursa between teres major and triceps brachii long head

Axillary artery   Teres major

Fig. 15.5: Sagittal section of shoulder joint showing related muscles and bursae

Coracohumeral Ligament

The coracohumeral ligament extends from the base of coracoid process to the upper surface of greater tubercle of humerus. A few tendinous fibres from the insertion of pectoralis minor may become continuous with coracohumeral ligament.

Transverse Humeral Ligament

The transverse humeral ligament bridges the gap between the greater and lesser tubercles, thus converting the intertubercular sulcus into a canal for the passage of the tendon of long head of the biceps brachii.

Synovial Membrane

The synovial membrane lines the fibrous capsule internally and covers intracapsular part of the anatomical neck of humerus. The intracapsular part of the long tendon of biceps brachii is enveloped in a tubular synovial sheath, which is carried outside the joint through the intertubercular sulcus up to the level of the surgical neck of humerus. The synovial sheath also protrudes through an opening in the anterior part of the capsule to communicate with the subscapular bursa.

Bursae Around Shoulder Joint (Fig 15.5)

- *Subscapular bursa* is the only communicating bursa, which is always present. Its opening in the joint is located between middle and superior glenohumeral ligaments.

- *Infraspinatus bursa* may occasionally open into the joint.
- *Subacromial (subdeltoid) bursa* is located between the supraspinatus tendon below and the coracoacromial arch and deltoid muscle above. It is a non-communicating bursa. It is the largest bursa in the body. This bursa acts as a secondary socket for humeral head during hyper-abduction when the bursa shifts its position under the acromion.
- *Supraacromial bursa* lies above the acromion.
- *Subcoracoid bursa* is below the coracoid process.
- A bursa may be present deep to coracobrachialis tendon.

Relations of Shoulder Joint (Fig 15.5)

The muscles wrap the shoulder joint snugly on almost all sides. Both communicating and non-communicating bursae are located close to the joint. These bursae are necessary to facilitate frictionless movements of various musculoskeletal structures around the joint.

- The massive deltoid muscle covers the joint anteriorly, superiorly, posteriorly and laterally.
- *Superiorly*, the coracoacromial arch covers the joint. The subacromial bursa lies below the arch and the adjoining deltoid muscle. It separates the coracoacromial arch from the underlying supraspinatus tendon.
- *Posteriorly*, the joint is related to the infraspinatus and teres minor muscles.
- Immediately *anterior* to the joint there is the subscapularis tendon. The coracoid process and the origin of conjoint tendon of coracobrachialis and

short head of biceps brachii are located in front of the subscapularis.

- **Inferiorly**, the capsule is closely related to the axillary nerve and posterior circumflex humeral vessels in the quadrangular space. The long head of triceps offers the only support for the capsule inferiorly. Hence, the head of humerus is more prone to subglenoid and subcoracoid dislocation.

Stability of Shoulder Joint

- **The musculotendinous rotator cuff** provides dynamic stability as its component muscles undergo tonic contractions. The rotator cuff is composed of the tendons of supraspinatus above, infraspinatus and teres minor behind and subscapularis in front. These muscles are known as **SITS muscles**. The cuff blends with the fibrous capsule. The inferomedial part of the capsule sags down in the quadrangular space, when the arm hangs by the side. This part is the weakest and is maximally stretched during abduction. Rotator cuff syndrome is due to the complete or partial rupture of one or more tendons (usually supraspinatus) of the rotator cuff.
- The **coracoacromial arch** provides a secondary socket for the joint superiorly. The arch is composed of the tip of the acromion, coracoacromial ligament and the lateral surface of coracoid process. The subacromial bursa intervenes between the arch and the tendon of supraspinatus. The movements of the upper end of humerus in abduction of the arm are smoothened by the presence of this bursa. The coracoacromial arch prevents the upward dislocation of shoulder joint during abduction.

Blood Supply

The articular branches of anterior and posterior circumflex humeral, suprascapular and circumflex scapular arteries supply the joint.

Nerve Supply

The articular branches of suprascapular, axillary and lateral pectoral nerves supply the joint.

Movements

The shoulder joint is multiaxial hence movements take place along three mutually perpendicular mechanical axes (Table 15.1).

TABLE 15.1: Muscles Producing Movements of Shoulder Joint

Movement	Muscles responsible for movement
Flexion	Clavicular head of pectoralis major, anterior fibers of deltoid and coracobrachialis
Extension	Posterior fibers of deltoid, teres major and latissimus dorsi
Abduction	Supraspinatus and deltoid
Adduction	Pectoralis major, latissimus dorsi and teres major
Medial rotation	Pectoralis major, teres major, latissimus dorsi, subscapularis
Lateral rotation	Infraspinatus, teres minor and posterior fibers of deltoid

- In **flexion** the arm crosses the front of the chest.
- In **extension** the arm moves backwards and laterally.
- In **adduction** the arm is by the side of the body.
- In **abduction** the arm moves away from the side of the body in lateral and forward direction.
- Circumduction is a succession of flexion-extension and adduction-abduction in an order.
- The rotation of humerus is best seen in flexed elbow. In **medial rotation** the hand is carried medially whereas in **lateral rotation** the hand is carried laterally.

Stages in Movement of Abduction (Figs 15.6A to C)

In abduction movement, the arm is carried away from the trunk laterally till it comes in horizontal position at right angles to the trunk. The abduction is further continued to raise the arm to a vertical position above the head so that the arm moves a total of 180°.

- In the **first stage**, the arm is abducted from neutral position to 15–30° at shoulder joint by contraction of supraspinatus (Fig. 15.6A).
- In the **second stage**, further abduction to 90–120° occurs at the shoulder joint by contraction of acromial fibers of deltoid (Fig. 15.6B).
- The hyperabduction (overhead abduction) from 90–120 to 180° takes place at the sternoclavicular and acromioclavicular joints by the contraction of trapezius and serratus anterior muscles. The subacromial bursa facilitates abduction above 90°. The greater tuberosity of humerus slips below the bursa deep to the acromion (Fig. 15.6C).

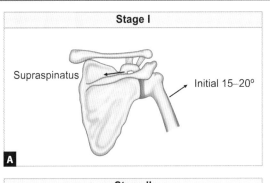

Stage I

Supraspinatus — Initial 15–20°

A

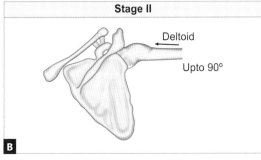

Stage II

Deltoid — Upto 90°

B

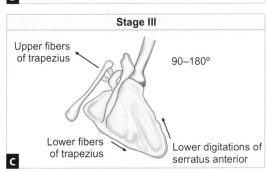

Stage III

Upper fibers of trapezius — 90–180°

Lower fibers of trapezius — Lower digitations of serratus anterior

C

Figs 15.6A to C: Movement of abduction of arm at shoulder joint and of hyperabduction at girdle joints

Contd…

⚭ CLINICAL CORRELATION

- The painful arc syndrome is also known as ***impingement syndrome***. The condition occurs usually in elderly, who complain for pain in the shoulder (aggravated on attempting certain activities like putting on a jacket). This condition is characterized by mid-abduction pain. The abduction movement up to 60° is painless. Further abduction up to 120° is acutely painful while beyond it is painless. The pain in midabduction is due to impingement of the swollen supraspinatus tendon or of inflamed subacromial bursa under the coracoacromial arch.
- The anterior or subglenoid dislocation of head of humerus is common in volleyball players, swimmers and badminton players. When the arm is forcefully abducted and laterally rotated the head is driven through the inferior weak part of capsule and dislocated anterior to the infraglenoid tubercle.

Contd…

Contd…

⚭ CLINICAL CORRELATION

This causes intense pain. The axillary nerve is in great danger of injury. The radiograph confirms the dislocation of the head (Fig. 15.7).

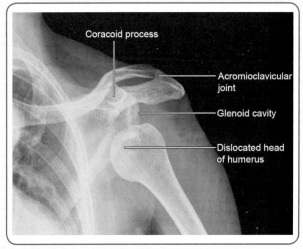

Coracoid process — Acromioclavicular joint — Glenoid cavity — Dislocated head of humerus

Fig. 15.7: Radiograph showing anterior dislocation of head of humerus

- Aspiration of fluid from the joint cavity is done by introducing the needle either anteriorly through the deltopectoral groove (lateral to the tip of coracoid process) or from lateral aspect between the acromion and greater tubercle of humerus.
- The steps in anterior or deltopectoral approach to the shoulder joint (Fig. 15.8) are easy to follow with the help of the diagram of the relations of the joint. The skin incision is placed along the anterior margin of the deltoid muscle to expose the deltopectoral groove, in which the cephalic vein is isolated. The pectoralis major and deltoid muscles are retracted from each other to expose the coracoid process and the conjoint tendon (pectoralis minor and short head of biceps brachii) attached to its tip. The conjoint tendon is divided about 2 cm below the coracoid process to expose the subscapularis tendon, which is cut to reach the capsule of the shoulder joint.

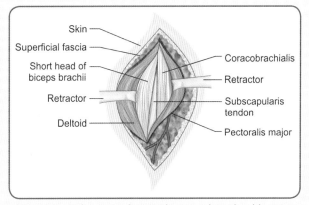

Skin — Superficial fascia — Short head of biceps brachii — Retractor — Deltoid — Coracobrachialis — Retractor — Subscapularis tendon — Pectoralis major

Fig. 15.8: Deltopectoral surgical approach to shoulder joint

16

Upper Limb (Cutaneous Nerves, Dermatomes, Superficial Veins, Lymph Vessels and Lymph Nodes)

Chapter Contents

INTRODUCTION

The upper limb is a segmented lever. It consists of upper arm (arm), elbow, forearm, wrist, hand and digits. It consists of groups of muscles, nerves and blood vessels enclosed within fascial compartments. The deep fascia and the intermuscular septa help in defining the boundaries of the fascial compartments. The superficial fascia contains the cutaneous nerves and the superficial veins.

CUTANEOUS NERVES

There are three sources from which cutaneous nerves originate:
1. **Supraclavicular nerves** (medial, intermediate and lateral) from the cervical plexus.
2. **Intercostobrachial nerve** (lateral cutaneous branch of the second intercostal nerve).
3. **Direct cutaneous nerves** from brachial plexus and cutaneous nerves from branches of brachial plexus.

Cutaneous Nerves of Arm

- The **lateral supraclavicular nerve** (C4) supplies the tip of shoulder and the skin overlying the upper part of the deltoid.
- The **intercostobrachial nerve** (T2) gives branches to the skin of the floor of axilla and the upper part of the medial side of arm.

- The **upper lateral cutaneous nerve of arm** (C5, C6), a branch of axillary nerve, supplies the skin overlying the lower half of deltoid.
- The **lower lateral cutaneous nerve of arm** (C5, C6), a branch of radial nerve in spiral groove, supplies the skin on the lateral side of arm below the insertion of deltoid.
- The **posterior cutaneous nerve of arm** (C5), branch of radial nerve in the axilla, supplies the skin of the back of arm from the insertion of deltoid to the olecranon.
- The **medial cutaneous nerve of arm** (T1) is a branch of medial cord of brachial plexus. It pierces the deep fascia at the middle of the medial side of arm to supply the skin on the lower half of arm.

Cutaneous Nerves of Forearm

- The **posterior cutaneous nerve of forearm** (C6, C7, C8), a branch of the radial nerve in the spiral groove, supplies the skin of posterior aspect of forearm. It travels in the superficial fascia of the middle of the back of the forearm.
- The **lateral cutaneous nerve of forearm** (C5, C6) is the continuation of musculocutaneous nerve. It supplies the skin covering the anterolateral and posterolateral surfaces of the forearm (extending up to the ball of thumb).
- The **medial cutaneous nerve of forearm** (C8, T1) is a branch of medial cord of brachial plexus. It pierces

the deep fascia with the basilic vein at the level of insertion of coracobrachialis and supplies the skin of the anteromedial and posteromedial surfaces of the forearm.

Cutaneous Nerves of Hand

- The superficial branch of radial nerve (C6, C7, and C8) is one of the terminal branches of radial nerve. It supplies the lateral two-thirds of the dorsum of the hand and dorsal aspects of thumb and lateral 2 ½ fingers through five dorsal digital nerves (Fig. 21.1). There is considerable variation in the area of supply of the radial nerve on the dorsum of hand and digits.
- The palmar cutaneous and palmar digital branches of median nerve (C6, C7, C8) supply the skin of the palm and the palmar aspect of lateral 3 ½ fingers including the skin on the dorsal aspect of the terminal phalanges of the corresponding fingers.
- The dorsal and palmar cutaneous branches of ulnar nerve (C7, C8, and T1) supply the medial side of the hand and the medial one and half fingers on both aspects.

From the areas of the cutaneous supply of various nerves, it is evident that the radial nerve supplies the maximum area. However, it is observed that, the areas of sensory loss due to injury to the individual nerve do not coincide with the areas of their cutaneous supply. The reason for this discrepancy is that the cutaneous nerves supplying adjacent areas of skin overlap to a considerable extent. To cite an example, if the radial nerve is injured in the axilla or in the spiral groove, the area of sensory loss is confined to a small area on the dorsum of hand between the thumb and index finger (Fig. 22.9). If axillary nerve is injured the sensory loss is found on a small patch of skin on the lower half of deltoid (Fig. 14.7).

🏛 STUDENT INTEREST

Cutaneous or sensory innervation of hand is extremely important clinically hence, one has to learn it by drawing diagrams repeatedly.

DERMATOMES

A dermatome is an area of skin supplied by a single spinal segment through its dorsal root.

- In the **case of the trunk**, the dermatomes extend from the posterior to anterior median lines of the trunk. There is a marked overlap in adjacent dermatomes so that injury to a single spinal nerve produces very little sensory loss in the corresponding dermatome.

- In the **case of the upper limb**, the innervation is through the brachial plexus. So a limb dermatome can be defined as an area of skin supplied by the ventral ramus of a single spinal nerve through the branches of the plexuses. There is a marked overlap in the adjacent dermatomes because of the presence of fibers of more than one ventral ramus in branches of the brachial plexus. Thus, it can be inferred that the area of distribution of any one cutaneous nerve cannot be equated to any one dermatome.

Dermatomes of Upper Limb (Fig. 16.1)

The dermatomes of the upper limb can be understood better if we know the development of the limb. In the embryo, the upper limb bud carries within it the ventral rami from C5 to T1 segments of the spinal cord. Each limb bud has ventral and dorsal surfaces and preaxial (cranial) and postaxial (caudal) borders. The upper limb bud undergoes lateral rotation as a result of which the preaxial or cranial border becomes the lateral border and postaxial or caudal border becomes the medial border of the limb. Consequently the thumb becomes the preaxial digit and little finger the postaxial digit. The proximal two dermatomes (C5 and C6) are arranged in numerical sequence along the preaxial border up to the preaxial digit. Similarly distal two dermatomes (C8 and T1) are arranged along the postaxial border from the little finger upwards. The middle dermatome (C7) is present only in the hand and it includes the middle three digits. The C4 dermatome

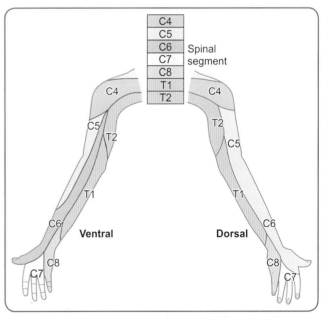

Fig. 16.1: Dermatomes of upper limb from ventral and dorsal aspects

TABLE 16.1: Dermatomes of upper limb

Spinal segment	Dermatomal area
C5	Lateral aspect of arm
C6	Lateral aspect of forearm & thumb
C7	Middle three fingers
C8	Little finger & medial side of hand
T1	Medial aspect of forearm & of lower part of arm
T2	Medial aspect of upper part of arm & floor of axilla

overlies the shoulder and T2 dermatome covers the base of axilla. Thus the dermatomes are arranged in such a way that the discontinuous dermatomes come side by side on the surfaces of the limbs along the ventral and dorsal axial lines (Table 16.1).

CLINICAL CORRELATION

Damage to the cutaneous nerves results in sensory loss in the skin (inability to feel the exteroceptive sensations like touch, pain and temperature). A dermatomal sensory loss results if the dorsal roots of a spinal nerve are damaged. The neurological examination of the patient with nerve root lesion, for example, compression of C7 root (in acute disc lesion) is incomplete without a thorough examination of dermatomes and areas of cutaneous distribution of upper limb. This is very crucial in differentiating the disease of the nerve root from that of a peripheral nerve. Therefore, a clinician must have a working knowledge of the dermatomes of the body. In herpes zoster (shingles) infection, the virus affects the dorsal root ganglion. This typically gives rise to a crop of cutaneous blisters in the dermatome of that particular nerve.

VEINS OF UPPER LIMB

The upper limb has two sets of veins—(1) superficial or subcutaneous and (2) deep.

Superficial Veins (Fig. 16.2)

The *superficial veins* are located in the superficial fascia and being easily accessible, are often used for drawing blood sample or for giving intravenous injection.

There are two major superficial or subcutaneous veins in upper limb:
1. Cephalic vein
2. Basilic vein

These veins begin at the dorsal venous network (Fig. 16.3). Other named veins like median cubital vein and the median vein of the forearm are the tributaries of these major veins.

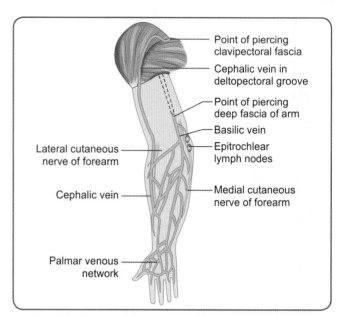

Fig. 16.2: Course of the main superficial veins of upper limb (cephalic vein on lateral side and basilic vein on medial side) Note the cutaneous nerves that are closely related to the main superficial veins

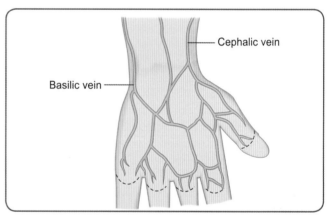

Fig. 16.3: Formation of cephalic and basilic veins from dorsal venous arch

Dorsal Venous Network

The dorsal venous network or arch is located in the superficial fascia on the dorsum of the hand. The dorsal digital veins draining the adjacent sides of the four fingers unite to form three dorsal metacarpal veins, which form the dorsal venous network (Fig. 16.3).

Cephalic Vein

Formation

The cephalic vein is formed by the union of dorsal digital vein from the radial side of the index finger and the veins from either side of the thumb with the lateral end of dorsal venous arch.

Extent

The cephalic vein extends from the lateral end of the dorsal venous network to its termination into the axillary vein in the axilla.

Course

- *In the wrist*, at lies in the roof of anatomical snuffbox, where it is posterior to the styloid process of radius.
- *In the forearm*, it ascends along the posterolateral side and then turns anteriorly to reach the lateral part of cubital fossa. In this location, the cephalic vein is closely related to lateral cutaneous nerve of forearm.
- *In the arm*, cephalic the vein ascends along the lateral side of biceps brachii. At the upper part of the arm (at the level of lower margin of pectoralis major muscle) the cephalic vein pierces the deep fascia and enters the deltopectoral groove, where it is related to the deltoid branch of the thoracoacromial artery and the deltopectoral lymph nodes.
- At the deltopectoral groove or triangle, the vein takes a sharp turn backwards to pierce the clavipectoral fascia and enters the axilla to terminate in to the axillary vein.

Tributaries

- A large number of tributaries, which collect blood from the hand, forearm and arm open into the cephalic vein.
- The median cubital vein is a large and named tributary. It passes in the superficial fascia of the cubital fossa, upwards and medially from the cephalic vein to the basilic vein (the blood flows from the cephalic to the basilic vein). This venous pattern in front of the elbow resembles the letter H. There may be an M pattern of veins, in which the median forearm vein bifurcates just distal to the cubital fossa, one limb passing to the basilic vein and the other to cephalic vein. The median cubital vein rests on the platform provided by the bicipital aponeurosis, which separates it from brachial artery and the median nerve. The deep median vein arising from the deep aspect of the median cubital vein pierces the bicipital aponeurosis and joins the veins accompanying the brachial artery.
- Occasionally, a small communicating vein, which crosses the clavicle superficially, may join the terminal part of the cephalic vein to the external jugular vein.

Basilic Vein

Formation

The basilic vein is formed by the union of dorsal digital vein of the ulnar side of the little finger with the medial end of the dorsal venous arch.

Extent

The basilic vein extends from the medial end of dorsal venous arch at the level of wrist to the lower margin of teres major muscle. It is shorter than cephalic vein.

Course in forearm

The basilic vein ascends on the medial side of posterior surface of the forearm. Just below the elbow, it moves to the anterior surface of the forearm and courses on the medial part of the front of elbow to enter the arm. The medial cutaneous nerve of the forearm is closely related to it in front of the elbow. The epitrochlear (supratrochlear) or superficial cubital lymph nodes lie by the side of basilic vein just above the elbow.

Course in arm

In the arm, the basilic vein runs along the medial margin of biceps brachii muscle and at the mid-arm level it pierces the deep fascia of the arm to enter the anterior compartment, where it lies medial to the brachial artery.

Termination

At the lower border of teres major, the basilic vein unites with the brachial veins (venae comitantes of the brachial artery) to form the axillary vein. However, in some cases, it is observed that basilic vein continues as axillary vein at the lower margin of teres major. In that case the brachial veins open into the axillary vein at the lower margin of subscapularis.

Tributaries

- The basilic vein collects blood from the medial aspect of hand, forearm and arm by numerous tributaries.
- The median cubital vein is its large tributary.
- It may receive median forearm vein in cases where the latter does not join the median cubital vein.

Median Vein of Forearm

This vein on the front of the forearm is also called *antebrachial vein*. It drains the superficial palmar plexus and travels in the superficial fascia of the front of forearm upward to open into the median cubital vein or the basilic vein.

CLINICAL CORRELATION

- For routine purposes like drawing blood sample for laboratory investigations or for giving intravenous medicines or saline or for blood transfusion, the preferred sites for venipuncture are the median cubital vein (Fig. 16.4) in front of the elbow, median vein of forearm and the cephalic vein behind styloid process of radius.
- The cephalic vein cut-down at deltopectoral groove is preferred, when superior vena caval infusion is necessary.
- The basilic vein is preferred for inserting a cardiac catheter to reach the right side of the heart. To enter the right atrium the catheter passes on succession through the basilic vein,

Contd...

Contd...

♪ **CLINICAL CORRELATION**

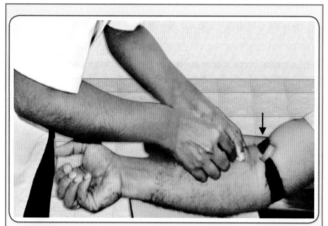

Fig. 16.4: Venipuncture of median cubital vein in the cubital fossa (arrow showing)

axillary vein, subclavian vein, brachiocephalic vein and finally the superior vena cava. The sharp curve at cephalo-axillary junction and presence of valves at this junction are the factors against preferring cephalic vein for this purpose.

- Patients with chronic renal failure are subjected to hemodialysis at regular intervals to remove accumulated waste products from the blood. For this purpose the superficial veins are arterialized by surgically creating arteriovenous fistula (A-V fistula). The cephalic vein is arterialized at the wrist by anastomosing the cephalic vein to the radial artery. The cephalic vein gradually shows distension and thickening as it is subjected to arterial pressure. This structural change in the cephalic vein is called its ***arterialization***. This enables repeated punctures in it with a wide bored needle. The arterial line of the dialysis machine is introduced into the cephalic vein, by which the impure blood is drawn in to the dialysis machine. The purified blood is returned back to the circulation by venous line inserted into the median cubital vein (Figs 16.5A and B). The basilic vein similarly is connected to ulnar artery (ulnobasilic fistula) to use the arterialized basilic vein for hemodialysis (Fig. 16.6).

🏆 **STUDENT INTEREST**

Superficial veins of upper limb are useful for venous access in clinical practice. Apart from their day to day use in blood banks and laboratories or in wards for intravenous injections or glucose infusion they are used in hemodialysis units for creating an arteriovenous fistula on regular basis in nephrology wards. Therefore, anatomical knowledge of the veins of upper limb is a must know.

Deep Veins

The ***deep veins*** are located deep to deep fascia and they accompany the arteries as venae comitantes.

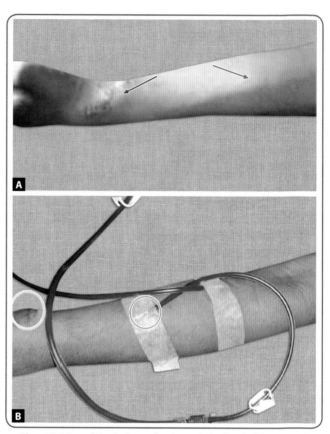

Figs 16.5A and B: A. Scar of radiocephalic fistula (blue arrow) and cephalic vein (red arrow); **B.** Patient of chronic renal failure with radiocephalic fistula (yellow circle) undergoing hemodialysis

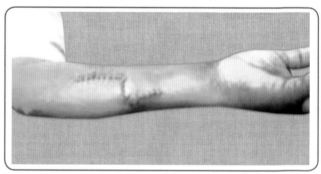

Fig. 16.6: Scar of ulnobasilic fistula (Note that ulnar artery is anastomozed with basilic vein to arterialize the latter)

LYMPHATIC DRAINAGE OF UPPER LIMB

The lymphatic vessels are disposed as two groups—(1) superficial and (2) deep.

Superficial Lymph Vessels (Fig. 16.7)

The superficial lymph vessels from the lateral side of the limb and lateral two digits follow the cephalic vein whereas those of the medial side of the limb and medial three digits follow the basilic vein. Some of the medial

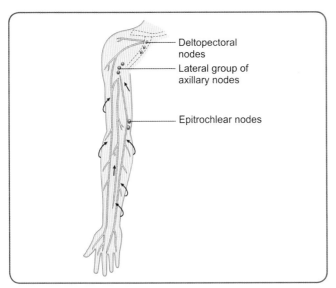

Fig. 16.7: Superficial lymph vessels and lymph nodes of upper limb

vessels terminate in the supratrochlear or epitrochlear lymph nodes, which are situated just above the medial epicondyle. These nodes are palpated in a patient, when enlarged (Fig. 16.8).

Termination of Superficial Lymphatics

- The lateral group of axillary nodes receive majority of the superficial lymphatics of the upper limb.
- A few lymphatics that travel along the cephalic vein (draining the thumb and lateral side of upper limb)

drain in to deltopectoral lymph nodes. The lymphatics from deltopectoral nodes pierce the clavipectoral fascia to terminate into the apical group. A few lymphatics that circumvent the deltopectoral nodes directly pierce the clavipectoral fascia to empty into apical nodes.

STUDENT INTEREST

Inflammation of lymph vessels is known as **lymphangitis**. In acute lymphangitis, superficial lymph vessels are seen through the skin as red and painful streaks.

The superficial lymphatic draining the thumb and lateral side of upper limb travel along the cephalic vein and pierce the clavipectoral fascia to terminate in to the apical lymph nodes. The major portion of superficial lymphatic and all deep lymphatics join the lateral or brachial group of axillary lymph nodes.

CLINICAL CORRELATION

- **Lymphadenopathy** is an enlargement of lymph nodes. The infections affecting the medial side of hand and forearm may cause painful enlargement of the supratrochlear lymph nodes at first. The lateral axillary nodes are enlarged and painful in infection of any part of the upper limb.
- Lymphaedema of upper limb is due to blockage to lymph flow from the upper limb. This gives rise to swelling of the upper limb. A commonly encountered cause is **postmastectomy edema** due to removal of axillary nodes (Fig. 16.9). Another common cause in tropical countries is obstruction of lymph vessels by filarial microorganisms (Wuchereria Bancrofti) causing elephantiasis.

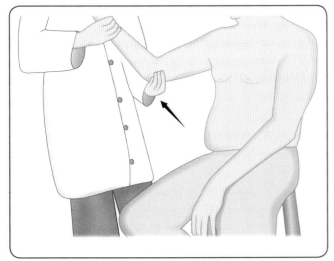

Fig. 16.8: Method of palpation of epitrochlear lymph nodes (arrow showing)

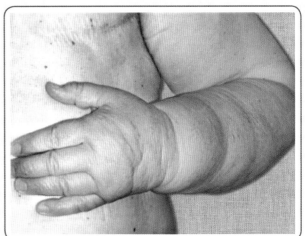

Fig. 16.9: Postmastectomy lymphaedema of left upper limb in a patient

Compartments of Arm

Chapter Contents

INTRODUCTION

The arm is the part of the free upper limb, which extends between the shoulder and the elbow. The deep fascia of the arm surrounds it on all sides like a sleeve. The lateral and medial intermuscular septa extend from the deep fascia to the humerus to divide the arm into anterior and posterior compartments (Fig. 17.1). The septa are attached to the margins of supracondylar ridges of the humerus. The ulnar nerve and superior ulnar collateral artery pierce

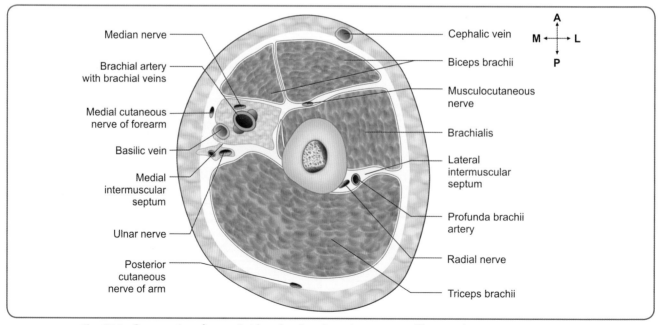

Fig. 17.1: Cross section of arm at (midarm level) to show the contents of flexor and extensor compartments

the medial intermuscular septum to enter the posterior compartment of arm. The radial nerve and radial collateral artery pierce the lateral intermuscular septum to enter anterior compartment of arm.

ANTERIOR COMPARTMENT

Contents

Muscles

The (1) coracobrachialis, (2) brachialis and (3) biceps brachii are the three main muscles. In addition, the brachioradialis and extensor carpi radialis longus take origin here.

Nerves

This is the nerve of the anterior compartment as it supplies the three main muscles mentioned above:
- The **median nerve** passes through the entire extent.
- The **ulnar nerve** travels in the upper half medially.
- The **radial nerve** travels in the lower half laterally.
- The **medial cutaneous nerves** of arm and of forearm travel in the compartment until they pierce the deep fascia of the arm.

Vessels

The **brachial artery** and the **brachial veins** (venae comitantes) are present throughout, whereas the basilic vein enters the compartment by piercing the deep fascia at the level of insertion of coracobrachialis.

Coracobrachialis (Fig. 17.2)

Origin

From the tip of coracoid process of scapula along with short head of biceps brachii.

Insertion

Into the middle of medial margin of humerus

Nerve Supply

By which pierces it.

Action

A weak flexor of the arm.

Biceps Brachii

This muscle being a strong supinator of forearm is described in chapter 20 along with muscles of supination.

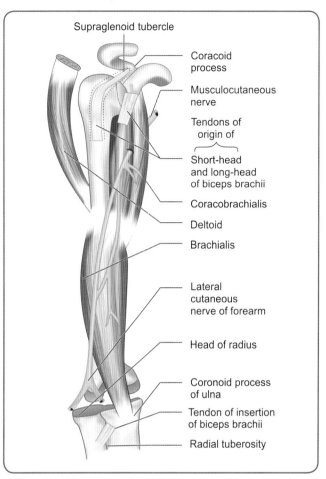

Fig. 17.2: The muscles of anterior compartment of arm and the musculocutaneous nerve

Brachialis

Origin

From lower half of the anteromedial and anterolateral surfaces of the humerus.

Insertion

On the anterior surface of the coronoid process of ulna.

Nerve Supply

Dual nerve supply by musculocutaneous and by proprioceptive fibers of radial nerve.

Action

Chief flexor of elbow joint. It flexes the elbow joint in any position of the forearm.

Testing Function of Brachialis

The subject is asked to flex the elbow against resistance in any position of the forearm.

Brachial Artery (Fig. 17.3)

The brachial artery begins at the level of lower border of teres major muscle as the continuation of axillary artery. It terminates at the level of the neck of radius in the cubital fossa by dividing into radial and ulnar arteries.

Variations

The brachial artery may show high division into two or three branches. It may be absent when an axillary artery itself divides into radial and ulnar arteries.

Relations in Arm

The brachial artery is accompanied by venae comitantes (also called **brachial veins**), which are connected by transverse channels.

- **Anteriorly**, the brachial artery is easily accessible because only the skin and fasciae cover it. At the level of mid- arm, the median nerve crosses anterior to the brachial artery from lateral to medial side (Fig. 17.4).
- **Posteriorly**, from above downwards, the brachial artery rests on the long head of triceps, medial head of triceps, coracobrachialis and brachialis muscles. The level of insertion of coracobrachialis is the best place to apply pressure by squeezing the artery against the shaft

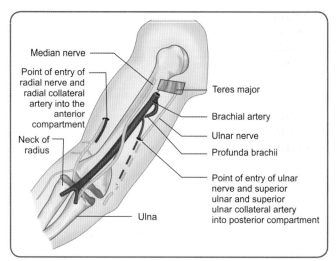

Fig. 17.4: Median nerve crossing the brachial artery from lateral to medial side (also note the ulnar nerve piercing the medial intermuscular septum at midarm level along with superior ulnar collateral branch of brachial artery to enter the posterior compartment of arm and radial nerve piercing the lateral intermuscular septum along with radial collateral branch of profunda brachii to enter the anterior compartment of arm)

of the humerus (Fig 17.5). This is necessary if severe hemorrhage takes place from any artery distal to the brachial artery and direct pressure on the bleeding artery fails to stop the hemorrhage (for example in bleeding wounds of the palmar arches).

- **Laterally**, the proximal part of brachial artery is related to the median nerve (before it crosses the artery) and coracobrachialis muscle, whereas its distal part is in relation to biceps brachii muscle.

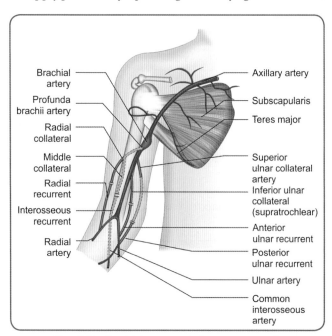

Fig. 17.3: Brachial artery and elbow anastomosis

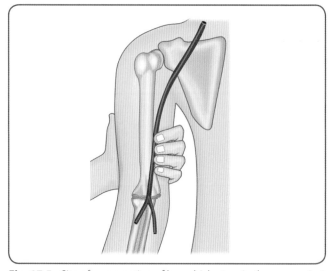

Fig. 17.5: Site of compression of branchial artery in the arm against the shaft of humerus

- **Medially**, its proximal part is in relation to the ulnar nerve, medial cutaneous nerve of forearm and the basilic vein, whereas its distal part is related to median nerve.

Relations in Cubital Fossa

- **Laterally:** Biceps tendon
- **Medially:** Median nerve
- **Posteriorly:** Brachialis muscle
- **Anteriorly:** Bicipital aponeurosis (which separates it from median cubital vein).

 STUDENT INTEREST

The changing relations of median nerve to brachial artery are to be noted (Fig. 17.4 and 22.1). In the upper part of arm, the median nerve is lateral to the brachial artery. In the middle of the arm, the median nerve crosses anterior to the branchial artery. In the lower part of arm, the median nerve lies medial to the brachial artery and retains this relation in the cubital fossa also.

 CLINICAL CORRELATION

Recording Blood Pressure (Figs 17.6A and B)

While taking blood pressure, the cuff of the sphygmoma-nometer is tied around the arm and is inflated (to compress brachial artery) until the radial pulse disappears. Then the diaphragm of stethoscope is placed on the brachial artery in the cubital fossa and the cuff is gradually deflated until the sound is heard. The reading on the manometer at this point is the systolic pressure. On further deflating the sound muffles (disappears). The reading at this point is the diastolic pressure.

Brachial Pulse (Fig. 17.7)

The brachial pulse is felt medial to the tendon of biceps brachii in the cubital fossa.

Branches of Brachial Artery (Fig. 17.8)

- **Profunda brachii** is the largest and the first branch to arise from the posteromedial aspect of brachial artery just below its beginning. It immediately leaves along with the radial nerve through the lower triangular

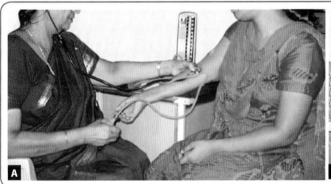
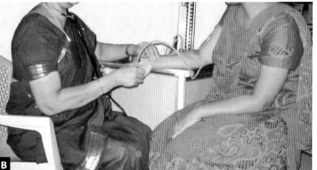

Figs 17.6A and B: Auscultation of branchial artery while recording blood pressure

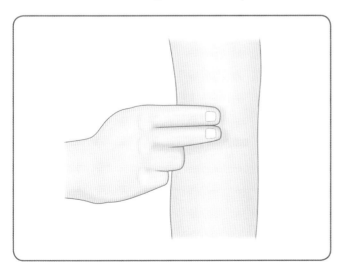

Fig. 17.7: Palpation of brachial artery in cubital fossa

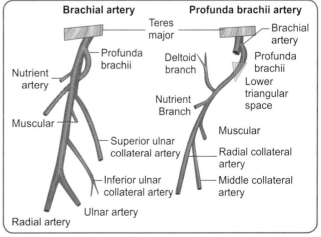

Fig. 17.8: Schematic diagrams to depict branches of brachial artery and profunda brachii artery

space to enter the spiral groove on the posterior surface of humerus.

- **Nutrient artery** to the humerus enters the nutrient foramen located near the insertion of coracobrachialis. It is directed downwards towards the non-growing end of the humerus.
- **Superior ulnar collateral artery** follows the ulnar nerve into the posterior compartment.
- **Inferior ulnar collateral artery** (also known as supratrochlear artery) divides into anterior and posterior branches.
- **Muscular branches** supply the muscles in the anterior compartment.

Surface Marking

The brachial artery corresponds to the lower two third of the line connecting the midclavicular point to the point 1cm below the midpoint of the interepicondylar line of humerus (position of arm being abducted to 90° with palm facing upwards).

🔖 CLINICAL CORRELATION

- The lack of blood supply to flexor muscles of forearm (due to compression or spasm of brachial artery) leads to necrosis and muscle contracture. In **supracondylar fracture of the humerus**, the anteriorly displaced upper bony fragment compresses the brachial artery. This results in inadequate blood supply to the flexor muscles. Initially this gives rise to pallor, pain, puffiness, pulselessness and paralysis. Further reduction in blood supply results in necrosis and fibrosis of the muscles leading to Volkmann's ischemic contracture, in which there is flexion contracture of the metacarpophalangeal and interphalangeal joints.
- **Brachial artery aneurysm** (Fig. 17.9) is a rare condition. If present, it causes symptoms of vascular insufficiency in the forearm and hand.
- The brachial artery is sometimes anastomozed with cephalic vein in the cubital fossa to create an **AV fistula**. The brachial artery can also be anastomozed with basilic vein in the arm to create AV fistula in the arm. This is necessary for hemodialysis in renal failure in case the more common cephaloradial fistula fails to function.

Musculocutaneous Nerve

The musculocutaneous nerve (C5, C6, C7) is the nerve of the anterior compartment of arm (Fig. 17.2).

Course

- It arises in the axilla as a branch of the lateral cord of the brachial plexus. It leaves the axilla by piercing the coracobrachialis muscle and then enters the front of the arm.

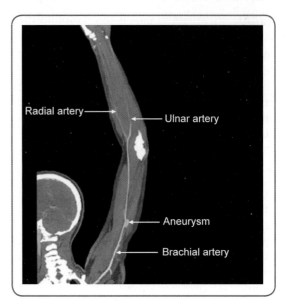

Fig. 17.9: Radiographic depiction of aneurysm of brachial artery (a rare cause of ischemia of distal limb)

- It courses down lying between the biceps brachii and brachialis muscles and comes out of the intermuscular plane laterally. In the lower part of arm it passes in front of the elbow, where it pierces the deep fascia and continues down as the lateral cutaneous nerve of forearm.

Distribution

- It supplies the coracobrachialis, biceps brachii and brachialis muscles.
- The lateral cutaneous nerve of forearm supplies the skin along the lateral side of the forearm as low down as the ball of the thumb.

🔖 CLINICAL CORRELATION

Injury to though rare, produces inability to flex and supinate the forearm strongly. There is loss of biceps tendon reflex and loss of sensation along the lateral aspect of forearm.

⚖ STUDENT INTEREST

The brachial artery travels in the anterior compartment from upper to lower limit. The musculocutaneous nerve is the nerve of anterior compartment as it supplies the three muscles of the compartment, namely coracobrachialis, biceps brachii and brachialis.

Median Nerve in Arm

The median nerve is formed in the axilla. It enters the arm at the level of the lower margin of the teres major muscle.

In its initial course, it is in lateral relation of the brachial artery. The median nerve crosses in front of the brachial artery at the level of insertion of coracobrachialis. Below this level, it travels downwards to the front of the elbow in medial relation of the artery. The median nerve gives vascular branches to the brachial artery and may supply muscular branch to the pronator teres muscle just above the elbow.

Ulnar Nerve in Arm

The ulnar nerve arises in the axilla. After entering the arm it is in medial relation to the brachial artery till the midshaft level where it pierces the medial intermuscular septum and leaves the anterior compartment (along with superior ulnar collateral branch of brachial artery) to enter the posterior compartment. Here, it descends to reach the back of medial epicondyle. It leaves the arm between the humeral and ulnar heads of flexor carpi ulnaris.

POSTERIOR COMPARTMENT OF ARM

The triceps brachii is the only muscle in the posterior compartment of arm. In addition, the compartment contains the radial nerve and profunda brachii vessels in the spiral groove and the ulnar nerve in the lower half medially.

Triceps Brachii

Origin

Origin by three heads as follows:
1. **Long head** from infraglenoid tubercle of scapula.
2. **Lateral head** from a linear oblique ridge on the posterior surface of the shaft of humerus above the level of spiral groove.
3. **Medial head** from posterior surface of shaft of humerus below the level of spiral groove.

Note: Nerve to anconeus and middle collateral artery descend inside the medial head.

Insertion

By common tendon in to olecranon process of ulna.

Note: A few fibers of the medial head (which are known as **articularis genu** or **subanconeus**) are inserted into the fibrous capsule of the elbow joint.

Nerve Supply

Each head of the triceps receive a separate twig from the radial nerve as follows.
• The long head receives a branch in the axilla.

• Before entering the spiral groove, the radial nerve gives off ulnar collateral nerve that supplies the medial head.
• The branches for the medial and lateral heads arise in the spiral groove.

It is to be noted that the medial head receives two separate branches at two levels.

Actions

• The triceps brachii is the main extensor of the elbow joint.
• The long head provides support to the inferior part of the shoulder joint.

Testing Function of Triceps Brachii

The subject is asked to extend the elbow against resistance.

Spiral or Radial Groove (Fig 17.10)

The spiral groove is present on the back of the shaft of the humerus

Boundaries

• **Anteriorly**, by the middle third of the posterior surface of the shaft of the humerus.
• **Posteriorly**, by the lateral head of triceps
• **Superiorly**, by the origin of lateral head
• **Inferiorly**, by the origin of medial head of triceps brachii.

Contents

• Radial nerve
• Profunda brachii vessels.

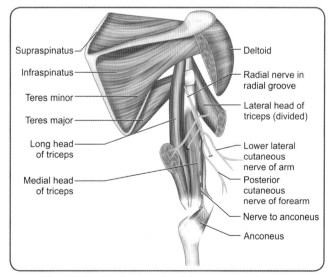

Fig. 17.10: Distribution of radial nerve in spiral groove

Profunda Brachii Artery

The profunda brachii artery is the first and the largest branch of the brachial artery (Fig. 17.8). It rises immediately below the lower border of teres major muscle. It enters the spiral groove through the lower triangular space along with the radial nerve and terminates by dividing into middle collateral and radial collateral arteries at the lower end of the spiral groove.

Branches (Fig. 17.8)

- *Muscular branches* to triceps brachii muscle
- *Nutrient branch* to the humerus
- *Deltoid branch* ascends to anastomose with a branch of posterior circumflex humeral artery.
- *Middle collateral artery* (posterior descending) descends through the substance of medial head of triceps and takes part in elbow anastomosis behind the lateral epicondyle.
- *The radial collateral artery* (anterior descending) pierces the lateral intermuscular septum along with radial nerve to enter the anterior compartment, where it travels down to take part in elbow anastomosis in front of the lateral epicondyle.

Radial Nerve (Fig. 17.10)

The radial nerve arises in the axilla.

- *In the arm*, it is in posterior relation to the initial part of the brachial artery. It soon leaves the medial part of the arm accompanying profunda brachii artery to enter the spiral groove at the back of the humerus.
- *While in the spiral groove* (in direct contact with the bone), it lies between the lateral and medial heads of triceps. At the lower end of the spiral groove, it pierces the lateral intermuscular septum along with radial collateral artery to enter the anterior compartment of arm.
- *In the lower part of anterior compartment*, the radial nerve is placed between the brachialis medially and brachioradialis and extensor carpi radialis longus muscles laterally. The radial nerve passes in front of the lateral epicondyle under cover of brachioradialis to enter the cubital fossa.

Branches in the Arm

In the spiral or radial groove

- Lower lateral cutaneous nerve of arm
- Posterior cutaneous nerve of forearm
- Muscular branch to the lateral head of triceps
- Muscular branch to medial head of triceps
- Muscular branch to anconeus through the substance of medial head.

In the anterior compartment

- Muscular branch to brachioradialis
- Muscular branch to extensor carpi radialis longus
- Proprioceptive fibers to brachialis.

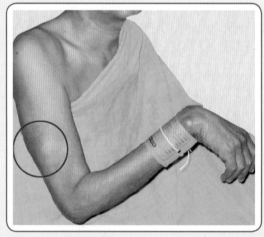
Contd...

Contd…

🕭 CLINICAL CORRELATION

Surgical Exposure of Radial Nerve

The radial nerve is surgically exposed at spiral groove by dividing the lateral head of triceps as shown in the intraoperative photograph (Fig. 17.12) in a patient who had pathology of radial nerve at spiral groove .

Sensory loss on the dorsum of hand at the first interosseous space.

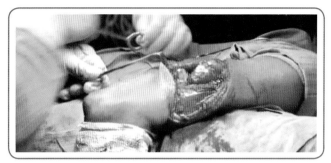

Fig. 17.12: Surgical exposure of radial nerve to remove the pathological mass arising from it

18

Cubital Fossa and Elbow Joint

Chapter Contents

CUBITAL FOSSA

The cubital fossa is a triangular intermuscular space seen as a shallow surface depression in front of the elbow.

BOUNDARIES (FIG. 18.1)

Base

It is the imaginary line on the anterior aspect of elbow joining the medial and lateral epicondyles of humerus.

Medial Boundary

It is formed by the lateral margin of pronator teres muscle.

Lateral Boundary

It is formed by medial margin of brachioradialis muscle.

Apex

It is directed downwards and laterally, where pronator teres and brachioradialis meet.

Floor

The floor consists of brachialis muscle of arm in the upper part and supinator muscle of forearm in the lower part.

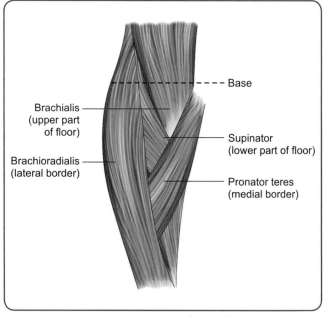

Fig. 18.1: Boundaries of cubital fossa

Roof

The roof consists of skin, superficial fascia and deep fascia. The superficial fascia is characterized by median cubital vein connecting to the cephalic and basilic veins.

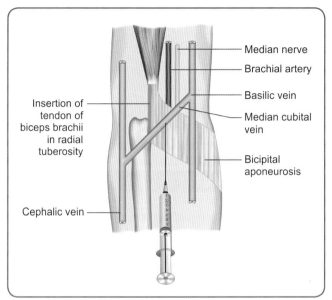

Fig. 18.2: Showing bicipital aponeurosis in the roof of cubital fossa (Note that bicipital aponeurosis provides a supporting platform to the median cubital vein during venipuncture and protects the underlying artery and nerve)

It also contains cutaneous nerves, lateral cutaneous nerve of forearm lying along the cephalic vein and medial cutaneous nerve of forearm along the basilic vein (Fig. 18.2). The deep fascia in the roof is strengthened by the bicipital aponeurosis which is crossed superficially by median cubital vein. The bicipital aponeurosis provides a firm platform to steady this vein during venipuncture (Fig. 18.2) and to protect the underlying brachial artery and the median nerve.

CONTENTS (FIG 18.3)

The three main contents from lateral to medial side are—(1) *tendon of biceps brachii,* (2) *brachial artery and* (3) *median nerve* (TAN). The radial nerve is present in the superolateral part of the fossa under cover of brachioradialis.

Details About the Contents

- The *tendon of biceps brachii* is the midline structure in the cubital fossa. It is inserted into the radial tuberosity from where it sends bicipital aponeurosis towards the deep fascia.
- The *brachial artery* lying between the median nerve medially and biceps tendon laterally, terminates in to the radial and ulnar arteries at the level of neck of radius. The radial artery leaves the cubital fossa through its apex to enter the front of forearm. It gives

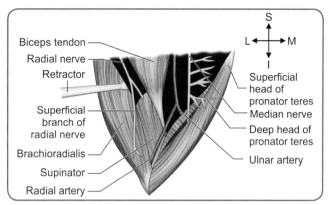

Fig. 18.3: Three main contents of cubital fossa from lateral to medial side are- biceps **t**endon, brachial **a**rtery and median **n**erve (TAN)

one branch called *radial recurrent artery*. The ulnar artery leaves the cubital fossa deep in the deep (ulnar) head of pronator teres. It gives off anterior ulnar recurrent, posterior ulnar recurrent and common interosseous branches. The latter divides into anterior and posterior interosseous arteries. The interosseous recurrent artery is branch of the posterior interosseous artery.

- The *median nerve* is the medial most content. It gives medially direct muscular branches to pronator teres, flexor carpi radialis, palmaris longus and flexor digitorum superficialis muscles. It leaves the fossa between the ulnar (deep) and humeral (superficial) heads of pronator teres.

- The *radial nerve* (Fig. 18.3) appears under cover of the brachioradialis, hence is the lateral most structured. It supplies extensor carpi radialis brevis and terminates in to superficial and deep (posterior interosseous nerve) branches just below the level of lateral epicondyle. The superficial branch of the radial nerve enters the anterior compartment of forearm. The deep branch or posterior interosseous nerve enters the supinator muscle to reach the posterior compartment of forearm.

CLINICAL CORRELATION

- For routine purposes, like drawing blood sample for laboratory investigations or for giving intravenous medicines or saline or for blood transfusion, the preferred site for venipuncture is the median cubital vein (Fig. 18.2) in front of the elbow. Care must be exercised not to injure the median nerve and the brachial artery.
- The blood pressure is recorded by auscultating the brachial artery in the cubital fossa.

Mnemonic

For remembering the contents – *My Best Buddy Rasputin.*
The contents of cubital fossa from medial to lateral side are, Median nerve—Brachial artery—Biceps tendon—Radial nerve.

ANASTOMOSIS AROUND ELBOW (FIG. 17.3)

The articular branches of following four arteries—1. brachial, 2. profunda brachii, 3. ulnar and 4. radial take part in this anastomosis.

- The articular branches of brachial and profunda brachii arteries are given off in the arm and are referred to as *collateral arteries.*
- The articular branches of radial and ulnar arteries are given off in cubital fossa and are referred to as *recurrent arteries.*

The collateral and recurrent arteries anastomose with each other in front and behind the epicondyles of the humerus as follows:

Anterior anastomosis medially
- Anterior branch of inferior ulnar collateral (branch of brachial artery).
- Anterior ulnar recurrent (branch of ulnar artery).

Posterior Anastomosis Medially
- Superior ulnar collateral (branch of brachial artery).
- Posterior ulnar recurrent (branch of ulnar artery).

Anterior Anastomosis Laterally
- Radial collateral (branch of profunda brachii artery).
- Radial recurrent (branch of radial artery).

Posterior Anastomosis Laterally
- Middle collateral (branch of profunda brachii artery).
- Interosseous recurrent (branch of posterior interosseous artery).

Functional Importance

This arterial anastomosis ensures the normal circulation to forearm and hand, when the elbow is flexed and the brachial artery is compressed temporarily.

ELBOW JOINT (FIGS 18.4 AND 18.5)

The elbow joint is a hinge variety of synovial joint permitting movements of flexion and extension around a transverse axis. It is a compound joint as three bones—(1) humerus, (2) ulna and (3) radius take part in this articulation.

Articulating Bones

The lower end of humerus presents—laterally placed capitulum and medially placed trochlea (pulley like in shape). Both are covered with articular cartilage.

- The capitulum articulates with the disc-shaped head of the radius to form humeroradial articulation.
- The trochlea articulates with the trochlear notch of the ulna (formed by articular areas of coronoid and olecranon processes) to form humeroulnar articulation Thus elbow joint consists of two articulations.

Articular Surfaces

- The articular surfaces of the *humeroradial* articulation are reciprocally curved. The closest contact between

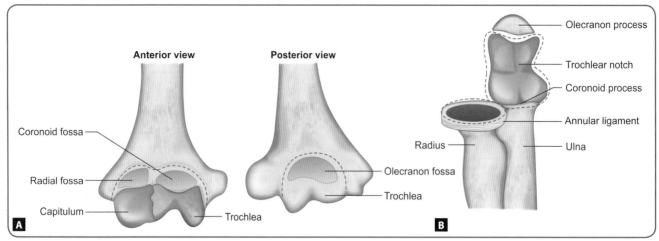

Figs 18.4A and B: Bones taking part in elbow joint and capsular attachments of elbow joint. **A.** Upper attachment of fibrous capsule; **B.** Lower attachment of fibrous capsule

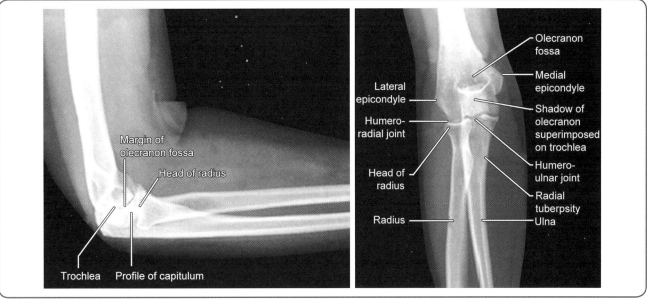

Fig. 18.5: Anatomical features of elbow joint as seen in radiographs

the head of radius and capitulum of humerus occurs in semi-flexed and mid-prone position of the forearm.

- The articular surfaces of **humeroulnar** articulation are not reciprocally congruent because the trochlea of the humerus is not a simple uniform pulley, as its medial flange projects downwards for a longer distance than its lateral counterpart. Moreover the trochlea is widest posteriorly, where its lateral edge is sharp. This is the reason why the humerus and ulna are not in the same plane in extended and supinated position of forearm. The angulation between the arm and forearm is called **carrying angle**. On the contrary, in pronated position of an extended forearm they are in the same plane. This is for functional needs of human hand, as extended and semi prone forearm and hand are essential for optimum precision.

💡 ADDED INFORMATION

The **carrying angle** is the angulation between the long axis of arm and forearm, when the forearm is extended and supinated. The angle obliterates in pronated and extended forearm because in this position the human hand has optimum functional capacity. It also obliterates in flexed forearm. The carrying angle facilitates the movements of the forearm in relation to the hip and thigh. It is present mainly because the medial flange of trochlea of humerus projects downward 6 mm longer than the lateral flange. There are differing views regarding normal value of carrying angle. If one defines carrying angle as angle of deviation of forearm from the axis of arm then its normal value ranges from 10–15 degrees (slightly more in female). If one defines the carrying angle as the angulation (which is open laterally) between the long axis of the arm and that of the forearm then the normal value ranges from 160–170 degrees.

Ligaments

Fibrous Capsule

Being a hinge joint the articular capsule is lax and thin anteriorly and posteriorly, but is strengthened by collateral ligaments on either side.

Upper attachment of capsule (Fig. 18.4A)

- **Anteriorly**, it is attached to the margins of articular surfaces covering capitulum and trochlea, and to the margins of radial and coronoid fossae.
- **Posteriorly**, it is attached to the lateral trochlear margin and to the edge of olecranon fossa.

Lower attachment of capsule (Fig. 18.4B)

- **Anteriorly**, it is attached to the edges of coronoid process of the ulna and to the front of the annular ligament of radius.
- **Posteriorly**, it is attached to the superior and lateral margins of olecranon process and to the back of annular ligament.

Intra-articular Fossae

At the lower end of the humerus there are three fat filled intra-articular fossae.

1. The **coronoid fossa**, lies above the trochlea on the anterior aspect.
2. The **radial fossa**, lies above the capitulum on the anterior aspect.
   During flexion of elbow, coronoid and radial fossae are occupied with upper border of coronoid process and head of radius respectively.

3. The **olecranon fossa**, lies on posterior aspect. During extension of elbow, the tip of the olecranon process occupies the olecranon fossa.

Synovial Membrane

It lines the fibrous capsule and all the intra-articular parts of the joint, which are not covered with articular cartilage. The fat pads in the fossae are intra-capsular but extra-synovial. The synovial membrane projects under the annular ligament to surround the neck of the radius. Thus the elbow and superior radioulnar joints share a common synovial sheath.

Collateral Ligaments (Figs 18.6A and B)

- The **ulnar collateral ligament** is triangular in shape. It extends from medial epicondyle of humerus to the upper end of ulna. It consists of three parts—(1) anterior, (2) posterior and (3) oblique (inferior). These parts share a common upper attachment to the medial epicondyle. However, their lower attachments are separate. The anterior thick band is attached to the medial margin of the coronoid process. The posterior band is attached to the medial margin of olecranon process. The oblique band stretches between coronoid and olecranon processes connecting the lower ends of the anterior and posterior bands. The ulnar nerve is in contact with the medial surface of this ligament (Fig. 18.6A).
- The **radial collateral ligament** extends from lateral epicondyle of humerus to the lateral part of annular ligament surrounding the head of radius. Some of its posterior fibers cross the annular ligament to get attached to the upper end of supinator crest of ulna (Fig. 18.6B).

Relations

- **Anteriorly:** Structures in the cubital fossa, namely, brachialis, biceps tendon, median nerve and brachial artery.
- **Posteriorly:** Insertion of the triceps brachii in olecranon process.
- **Medially:** Ulnar nerve and common origin of superficial flexor muscles of forearm.
- **Laterally:** Common origin of extensor muscles of forearm.

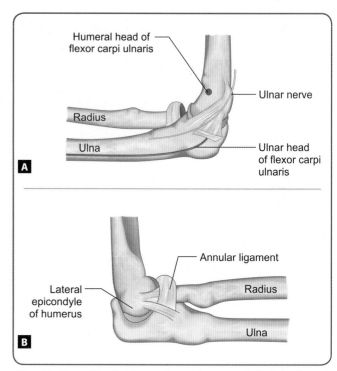

Figs 18.6A and B: A. Ulnar collateral ligament; **B.** Radial collateral ligament

Arterial Supply

The arterial anastomosis around the elbow provides twigs to the joint.

Nerve Supply

The articular branches are given from the radial nerve (through its branch to anconeus), musculocutaneous nerve (through a branch to brachialis), ulnar nerve and median nerve.

Movements

- **Flexion** is produced by brachialis, biceps brachii and brachioradialis muscles. The biceps brachii flexes the elbow in the supinated position of forearm and the brachioradialis in the midprone position.
- **Extension** is produced by triceps brachii and anconeus assisted by gravity.

⌀ CLINICAL CORRELATION

- At the back of the elbow, there are three palpable bony points namely, (1) medial epicondyle of humerus, (2) lateral epicondyle of humerus and (3) the tip of olecranon process of ulna. In the extended elbow these points lie in a straight horizontal line (Fig. 18.7A). In flexed elbow, they form an equilateral triangle (Fig. 18.7B). These bony points are examined in patient to differentiate supracondylar fracture of humerus (Fig. 18.7C) from posterior dislocation of elbow joint (Fig. 18.8). In supracondylar fracture, normal bony relation at the back of elbow is retained since the olecranon process of ulna along with lower end of humerus shifts backwards as shown in figure 18.6. In posterior dislocation of elbow joint, the olecranon process moves backwards from the lower end of humerus resulting in loss of normal relation of the three bony points as shown in the radiograph of dislocated elbow joint (Fig. 18.8). The brachial artery is in danger of compression by the proximal fragment in supracondylar fracture of humerus as this fragment is displaced forwards.

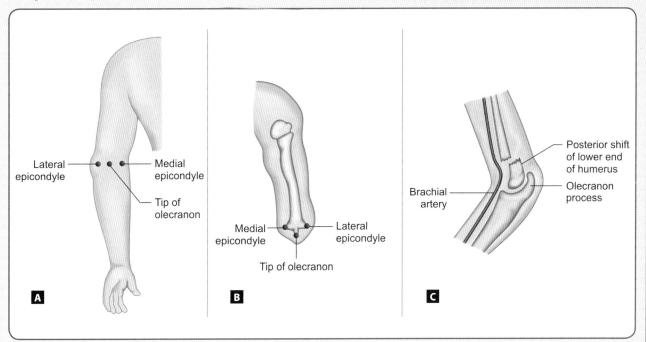

Figs 18.7A to C: A. Three bony points in a straight line behind the elbow in extended elbow; **B.** Equilateral triangle formed by the three bony points in flexed elbow; **C.** In posterior dislocation of elbow joint the equilateral triangle is disrupted due to posterior shift of the olecranon process of ulna

- ***Pulled elbow*** is the condition in which the radial head escapes downward from the annular ligament. Children are more prone to pulled elbow ***(nursemaid's elbow)*** because the shape of annular ligament is tubular and the head of radius is not fully developed.
- ***Tennis elbow*** is due to inflammation of the radial collateral ligament and of the periosteum around its attachment to the lateral epicondyle.

Contd...

Contd…

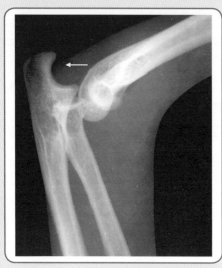

Fig. 18.8: Radiograph showing posterior dislocation of elbow joint (see arrow)

- **Golfer's elbow** is due to inflammation at the site of common flexor origin from the anterior surface of medial epicondyle.
- **Students elbow** is due to inflammation of the subcutaneous olecranon bursa, caused by friction between the overlying skin and the hard surface of the desk.
- In acute synovitis of the elbow joint the swelling is more conspicuous around the olecranon. This is because the capsule is lax and the deep fascia is thin posteriorly.
- In **cubitus valgus deformity**, the forearm is deviated laterally more than normal due to increase in the carrying angle. The cubitus valgus may gradually stretch the ulnar nerve behind the medial epicondyle leading to a clinical condition called **tardy ulnar palsy**.
- In **cubitus varus deformity**, the forearm is deviated medially due to reduction in the carrying angle as a consequence of which the ulnar side of the forearm touches the thigh.

19

Compartments of Forearm

Chapter Contents

FOREARM

The forearm extends from the elbow to the wrist. Like the arm it is enclosed in a sleeve of deep fascia. The two bones (radius and ulna) of the forearm and the intervening interosseous membrane divide the forearm into flexor compartment anteriorly and the extensor compartment posteriorly.

ANTERIOR COMPARTMENT (FIG. 19.1)

Note: That flexor carpi radialis has an oblique course in forearm and flexor carpi ulnaris has a straight course along the medial margin of forearm.

This compartment contains muscles, vessels and nerves. The muscles are arranged in three strata.

Superficial stratum

The muscles in this stratum have common origin from anterior aspect of medial epicondyle and they consist of pronator teres, flexor carpi radialis, palmaris longus and flexor carpi ulnaris.

Intermediate stratum

This stratum consists of only the flexor digitorum superficialis (arising from common flexor origin from anterior aspect of medial epicondyle of humerus).

Deep stratum

This stratum has three muscles consisting of flexor pollicis longus, flexor digitorum profundus and pronator quadratus.

Pronator Teres

The pronator teres muscle is described in chapter 20 (Fig. 20.4).

Flexor Carpi Radialis

Origin

From common flexor origin on the anterior aspect of the medial epicondyle of humerus.

The muscle belly ends in a tendon about halfway down the middle of forearm. Near the wrist its tendon is related medially to the radial artery (Fig. 19.1). The tendon passes deep to the flexor retinaculum in a separate osseofibrous canal, produced by the groove on the trapezium and the flexor retinaculum.

Insertion

Into the palmar surfaces of the bases of second and third metacarpal bones.

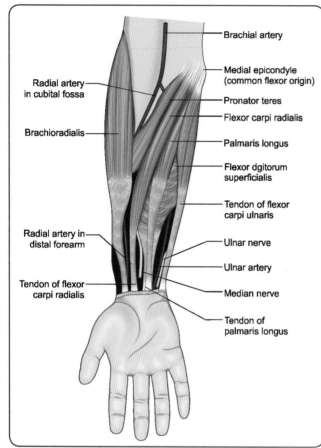

Fig. 19.1: Four superficial muscles in the anterior compartment of forearm arising from common flexor origin on medial epicondyle (muscles disposed in lateromedial order are—pronator teres, flexor carpi radialis, palmaris longus and flexor carpi ulnaris)

Nerve Supply

By the median nerve in the cubital fossa

Actions

Acting singly it is the flexor of wrist joint but acting synergistically with radial extensors of the carpus (extensor carpi radialis longus and brevis) it produces abduction of wrist (radial deviation).

Palmaris Longus

This muscle is not always present. It has a short belly and a long tendon.

Origin

Common origin from medial epicondyle of humerus. Distally, its tendon passes in front of the flexor retinaculum with which its fibers mingle and beyond this it becomes continuous with the apex of palmar aponeurosis. The median nerve lies just behind the thin palmaris longus tendon above the wrist and hence is likely to be mistaken for the tendon.

Nerve Supply

By median nerve in the cubital fossa.

Action

A weak flexor of wrist joint.

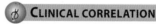

CLINICAL CORRELATION

The palmaris longus tendon is used as a graft in surgical repair of damaged flexor tendons in the hand.

Flexor Carpi Ulnaris

Origin

- **Origin of humeral head:** From anterior aspect of medial epicondyle.
- **Origin of ulnar head:** From medial margin of olecranon process and the upper two-thirds of the posterior margin of ulna.

The ulnar nerve enters the forearm between two heads of origin of flexor carpi ulnaris. The compression of ulnar nerve in this location is known as **cubital tunnel syndrome**. At the wrist the tendon of flexor carpi ulnaris lies medial to the ulnar nerve (Fig. 19.1).

Insertion

Into pisiform bone.

The insertion is prolonged through the pisohamate ligament to the hamate and through pisometacarpal ligament to the base of fifth metacarpal bone.

Nerve Supply

By ulnar nerve

Actions

Acting singly it is a flexor of wrist but acting synergistically with extensor carpi ulnaris it produces adduction of wrist (ulnar deviation).

Note: Flexor carpi ulnaris is the only muscle of common flexor origin not supplied by ulnar nerve and pisiform is the sesamoid bone in its tendon.

Flexor Digitorum Superficialis (FDS)

This is a broad muscle that takes origin by two heads (Fig. 19.2).
- ***Origin of humeroulnar head:*** From common flexor origin, ulnar collateral ligament and medial margin of coronoid process of ulna.
- ***Origin of radial head:*** From anterior oblique line of radial shaft.

The two heads of origin are joined by a fibrous band and the median nerve and ulnar artery pass downwards deep to this band. The muscle belly ends into four tendons, which are bunched together, in such a way that the tendons for middle and ring fingers lie anterior to those for index and little fingers. The tendons pass deep to the flexor retinaculum within the carpal tunnel, where they are enclosed in a common synovial sheath (ulnar bursa) along with tendons of flexor digitorum profundus and flexor pollicis longus.

Insertion

On reaching the base of proximal phalanx, each digital tendon enters the fibrous flexor sheath along with respective tendon of flexor digitorum profundus. The superficialis tendon splits into two slips, which pass posteriorly around the profundus tendon (Fig. 19.3). The slips join behind the profundus tendon and then insert into the palmar aspect of the sides of middle phalanx of the medial four digits.

Note: The tendon of flexor digitorum profundus perforates the tendon of FDS on way to its insertion)

Nerve Supply

By median nerve

Note: The part of muscle giving origin to tendons of medial three digits is supplied by a branch in the cubital fossa and the part giving origin to tendon of index finger is supplied by a branch given off in the forearm.

Actions

- These are as follows
  - Flexion of middle phalanx at the proximal interphalangeal joint

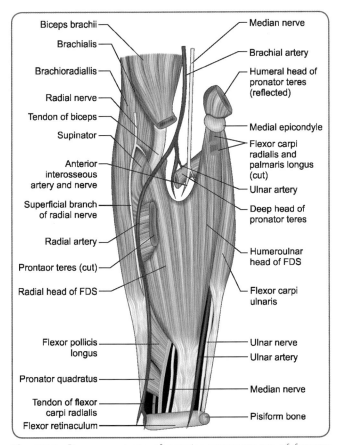

Fig. 19.2: Deeper contents of anterior compartment of forearm after reflection of superficial muscles (Note the posterior relations of radial artery from above downwards—tendon of biceps brachii, supinator (in cubital fossa), pronator teres, radial head of flexor digitorum superficialis, flexor pollicis longus, lower end of radial shaft and pronator quadratus).

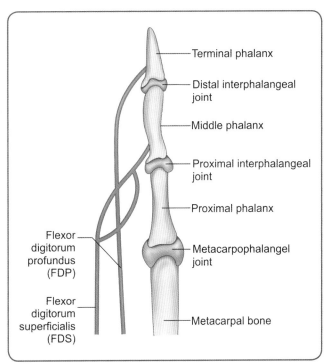

Fig. 19.3: Insertion of flexor digitorum superficialis and of flexor digitorum profundus respectively in to middle phalanx and distal phalanx

– Weak flexor of proximal phalanx at the metacarpophalangeal joint
– Weak flexor of wrist joint.

Note: Each tendon of FDS can act independently of others.

Testing Function of Flexor Digitorum Superficialis (Fig. 19.4A)

The subject is asked to flex the middle phalanx of the finger (to be examined) while holding down the adjoining fingers in extension (to eliminate action of flexor digitorum profundus). If the subject is able to flex the middle phalanx, the FDS is intact.

Flexor Digitorum Profundus (FDP) (Fig. 19.3)

Origin

From anterior and medial surfaces of upper three fourth of shaft of ulna, from adjacent interosseous membrane and upper three fourth of the posterior border of ulna by an aponeurosis.

About halfway down the forearm, four tendons are formed. The tendons pass deep to the flexor retinaculum in the carpal tunnel where they are enclosed in a common synovial sheath (ulnar bursa). After entering the palm, each tendon gives origin to the lumbrical muscle and proceeds towards respective digit.

Insertion

Each tendon enters the fibrous flexor sheath, where it perforates the tendon of flexor digitorum superficialis. Finally, it is inserted into the base of respective terminal phalanx.

Nerve supply

Double nerve supply by ulnar nerve (medial half) and median nerve via anterior interosseous nerve (lateral half).

Actions

• Only flexor of terminal phalanges of the medial four fingers (when the middle phalanges are flexed)
• Flexion of other joints of fingers and of the wrist joint.

Testing Function of Flexor Digitorum Profundus (Fig. 19.4B)

The subject is asked to flex the finger (to be examined) while holding down the proximal and middle phalanges of the same finger. If the subject can flex the terminal phalanx the FDP is intact.

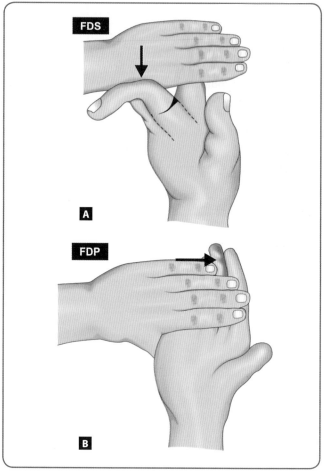

Figs 19.4A and B: A. Testing the function of flexor digitorum superficialis (FDS); **B.** Testing the function of flexor digitorum profundus (FDP)

Flexor Pollicis Longus (FPL)

Origin

From anterior surface of radius (below the anterior oblique line up to the upper attachment of pronator quadratus) and adjacent interosseous membrane.

It ends in a tendon just above the wrist. The tendon (wrapped in a separate synovial sheath called radial bursa) passes deep to the flexor retinaculum in the carpal tunnel. In the palm, it passes distally between the opponens pollicis and oblique head of adductor pollicis.

Insertion

It enters the fibrous flexor sheath at the base of the proximal phalanx and is inserted into the base of distal phalanx of thumb.

Nerve Supply

By anterior interosseous branch of median nerve supplies the muscle in the forearm.

Action

Flexion of terminal phalanx of thumb.

Testing Function of Flexor Pollicis Longus

The subject is asked to flex the distal phalanx of thumb against resistance, while the proximal phalanx is held stationary.

 CLINICAL CORRELATION

Injury to Flexor Tendons

- In *traumatic injuries* to the distal forearm, the cut tendons are often repaired surgically. The tendon grafting can be done using the tendon of palmaris longus muscle.
- *Avascular necrosis* of the tendon is a complication of tenosynovitis (inflammation of synovial sheath surrounding the tendon) and pus formation. This results due to pressure on the arteries supplying the tendons by accumulated pus. These delicate arteries reach the tendons inside the digital synovial sheath via the vincula brevia (located near the insertion of the tendon) and vincula longa (located closer to the base of the finger).

Pronator Quadratus

This muscle is described in chapter 20 along with muscles of supination and pronation.

Superficial Branch of Radial Nerve

It is one of the terminal branches of the radial nerve given off in the cubital fossa under cover of brachioradialis muscle. The superficial branch of the radial nerve is purely sensory.

Course and relations in front of forearm

During its downward course in the lateral part of the forearm, it is placed successively on the supinator, pronator teres, and radial head of flexor digitorum superficialis and flexor pollicis longus muscles. The radial nerve is in close lateral relation to the radial artery in the middle third of its course. It leaves the radial artery about 7 cm above the wrist, passes deep to the tendon of brachioradialis and curves round the lateral side of radius as it descends.

Course in dorsum of hand

On the dorsum of the hand, the superficial branch of radial nerve gives four to five digital branches after piercing the deep fascia.

Distribution (Fig. 21.1)

It supplies a variable area of the dorsum of hand and its digital branches supply the lateral three and half digits (excluding the nail beds). Therefore, there will be sensory loss on the dorsum of the hand if radial nerve is injured anywhere from its origin upto it's termination in the cubital fossa or if the superficial branch of radial nerve is injured.

Ulnar Nerve

The ulnar nerve enters the forearm from the back of the medial epicondyle between the humeral and ulnar heads of flexor carpi ulnaris.

Course and relations in front of forearm

The ulnar nerve descends along the medial side of forearm lying on flexor digitorum profundus and covered with flexor carpi ulnaris. In the lower part of forearm, it becomes superficial, covered only by skin and fasciae. Anterior or superficial to flexor retinaculum it is inside a fascial canal called **Guyon's canal** lateral to the pisiform bone.

The ulnar artery is separated from it in the upper third of its course in forearm but in the distal two-third they form a close neurovascular unit.

Termination

The ulnar nerve terminates under cover of the palmaris brevis muscle into superficial and deep branches.

Surface Marking of Ulnar Nerve

A line joining the back of the medial epicondyle of the humerus to the pisiform bone represents the ulnar nerve in the forearm.

Branches in forearm

- Articular branch to the elbow joint
- Muscular branches to the flexor carpi ulnaris and medial half of flexor digitorum profundus
- Palmar cutaneous and dorsal cutaneous branches nearer the wrist.

Median Nerve

The median nerve leaves the cubital fossa to enter the forearm between the humeral and ulnar heads of pronator teres muscle.

Course and relations in front of forearm

The median nerve passes downward behind the tendinous bridge connecting the humeroulnar and radial heads of flexor digitorum superficialis and remains adherent to the deep surface of the same muscle. It is accompanied by median artery (which supplies blood to median nerve and is a branch of anterior interosseous artery) in the middle part of forearm. About 5 cm proximal to the flexor retinaculum, the median nerve comes to lie anterior to the tendons of flexor digitorum superficialis. Here, it is very close to the surface being posterior to palmaris longus tendon (Fig. 19.1). It enters the carpal tunnel along with the long flexor tendons of digits.

Branches in forearm

- Anterior interosseous nerve
- Muscular branch to part of FDS giving origin to tendon of index finger
- Palmar cutaneous branch just proximal to the flexor retinaculum (it supplies the skin of the palm overlying the thenar eminence).

Anterior Interosseous Nerve

This nerve arises as the median nerve leaves the cubital fossa. It soon joins company with the anterior interosseous artery and the two descend on the anterior surface of the interosseous membrane. It passes posterior to the pronator quadratus muscle to end in front of the wrist

Distribution

The anterior interosseous nerve supplies lateral half of the flexor digitorum profundus, flexor pollicis longus and pronator quadratus muscles.

Its articular branches supply the distal radioulnar, radiocarpal (wrist) and intercarpal joints.

 CLINICAL CORRELATION

Anterior Interosseous Nerve Syndrome

There is paralysis of flexor pollicis longus, flexor digitorum profundus for index and middle fingers and pronator quadratus in the lesion of this nerve. There is inability to pinch the thumb and index finger together to make **OK sign** (Fig. 19.5A). Instead the patient will make triangular sign (Fig. 19.5B) in which the terminal phalanges of thumb and index finger are in close approximation due to inability to flex distal IP joints. The patient will have difficulty in picking up small objects (like coin, needle or grain) from the flat surface.

 STUDENT INTEREST

The ulnar and median nerves are at the risk in traumatic injuries to distal forearm. The median nerve passes deep to flexor retinaculum and ulnar nerve passes superficial to flexor retinaculum. The ulnar nerve is easily injured at distal forearm and proximal hand while median nerve is easily injured in distal forearm.

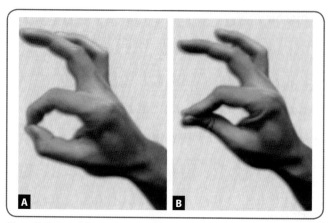

Figs 19.5A and B: A. OK sign (by pinching thumb and index finger together). Positive OK sign indicates integrity of anterior interosseous nerve which supplies flexor pollicis longus and lateral half of flexor digitorum profundus; **B.** Triangular sign indicates inability to flex the distal phalanx hence the distal phalanges of thumb and index finger are approximated to each other so that OK sign (a circle) is changed in to a triangle suggesting injury to anterior interosseous nerve.

Radial Artery

The radial artery (Fig. 19.2) is one of the terminal branches of the brachial artery.

Extent in forearm and dorsum

It extends from the level of the neck of the radius in the cubital fossa to the proximal end of the first inter-metacarpal space on the dorsum of the hand.

Exit from dorsum

The artery enters the palm between the heads of first dorsal interosseous muscle to continue as the deep palmar arch. The course of the radial artery can be divided into three parts, in the forearm, at the wrist and in the palm.

Relations in forearm

- *Anteriorly*, in the proximal part the radial artery is related to the fleshy belly of brachioradialis and in the distal part to the skin and fasciae. Therefore, in the distal forearm the artery is accessible for arterial puncture (Fig. 19.7).
- *Posteriorly*, the radial artery is related from above downwards (Fig. 19.2) to tendon of biceps brachii, supinator, pronator teres, flexor digitorum superficialis, flexor pollicis longus, pronator quadratus and the lower end of radius.
- *Laterally*, it is related proximally to the fleshy belly of brachioradialis and distally to the tendon of

brachioradialis. In its middle third, the radial nerve comes in close lateral relation of the radial artery.

- *Medially*, it is related to pronator teres proximally and to tendon of flexor carpi radialis distally (where the radial pulse is felt lateral to this tendon).

Course at wrist

The radial artery takes a curve from the styloid process of radius backwards across the anatomical snuffbox. At first it passes deep to the two tendons (abductor pollicis longus and extensor pollicis brevis), which form the anterior boundary of the anatomical snuffbox. Then the artery lies on the scaphoid and the trapezium in the floor of the snuffbox where, the cephalic vein is superficial to the radial artery. Lastly the artery passes deep to the extensor pollicis longus tendon and approaches the proximal end of the first intermetacarpal space, where it enters the palm between the two heads of first dorsal interosseous muscle.

Course in palm

The radial artery in the palm takes a transverse course medially to anastomose with the deep branch of ulnar artery to complete the deep palmar arch at the base of fifth metacarpal bone.

> ### Surface Marking in Forearm
> A line drawn from a point 1 cm below the midpoint of the interepicondylar line at the elbow to the point of the radial pulse represents the radial artery.

Branches

- Radial recurrent artery in the cubital fossa.
- Muscular, anterior radial carpal or palmar carpal branches and superficial palmar branch in the forearm.
- Posterior radial carpal branches or dorsal carpal and the first dorsal metacarpal artery at the wrist.

CLINICAL CORRELATION

Radial Pulse

The radial pulse is felt on the anterior surface of the distal end of radius lateral to the tendon of flexor carpi radialis (Fig. 19.6).
- For *arterial puncture* (Fig. 19.7), the radial artery is chosen since it is superficial in the distal forearm. In this procedure blood is withdrawn for the purpose of arterial blood gas (ABG) analysis.

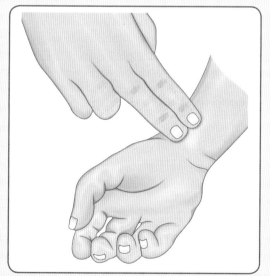

Fig. 19.6: Site of feeling radial pulse against lower end of radius lateral to tendon of flexor carpi radialis

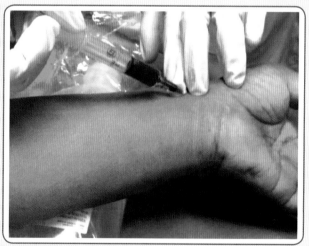

Fig. 19.7: Radial artery puncture at distal forearm to draw sample of arterial blood

- The radial artery graft is used in coronary artery bypass surgery.
- *Allen test* is performed to find out the patency or arterial sufficiency of radial artery (for example when it is used as coronary artery graft). The steps are illustrated in figure 19.8A.
- The radial artery is often used for creating arteriovenous fistula like radio-cephalic fistula (Fig.16.5A and B) for dialysis purposes in patients of chronic renal failure.

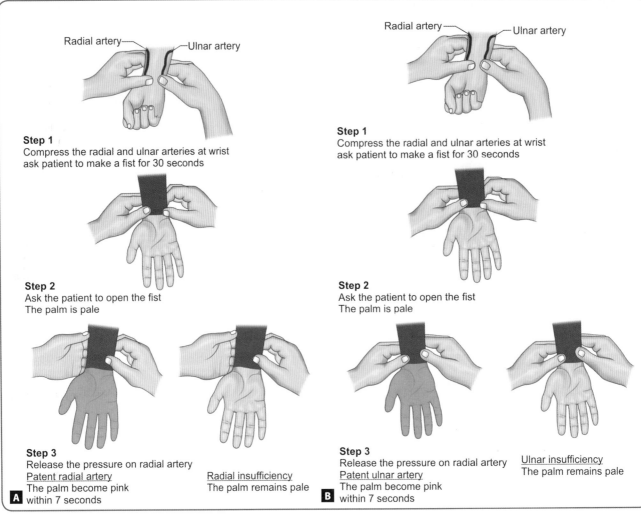

Figs 19.8A and B: A. Steps in Allen's test to ascertain patency of radial artery; **B.** Steps in Allen's test to ascertain patency of ulnar artery

- Radialis indicis, princeps pollicis and deep palmar arch in the palm.

Ulnar Artery

The ulnar artery is the larger of the two terminal branches of the brachial artery.

Extent

It begins at the level of neck of radius in the cubital fossa and terminates in front of the flexor retinaculum at the pisiform bone.

Exit from cubital fossa

The ulnar artery leaves the cubital fossa deep to the deep (ulnar) head of pronator teres, to enter the forearm.

Course in forearm

Its course in the forearm can be divided into upper oblique part and lower vertical part.

In the upper third of the forearm the ulnar artery takes as oblique course to reach the medial margin of the forearm.

In the lower two-thirds the artery passes vertically down along the medial margin of forearm to reach the wrist.

At the wrist, it crosses the flexor retinaculum superficially (Fig. 19.2) and at the pisiform it terminates by dividing into deep and superficial branches.

Course in palm

The deep branch of ulnar artery takes part in the completion of deep palmar arch medially by uniting with radial artery.

The superficial branch of ulnar artery runs laterally across the palm to meet the superficial palmar branch of radial artery or one of its branches to complete the superficial palmar arch.

Surface Marking in Forearm

The oblique part of ulnar artery is indicated by a line joining the point (1 cm below the midpoint of interepicondylar line) to a point coinciding with the junction of upper one third and lower two third of a line from medial epicondyle to the pisiform. The vertical part is indicated by a line starting from the lower end of the oblique part to the pisiform bone.

Relations

The oblique part is situated deeply compared to the vertical part of the artery.

- *Anteriorly*, the oblique part is related to the muscles that arise from medial epicondyle, namely, pronator teres, flexor carpi radialis, palmaris longus and flexor digitorum superficialis. The deep head of pronator teres intervenes between the ulnar artery and median nerve at the apex of cubital fossa.
- *Laterally*, the vertical part is related to flexor carpi ulnaris in upper extent but towards the wrist it is covered with the skin and fasciae. Distally it lies between flexor carpi ulnaris medially and flexor digitorum superficialis laterally before piercing the deep fascia along with the ulnar nerve. Thus, it passes in front of the flexor retinaculum.
- *Posteriorly*, the ulnar artery is related from above downward, to brachialis, flexor digitorum profundus and flexor retinaculum.
- *Medially*, the ulnar nerve is in close relation in its lower two- third.

Branches of ulnar artery

- *Anterior ulnar recurrent artery* anastomoses with inferior ulnar collateral branch of brachial artery.
- *Posterior ulnar recurrent artery* anastomoses with inferior ulnar collateral branch of brachial artery.
- Muscular branches
- *Common interosseous artery* which soon divides in to larger anterior interosseous artery and smaller posterior interosseous artery in the cubital fossa.
- *Anterior or palmar ulnar carpal branch*.
- *Posterior or dorsal ulnar carpal branch*.
- Terminal branches (superficial and deep).

 CLINICAL CORRELATION

- Ulno-basilic fistula (Fig. 16.6) is created in forearm by anastomosing ulnar artery with basilic vein to arterialize the basilic vein. Once successfully arterialized, a bruit is heard on auscultation on the dilated basilic vein. The arterialized basilic vein is then connected to dialysis machine in chronic renal failure patients and when needed.
- Allen test is performed to test the patency or sufficiency of ulnar artery (in cases where radial artery is used as coronary graft). Then the ulnar artery is the only supply of the palm. The steps of the test are illustrated in figure 19.8B.

Anterior Interosseous Artery

The anterior interosseous artery descends lying deeply in the anterior compartment on the interosseous membrane along with anterior interosseous nerve. It pierces the interosseous membrane at the upper margin of pronator quadratus muscle to gain entry into the posterior compartment where it almost takes the place of the thinned out posterior interosseous artery. The anterior interosseous artery in its small course in posterior compartment travels with posterior interosseous nerve in the fourth compartment deep to extensor retinaculum and takes part in the dorsal carpal arch.

Branches in anterior compartment

- Median artery arises high up and it accompanies the median nerve. It is an example of axis artery of upper limb.
- Muscular branches to deep muscles of front of forearm
- Nutrient arteries to radius and ulna.
- Carpal branch, which takes part in palmar carpal arch.

Note: For course of anterior interosseous artery in the posterior compartment refer to posterior compartment.

Posterior Interosseous Artery

After giving origin to interosseous recurrent artery near its origin in the cubital fossa, the posterior interosseous artery enters the posterior compartment of forearm by passing through the gap between the upper margin of interosseous membrane and the oblique cord. Its further course and branches are described in posterior compartment.

STUDENT INTEREST

Both radial and ulnar arteries are of use in clinical practice. Hence, students should be serious while studying their course and branches in forearm and hand.

POSTERIOR COMPARTMENT OF FOREARM

The posterior compartment of the forearm contains extensor muscles, posterior interosseous nerve and both posterior and anterior interosseous arteries. A total of twelve muscles belong to the posterior compartment. They are divided into two sets—(1) superficial and (2) deep.

Superficial Muscles of Posterior Compartment

- Anconeus
- Brachioradialis
- Extensor carpi radialis longus
- Extensor carpi radialis brevis
- Extensor digitorum
- Extensor digiti minimi
- Extensor carpi ulnaris.

Anconeus (Fig 19.9A)

This is a triangular muscle with narrow origin and broad insertion.

Origin

From posterior surface of lateral epicondyle of humerus.

Insertion

Into olecranon process and posterior surface of upper fourth of ulna.

Nerve Supply

By nerve to anconeus (branch of radial nerve in the spiral groove).

Action

Extensor of elbow joint.

Brachioradialis (Fig. 19.1)

This is regarded as a borderline muscle since developmentally it is an extensor muscle, but functionally and topographically it is a flexor muscle.

Origin

From upper two thirds of lateral supracondylar ridge of humerus (above the elbow).

Insertion

Into radius just above the styloid process (above the wrist).

Nerve Supply

By the radial nerve in the anterior compartment of arm.

Actions

- Flexor of elbow joint in midprone position of forearm.
- Pronation of supinated forearm to midprone position and supination of fully pronated forearm to midprone position.

Testing Function of Brachioradialis

The elbow of the subject is flexed to 90° and the forearm is kept in midprone position. Now the subject is instructed to flex the elbow against resistance. A normal muscle can be seen and felt.

Supinator Jerk or Reflex

When the distal end of radius is tapped there is reflex flexion of the forearm. Positive response indicates the integrity of spinal segments C7–C8. It is the brachioradialis that contracts and not the supinator.

Extensor Carpi Radialis Longus (ECRL)

Origin

From lower third of lateral supracondylar ridge of humerus.

It passes downward under cover of brachioradialis and superficial to the extensor carpi radialis brevis. At the wrist, its tendon passes deep to extensor retinaculum in the second compartment.

Insertion

Into the base of second metacarpal bone.

Nerve Supply

By radial nerve in the arm just above the elbow.

Extensor Carpi Radialis Brevis (ECRB)

Origin

From common extensor origin on anterior aspect of lateral epicondyle of humerus.

It passes downward deep to the extensor carpi radialis longus muscle lying in direct contact with radial shaft. At the wrist, its tendon passes deep to extensor retinaculum in second compartment.

Insertion

Into the bases of second and third metacarpal bones.

Nerve Supply

By deep branch of radial nerve (posterior interosseous nerve) above the proximal margin of supinator in the cubital fossa.

Actions of Radial Extensors of Carpus

- Both extensor carpi radialis longus (ECRL) and extensor carpi radialis brevis (ECRB) along with extensor carpi ulnaris produce extension or dorsiflexion of the wrist.
- Both ECRL and ECRB muscles along with flexor carpi radialis act synergistically to produce abduction or radial deviation of wrist.

Testing Function of Extensor Carpi Radialis Longus (ECRL) and Extensor Carpi Radialis Brevis (ECRB)

The subject clenches the fist and dorsiflexes the wrist on the radial side against resistance. The ECRL and ECRB muscles can be palpated and their tendons can be felt near the insertion.

Extensor Digitorum

Origin

From common extensor origin on anterior aspect of lateral epicondyle of humerus.

It ends into four tendons in mid-forearm. The tendons of extensor digitorum and the tendon of extensor indicis are lodged in the fourth compartment deep to the extensor retinaculum. On the dorsum of the hand the tendons are connected by tendinous interconnections, which restrict the independent actions on the fingers.

Insertion

Each tendon expands into the extensor expansion over the proximal phalanx and is inserted through it into the base of the middle phalanx and that of the terminal phalanx. The parts and attachments of the extensor expansion are described with the interossei and lumbrical muscles of the hand in chapter 21 and depicted in figure 21.17.

Nerve Supply

By posterior interosseous nerve.

Action

Extension of metacarpophalangeal joints.

Note: Extension at interphalangeal joints is produced by lumbricals and interossei

Testing Function of Extensor Digitorum

The subject is asked to keep the elbow and the anterior aspect of forearm and the palm on the table. After the examiner stabilizes the wrist of the subject with one hand, the subject extends the (metacarpophatangeal) MCP joint of each finger against resistance.

Extensor Digiti Minimi

This is a separate extensor of the little finger.

Origin

From common extensor origin on the front of lateral epicondyle.

It passes downwards along the medial side of extensor digitorum. It passes deep to the extensor retinaculum in the fifth compartment. On the dorsum of the hand, it usually splits into two slips. Insertion—into the extensor expansion of little finger.

Nerve Supply

By posterior interosseous nerve.

Action

Extension at metacarpophalangeal joint of little finger.

Extensor Carpi Ulnaris (ECU)

Origin

From common extensor origin on the front of lateral epicondyle and from the posterior subcutaneous border of ulna (in common with origin of flexor carpi ulnaris).

Its tendon passes deep to the extensor retinaculum in the sixth compartment, where it lies in a groove between head and styloid process of ulna.

Insertion

Into the base of fifth metacarpal bone.

Nerve Supply

By posterior interosseous nerve.

Actions

- Extension of wrist joint along with the two radial extensors of the carpus (ECRB and ECRL).
- Adduction or ulnar deviation of wrist joint by acting synergistically with flexor carpi ulnaris.

Testing Function of ECU

The subject is asked to keep the closed fist in position of ulnar deviation against resistance.

Deep Muscles of Posterior Compartment (Figs 19.9A and B)

- Supinator
- Abductor pollicis longus
- Extensor pollicis brevis
- Extensor pollicis longus
- Extensor indicis.

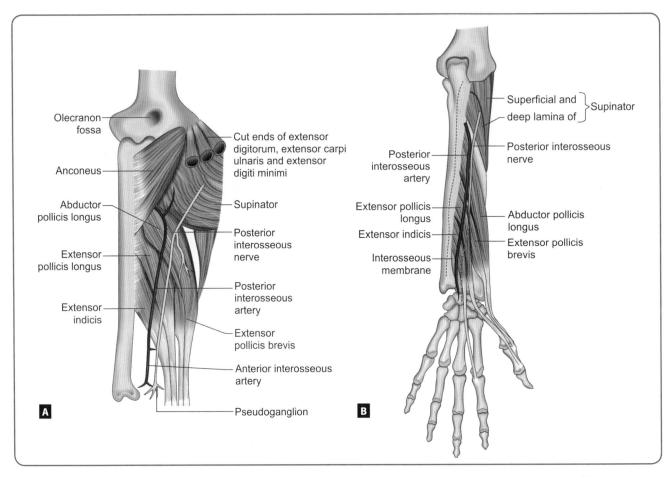

Figs 19.9A and B: A. Contents of posterior (extensor) compartment of forearm; **B.** Details of deep muscles of the extensor compartment of forearm

Supinator

The supinator muscle is described in chapter 20 along with muscles of supination and pronation.

Abductor Pollicis Longus (APL)

Origin

From posterior surface of both radius and ulna and from the interosseous membrane.

Its long tendon spirals round the tendons of brachioradialis and the radial extensors of the carpus. The tendons of abductor pollicis longus and extensor pollicis brevis enclosed in common synovial sheath pass deep to the extensor retinaculum in the first compartment.

Insertion

Into radial side of the base of first metacarpal bone.

Nerve Supply

By posterior interosseous nerve.

Actions

Abduction and extension of thumb at the first carpometacarpal joint.

Testing Function of Abductor Pollicis Longus (APL)

The subject holds the forearm in midprone position and is then asked to abduct the thumb against resistance. The tendon of APL stands out in the margin of anatomical snuffbox.

Extensor Pollicis Brevis (EPB)

Origin

From posterior surface of radius below the origin of abductor pollicis longus as well as from the adjacent interosseous membrane.

Its tendon closely follows the tendon of abductor pollicis longus.

Insertion

Into the dorsal surface of proximal phalanx of thumb.

Nerve Supply

By posterior interosseous nerve.

Actions

Extension of proximal phalanx of thumb and of the first metacarpal bone.

Testing Function of Extensor Pollicis Brevis (EPB)

Ask the subject to extend the proximal phalanx of thumb at the metacarpopharyngeal joint against resistance (while the forearm is resting on the table in prone position).

 CLINICAL CORRELATION

> **De Quervain's Tenosynovitis**
>
> It is the inflammatory condition of the common synovial sheath which wraps around the tendons of abductor pollicis longus and extensor pollicis brevis. This produces swelling and pain along the lateral aspect of the wrist. Symptoms usually subside after incising the tendon sheath.

Extensor Pollicis Longus (EPL)

Origin

From posterior surface of ulna below the origin of abductor pollicis longus and from the interosseous membrane.

Its long tendon hooks round the Lister's tubercle of radius deep to extensor retinaculum in the third compartment.

Insertion

Into the base of terminal phalanx of thumb. On the dorsum of the proximal phalanx (in the absence of extensor expansion proper), the sides of the extensor pollicis longus tendon receive connections from the tendon of extensor pollicis brevis on the lateral side and from the insertion of adductor pollicis and first palmar interosseous muscles on the medial side.

Nerve Supply

By posterior interosseous nerve.

Arterial supply

Muscle belly by arterial twigs from posterior interosseous artery but tendon mainly from anterior interosseous artery.

Actions

Extension of thumb at interphalangeal and first carpometacarpal joints.

Testing Function of Extensor Pollicis Longus (EPL)

The subject is asked to extend the distal phalanx of thumb against resistance.

 CLINICAL CORRELATION

> **Rupture of EPL Tendon**
>
> The spontaneous rupture of EPL tendon may occur due to ischemia as a result of injury to anterior interosseous artery. This artery or its branches may be injured in Colles fracture. The tendon ruptures, where it changes direction around the Lister's tubercle. The patient feels that the thumb has **dropped** as the interphalangeal joint of the thumb cannot extend (hammer thumb deformity).

Extensor Indicis

Origin

From posterior surface of ulna below the origin of extensor pollicis longus.

Its tendon passes along with extensor digitorum tendons deep to the extensor retinaculum in the fourth compartment.

Insertion

Into dorsal digital expansion of index finger.

Nerve Supply

By posterior interosseous nerve.

Action

Extension of index finger.

Posterior Interosseous Nerve (Figs 19.10A and B)

This is the only nerve inside the posterior compartment of forearm. It is a purely motor nerve. It is the continuation of the deep branch of radial nerve in the cubital fossa.

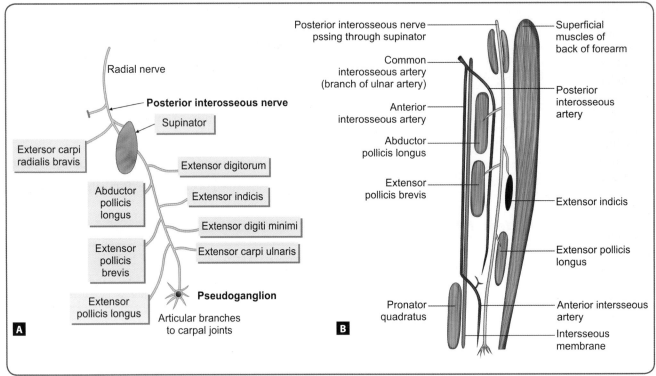

Figs 19.10A and B: A. Schematic diagram to show the distribution posterior interosseous nerve; **B.** Schematic diagram to show posterior interosseous nerve accompanied by posterior interosseous artery above and anterior interosseous artery below in the posterior compartment of forearm

As the nerve passes through the supinator it is closely related to the lateral aspect of the neck of radius. Then it enters the back of forearm by piercing the distal part of the supinator.

Course in Posterior Compartment

At first the posterior interosseous nerve lies between the superficial and deep extensor muscles. At the distal border of extensor pollicis brevis, it passes deep to extensor pollicis longus and directly rests on the interosseous membrane.

In its upper part, the posterior interosseous artery accompanies the nerve, but distally the anterior interosseous artery accompanies it.

The posterior interosseous nerve and anterior interosseous artery reach the dorsum of the carpus, where they occupy the fourth compartment deep to the extensor retinaculum. Here, the nerve terminates in a pseudoganglion.

Branches

- Before the posterior interosseous nerve enters the supinator it supplies extensor carpi radialis brevis and supinator in the cubital fossa.

- While passing through the supinator it gives additional branches to supinator.
- In its initial course at the back of forearm it gives three short branches to the extensor digitorum, extensor digiti minimi and extensor carpi ulnaris muscles of superficial set.
- Then it gives longer branches to extensor pollicis longus, extensor indicis, abductor pollicis longus and extensor pollicis brevis.
- It ends in to a pseudoganglion from which branches arise to supply the carpal joints.

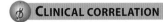 **CLINICAL CORRELATION**

PIN Syndrome

Posterior interosseous nerve (PIN) syndrome occurs if the nerve is compressed deep to the arcade of Frohse, which is a musculotendinous structure at the proximal edge of supinator muscle. The extensor carpi ulnaris is usually affected first so wrist extension causes radial deviation due to over-action of radial extensors. There is weakness of extension and abduction of thumb (thumb drop) besides weak extension of fingers (finger drop).

Posterior Interosseous Artery (Fig. 19.10B)

It is one of the terminal branches of the common interosseous artery, which arises from the ulnar artery in cubital fossa. It enters the posterior compartment through the gap between the upper margin of interosseous membrane and the oblique cord. It passes downwards between the supinator and abductor pollicis longus and accompanies the posterior interosseous nerve. It provides muscular branches and ends by anastomosing with a branch of anterior interosseous artery and by contributing a slender carpal branch to the dorsal carpal arch.

Anterior Interosseous Artery

The anterior interosseous artery enters the posterior compartment by piercing the interosseous membrane in the lower part of forearm. It accompanies the lower part of the posterior interosseous nerve up to the fourth compartment of the extensor retinaculum (Fig. 19.10B). It terminates by sending carpal branches to dorsal carpal arch.

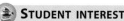 **STUDENT INTEREST**

The *posterior interosseous nerve* is the deep terminal branch of radial nerve in the cubital fossa. It enters the supinator muscle and travels downwards and backwards to enter the posterior compartment at the distal margin of supinator. It supplies three superficial muscles (extensor digitorum, extensor digiti minimi and extensor carpi ulnaris) and four deep muscles (abductor pollicis longus, extensor pollicis longus, extensor pollicis brevis and extensor indicis). The posterior interosseous nerve ends in the fourth compartment deep to the extensor retinaculum as a pseudoganglion from which branches arise to supply carpal and wrist joints. One peculiar feature of this nerve is that it is accompanied in its upper part by slender posterior interosseous artery and in its lower part by anterior interosseous artery. In summary, the posterior interosseous nerve supplies nine muscles of extensor compartment of forearm except anconeus, brachioradialis and extensor carpi radialis longus (which are supplied by radial nerve directly).

20

Radioulnar Joints and Wrist Joint

Chapter Contents

RADIOULNAR JOINTS

The radius and ulna articulate with each other by two synovial joints, the superior and inferior radioulnar joints and by the middle radioulnar joint, which is of fibrous variety (Fig. 20.1).

Superior Radioulnar Joint

This is the pivot type of synovial joint between the circumference of radial head and the radial notch on the upper end of the ulna (Fig. 20.1). The fibrous capsule of the elbow joint covers the superior radioulnar joint. The synovial membrane lines the annular ligament and the fibrous capsule internally and is continuous with that of the elbow joint.

Ligaments

- The **annular ligament** holds the head of radius against the radial notch of ulna. This strong ligament encircles the head of the radius and is attached to anterior and posterior margins of the radial notch of ulna. The annular ligament and the radial notch together form an osseofibrous ring (Fig. 20.2) for the head of the radius to rotate during pronation and supination.

- The **quadrate ligament** is a weak bond between the neck of radius and lower margin of radial notch of ulna.

CLINICAL CORRELATION

Pulled elbow (nursemaid's elbow)

There is a difference in the shape of the annular ligament in adults and children. In adults, the cup shaped ligament firmly grips the neck of radius (thus preventing its downward displacement). On the contrary, in children (below five years) the head tends to slip out of the ring due to the tubular shape of the ligament and the smaller circumference of the head of radius resulting in a pulled elbow or nursemaid's elbow.

Inferior Radioulnar Joint

This is the **pivot type of synovial joint** between the head of ulna and the ulnar notch on the lower end of radius. The fibrous capsule surrounds the joint cavity (Fig. 20.1). The synovial membrane lines the capsule and projects upwards between the interosseous membrane and the pronator quadratus as a narrow recess.

The articular disc is attached medially to a pit between the styloid process and the head of the ulna and laterally

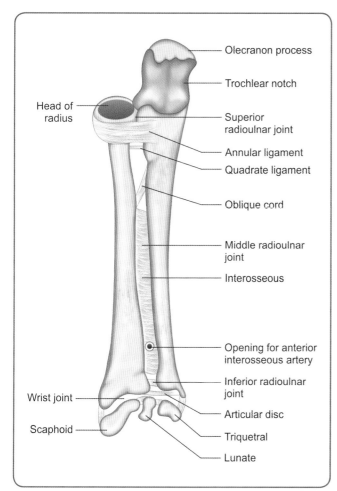

Fig. 20.1: Showing superior, middle and inferior radioulnar joints

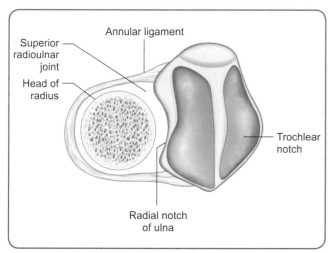

Fig. 20.2: Showing annular ligament encircling head of radius but attaching only to margins of radial notch of ulna

to the inferior margin of the ulnar notch of the radius. The disc excludes the ulna from the wrist joint.

Middle Radioulnar Joint

This is a longitudinally oriented joint between the shafts of the radius and ulna (Fig. 20.1). This is a syndesmosis type of fibrous joint. The oblique cord and the interosseous membrane are the connecting bonds between the two bones. The oblique cord extends from the lateral side of ulnar tuberosity to the lower limit of radial tuberosity.

Interosseous Membrane

The interosseous membrane is a thick sheet of collagenous tissue between the interosseous borders of radius and ulna. The fibers in the membrane are directed downwards and medially from radius to ulna. Proximally the membrane starts about 2–3 cm below the radial tuberosity and distally it reaches up to the level of distal radioulnar joint, where it fuses with the capsule of this joint.

Attachments and Relations of Anterior Surface

- Origin to flexor digitorum profundus, flexor pollicis longus and pronator quadratus.
- Anterior interosseous nerve and vessels are closely related to this surface.
- The anterior interosseous vessels pass through the interosseous membrane at the upper margin of the pronator quadratus to enter the posterior compartment. The anterior interosseous nerve descends up to the lower limit of the membrane.

Attachments and Relations of Posterior Surface

- Origin to abductor pollicis longus, extensor pollicis brevis, extensor pollicis longus and extensor indicis.
- Lower part of the posterior surface is closely related to the posterior interosseous nerve and anterior interosseous vessels.

Functions

- The interosseous membrane transmits the compression forces from radius to ulna.
- It increases the area of origin of deep muscles of the forearm.

Supination and Pronation (Figs 20.3A and B)

The superior and inferior radioulnar joints permit the movements of supination and pronation. The movements take place around a mobile vertical axis passing through

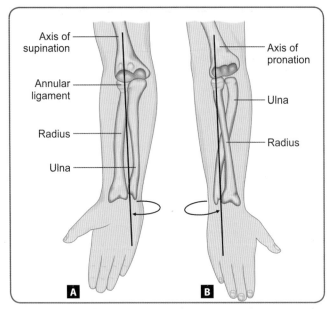

Figs 20.3A and B: Movements of supination and pronation of forearm. **A.** Supination and forearm **B.** Pronation of forearm

the center of the head of the radius and the lower end of ulna. The head of the radius rotates within the osseofibrous ring.

- In the *movement of pronation (Fig. 20.3B)*, the radius carrying the hand with it, turns anteromedially across the ulna with the result that the lower part of radius comes to lie medial to the ulna and the palm faces posteriorly.
- In the *movement of supination (Fig. 20.3B)*, the radius comes back to its position, lateral to ulna so that the palm faces anteriorly. The supination is a more powerful movement as is evident from the design of the screws. The supination is equated to the screwing movement while pronation to the unscrewing movement. The opening of a lock with the key in right hand is an example of supination while the action of locking with the key in right hand is an example of pronation.

🐾 STUDENT INTEREST

For eating food we need both supination and pronation (picking up food from the plate by pronation and putting it in mouth by supination). To make supination and pronation easier of students, the teachers in past used to bring in some humor by quoting such examples as—supination is the position of forearm and hand for begging and pronated forearm and hand are necessary to give blessings.

Muscles of Pronation (Fig. 20.4)

Pronator Teres

It takes origin by two heads. The humeral head is larger and more superficial than the ulnar head.

1. *Origin of humeral head:* From lower part of medial supracondylar ridge and from the common flexor origin on the front of medial epicondyle.
2. *Origin of ulnar head:* From medial margin of coronoid process of ulna.

   The two heads of origin unite with each other and the combined muscle passes obliquely across the proximal forearm.

- *Insertion:* Into area of maximum convexity on the lateral surface of radius.
- *Nerve supply:* By median nerve
- *Actions:* Pronator of forearm and weak flexor of forearm at elbow joint.

Note: The median nerve leaves the cubital fossa between the two heads of pronator teres. The ulnar artery passes deep to the deep head. Thus, the ulnar head of pronator teres is sandwiched between the median nerve and the ulnar artery.

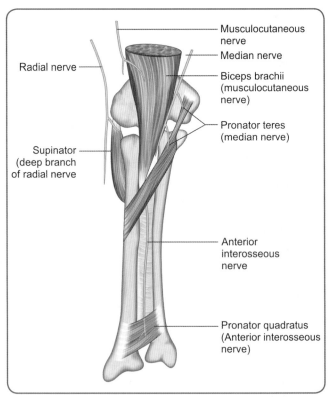

Fig. 20.4: Muscles of supination and pronation (Note all four muscles shown in the figure are inserted in to radius)

Testing Function of Pronator Teres

After flexing the elbow roughly to 20°, the subject is asked to supinate the forearm fully. After this the subject attempts to pronate the forearm against resistance. If normal, the contraction of the muscle is felt in upper part of forearm.

Pronator Quadratus

It is a quadrilateral and flat muscle, which is located deeply in the distal part of the forearm.

Origin

From the bony ridge on anterior surface of lower one fourth of the shaft of ulna.

Insertion

On the anterior surface of lower fourth of radius.

The muscle lies in contact with the anterior surface of the lower part of the interosseous membrane. The anterior interosseous nerve descends behind the posterior surface of the muscle. The space of Parona or deep forearm space lies between the long flexor tendons and the anterior surface of the pronator quadratus.

Nerve supply

By anterior interosseous branch of the median nerve.

Actions

Chief pronator of forearm (assisted by pronator teres only in rapid and forceful pronation).

Muscles of Supination (Fig. 20.4)

Biceps Brachii

This muscle is a powerful supinator. It is a muscle of the anterior compartment of arm (Fig. 17.2).

Origin of short head

From tip of coracoid process of scapula along with coracobrachialis.

Origin of long head

From supraglenoid tubercle of scapula.

The tendon of the long head is intracapsular but extrasynovial in position. It leaves the shoulder joint by passing beneath the transverse humeral ligament to enter the intertubercular sulcus. The synovial sheath covers the tendon up to the level of surgical neck of humerus.

The two heads fuse to form a fusiform belly, which ends in a flat tendon about 6–7 cm above the elbow. In the cubital fossa the tendon is in lateral relation to the brachial artery.

Insertion

Into the posterior part of the radial tuberosity. The extension from the medial border of the tendon is called **bicipital aponeurosis**. This extends medially in front of the brachial artery and median nerve to get attached to the deep fascia of the forearm and through it to the subcutaneous posterior border of ulna.

Nerve supply

By musculocutaneous nerve.

Actions

Acts on three joints (shoulder, elbow and superior radioulnar) since it crosses them:
1. On the **radioulnar joint** it acts as powerful supinator of the forearm. The biceps has its maximum supination power, when the elbow is flexed at right angle. In this position of the elbow the insertion of the biceps is in line with the rest of the muscle.
2. On the **elbow joint** its action is flexion.
3. On the **shoulder joint** it acts as flexor. The long head helps in stabilizing the head of humerus during movements of the shoulder joint.

Testing function of biceps

The subject flexes the elbow against resistance, when the forearm is supinated and extended.

CLINICAL CORRELATION

Biceps Reflex

A tap on the tendon of biceps at the cubital fossa by a tendon hammer produces brisk flexion of elbow joint. This tests the C5 spinal segment.

Popeye Sign and Deformity

When the biceps contracts to flex the elbow joint there is a prominent bulge of muscle belly (especially in body builders). This is called **Popeye sign**. When the tendon of long head of biceps ruptures (as in weight lifters or in swimmers) it causes a sudden appearance of a swelling in the lower part of the front of arm (Fig. 20.5). This is due to the detached muscle belly taking the shape of a ball. This appearance resembles the arm of a cartoon character named Popeye (hence called **Popeye deformity**).

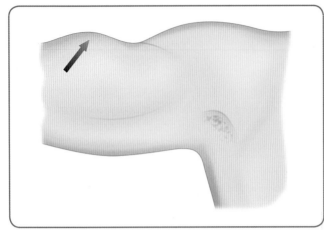

Fig. 20.5: Popeye deformity (indicated by arrow) in rupture of tendon of long head of biceps brachii

Supinator

The supinator belongs to the extensor compartment of forearm (Figs 20.6A and B). It is composed of two laminae (superficial and deep).

Origin of superficial lamina

By tendinous fibers from the lateral aspect of lateral epicondyle of humerus, radial collateral ligament of elbow joint and annular ligament (Fig. 20.6A).

Origin of deep lamina

By muscular fibers from supinator crest of ulna.

Insertion

Into the lateral surface of proximal third of radius between the anterior and posterior oblique lines (Fig. 20.6A).

Relations (Fig. 20.6B)

The supinator muscle lies deep in the distal part of the floor of cubital fossa. The deep branch of the radial nerve (posterior interosseous nerve) leaves the cubital fossa by entering the substance of the supinator at its proximal edge. The nerve travels between the two laminae and enters the posterior compartment just above the distal border of the supinator. The proximal edge of the superficial lamina is fibro-tendinous (called **arcade of Frohse**) in some

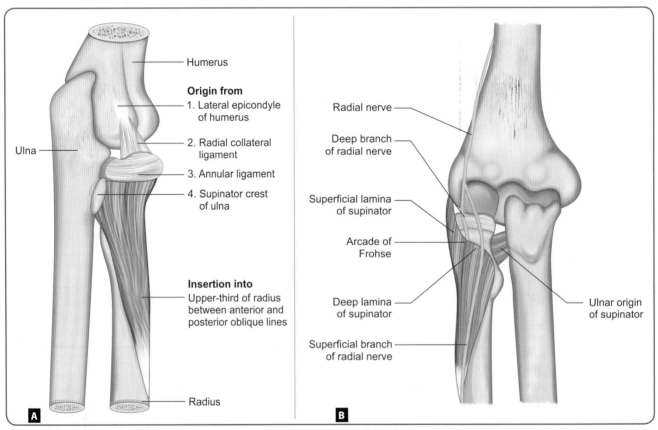

Figs 20.6A and B: A. Origin and insertion of supinator muscle; B. Relation of deep branch of radial nerve (posterior interosseous nerve) to supinator muscle

percentage of population. This is a site of compression of the posterior interosseous nerve, producing posterior interosseous nerve (PIN) syndrome.

Nerve supply

By posterior interosseous nerve usually before it enters the muscle and also as it passes through the muscle.

Actions

- Supination of the forearm in extended forearm.
- In flexed forearm the role of supinator is to fix the radius (the prime supinator being biceps brachii).

Testing Function of Supinator

The subject is asked to supinate forearm against resistance in extended and fully pronated position.

 STUDENT INTEREST

Movements of supination and pronation, muscles producing supination and pronation, radioulnar joints and interosseous membrane between radius and ulna must be studied by every student.

WRIST OR RADIOCARPAL JOINT

The wrist joint is an ellipsoid type of synovial joint permitting movements along two axes. The wrist joint is called the **radiocarpal joint** suggestive of the fact that among the forearm bones only the radius (and not the ulna) articulates with the carpus. This is a functional necessity as the radius alone carries the hand with it during pronation and supination.

Articulating Bones (Fig. 20.7)

- The **proximal articular surface** is formed by the concave area on the inferior surface of the lower end of the radius and the inferior surface of the articular disc of the inferior radioulnar joint.
- The **distal articular surface** is reciprocally convex. It is formed by the proximal surfaces of the scaphoid, lunate and triquetral bones from lateral to medial side.

Note: In anatomical position of the wrist, only the scaphoid and lunate are in contact with the radius and articular disc. In adduction or ulnar deviation of wrist, the triquetral comes in contact with the articular disc.

Surface Marking of Cavity of Wrist Joint

A line that is convex upward joining the tips of styloid processes of radius and ulna represents the wrist joint.

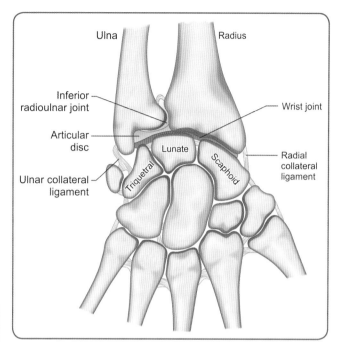

Fig. 20.7: Articulating bones of wrist joint (Note that articular disc of inferior radioulnar joint excluding head of ulna from taking part in wrist joint)

Ligaments

The joint is surrounded by the fibrous capsule, which is strengthened by the palmar and dorsal radiocarpal ligaments and the carpal collateral ligaments.

Fibrous Capsule

The fibrous capsule is attached to the articular margins of the proximal and distal articular areas, including the articular disc. It is lined by synovial membrane.

Radiocarpal Ligaments

- **Palmar radiocarpal ligament** is the thickening of anterolateral part of the capsule.
- **Palmar ulnocarpal ligament** is the thickening of anteromedial part of the capsule.
- **Dorsal radiocarpal ligament** is the thickening of dorsal aspect of the capsule.

  These ligaments are attached distally mainly to the proximal row of carpal bones and also to the capitate (a bone of distal row).

Collateral Carpal Ligaments

- **Radial collateral carpal ligament** extends from the styloid process of the radius to the scaphoid and trapezium.

- *Ulnar collateral carpal ligament* extends from the ulnar styloid process to the triquetral and pisiform.

Relations

- *Anteriorly:* Tendons of long flexor muscles (flexor pollicis longus, flexor digitorum superficialis and flexor digitorum profundus) and the median are close relations.
- *Posteriorly:* Tendons of long extensors of digits (extensor digitorum, extensor indicis and extensor digiti minimi) and the carpal extensors (extensor carpi ulnaris, extensor carpi radialis longus and brevis) along with extensor pollicis longus.
- *Laterally:* The radial artery in the anatomical snuffbox crosses the radial carpal collateral ligament between the tendons of abductor pollicis longus and extensor pollicis brevis.

Nerve Supply

The articular branches of anterior and posterior interosseous nerves supply the joint.

Arterial Supply

The palmar and dorsal carpal arches are the source of arterial supply. The carpal arches are the arterial anastomoses on the front and back of the wrist deep to the long tendons.

 ADDED INFORMATION

Arteries forming palmar carpal arch
- Palmar carpal branch of radial artery
- Palmar carpal branch of ulnar artery
- Descending branch of anterior interosseous artery
- Recurrent branches of deep palmar arch.

Arteries forming dorsal carpal arch
- Dorsal carpal branch of radial artery
- Dorsal carpal branch of ulnar artery
- Carpal branches of anterior interosseous artery
- Carpal branches of posterior interosseous artery.

Note: Anterior interosseous artery takes part in both palmar and dorsal carpal arches.

Movements of Wrist Joint

Flexion (Palmar Flexion or Upward Bending of Wrist)

- *Main flexor muscles:* Flexor carpi radialis and flexor carpi ulnaris.

- *Accessory flexor muscles:* Flexor digitorum superficialis, flexor digitorum profundus and flexor pollicis longus.

Extension (Dorsal Flexion or Backward Bending of Wrist)

- *Main extensor muscles:* Extensor carpi radialis longus, extensor carpi radialis brevis and extensor carpi ulnaris.
- *Accessory extensor muscles:* Extensor digitorum, extensor digiti minimi, extensor indicis, and extensor pollicis longus.

 ADDED INFORMATION

The extensor muscles of the wrist joint are synergistic with the flexor muscles of the digits. Therefore, one can make a tight fist only in the extended position of the wrist and conversely by flexing the wrist one can open the tight fist.

Adduction (Ulnar Deviation)

Adduction is the combined action of extensor carpi ulnaris and flexor carpi ulnaris muscles.

Abduction (Radial Deviation)

Abduction is the combined action of extensor carpi radialis longus and brevis and flexor carpi radialis muscles. The abductor pollicis longus and extensor pollicis brevis also assist.

 CLINICAL CORRELATION

Ganglion of wrist Joint
The ganglion is a localized cystic swelling on the dorsum of the wrist arising from either the capsule of the joint or from the synovial sheath surrounding the extensor tendons of the intercarpal joints. It usually presents as a painful lump and causes discomfort during the movements of the wrist.

Anatomical Snuffbox (Fig. 20.8)

This is a hollow space, which appears on the posterolateral side of the wrist in the fully extended position of the thumb.

Boundaries

- On the *ulnar side* (posteriorly) by the extensor pollicis longus tendon.
- On the *radial side* (anteriorly) by the tendons of abductor pollicis longus and extensor pollicis brevis.

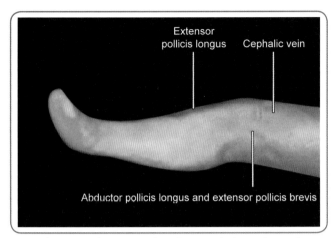

Fig. 20.8: Showing tendons forming the boundaries of anatomical snuff box

- The floor consists of four bony parts. In the proximal to distal order the bones are styloid process of radius, scaphoid, trapezium and base of the first metacarpal (Fig. 20.7).
- The superficial fascia forms the fascial roof, which is crossed by the cephalic vein and superficial branch of radial nerve.

Content

The radial artery passes via the anatomical snuffbox to the dorsum of the hand. Light pressure applied in the floor, pulsations of the radial artery are felt.

Retinacula at Wrist

The wrist is a junctional zone between the forearm and the hand. The tendons of the extensor muscles of the forearm cross the wrist from behind whereas the tendons of the flexor muscles cross in front. The deep fascia of the wrist is modified to form flexor and extensor retinacula to strap down these tendons.

Flexor Retinaculum

It is a square-shaped dense thickening of the deep fascia. Its size is 2.5 × 2.5 cm.

Medial and lateral attachments (Fig. 20.9)

- *Medially:* To pisiform bone and hook of hamate.
- *Laterally:* To tubercle of scaphoid and crest of trapezium.

Proximal and distal continuity

- *Proximally:* Continuous with the deep fascia of forearm.
- *Distally:* Continuous with palmar aponeurosis.

Surface Marking

Cup the palm of the hand by spreading the fingers (as though to grasp a large ball). The hollow between the proximal parts of the thenar and hypothenar eminences marks the position of flexor retinaculum distal to the distal flexure crease of the wrist.

Note: The flexor retinaculum is quite deep from the skin because its anterior surface is covered with origin of thenar and hypothenar muscles. The surgeon operating on flexor retinaculum for the first time must be aware of this fact.

Relations (Fig. 20.9)

Anterior or superficial to the retinaculum, five structures are related as follows—

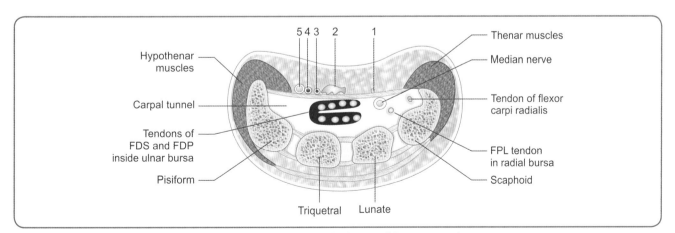

Fig. 20.9: Attachments and relations of flexor retinaculum

Key: (1) Palmar cutaneous branch of median nerve; (2) Tendon of palmaris longus; (3) Palmar cutaneous branch of ulnar nerve; (4) Ulnar artery; (5) Ulnar nerve

FDS, flexor digitorum superficialis; FDP, flexor digitorum profundus; FPL, flexor pollicis longus.

From medial to lateral:
1. Ulnar nerve
2. Ulnar vessels
3. Palmar cutaneous branch of ulnar nerve
4. Palmaris longus tendon
5. Palmar cutaneous branch of median nerve.

Special note: Ulnar nerve and vessels are protected in Guyon's canal inside the substance of the flexor retinaculum. The thenar and hypothenar muscles take origin from the anterior surface of the retinaculum.

- Posterior or deep to the retinaculum are the contents of the carpal tunnel as follows:
- Four tendons of flexor digitorum superficialis
- Four tendons of flexor digitorum profundus
- One tendon of flexor pollicis longus
- Median nerve

Tendon of flexor carpi radialis lies in a separate tunnel formed by the groove of trapezium posterior to the retinaculum.

 CLINICAL CORRELATION

Carpal tunnel syndrome (CTS)

This syndrome results due to compression of median nerve in the carpal tunnel. A few causes of CTS are chronic tenosynovitis (inflammation of the synovial sheath around tendons in the carpal tunnel), anterior dislocation of lunate bone and hypothyroidism.

Effects of median nerve compression

- The early symptoms are numbness, tingling and burning pain in lateral three and half fingers. The sensory loss develops in the same fingers in due course of time.
- Weakness of thenar muscles and flattening of thenar eminence are the symptoms and signs of loss of motor function. Gradually, it will lead to ape thumb deformity if left untreated.

Surgical treatment

Cutting of flexor retinaculum is one of the methods of relieving pressure on the median nerve.

Extensor Retinaculum (Fig. 20.10)

This is the rectangular thickening of deep fascia (about 3.5 cm long) on the back of the wrist.

Medial and lateral attachments

- *Medially:* To pisiform and triquetral.
- *Laterally:* To anterior border of lower end of radial shaft.

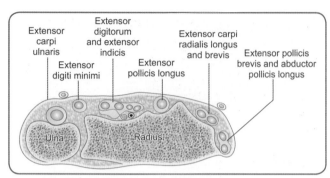

Fig. 20.10: Attachments and relations of extensor retinaculum

Proximal and distal continuity

- *Proximally:* Continuous with the deep fascia at the back of forearm.
- *Distally:* Continuous with deep fascia on the dorsum of hand.

Relations (Fig. 20.10)

- The posterior or superficial relations are the superficial branch of the radial nerve and the dorsal cutaneous branch of the ulnar nerve.
- From its anterior or deep aspect septa arise, which attach to the back of radius and ulna so that six osseofibrous compartments are formed for the passage of the extensor tendons. The compartments are numbered from lateral to medial side.

Contents of compartments

- Abductor pollicis longus and extensor pollicis brevis
- Extensor carpi radialis longus (ECRL) and extensor carpi radialis brevis (ECRB)
- Extensor pollicis longus
- Extensor digitorum and extensor indicis (along with posterior interosseous nerve and anterior interosseous artery).
- Extensor digiti minimi
- Extensor carpi ulnaris

STUDENT INTEREST

Flexor and extensor retinacula, their attachments and relations and carpal tunnel must be studied with full focus in mind. The carpal tunnel has nine tendons inside it (4 flexor digitorum superficialis (FDS), 4 flexor digitorum profundus (FDP) and 1 flexor pollicis longus (FPL)) and median nerve, which is the most important content. The long flexor tendons are covered with synovial sheath. In inflammation of synovial sheath in carpal tunnel the median nerve may be compressed producing symptoms and signs of carpal tunnel syndrome.

21

Hand

Chapter Contents

INTRODUCTION

The hand is the most functional part of the upper limb distal to the forearm. The skeleton of hand consists of the carpal bones, metacarpal bones and the phalanges in the digits. The digits are numbered from lateral to medial side. So the thumb is the first digit and little finger is the fifth digit. The dorsal and palmar aspects of hand have characteristic features.

DORSUM OF HAND

In striking contrast to the skin of palm, the skin on the dorsum is very thin and can be very easily pinched. The subcutaneous veins including the dorsal venous arch show through it clearly. If there is a deep-seated abscess in the palm, its outer sign in the form of swelling appears on the dorsum. This is due to availability of subcutaneous space on the dorsum for the lymph to accumulate. It is noteworthy that lymph flows from palmar to the dorsal aspect.

Spaces on Dorsum

The deep fascia of the dorsum is extremely thin and is attached to the extensor tendons, which are devoid of the synovial sheaths here. An aponeurotic layer is formed under the skin by inter-tendinous connections. So, the dorsum presents dorsal subcutaneous space and dorsal subaponeurotic space. The infection of the subaponeurotic space usually results from laceration of the knuckles, as for example in tooth bite on the fist.

Structures on Dorsum

- Dorsal venous network or arch (Fig. 16.3).
- Cutaneous (sensory) nerves (Fig. 21.1) and vessels.
- Long extensor tendons of the digits (Fig. 21.2).

Dorsal Venous Arch (Fig. 16.3)

For description of dorsal venous arch, refer to chapter 16.

Sensory Nerves on Dorsum (Fig. 21.1)

- **Dorsal digital branches** of superficial branch of radial nerve supply the skin of the radial side of the hand as well as the lateral three and half digits up to the level of approximately the middle of middle phalanx.
- **Dorsal cutaneous branches** of ulnar nerve supply the ulnar side of dorsum and medial one and half digits up to the level of distal interphalangeal joint.
- **Palmar digital branches** of median nerve reach the dorsal aspect over the tips of digits to supply the nail beds of lateral three and half digits.

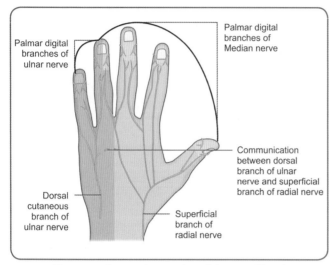

Fig. 21.1: Sensory innervation of dorsum of hand

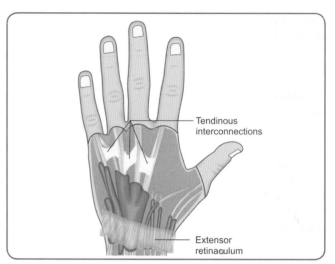

Fig. 21.2: Extensor tendons surrounded by synovial sheath on the dorsum of hand

- *Palmar digital branches* of ulnar nerve supply the nail beds of medial one and half digits.

Arteries of Dorsum

The dorsal metacarpal arteries are the main supply of the dorsum. Corresponding to the four interosseous spaces there are four metacarpal arteries. On reaching the bases of the digits the metacarpal arteries divide into dorsal digital arteries for the supply of the adjacent fingers.

- The first dorsal metacarpal artery is a branch of radial artery, which is given off before leaving the dorsum between the two heads of first dorsal interosseous muscle.
- The second, third and fourth dorsal metacarpal arteries are the branches of dorsal carpal arch.

Connections of Dorsal Metacarpal Arteries

- *Proximally*, the proximal perforating arteries from the deep palmar arch reinforce the medial three metacarpal arteries.
- *Distally*, the distal perforating arteries connect the dorsal metacarpal arteries to the common palmar digital arteries (arising from superficial palmar arch).

Extensor Tendons on Dorsum (Fig. 21.2)

The long extensor tendons enter the dorsum after passing deep to the extensor retinaculum. All the tendons are covered with synovial sheath. They cross the dorsum to reach the digits for insertion.

- *The extensor digitorum tendons* of the medial four digits are connected by tendinous interconnections, which restrict the independent movements of the digits.

- The tendon of *extensor digiti minimi usually* splits in two on the dorsum. The extensor digiti minimi and extensor indicis tendons fuse with the respective tendons of the extensor digitorum distal to the tendinous interconnection.
- The *extensor tendons form a dorsal expansion* over the respective metacarpophalangeal (MCP) joints and the proximal phalanges. The extensor expansion provides insertion not only to the extensor tendons but also to the interosseous and lumbrical muscles. The details of the parts of extensor expansion are described along with interossei and lumbrical muscles.
- The *extensor expansion is not* present in the thumb. The abductor pollicis longus does not reach the thumb phalanx. The tendon of extensor pollicis longus reaches the terminal phalanx. The tendon of extensor pollicis brevis sends a connection to the tendon of extensor pollicis longus on the proximal phalanx from the lateral aspect. The tendon of extensor pollicis longus receives similar connection from the insertion of first palmar interosseous and the adductor pollicis on medial aspect.

PALM

The palm houses twenty intrinsic muscles of the hand, nine long flexor tendons, ulnar and median nerves and the palmar arterial arches. These structures are wrapped in fascial layers of palm in four definite compartments.

External Appearance

The skin of the palmar aspect of hand is of thick glabrous type with abundant sweat glands. The skin presents characteristic papillary ridges, which are responsible for the fingerprints.

Flexure Lines

The palmar skin is firmly anchored to the deep fascia at the skin creases (flexure lines) of palm.

Transverse Palmar Creases

- The *distal palmar crease* (heart line) lies just proximal to the metacarpophalangeal joints (MCP joints).
- The *proximal palmar crease* is called the *headline*.
  In Down syndrome (Trisomy-21), there is a single transverse crease on the palm (simian crease).

Longitudinal Palmar Crease

There is one longitudinally oriented crease laterally. On its lateral side there is an elevated area called *thenar eminence*. A less well-marked area on the medial side is known as hypothenar eminence.

Flexure Creases on Fingers

- The *proximal crease* at the root of the finger is situated about 2–3 cm distal to the heart line.
- The *middle crease* of each finger lies at the level of proximal interphalangeal (PIP) joint.
- The *distal crease* of each finger lies proximal to distal interphalangeal (DIP) joint.

Superficial Fascia of Palm

The superficial fascia contains subcutaneous fat interspersed with dense fibrous tissue. This connects the skin of palm firmly to palmar aponeurosis (modified deep fascia). The superficial transverse metacarpal ligament at the web margins of the hand is a modification of superficial fascia. The palmaris brevis muscle is located in the superficial fascia.

Palmaris Brevis (Fig. 21.3)

The palmaris brevis is a subcutaneous muscle (representing panniculus carnosus of quadrupeds) seen on the medial side across the base of hypothenar eminence.

Origin

From flexor retinaculum and palmar aponeurosis near its apex.

Insertion

Into the dermis of medial margin of hand.

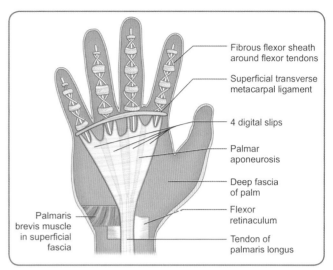

Fig. 21.3: Palmar aponeurosis and its four digital slips for medial four digits

Nerve supply

By superficial branch of ulnar nerve.

Action

Improving the grip of the hand.

Palmar Aponeurosis (Fig. 21.3)

The palmar aponeurosis is a triangular thickening of deep fascia in the central region of the palm. It has an apex pointed proximally and a base pointed distally.

- The apex is continuous with flexor retinaculum and the tendon of palmaris longus.
- The base extends distally to the level of distal palmar crease, where it splits into four digital slips for the medial four digits. Each slip divides into two slips.
- The deep slip is attached to deep transverse metacarpal ligament, capsule of corresponding MCP joint, base of proximal phalanx and to fibrous flexor sheath of corresponding digit.
- The superficial slip is attached to the superficial transverse metacarpal ligament and the skin.
- The medial palmar septum connects the medial margin of palmar aponeurosis to the fifth metacarpal bone.
- The lateral palmar septum arises from lateral margin of palmar aponeurosis and is attached to first metacarpal bone.
  These septa divide the palm into fascial compartments.

Functions

- The palmar aponeurosis protects the nerves and vessels inside the palm.
- It helps to improve the grip of the hand.

Dupuytren's Contracture

The medial part of the palmar aponeurosis undergoes progressive shortening in this condition. This exerts pull on the little and ring fingers causing flexion deformity in them. The surgical cutting of the shortened part of the aponeurosis (fasciotomy) is done to straighten the bent fingers.

Fibrous Flexor Sheath (Fig. 21.3)

The fibrous flexor sheath is the thickened deep fascia on all five digits. It has a very thick and unique structure (consisting of five dense and stiff annular pulleys and three thin and lax cruciform pulleys). The sheath is attached to the margins of the phalanges.

Extent

The sheath extends from the level of head of metacarpal bone to the base of distal phalanx. Thus, the phalanges and the sheath together form an osseofibrous tunnel in each digit. The tunnel is closed distally by the attachment of the sheath to the phalanx beyond the insertion of flexor pollicis longus in thumb and flexor digitorum profundus in other fingers.

Contents

The sheath for the thumb houses one tendon of flexor pollicis longus whereas the sheaths for the other digits house two tendons, one each of flexor digitorum superficialis and flexor digitorum profundus. The tendons are surrounded by synovial sheath to allow their frictionless movements inside the tunnel. The arteries are carried to the tendon by the synovial folds, the vincula longa and

brevia. The vincula longa are located near the roots of the fingers whereas the vincula brevia are found closer to the insertion of the tendons.

Fascial Compartments of Palm (Fig 21.4)

The deep fascia of the palm is disposed in two layers, which wrap the intrinsic muscles, the long flexor tendons, the nerves and vessels of the palm. The deep fascia of palm covering the thenar and hypothenar areas turns posteriorly around the margins of these areas to become continuous with the deeper layer of fascia covering the anterior surfaces of the metacarpals, the interosseous muscles between them, and the adductor pollicis muscle. These two layers (superficial and deep) of deep fascia are connected to each other by means of medial and lateral palmar septa. In this way the palm is divided into four fascial compartments—thenar, hypothenar, intermediate and adductor.

1. The ***thenar compartment*** contains abductor pollicis brevis, flexor pollicis brevis and opponens pollicis.
2. The ***hypothenar compartment*** contains abductor digiti minimi, flexor digiti minimi, and opponens digiti minimi.
3. The ***intermediate compartment*** contains the long flexor tendons surrounded by synovial sheaths, lumbricals, palmar arterial arches and the branches of median and ulnar nerves.
4. The ***adductor compartment*** contains only the adductor pollicis muscle.

Palmar Spaces (Fig. 21.4)

The ***palmar spaces*** are known as the fascial spaces of palm. Under normal conditions there are no well-defined fascial spaces inside the fascial compartments of palm. However,

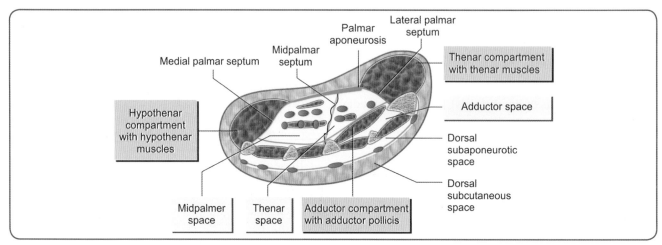

Fig. 21.4: Cross section of hand to show fascial compartments (labeled in pink boxes) and fascial spaces (labeled in blue boxes)

these fascial spaces become apparent in the intermediate fascial compartment only if there is collection of pus. A new septum called ***midpalmar septum*** (or intermediate palmar septum) develops in this compartment to divide it into thenar and midpalmar spaces.

The following spaces are included under the term palmar spaces.
- Midpalmar space
- Thenar space
- Web spaces
- Pulp spaces
- Forearm space of parona.

Boundaries of Midpalmar Space

- ***Anteriorly (from superficial to deep):*** Palmar aponeurosis, superficial palmar arch, flexor tendons of medial three digits covered with common synovial sheath (ulnar bursa) and medial three lumbrical muscles.
- ***Posteriorly:*** Deep layer of deep fascia covering 3rd and 4th interossei and 3rd to 5th metacarpal bones.
- ***Medially:*** Medial palmar septum.
- ***Laterally:*** Midpalmar septum.
- ***Proximally:*** Midpalmar space extends up to the level of distal margin of flexor retinaculum, where normally it is closed (but sometimes may extend deep to the retinaculum).
- ***Distally:*** Midpalmar space extends up to the level of distal palmar crease beyond which it communicates with fourth and third lumbrical canals (Fig. 21.5).

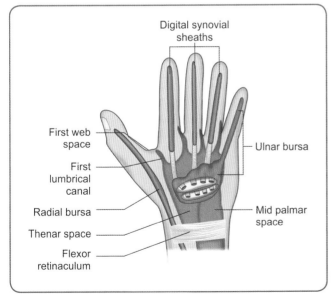

Fig. 21.5: Synovial sheath around flexor pollicis longus (radial bursa), Synovial sheath around long flexor tendons of medial 4 digits (ulnar bursa) and digital synovial sheaths of middle three digits

Boundaries of Thenar Space

- ***Anteriorly (from superficial to deep):*** Palmar aponeurosis, superficial palmar arch, flexor tendons of flexor pollicis longus covered with a synovial sheath (radial bursa) and the first lumbrical muscle.
- ***Posteriorly:*** Deep layer of deep fascia covering the adductor pollicis muscle.
- ***Medially:*** Midpalmar septum.
- ***Laterally:*** Lateral palmar septum.
- ***Proximally:*** Thenar space extends up to the level of distal margin of flexor retinaculum, where normally it is closed (but sometimes may extend deep to the retinaculum).
- ***Distally:*** Thenar space extends up to the level of distal palmar crease beyond which it communicates with first lumbrical canal.

Relation of Palmar Spaces to Radial and Ulnar Bursae (Fig. 21.5)

- The ***radial bursa*** is the synovial sheath surrounding the flexor pollicis longus tendon. It extends from the forearm (2 cm proximal to the proximal margin of flexor retinaculum) to the level of the base of terminal phalanx of thumb. The radial bursa is closely related to thenar space.
- The ***ulnar bursa*** is the common synovial sheath surrounding the tendons of flexor digitorum superficialis and flexor digitorum profundus. It extends from the forearm (2 cm proximal to proximal margin of flexor retinaculum) to the mid-palm level where the ulnar bursa ends as a cul–de-sac but retains its continuity with the digital sheath around the flexor tendons of the little finger. The ulnar bursa and its distal extension in the little finger are closely related anteriorly to midpalmar space. Beyond the cul-de-sac, the tendons of index, middle and ring fingers are devoid of synovial sheath until they enter the fibrous flexor sheath.

🔊 CLINICAL CORRELATION

Tenosynovitis

Tenosynovitis means inflammation of synovial sheath surrounding a tendon. The tenosynovitis of little finger can infect the ulnar bursa. Similarly, tenosynovitis of thumb can infect the radial bursa. The inflamed ulnar bursa can burst into the midpalmar space and the inflamed radial bursa can burst into the thenar space causing abscesses in these spaces.
- With the current trend of liberal use of antibiotics to control infections, the occurrence of abscesses in palmar spaces is much reduced.

Contd…

Contd...

CLINICAL CORRELATION

Lumbrical Canals

If pus collects in the thenar or midpalmar spaces it is drained through lumbrical canals, which are spaces around lumbrical muscles. They open distally into web spaces.
- The midpalmar space communicates with third and fourth web spaces via corresponding lumbrical canals. Hence incision may be placed in the third or fourth web space to open the lumbrical canal to let out the pus.
- The thenar space communicates with first web space via first lumbrical canal. Hence first web space is incised to open the first lumbrical canal to let out the pus.

(**Note:** If midpalmar and thenar spaces are analogous to pus tanks then lumbrical canals are the pus taps, which can be opened in web spaces to let out the pus).

Web Spaces

There are four subcutaneous spaces within the folds of skin connecting the bases of the proximal phalanges. Each web space has a free margin. The web space extends from its free margin up to the level of metacarpophalangeal joint. The web space contains subcutaneous fat, superficial transverse metacarpal ligament, tendon of interosseous and lumbrical and digital nerves and vessels.

Pulp Space (Fig. 21.6)

The pulp space is a subcutaneous space between the distal phalanx and the skin of the terminal digit. It is closed proximally by the fusion of the fibrous flexor sheath (deep fascia) to the skin of the digit at the distal crease on the anterior aspect and by fusion of the deep fascia to the

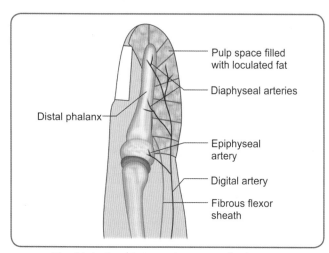

Fig. 21.6: Boundaries and contents of pulp space

periosteum of terminal phalanx on the posterior aspect. The pulp space contains subcutaneous fatty tissue (which is loculated by tough fibrous septa) and digital nerves and vessels.

Arterial Supply of Distal Phalanx

Before entering the pulp space the digital artery gives off its epiphyseal branch to the proximal one fifth of the distal phalanx. After entering the space the diaphyseal branches arise. They supply the distal four fifth of the phalanx.

CLINICAL CORRELATION

Whitlow or Felon

An abscess in the pulp space is **called whitlow** or **felon**. Being the most exposed part of the finger the pulp space is frequently injured and infected. When abscess forms in it there is throbbing pain due to increased tension in the closed space. The complication of whitlow is avascular necrosis of the distal four fifth of the distal phalanx due to thrombosis of the diaphyseal branches of the digital artery. This complication can be avoided if the abscess is drained at the right time by placing a small incision on the point of maximum tenderness.

ADDED INFORMATION

Forearm Space or Space of Parona

Though it is located in the forearm, the space of parona is included under palmar spaces because it is in continuity with the palmar spaces behind the flexor tendons through the carpal tunnel. The space of parona is bounded anteriorly by long flexor tendons wrapped in synovial sheaths and posteriorly by pronator quadratus muscle. Very rarely this space is filled with pus if the inflamed radial or ulnar bursa bursts here.

STUDENT INTEREST

The fascial spaces of hand (midpalmar, thenar, pulp spaces, web spaces, lumbrical canals etc) are of surgical importance. Learn by drawing cross section of hand showing compartments and fascial spaces. Remember that anatomy of hand including the interossei, lumbricals, adductor pollicis, thenar and hypothenar muscles, nerves, vessels and tendons is a must know topic.

ARTERIES OF HAND

The hand is provided with abundant blood supply through branches of the radial and ulnar arteries, which form the superficial and deep palmar arterial arches.

Superficial Palmar Arch (Fig. 21.7)

This arterial arch is located between the palmar aponeurosis and the long flexor tendons.

Modes of Completion

The superficial branch of the ulnar artery continues in the palm as superficial palmar arch. The completion of the arch on the lateral side is variable.

- In the most common mode, superficial palmar branch of radial artery joins the superficial branch of ulnar artery.
- Sometimes either the princeps pollicis or the radialis indicis (branches of radial artery) may complete the arch.
- Rarely the median artery, a branch of anterior interosseous artery completes the arch.

Branches

Three common palmar digital arteries and one proper digital artery arise from the convexity of the arch.

- Common palmar digital arteries are reinforced by palmar metacarpal arteries (branches of deep palmar arch), which join them nearer the webs. Each artery divides into two proper digital arteries. The six proper digital arteries thus formed supply the adjacent sides of the medial four fingers.
- Proper digital artery (arising directly from the arch, supplies medial side of little finger).

Surface Marking

A distally convex line drawn from the distal border of fully extended thumb across the palm to meet the hook of the hamate represents the superficial arch.

Deep Palmar Arch (Fig. 21.8)

This arterial arch is located deep in the palm between the flexor tendons in front and the interossei muscles and the metacarpal bones behind.

Formation

The continuation of the radial artery in the palm mainly forms the deep palmar arch, which is completed on the medial side by the deep branch of ulnar artery. The deep branch of the ulnar nerve lies in the concavity of the arch.

Branches

- Three palmar metacarpal arteries join the common palmar digital arteries (branches of superficial palmar arch).
- Three perforating arteries pass through the second, third and fourth interosseous spaces to anastomose with the dorsal metacarpal arteries.
- Recurrent arteries turn proximally and pass in front of the carpus to take part in the formation of palmar carpal arch.

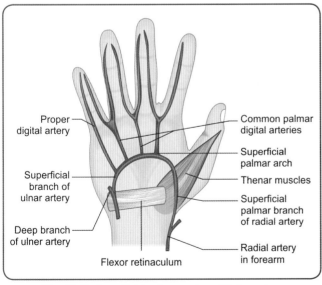

Fig. 21.7: Superficial palmar arch and its branches

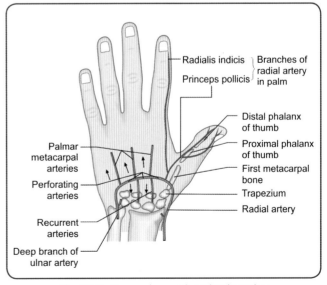

Fig. 21.8: Deep palmar arch and its branches

Surface Marking

A 4 cm-long horizontal line drawn across the palm from a point just distal to the hook of hamate represents the deep palmar arch. It is 1 to 1.5 cm proximal to the superficial palmar arch.

♪ CLINICAL CORRELATION

Bleeding Injury of Palmar Arterial Aches

Injury to palmar arterial arches causes uncontrollable bleeding. The compression of the brachial artery against the humerus (Fig. 16.5) is the most effective method to arrest bleeding. Tying or clamping the radial or ulnar or both radial and ulnar arteries proximal to the wrist fails to control the bleeding because of the communications between the palmar and dorsal carpal arches with the palmar arches.

Note: The anterior and posterior interosseous arteries arising from proximal part of ulnar artery contribute to carpal arches.

NERVES OF PALM

Median Nerve in Palm (Fig. 21.9)

The median nerve enters the palm under the distal margin of flexor retinaculum from the carpal tunnel. It divides almost immediately into six branches as follows:

- Recurrent branch is the most lateral branch and is short and thick. It turns proximally on the distal margin of the flexor retinaculum to enter the thenar muscles to supply abductor pollicis brevis, opponens pollicis and the superficial head of flexor pollicis brevis.
- First proper palmar digital branch supplies the radial side of the thumb.

- Second proper palmar digital branch supplies the medial side of the thumb.
- Third proper palmar digital branch supplies the radial side of the index finger and also gives a motor branch to the first lumbrical muscle (motor twig enters muscle from its superficial aspect).
- Lateral common palmar digital branch gives a motor twig to the second lumbrical muscle (motor twig enters the muscle from its superficial aspect). Then it divides into two proper palmar digital branches for the adjacent sides of index and middle fingers.
- Medial common palmar digital branch divides into two branches for the adjacent sides of middle and ring fingers.

All the proper palmar digital branches cross over the tips of the respective digits and supply the nail bed as well some variable area on the dorsal aspect of digits beyond the nail bed.

Ulnar Nerve in Palm

The ulnar nerve terminates on the anterior surface of the flexor retinaculum in close relation to the pisiform bone into a smaller superficial and a larger deep branch.

The superficial branch of ulnar nerve (Fig. 21.10) enters the palm under cover of the palmaris brevis muscle, which it supplies and then divides into one proper digital and one common digital branch. The proper digital branch supplies the medial side of little finger and the common digital branch divides to supply adjacent sides of little and ring fingers.

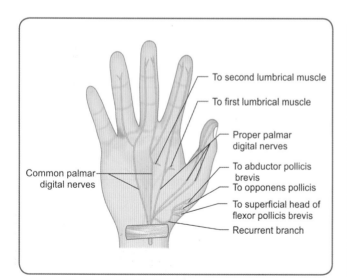

Fig. 21.9: Distribution of median nerve in palm

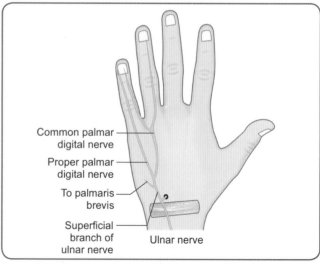

Fig. 21.10: Distribution of superficial branch of ulnar nerve in palm

The digital nerves cross over the tips of digits to supply the nail bed and adjacent area of terminal digit.

Digital Nerve Block (Fig. 21.11)

This procedure is necessary while draining abscesses on digits or repairing the tendons in digits to name a few. There are four digital nerves per digit (two palmar and two dorsal). To achieve full anesthesia, needle is inserted on either side of the base of the digit from dorsal aspect to inject anesthetic agent.

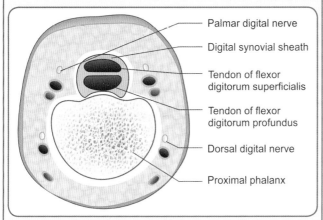

Palmar digital nerve

Digital synovial sheath

Tendon of flexor digitorum superficialis

Tendon of flexor digitorum profundus

Dorsal digital nerve

Proximal phalanx

Fig. 21.11: Cross section of base of proximal digit to show digital nerves (to be blocked during surgery on finger)

INTRINSIC MUSCLES OF HAND

There are twenty intrinsic muscles located inside the palm. They are described into four groups—(1) subcutaneous (palmaris brevis), (2) hypothenar muscles (muscles acting on little finger), (3) thenar muscles (muscles acting on thumb) including adductor pollicis, and (4) muscles acting on fingers (interossei and lumbricals).

Hypothenar Muscles

- Abductor digiti minimi medially (on superficial plane).
- Flexor digiti minimi laterally (on superficial plane).
- Opponens digiti minimi (on a deeper plane).

Abductor Digiti Minimi

Origin

From pisiform bone, pisohamate ligament and the tendon of flexor carpi ulnaris.

Insertion

Into ulnar side of the base of proximal phalanx of little finger.

Action

Abduction of the little finger away from the fourth finger.

Nerve supply

By deep branch of ulnar nerve.

Testing function of abductor digiti minimi

This is the first muscle to show weakness in ulnar nerve lesion, hence it is essential to know to test its function. The subject is asked to place the back of the hand on the table and to abduct the little finger against resistance.

Flexor Digiti Minimi (Flexor Digiti Minimi Brevis)

Origin

From the hook of hamate and adjoining flexor retinaculum.

Insertion

Into the ulnar side of the base of proximal phalanx of little finger.

Action

Flexion of little finger at MCP joint.

Nerve supply

By deep branch of ulnar nerve.

Testing function of flexor digiti minimi

The subject is asked to flex the MCP joint of little finger against resistance.

This muscle is tested clinically in suspected cases of ulnar nerve lesion, since the loss of function of this muscle may be the only sign initially.

Opponens Digiti Minimi

Origin

Common with flexor digiti minimi.

Insertion

Into ulnar side of the shaft of fifth metacarpal bone.

Actions

Flexion of fifth metacarpal bone as in the act of deepening the hollow of the palm.

Nerve supply

By deep branch of ulnar nerve.

Thenar Muscles

- Abductor pollicis brevis laterally (on the superficial plane).
- Flexor pollicis brevis medially (on the superficial plane).
- Opponens pollicis (on a deeper plane).

Abductor Pollicis Brevis

Origin

From tubercle of scaphoid, trapezium and the adjoining part of flexor retinaculum.

Insertion

Into lateral side of base of proximal phalanx of thumb.

Action

Abducts the thumb

Nerve supply

Recurrent branch of median nerve.

Testing function of abductor pollicis brevis

The subject is asked to abduct the thumb in a plane at right angles to the palmar aspect of index finger against the resistance of examiner's thumb.

This muscle is tested clinically, in case of median nerve compression in the carpal tunnel. It is the first muscle to show weakness in carpal tunnel syndrome.

Flexor Pollicis Brevis

Origin of superficial head

From flexor retinaculum and the tubercle of trapezium.

Origin of deep head

From capitate and trapezoid bones.

Insertion

Into the lateral side of the base of the proximal phalanx of thumb.

Action

Flexor to thumb.

Nerve supply

Superficial head by recurrent branch of median nerve and deep head by deep branch of ulnar nerve.

Note: There is usually a sesamoid bone at the site of insertion flexor pollicis brevis.

Opponens Pollicis

Origin

From the tubercle of trapezium and the adjacent part of flexor retinaculum.

Insertion

Into lateral half of palmar surface of first metacarpal bone.

Action

Flexion and medial rotation of first metacarpal bone so as to help in opposition of the thumb.

Nerve supply

By recurrent branch of median nerve.

Testing function of opponens pollicis

This muscle is tested by asking the subject to touch the tip of little finger with the point of thumb or by asking the subject to make a circle with the thumb and index finger.

 STUDENT INTEREST

Remember that flexor pollicis brevis is a composite muscle as each head is supplied by separate nerve.

Adductor Pollicis (Fig. 21.12)

This muscle has two heads of origin.

Origin of oblique head

From capitate bone and bases of the second and third metacarpal bones. Origin of transverse head—from palmar aspect of third metacarpal bone.

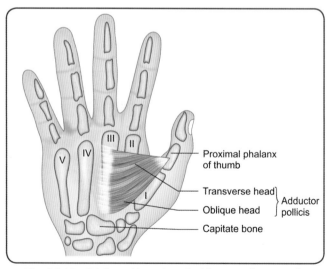

Fig. 21.12: Origin and insertion of adductor pollicis muscle

Insertion

By a common tendon into medial side of base of proximal phalanx of thumb.

Action

Adduction of thumb (from the abducted position).

Nerve supply

By deep branch of ulnar nerve.

Testing function of adductor pollicis

When the patient pinches a piece of paper between thumb and index finger (or grasps a book firmly between the thumbs and other fingers of both hands), the thumb on the affected side flexes at interphalangeal (IP) joint. This is due to weakness of adductor pollicis muscle (supplied by ulnar nerve), which permits uncontrolled contraction of flexor pollicis longus (supplied by anterior interosseous nerve).

Lumbrical Muscles (Fig. 21.13)

Lumbrical is a Latin word, which means earthworm. The shape of the lumbrical muscle is like that of earthworm. The lumbricals are four tiny muscles, which are numbered one to four from lateral to medial side.

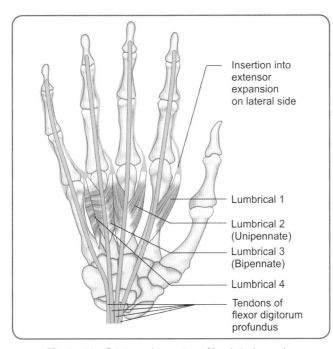

Insertion into extensor expansion on lateral side

Lumbrical 1

Lumbrical 2 (Unipennate)

Lumbrical 3 (Bipennate)

Lumbrical 4

Tendons of flexor digitorum profundus

Fig. 21.13: Origin and insertion of lumbrical muscles

TABLE 21.1: Comparative Features of Lateral and Medial Lumbricals

Features	Lateral lumbricals	Medial lumbricals
Number	First and second	Third and fourth
Type	Unipennate	Bipennate
Nerve supply	Digital branches of median nerve	Deep branch of ulnar nerve
Point of nerve entry	Superficial surface	Deep surface

Origin of:

- *The first and second lumbricals:* From lateral side of the respective tendons of flexor digitorum profundus (FDP).
- *The third and fourth lumbricals:* From adjacent sides of the tendons of FDP going to the middle and ring fingers and of FDP tendons going to ring and little fingers respectively.
- Each lumbrical muscle ends in a tendon which enters its corresponding web space and turns dorsally along the lateral side of MCP joint.

Insertion

- Into lateral basal angle of corresponding extensor expansion.
  The lumbricals are the connecting link between the flexor and extensor tendons of the digits (Fig. 21.14). A connective tissue sheath called *lumbrical canal* surrounds each lumbrical tendon (for clinical importance of these canals read palmar spaces).

Actions

Flexion of metacarpophalangeal joints and extension of interphalangeal joints.

Nerve supply

Lateral two lumbricals by median nerve and medial two lumbricals by deep branch of ulnar nerve.

Testing function of lumbricals

The subject is asked to flex the metacarpophalangeal joint of the extended finger (being tested) against resistance.

Palmar Interossei (Fig. 21.15A) and Dorsal Interossei (Fig. 21.15B)

Both palmar and dorsal interossei consist of four muscles. The interossei are numbered one to four from lateral to medial side. The first palmar interosseous is not well developed. It works in unison with adductor pollicis. The

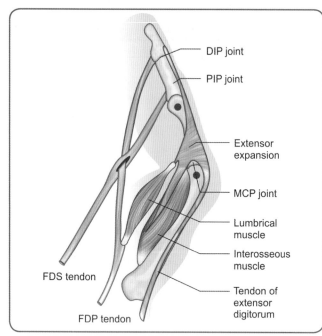

Fig. 21.14: Insertion of flexor digitorum superficialis and flexor digitorum profundus on ventral aspect of phalanges and attachment of extensor digitorum, interossei and lumbricals on dorsal aspect via extensor expansion
Key: DIP–Dorsal Interphalangeal Joint; PID–Proximal Interphalangeal Joint

palmar interossei are unipennate whereas the dorsal interossei are bipennate muscles. The palmar interossei are adductors of fingers and dorsal interossei are abductors. The central axis of adduction and abduction passes through the middle finger.

Nerve Supply

By deep branch of the ulnar nerve.

Adduction of Fingers

The palmar interossei are adductors as they adduct the finger to which they are attached towards the middle finger as follows:
• Second palmar interosseous adducts the index finger.
• Third palmar interosseous adducts the ring finger.
• Fourth palmar interosseous adducts the little finger.

Abduction of Fingers

The dorsal interossei are abductors of the middle three fingers. They move the fingers away from the central axis passing through middle finger as follows:
• First dorsal interosseous abducts the index finger away from the middle finger.
• Second dorsal interosseous abducts the middle finger on the radial side.
• Third dorsal interosseous abducts the middle finger on the ulnar side.
• Fourth dorsal interosseous abducts ring finger away from the middle finger.

Note: That there are two dorsal interossei for middle finger but the little finger has no dorsal interosseous muscle (since it is having its own abductor digiti minimi).

⚖ Student interest

The *interossei* and *lumbricals* produce flexion of metacarpophalangeal joints and extension of interphalangeal joints. When all interossei and lumbricals act together they produce Z movement (Practice Z movement on your own hand). A mnemonic to remember the actions of palmar and dorsal interossei—PAD and DAB = palmar adductors and dorsal abductors

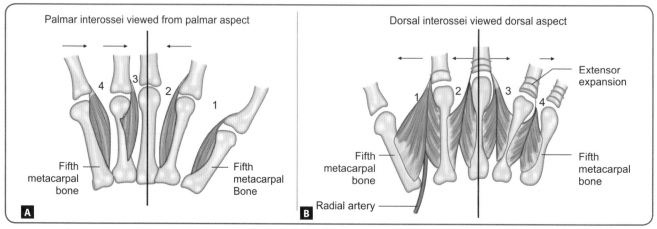

Figs 21.15A and B: A. Palmar interossei viewed from palmar aspect; **B.** Dorsal interossei viewed from dorsal aspect

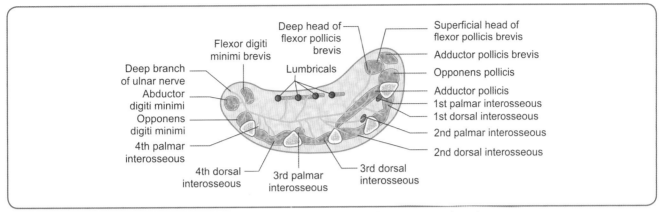

Fig. 21.16: Distribution of deep branch of ulnar nerve in the palm

Deep Branch of Ulnar Nerve (Fig. 21.16)

The deep branch of ulnar nerve begins near the pisiform bone and enters the hypothenar compartment of palm. It turns laterally around the hook of the hamate and crosses the palm. It travels in mediolateral direction across the palm lying in the concavity of deep palmar arch and posterior to the flexor tendons.

Distribution

Hypothenar muscles—3
Lumbrical muscles—2
Palmar and dorsal interossei—8
Adductor pollicis—1
Deep head of flexor pollicis brevis—1/2

The deep branch of ulnar nerve supplies muscles involved in precision and fine movements of digits. Therefore, it is aptly called the ***musician's nerve***.

Note: That the deep branch of ulnar supplied fourteen and half muscles in the palm

Extensor Expansion (Fig 21.17)

Each extensor digitorum tendon flattens into the extensor expansion over the dorsal aspect of the metacarpophalangeal joint.

Parts of Extensor Expansion

The extensor expansion is triangular in shape. Its base encircles the MCP joint on all sides except the palmar aspect. Each basal angle is fixed to the deep palmar metacarpal ligament. Its thickened lateral margin receives the insertion of a single lumbrical muscle. The attachment of interossei is as shown in figure 21.15. The thick axial part of the expansion carries the insertion of the extensor digitorum tendon (and of additional tendon in case of little finger and index finger). The axial part and the margins are interconnected by fibrous tissue nearer the base in order to ensure the firm anchorage of the extensor expansion to the back of MCP joint. Closer to the PIP joint the axial slip splits into three slips, of which the central one is attached to the base of the middle phalanx. Each collateral slip joins the lateral margin of its side and then unites with the fellow of the other side on the dorsal aspect of the middle phalanx. The united collateral slips cross the DIP joint to gain attachment to the base of the terminal phalanx. The central and collateral slips function independently. The

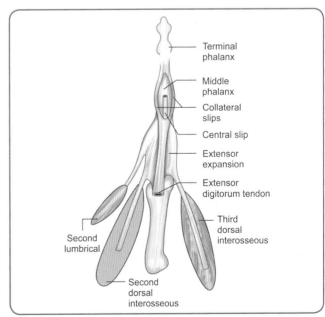

Fig. 21.17: Formation and attachments of extensor expansion or dorsal digital expansion of middle finger of right hand

TABLE 21.2: Composition of Extensor Expansion or Dorsal Digital Expansion of Each Finger

No.	Finger	Extensor tendon or tendons	Lumbrical	Palmar	Dorsal
I	Index	2	First	Second	First
II	Middle	1	Second	Nil	Second & Third
III	Ring	1	Third	Third	Fourth
IV	Little	2	Fourth	Fourth	Nil

Note: Palmar and dorsal indicate palmar and dorsal interossei.

central slip carrying the insertion of the extensor digitorum tendon acts on the MCP joint while the collateral slips carrying the insertions of lumbricals and interossei act on MCP, PIP and DIP joints

The slips of extensor expansion are closely applied to the dorsal aspects of the interphalangeal joints. In fact, they replace the fibrous capsule of IP and MCP joints on the dorsal aspect.

Combined Actions of Interossei and Lumbricals

The interossei and lumbricals together flex the metacarpophalangeal joints and simultaneously extend the interphalangeal joints. They can perform this unusual combination of actions due to their relations to the axes of movements of MCP and IP joints (Fig. 21.14). These muscles cross the metacarpophalangeal joints on palmar aspect therefore they are able to flex MCP joints. Through the extensor expansion, the muscles cross the interphalangeal joints on dorsal aspect. Accordingly, the pull of the muscles is transferred to the dorsal side of the axes of the interphalangeal joints, which they extend.

Testing Function of Dorsal Interossei

The principle of testing the dorsal interossei is to assess the capacity of middle three fingers to abduct against resistance after placing the hand flat on the table.

- To test first dorsal interosseous muscle, the index finger is abducted against resistance. The examiner can feel the contracted muscle in the first intermetacarpal space.
- To test the second muscle, the extended middle finger is crossed dorsally over the extended index finger (good luck sign) against resistance.
- To test the third muscle, the middle finger is abducted towards the ring finger against resistance.
- To test the fourth muscle, the ring finger is abducted away from middle figer against resistance.

Testing Function of Palmar Interossei

The principle of testing the palmar interossei is to assess the capacity of index, ring and little fingers to adduct against resistance after placing the hand of the patient on the table.

- To test the second palmar interosseous muscle the index finger is adducted towards the middle finger against resistance.
- To test the third muscle the ring finger is adducted towards the middle finger against resistance.
- To test the fourth muscle the little finger is adducted towards middle finger against resistance.

CLINICAL CORRELATION

Complete Claw Hand

Paralysis of all the interossei and lumbricals produces complete or true claw hand deformity (Fig. 13.5B) in which there is hyperextension of MCP and hyperflexion of PIP and DIP joints of all fingers.

STUDENT INTEREST

Testing function of interossei muscles is a must know topic. Don't give up until you learn the clinical significance of these very important muscles in the hand.

Movements of Thumb and Fingers

The thumb enjoys free mobility compared to the other fingers hence functionally it is regarded as one half of the hand. An opposable thumb is a human character. It is designed for grasping objects. The anatomical peculiarity of the thumb is that it has two phalanges and one modified metacarpal bone. Its metacarpal is at right angles to the plane of other metacarpals. The base of this metacarpal articulates with the trapezium to form the first carpometacarpal joint. It is a saddle variety of synovial joint, which confers great mobility to the thumb.

Movements of Thumb (Fig. 21.18)

The movements of the thumb take place in the first carpometacarpal joint.

- In *flexion*, the palmar surface of the thumb moves across the palm towards the ulnar border till the thumb comes in contact with the palm. Flexion is always accompanied by conjunct (automatic) medial rotation.
- In *extension*, the thumb moves away from the palm so that its dorsal surface comes to face the dorsum of hand. Extension is necessarily accompanied by lateral rotation of thumb.

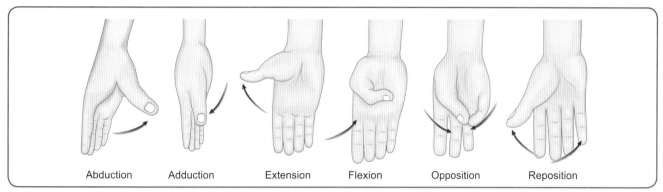

| Abduction | Adduction | Extension | Flexion | Opposition | Reposition |

Fig. 21.18: Movements of thumb

- In **abduction**, the thumb moves away from the index finger at right angles to the plane of the palm.
- In adduction, the thumb is brought back to the resting position (in front of and in contact with the palmar surface of the index finger).
- In **opposition**, the tip of the thumb is brought in contact with the base or tip of any other finger. It is a composite movement consisting of abduction, flexion and medial rotation. It can be defined as the movement of flexion with medial rotation of abducted thumb.
- In **reposition**, the opposed thumb is brought back to the resting position. In this movement, there is extension, lateral rotation and adduction of abducted thumb.
- Circumduction is an angular motion of the thumb consisting of flexion, abduction, extension and adduction.

First Carpometacarpal Joint

It is the trapeziometacarpal joint. It is a saddle type of synovial joint. The articulating ends consist of—the distal articular surface of trapezium and the proximal articular surface of the base of first metacarpal bone. Both the articulating surfaces are reciprocally concavo-convex. The fibrous capsule lined with synovial membrane encircles the joint. The carpometacarpal ligaments reinforce the joint.

Muscles Acting on Thumb

A total of nine muscles act on the thumb. The long muscles are—extensor pollicis longus, extensor pollicis brevis, abductor pollicis longus and flexor pollicis longus. The short muscles are the three thenar muscles, adductor pollicis and the first palmar interosseous.
- Flexion is produced by flexor pollicis longus and flexor pollicis brevis.
- Extension is produced by extensor pollicis brevis, extensor pollicis longus and abductor pollicis longus.

- Adduction is produced mainly by adductor pollicis assisted by first palmar interosseous.
- Abduction is produced mainly by abductor pollicis brevis assisted by abductor pollicis longus.
- Opposition movement is the result of synergistic actions of abductor pollicis longus and brevis, opponens pollicis and flexor pollicis brevis.
- Reposition (reverse of opposition) is by synergistic actions of extensor pollicis brevis and longus, abductor pollicis longus and brevis (for extension and lateral rotation) and adductor pollicis muscles.

Metacarpophalangeal (MCP) Joints

The knuckles indicate the positions of the MCP joints. These joints are condyloid types of synovial joints. The articulating ends are the convex metacarpal head and the spherical fossa on the base of the proximal phalanx. The fibrous capsule covers the joint except dorsally where it is replaced by extensor expansion. The collateral ligaments support the joints on either side. The palmar ligament is very strong. It is in the form of a fibrous plate attached firmly to the base of proximal phalanx, but loosely to the neck of the metacarpal. This plate undergoes excursions relative to the movements of the joint. The margins of the palmar ligament give attachment to deep transverse ligament, fibrous flexor sheath, and slips of palmar aponeurosis, collateral ligaments and transverse fibers of extensor expansion.

Movements

The movements of flexion, extension and adduction, abduction take place at these joints.

Flexion

- Flexor digitorum superficialis assisted by flexor digitorum profundus flex the joints in power grip.
- Interossei and lumbricals flex these joints in precision grip.

Extension

The extensor digitorum is the main extensor. Extensor digiti minimi and extensor indicis assist the extension of respective fingers.

Interphalangeal (IP) Joints

IP joints are of two types—the proximal interphalangeal (PIP) joints and the distal interphalangeal (DIP) joints. The PIP and DIP joints are simple hinge types of synovial joints. The thumb has only one interphalangeal joint. On the dorsal aspect, the capsule of these joints is replaced by the extensor expansion. Collateral ligaments, which are slack, support the joints, when the fingers are extended.

Movements

IP joints permit movements of flexion and extension.
- Flexor digitorum superficialis is the main flexor at the PIP joint.
- Flexor digitorum profundus alone causes flexion of DIP joint.
- Interossei and lumbricals produce extension at PIP and DIP joints.

In fully extended position of MCP joints, the distal part of extensor digitorum is slackened, due to which it becomes ineffective at IP joints.

 CLINICAL CORRELATION

Deformities of Fingers
- *In swan neck finger*, there is hyperextension of PIP and flexion at DIP joints due to degeneration of the flexor digitorum superficialis tendon and of the insertion of extensor expansion in the terminal digit.
- *In buttonhole finger* (Boutonniere deformity) there is flexion at PIP and hyperextension at DIP joint due to rupture of the central slip of extensor expansion.
- *The mallet finger* (baseball finger) is due to injury to attachment of extensor expansion in distal phalanx so the terminal phalanx is flexed.

 EMBRYOLOGIC INSIGHT

Development of Arteries of Upper Limb
The seventh cervical intersegmental artery enters the embryonic limb bud as axis artery. The following definitive arteries are the remnants of the embryonic axis artery of upper limb.
- Axillary artery
- Brachial artery
- Anterior interosseous artery
- Median artery
- Deep palmar arch

22

Long Nerves of Upper Limb

Chapter Contents

MEDIAN NERVE

The median nerve originates from the brachial plexus in the axilla by two roots.

- *Lateral root* arises from the lateral cord and carries C(5), C6, and C7 fibers in it.
- *Medial root* arises from the medial cord and carries C8 and T1 fibers in it.

Union of Roots

The medial root crosses the third part of the axillary artery and unites with the lateral root either in front of or on the lateral side of the artery, to form the median nerve. So, the root value of the median nerve is (C5), C6, C7, C8 and T1.

Course and Relations (Fig. 22.1)

In the Axilla

In the axilla, the median nerve is located on the lateral side of the third part of the axillary artery. It enters the arm at the lower border of teres major muscle along with other nerves and vessels in the axilla.

In the Arm

Initially, the median nerve travels downward in lateral relation to the brachial artery. It crosses in front of the brachial artery at the level of mid-arm (at insertion of the coracobrachialis) and travels downwards in medial relation to the brachial artery in the cubital fossa.

In the Cubital Fossa

In the cubital fossa, the median nerve is located medial to the brachial artery. The nerve and the artery are protected anteriorly by the bicipital aponeurosis (which provides a platform for the median cubital vein). The median nerve leaves the cubital fossa between the humeral (superficial) and ulnar (deep) heads of pronator teres.

In the Anterior Compartment of Forearm

The median nerve passes downwards behind the tendinous bridge between the humeroulnar and radial heads of flexor digitorum superficialis. During its descent in the forearm it remains adherent to the deep surface of flexor digitorum superficialis. About five cm proximal to the flexor retinaculum the median nerve becomes superficial (hence vulnerable to laceration injuries) lying along the lateral edge of flexor digitorum superficialis tendons and immediately posterior to the palmaris longus tendon as it approaches the flexor retinaculum.

In the Carpal Tunnel

The median nerve leaves the distal forearm to enter the carpal tunnel which lies deep to the flexor retinaculum. Inside the tunnel it is placed anterior to the tendons of long flexors of digits (FDS and FDP) and to the tendon of

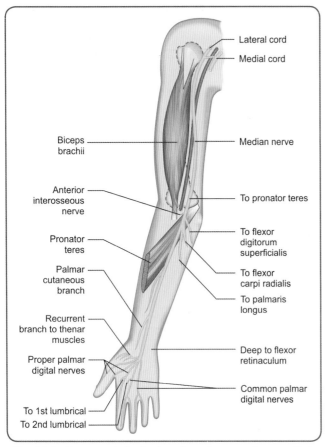

Fig. 22.1: Course and distribution of median nerve in upper limb

flexor pollicis longus (FPL). There is tight packing of nine tendons, their synovial sheaths and the median nerve in the carpal tunnel. Therefore, in case of narrowing of the carpal tunnel due to any cause median nerve is liable to compression.

Branches

Branches in Arm

The median nerve supplies a twig to the pronator teres just above the elbow in addition to supplying sympathetic fibers to the branchial artery.

Branches in Cubital Fossa

It gives muscular branches from its medial side to pronator teres, flexor carpi radialis, palmaris longus and flexor digitorum superficialis. It also gives articular branches to the elbow and superior radio-ulnar joints. At its point of exit the anterior interosseous branch arises from the median nerve.

Branches in Forearm

It supplies the part of flexor digitorum superficialis, which continues as the tendon for index finger. Before entering the carpal tunnel, the palmar cutaneous branch arises. This cutaneous branch supplies the skin overlying the thenar eminence and the lateral part of the palm.

Branches in the Palm

The median nerve flattens at the distal border of the flexor retinaculum and divides into six branches (Fig. 22.1) as follows:

- The recurrent branch is the most lateral branch. It is thick and short. It doubles back on the free margin of flexor retinaculum to gain entry into the thenar compartment. It supplies flexor pollicis brevis (superficial head), abductor pollicis brevis and opponens pollicis.
- The lateral three proper digital branches supply the sides of the thumb and radial side of index finger. The digital branch for the radial side of index finger also supplies the first lumbrical.
- There are two common digital branches. **The lateral common digital branch** after supplying second lumbrical divides into two proper digital branches for the adjacent sides of index and middle fingers. The medial common digital branch divides into two proper digital branches, which go to the adjacent sides of middle and ring fingers.

  All palmar digital branches supply the dorsal aspect of the distal one and half to two digits of the fingers including the nail beds,

Note: The median nerve is called **laborer's nerve** because it supplies flexor muscles that are responsible for baggage or hook grip.

⚡ **CLINICAL CORRELATION**

Effects of Lesion or Injury to Median Nerve
The effects of the lesion of the median nerve depend on the level of the site of lesion.

Injury at Elbow
The median nerve may be injured due to supracondylar fracture of humerus or pronator syndrome (entrapment of median nerve between two heads of pronator teres). This results in paralysis of all the muscles supplied by median nerve in forearm and palm and also the sensory loss.

Contd...

Contd…

Contd…

⌀ CLINICAL CORRELATION

Motor Effects

- Loss of pronation.
- Hand of Benediction deformity (Fig. 22.2A) which is due to paralysis of both superficial and deep flexors of the middle and index fingers (loss of flexion at proximal interphalangeal (PIP) and distal interphalangeal (DIP) joints). The ring and little fingers can be flexed due to retention of the nerve supply of their flexor digitorum (FDP).
- Paralysis of flexor pollicis longus results in loss flexion of thumb.
- Paralysis of lateral two lumbricals results in inability to flex lateral two metacarpophalangeal joints (MCP) joints.
- Ape thumb or simian hand deformity (Fig. 22.2B) is due to paralysis of thenar muscles. In this deformity the thumb comes to lie in line with other fingers and there is thenar atrophy producing ape thumb deformity.

Sensory Effects (Fig. 22.3A)

Injury to medial nerve above (the origin of palmar cutaneous branch) results in loss of sensation over the central part of palm; lateral half of palm and the lateral three and half digits in addition to loss of sensation on the dorsal aspects of the same digits (Fig. 22.3B).

Injury at Mid-forearm

- Pointing index deformity (Fig. 22.2C) due to paralysis of only the part of FDS that continues as the tendon of index finger and ape thumb deformity.
- Sensory loss is similar to that seen at lesion at previous level.

Injury at Wrist

The superficial laceration at wrist, usually, due to cut may damage the palmar cutaneous branch only. This results in sensory loss over the skin of lateral palm including the thenar eminence.

Injury at carpal tunnel results in carpal tunnel syndrome.

Sensory and Motor Effects in Carpal Tunnel Syndrome (Injury in Carpal Tunnel)

- Initially the patient experiences symptoms like, numbness, tingling and pins and needles sensations in the lateral three and half digits. In due course, there may be total sensory loss in lateral three and half digits and also on the dorsal aspect of the same digits. There is no sensory loss on the lateral part of palmar skin because of the sparing of palmar cutaneous branch in lesion at this level.
- There is ape thumb deformity due to paralysis of thenar muscles. There is loss of flexion of proximal IP joints of fingers and weakness of flexion of lateral two metacarpophalangeal joints (MCP) joints.

Injury in Palm

Injury to recurrent branch of the median nerve alone produces paralysis of thenar muscles, causing ape thumb but no sensory loss.

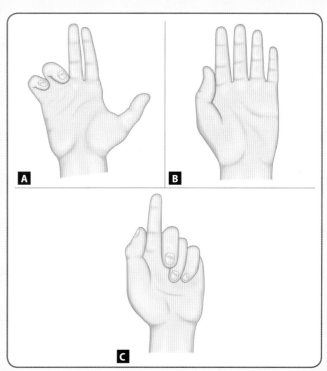

Figs 22.2A to C: A. Hand of Benediction deformity; **B.** Ape thumb; **C.** Pointing index (in injury to median nerve at the level of mid-forearm)

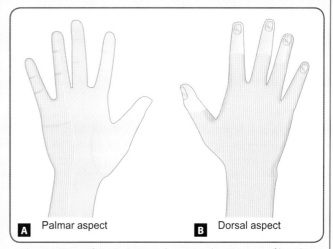

A Palmar aspect   **B** Dorsal aspect

Figs 22.3A and B: A. Sensory loss on palmar aspect of hand in median nerve lesion; **B.** Sensory loss on dorsal aspect of hand in median nerve lesion

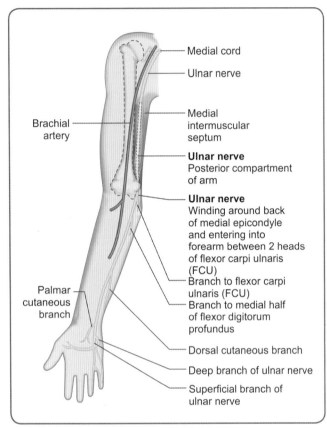

Medial cord

Ulnar nerve

Medial intermuscular septum

Ulnar nerve Posterior compartment of arm

Ulnar nerve Winding around back of medial epicondyle and entering into forearm between 2 heads of flexor carpi ulnaris (FCU)

Branch to flexor carpi ulnaris (FCU)

Branch to medial half of flexor digitorum profundus

Dorsal cutaneous branch

Deep branch of ulnar nerve

Superficial branch of ulnar nerve

Brachial artery

Palmar cutaneous branch

Fig. 22.4: Course and distribution of ulnar nerve in upper limb

ULNAR NERVE

The ulnar nerve arises in the axilla from the medial cord of brachial plexus. Its root value is C8 and T1.

Course and Relations (Fig. 22.4)

In the Axilla

The ulnar nerve is located medial to the third part of axillary artery between it and the axillary vein. It enters the arm as part of the main neurovascular bundle.

In the Anterior Compartment of Arm

The ulnar nerve is related medially to the brachial artery up to the level of insertion of coracobrachialis, where it pierces the medial intermuscular septum to enter the posterior compartment of the arm.

In the Posterior Compartment of Arm

The ulnar nerve courses downward on the medial head of the triceps along with the superior ulnar collateral artery.

At the back of the medial epicondyle, the ulnar nerve is lodged in a groove. The pressure on the ulnar nerve at this site produces *"funny bone" symptoms*, with tingling along the hypothenar eminence and little finger.

The ulnar nerve leaves the posterior compartment of arm (to enter the anterior compartment of forearm) between the humeral and ulnar heads of flexor carpi ulnaris, superficial to and ivn intimate contact with ulnar collateral ligament of the elbow joint.

In the Anterior Compartment of Forearm

The ulnar nerve travels downwards lying on the flexor digitorum profundus muscle under the coverage of the flexor carpi ulnaris in the upper third of forearm. In its initial course in the forearm the ulnar nerve and ulnar artery are widely separated from each other. In the lower two-thirds of forearm, the ulnar nerve is superficial as it less lateral to the flexor carpi ulnaris tendon. In this part of its course, the ulnar nerve and the ulnar artery descend together (the artery being on the lateral side of the nerve).

Note: Ulnar nerve gives no branches in the arm.

At the Wrist

The ulnar nerve passes on the superficial surface of the flexor retinaculum (in Guyon's canal) along with the accompanying ulnar artery is positioned lateral to the pisiform bone.

In the Palm

The ulnar nerve terminates under cover of palmaris brevis into superficial and deep branches.

Branches

In forearm:
- Articular branch to elbow joint.
- Muscular branches to medial half of flexor digitorum profundus and to the flexor carpi ulnaris.
- Palmar cutaneous branch arises at the mid-forearm level.
- Dorsal cutaneous branch arises 5 cm proximal to flexor retinaculum.

Distribution in Palm

Superficial Terminal Branch of Ulnar Nerve

The superficial branch supplies palmaris brevis and divides into one proper palmar digital branch for the medial side of little finger and the other common palmar digital branch for the adjacent sides of little and ring fingers. The palmar digital branches cross over to the dorsal side to supply the nail bed of the medial one and half digits (Fig. 22.4).

Deep Terminal Branch of Ulnar Nerve

The deep branch supplies the hypothenar muscles and turns deeply between the abductor digiti minimi and flexor digiti minimi. The deep branch of ulnar nerve (accompanied by deep branch of the ulnar artery) turns laterally on the base of the hook of hamate. While crossing the palm in medio-lateral direction, the deep branch lies in the concavity of the deep palmar arch. It supplies the dorsal and palmar interossei, medial two lumbricals (3rd and 4th lumbricals) and deep head of flexor pollicis brevis before it enters the adductor pollicis muscle to supply it.

Note: The deep branch of the ulnar nerve is called **musician's nerve** because it innervates all the small muscles of the hand involved in fine movements of hand).

♪ CLINICAL CORRELATION

Palpation of Ulnar Nerve

In leprosy, the ulnar nerve is thickened and hence palpable at behind the medial epicondyle in the early stages of the disease. In suspected cases of leprosy, the ulnar nerve is palpated at this site.

Lesions of Ulnar Nerve

Injury at Elbow

Being in exposed position the ulnar nerve is injured in cubital tunnel syndrome (compression between two heads of flexor carpi ulnaris), fracture of medial epicondyle, cubitus valgus, etc.

Motor Effects

- Weakness of flexor digitorum profundus muscle of ring and little fingers causes inability to flex the terminal phalanx of the aforementioned two fingers.
- Marked clawing at the medial two fingers due to paralysis of interossei and medial two lumbricals (Fig. 22.5).
- Atrophy of all interossei results in guttering on the dorsum of hand.
- Loss of adduction of thumb.

Positive Froment's Sign (Fig. 22.6)

The Froment's sign is positive in ulnar nerve injury. When the patient pinches a piece of paper between thumb and index finger (or grasps a book firmly between the thumbs and other fingers of both hands), the thumb on the affected side flexes at IP joint. This is due to weakness of adductor pollicis muscle (supplied by ulnar nerve), which permits uncontrolled contraction of flexor pollicis longus (supplied by anterior interosseous nerve).

Sensory Effects

There is sensory loss in the medial half of palmar and dorsal aspects of hand and medial one and half fingers (Figs 22.7A and B).

Injury at Wrist

The ulnar nerve is superficial to flexor retinaculum and hence vulnerable to compression **(Guyon's canal syndrome)** or laceration.

- This results in claw hand deformity of medial two digits and guttering of interosseous spaces.
- The sensory loss is limited only to medial one and half digits (palmar and dorsal cutaneous branches are spared).

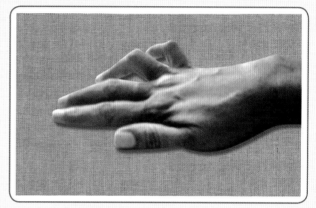

Fig. 22.5: Ulnar claw hand in a patient

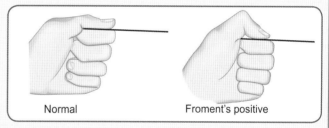

Normal   Froment's positive

Fig. 22.6: Froment's sign positive (due to loss of function of adductor pollicis muscle)

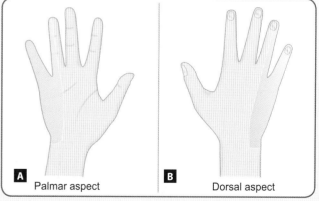

A Palmar aspect   **B** Dorsal aspect

Figs 22.7A and B: A. Sensory loss on palmar aspect of hand in lesion of ulnar nerve; **B.** Sensory loss on dorsal aspect of hand in lesion of ulnar nerve

Contd...

Contd...

 CLINICAL CORRELATION

Ulnar Nerve Paradox

The claw hand due to injury of ulnar nerve at the wrist is more obvious compared to the injury at the elbow. This is known as ***ulnar nerve paradox***. The reason of the ulnar paradox is that the lesion at the wrist spares the flexor digitorum profundus, which brings about powerful flexion at the interphalangeal joints causing marked clawing).

Injury in the Palm

In the palm, the deep branch of ulnar nerve may be compressed against the hamate bone, when the hand is used as a mallet or if a vibrating tool rubs against it. This gives rise to ulnar clawing of the hand but no sensory loss.

RADIAL NERVE

The radial nerve arises from the posterior cord of brachial plexus in the axilla. It is the largest branch of the brachial plexus. Theoretically, the nerve carries fibers from all the roots of brachial plexus but T1 fibers are not constant (C5), C6, C7, C8, (T1).

Course and Relations

In the Axilla

The radial nerve lies posterior to third part of the axillary artery and anterior to the three muscles forming the posterior wall of the axilla (subscapularis, teres major and latissimus dorsi). It leaves the axilla as a part of the principal neurovascular bundle to enter the arm at the level of lower border of teres major muscle.

In the Arm

The radial nerve is posterior to the brachial artery. Here it gives medial muscular branches to long and medial heads of the triceps brachii (the branch for the medial head of triceps lies very close to the ulnar nerve and hence is called the ***ulnar collateral nerve***).

In the Spiral or Radial Groove

The radial nerve soon passes between the long and medial heads of triceps to enter the lower triangular space, through which it reaches the spiral groove along with the profunda brachii vessels. This neurovascular bundle in the spiral groove lies in direct contact with the humerus, between the lateral and the medial heads of triceps. The radial nerve leaves the lower end of the spiral groove accompanied by radial collateral branch of the profunda artery.

In the Anterior Compartment of Arm

The radial nerve and radial collateral artery pierce the lateral intermuscular septum of the arm and enter the anterior compartment, where they descend between the brachialis (medially) and brachioradialis (laterally) and more distally between the brachialis and extensor carpi radialis longus muscles. In this location, the radial nerve supplies branches to brachioradialis and extensor carpi radialis longus. It also gives a few proprioceptive fibers to the brachialis.

In the Cubital Fossa

The radial nerve is hidden under cover of the brachioradialis muscle. At the level of lateral epicondyle of humerus, it terminates into superficial and deep branches in the lateral part of cubital fossa. The deep terminal branch (also otherwise described as ***posterior interosseous nerve***) gives branches to supinator and extensor carpi radialis brevis before entering the substance of supinator on way to the posterior compartment of forearm**.**

Branches

Branches in Axilla

- Posterior cutaneous nerve of arm
- A branch to long head of triceps brachii.

Branches in Spiral Groove

- The ***muscular branches*** supply the medial and lateral heads of triceps and the anconeus. The branch to anconeus lies in direct contact with the humerus as it passes downwards through the substance of the medial head (along with the middle collateral branch of profunda brachii artery).
- The ***cutaneous branches*** are posterior cutaneous nerve of forearm and lower lateral cutaneous nerve of arm.

Terminal Branches

The radial nerve terminates into the superficial branch and deep branch (posterior interosseous nerve) at the superolateral part of cubital fossa under cover of brachioradialis. The posterior interosseous nerve leaves the cubital fossa via the supinator muscle to enter the posterior compartment of forearm. Its further course is described in posterior compartment of the forearm.

Superficial Branch

The superficial branch of radial nerve is entirely sensory. It travels in the anterolateral part of the forearm under cover of brachioradialis. During its downward course, it lies successively on the pronator teres, flexor digitorum superficialis and flexor pollicis longus. The radial artery is on its medial side. About seven cm above the wrist the superficial branch of radial nerve passes deep to the tendon of brachioradialis and turns dorsally in the direction of the anatomical snuffbox. In this relatively unprotected position, the nerve is liable to be compressed by tight bracelets or watch straps. As it courses in the superficial fascia of the anatomical snuffbox the radial nerve divides into dorsal digital branches. It supplies a variable area of skin over the lateral side of the dorsum and lateral three and half digits. It may supply the proximal and middle phalanges or the proximal and half of the middle phalanges of the above digits.

Surface Marking

Mark the following three points. The ***first point*** is one cm lateral to the tendon of biceps brachii. The ***second point*** is at the junction of upper two-thirds and lower ***one-third*** of the lateral margin of the forearm. The ***third point*** is the anatomical snuffbox. A line joining the marked points represents the radial nerve in the forearm.

🎵 CLINICAL CORRELATION

Effects of Lesion of Radial Nerve at Different Levels

Injury at Axilla

In the axilla, the radial nerve may be injured due to pressure of the crutch (crutch palsy).

Motor Effects

All the muscles supplied by the radial nerve directly or indirectly through its posterior interosseous branch are paralyzed.

- Loss of extension at elbow (paralysis of triceps brachii).
- ***Wrist drop*** (Fig. 22.8) is due to paralysis of wrist extensors (extensor carpi radialis longus, extensor carpi radialis brevis and extensor carpi ulnaris).
- Loss of extension at metacarpophalangeal joints of fingers (finger drop due to paralysis of extensor digitorum) and thumb drop due to paralysis of extensor pollicis longus and brevis.

Sensory Effects

More often there is an isolated sensory loss on the dorsum of the hand at the base of the thumb (Fig. 22.9).

Injury in Mid-arm

The radial nerve may be injured due to fracture of shaft of humerus, inadvertent intramuscular injection in the triceps brachii or direct pressure on radial nerve as in Saturday night palsy. The long head of the triceps is spared hence extension of the elbow is not totally lost. Otherwise the effects of injury are similar to those found at injury in the axilla.

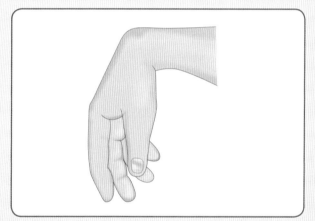

Fig. 22.8: Wrist drop in radial injury due to paralysis of extensor muscles of the wrist joint

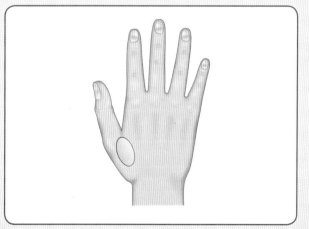

Fig. 22.9: Coin shaped area of sensory loss on dorsum of hand in injury to radial nerve

STUDENT INTEREST

- Median nerve is known as *"eye of the hand"* because it supplies sensory receptors in the tips of medial three and half fingers of the hand. The finger tips are highly sensitive.
- Median nerve by virtue of its motor supply to long flexor tendons (FDS, FPL, and lateral half of FDP) is known as *"laborer's nerve"* as these muscles are used in hook grip for holding the objects by flexing mainly the index finger and middle finger.
- Deep branch of the ulnar nerve is known as *"musician's nerve"* as it supplies the intrinsic muscles necessary for precision grip and fine movements of fingers.
- All long nerves of upper limb fall under must know topic.

TABLE 22.1: Segmental Innervation of Muscles of Upper Extremity	
Serratus anterior C5, C6,C7	Flexor carpi ulnaris C8, T1
Pectoralis major C5, C6, C7, C8, T1	Flexor pollicis longus C7, C8, T1
Pectoralis minor C5, C6, C7, C8, T1	Flexor digitorum profundus C8, T1
Latissimus dorsi C6, C7, C8	Supinator C6, C7
Deltoid C5, C6	Extensor carpi radialis longus and brevis C7, C8
Subscapularis C5, C6	Extensor pollicis longus and brevis C7, C8
Supraspinatus C5, C6	Abductor pollicis longus C7, C8
Infraspinatus C5, C6	Extensor digitorum C7, C8
Teres minor C5, C6	Hypothenar muscles C8, T1
Teres major C5, C6	Thenar muscles C8,T1
Triceps brachii C6, C7, C8	Adductor pollicis C8,T1
Biceps brachii and brachialis C5, C6	Interossei C8,T1
Brachioradialis C5, C6	Lumbricals C8, T 1
Flexor digitorum superficialis C8, T1	

23

Clinicoanatomical Problems and Solutions

CASE 1

An elderly man came to the hospital with the complaint of a pulsatile soft swelling in the left axilla. On examination, it was found that abduction movement of his left arm was restricted and there was sensory loss on the skin over lower half of deltoid muscle. There was slight swelling of the left upper limb.

Questions and Solutions

1. Which large blood vessel in the axilla is likely to give rise to a pulsatile swelling?

Ans. Axillary artery

2. What is dilatation of a blood vessel called?

Ans. Aneurysm

3. Give the extent of this vessel.

Ans. The axillary artery extends from the outer border of first rib to the lower margin of teres major.

4. Name the muscle that crosses this vessel anteriorly.

Ans. Pectoralis minor muscle

5. Which part/parts of this vessel is/are related to the cords of brachial plexus?

Ans. The first and second parts of axillary artery are related to the cords of branchial plexus.

6. Compression of which adjacent blood vessel will cause swelling of the upper limb. Give the formation and termination of this vessel.

Ans. Compression of axillary vein leads to swelling of upper limb. This vein is formed at the lower margin of teres major muscle in the anterior compartment of arm by the union of basilic vein and venae comitantes of brachial artery. The axillary vein continues as the subclavian vein at the outer margin of first rib.

CASE 2

A baby with a history of forceps delivery was brought to the pediatrician after four weeks for a routine checkup. On examination, it was observed that the baby's left arm was medially rotated and adducted and the left forearm was pronated and extended.

Questions and Solutions

1. Name the position of the upper limb seen in this baby.

Ans. Porter's tip position

2. Lesion at which site in the brachial plexus causes this position of the upper limb?

Ans. Lesion at upper trunk or Erb's point gives rise to Erb's palsy which causes this position of upper limb.

3. Paralysis of which muscles results in medial rotation of arm?

Ans. Infraspinatus and teres minor (lateral rotators of arm)

4. Paralysis of which muscles results in extended forearm?

Ans. Biceps brachii, brachialis and brachioradialis (flexors of forearm)

5. Paralysis of which muscles results in adducted arm?

Ans. Supraspinatus and deltoid (abductors of arm)

CASE 3

A 35-year-old woman came to the surgeon with complaint of hard, painless lump in the upper outer quadrant of the right breast. Examination revealed enlarged axillary lymph nodes on the right side and loss of mobility of the affected breast.

Questions and Solutions

1. What is the probable diagnosis?

Ans. Malignancy or cancer of right breast

2. Name muscles related to the base of the breast.

Ans. Pectoralis major, serratus anterior and aponeurosis of external oblique muscle

3. Which of the above muscles is utilized while testing the fixity of the breast?

Ans. Pectoralis major

4. Which part of the breast is in contact with the pectoral group of lymph nodes and how does this part enter the axilla?

Ans. Axillary tail of Spence enters the axilla by passing through foramen of Langer in axillary fascia.

CASE 4

A man involved in automobile accident was brought to the casualty in the hospital. On examination, it was found that his left shoulder was flattened and the head of humerus was palpable in the infraclavicular fossa. An AP X-ray of the shoulder confirmed the diagnosis of anterior dislocation of shoulder joint.

Questions and Solutions

1. Which nerve is in danger of injury in anterior dislocation of shoulder joint?

Ans. Axillary nerve

2. Describe the origin and distribution of this nerve.

Ans. The axillary nerve arises from posterior cord of brachial plexus in the axilla. Its root value is C5, C6.

Axillary nerve provides the following branches:

   i. Articular to shoulder joint

   ii. Sensory branches to upper lateral cutaneous nerve of arm (which supplies skin over lower half of deltoid muscle).

   iii. Motor branches to deltoid and teres minor

3. What is the peculiarity of branch to teres minor?

Ans. The branch to teres minor possesses a pseudoganglion on it.

4. Name the muscles in the rotator cuff of shoulder joint and give nerve supply of each.

Ans. The rotator cuff muscles are supraspinatus, infraspinatus, teres minor and subscapularis (subscapularis—subscapular nerves, teres minor—axillary nerve, supraspinatus and infraspinatus—suprascapular nerve)

5. What is the secondary socket of the shoulder joint?

Ans. The coracoacromial arch provides a secondary socket for the joint superiorly. The arch is composed of the tip of the acromion, coracoacromial ligament and the lateral surface of coracoid process. The subacromial bursa intervenes between the arch and the tendon of supraspinatus. The movements of the upper end of humerus in abduction of the arm are smoothened by the presence of this bursa. The coracoacromial arch prevents the upward dislocation of shoulder joint during abduction.

CASE 5

A gardener cut his right ring finger by a sharp edge of a broken glass piece while digging the soil. After about 3 to 4 days, he developed fever and his entire ring finger was swollen and painful.

Questions and Solutions

1. Name the structure in the pulp space of the ring finger that is likely to be inflamed.

Ans. Synovial sheath around flexor tendon (digital synovial sheath)

2. In what tubular structure is the digital synovial sheath protected?

Ans. Fibrous flexor sheath

3. Which flexor tendon is seen in the terminal digit?

Ans. Flexor digitorum profundus (FDP)

4. Give the nerve supply of the part of FDP that gives origin to the tendon in the ring finger?

Ans. This part of FDP is supplied by ulnar nerve in the forearm.

5. Name the palmar spaces in the intermediate compartment of the palm.

Ans. Midpalmar and thenar spaces (refer to figure 21.4 in chapter 21)

5. Name the canals that connect the palmar spaces to the web spaces.

Ans. Lumbrical canals

6. What is the surgical importance of these canals?

Ans. Lumbrical canals are opened up surgically in corresponding web spaces to drain the pus from the palmar spaces.

CASE 6

An elderly woman with a history of fall on the outstretched hand developed localized pain and swelling on the dorsal aspect of the wrist. When movements of wrist became painful, she came to the hospital. X-ray showed the fracture of the lower end of radius.

Questions and Solutions

1. What is the name of the fracture of the lower end of the radius and the typical deformity of the hand as a result of this fracture?

Ans. Colles' fracture-dinner fork deformity

2. Does the normal relationship of the styloid process of radius and ulna change consequent to this fracture?

Ans. Normally the radial styloid process is longer than the ulnar styloid process. In Colles' fracture the distal fragment of radius shifts posteriorly and upward carrying with it the styloid process. Hence both ulnar and radial styloid processes are either at the same level or the radial styloid process may be higher.

3. Name the space in which the styloid process of radius is felt.

Ans. Anatomical snuffbox

4. Which bones are found in the floor of this space?

Ans. From proximal to distal—styloid process of radius, scaphoid, trapezium, base of first metacarpal bone.

5. Which nerve crosses the roof of this space?

Ans. Superficial branch of radial nerve

CASE 7

While drawing a blood sample from the median cubital vein, the trainee nurse observed that blood in the syringe was bright red. She immediately withdrew the needle. Then she reinserted the needle slightly medial to the previous puncture site. Her patient experienced sharp pain, which radiated to the lateral three-and-a-half digits.

Questions and Solutions

1. Name the superficial veins that are connected by the median cubital vein giving direction of blood flow in this vein.

Ans. Cephalic vein laterally and basilic vein medially are connected by the median cubital vein. The blood flows from cephalic vein to basilic vein in the median cubital vein.

2. Which aponeurotic structure forms a platform for the median cubital vein?

Ans. Bicipital aponeurosis

3. Which nerve and artery lie deep to the aponeurotic structure?

Ans. Median nerve and brachial artery

5. Name the muscles of the forearm and palm, which are paralyzed if this nerve is cut in the cubital fossa.

Ans. The muscles supplied by median nerve in cubital fossa, forearm and in the palm are paralyzed.

In the cubital fossa—pronator teres, flexor carpi radialis, palmaris longus and flexor digitorum superficialis

In the forearm (via its anterior interosseous branch—flexor pollicis longus, pronator quadratus and lateral half of flexor digitorum profundus

In the palm—first and second lumbricals, abductor pollicis brevis, opponens pollicis and superficial head of flexor pollicis brevis.

CASE 8

A patient suffering from Hensen's disease (leprosy) came to the hospital with complaints of loss of sensation in the left hand. Examination revealed sensory loss in medial one-and-a-half fingers and medial side of palmar and dorsal aspects of the hand. In addition, there was flattening of hypothenar eminence and difficulty in holding a card between thumb and index finger.

Questions and Solutions

1. Name the nerve that is affected in this patient.

Ans. Ulnar nerve

2. Give reason for flattening of hypothenar eminence.

Ans. This is due to paralysis of muscles of hypothenar eminence (abductor digiti minimi, flexor digiti minimi and opponens digiti minimi).

3. Explain the inability of the patient to hold the card between thumb and index finger.

Ans. To hold the card between thumb and index finger, the adduction of thumb is necessary. The adduction of thumb is lost due to paralysis of adductor pollicis in this patient.

4. Name the cutaneous branches of the affected nerve (with their level of origin) that supply the skin of dorsal and palmar aspects of the hand.

Ans. Palmar cutaneous branch arises from ulnar nerve in middle of forearm.

Dorsal cutaneous branch of ulnar nerve arises a little above the wrist joint.

5. Name the deformity of hand if the roots of the affected nerve are cut.

Ans. Complete claw hand.

CASE 9

A patient was scheduled for cardiac bypass surgery. Preparatory to the operation, a vein was cannulated in the anatomical snuff box.

Questions and Solutions

1. Name the vein which is used for cannulation.

Ans. Cephalic vein

2. What is the termination of the above vein?

Ans. Cephalic vein pierces the clavipectoral fascia to enter the axilla to open in to the axillary vein.

3. Which nerve is closely related to this vein in front of the elbow?

Ans. Lateral cutaneous nerve of forearm, which is the continuation of musculocutaneous nerve.

4. How is this vein arterialized?

Ans. By creating radio-cephalic fistula (surgical connection between radial artery and cephalic vein at the wrist), the cephalic vein is subjected to high arterial pressure. Gradually it increases in size and can be used as an artery. Arterialization of cephalic vein is useful in dialysis in renal failure patients.

SINGLE BEST RESPONSE TYPE MULTIPLE CHOICE QUESTIONS

1. The following part of scapula forms the lateral most palpable landmark on the shoulder:
   a. Superior angle
   b. Glenoid cavity
   c. Coracoid process
   d. Acromion

2. Which of the following can extend, adduct and medially rotate the arm?
   a. Teres minor
   b. Subscapularis
   c. Latissimus dorsi
   d. Deltoid

3. What is the continuation of ventral ramus of 7th cervical spinal nerve called?
   a. Medial cord
   b. Upper trunk
   c. Middle trunk
   d. Lateral cord

4. A patient presents with loss of abduction and weakness of lateral rotation of arm. This is due to an injury to a nerve in fracture of humerus at:
   a. Anatomical neck
   b. Surgical neck
   c. Midshaft
   d. Medial epicondyle

5. Subacromial bursa separates coracoacromial arch from the tendon of:
   a Subscapularis
   b. Teres minor
   c. Infraspinatus
   d. Supraspinatus

6. Which of the following nerves gives rise to upper lateral cutaneous nerve of arm?
   a. Lateral supraclavicular
   b. Radial
   c. Intercostobrachial
   d. Axillary

7. On which aspect are the interphalangeal joints in hand devoid of capsule?
   a. Posterior
   b. Anterior
   c. Proximal
   d. Distal

8. Which of the following forms the anterior fold of axilla?
   a. Pectoralis major and pectoralis minor
   b. Pectoralis major alone
   c. Pectoral muscles and subclavius
   d. Clavipectoral fascia and subclavius

9. Epitrochlear lymph nodes are located along which vessel?
   a. Median cubital vein
   b. Cephalic vein above elbow
   c. Basilic vein above elbow
   d. Cephalic vein in the roof of cubital fossa

10. The opponens pollicis muscle is innervated by:
    a. Lateral common digital branch of median nerve
    b. Anterior interosseous nerve
    c. Recurrent branch of median nerve
    d. Deep branch of ulnar nerve

11. Which of the following nerves is known as "eye of the hand"?
    a. Anterior interosseous
    b. Ulnar
    c. Median
    d. Superficial branch of radial

12. Ligaments of Cooper are modifications of:
    a. Fibrous stroma of breast
    b. Pectoral fascia
    c. Fatty tissue of breast
    d. Axillary fascia

13. Which of the following is not a feature of ulnar nerve lesion at elbow?
    a. Total loss of flexion in middle and index fingers
    b. Total loss of flexion in ring and little fingers
    c. Guttering of intermetacarpal spaces
    d. Wasting of hypothenar muscles

14. In which of the following at elbow region does the secondary center of ossification appear first?
    a. Head of radius
    b. Capitulum
    c. Medial epicondyle
    d. Olecranon process

15. Froment's test is performed to assess the integrity of:
    a. Second palmar interosseous
    b. First dorsal interosseous
    c. Adductor pollicis
    d. First lumbrical

16. A sportsman with severe injury to the right leg had to use crutches for several months. Subsequently, his doctor found that he had restricted abduction of shoulder and extension of elbow. What is the site of injury in the branchial plexus?
    a. Middle trunk
    b. Posterior cord
    c. Lateral cord
    d. Medial cord

17. Which of the following is not the modification of deep fascia?
    a. Extensor retinaculum
    b. Palmar aponeurosis
    c. Extensor expansion
    d. Fibrous flexor sheath

18. Abduction of the middle finger is brought about by:
    a. Third dorsal interosseous
    b. Third lumbrical
    c. Second and third dorsal interossei
    d. Second and third lumbrical

19. Which dermatome overlies the thumb?
    A. T1
    B. C8
    C. C7
    D. C6

20. Which of the following pierces the interosseous membrane?

    a. Anterior interosseous artery

    b. Anterior interosseous nerve

    c. Posterior interosseous artery

    d. Posterior interosseous nerve

KEY TO MCQ

1. d	**2.** c	**3.** c	**4.** b	**5.** d	**6.** d	**7.** a	**8.** b
9. c	**10.** c	**11.** c	**12.** a	**13.** a	**14.** b	**15.** c	**16.** b
17. c	**18.** c	**19.** d	**20.** a				

Section 4

LOWER LIMB

Bones of Lower Limb

Chapter Contents

INTRODUCTION

The lower extremity or lower limb is specialized for weight transmission, balance and locomotion. The skeleton of lower extremity is subdivided into hip bone and the bones of free lower limb (Fig. 24.1). The right and left hip bones together form the skeleton of pelvic girdle. The lower limbs are connected to the vertebral column by bony pelvis (sacrum, coccyx and pelvic girdle). While in standing position, the weight of the body is transmitted from the vertebral column in succession to the hip bones, hip joints, femurs, knee joints, tibias, ankle joints and the bones of the feet.

HIP BONE OR INNOMINATE BONE OR COXAL BONE

The hip bone is an irregular bone made up of three components, the ilium, pubis and ischium, which are united to each other at the acetabulum.

Articulations

- Pubic symphysis between the pubic bones
- Sacroiliac joint between the sacrum and ilium

- Hip joint between the acetabulum and the head of femur

The hip bone forms the skeleton of not only the lower limb but also of pelvis and perineum due to its location in the body. Hence the attachments and relations of the hip bone are best appreciated only after familiarity with the anatomy of the lower limb, pelvis and perineum.

Anatomical Position

To hold the hip bone in anatomical position, one has to see that the pubic tubercle and anterior superior iliac spine lie in the same coronal plane. In this position, the pelvic surface of the body of pubis faces postero-superiorly and the medial surface of the body of pubis lies in the midline. The acetabulum faces inferolaterally and acetabular notch inferiorly.

Acetabulum

It is a large cup shaped cavity facing inferolaterally. It articulates with the head of femur. It is composed of the three parts of hip bone as follows—ilium (two fifth), ischium (two fifth) and pubis (one fifth). It presents a horse shoe shaped articular area (lunate surface) and a nonarticular acetabular fossa (where a pad of fat is located). The deficiency in the inferior part of acetabular margin is called acetabular notch. At birth, the acetabulum

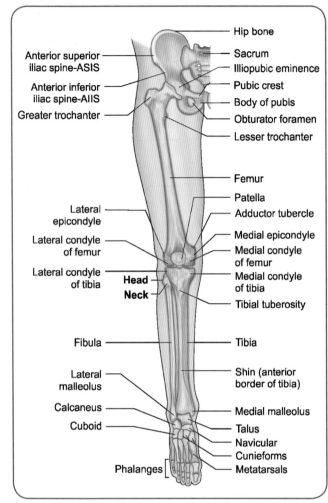

Anterior superior iliac spine-ASIS
Anterior inferior iliac spine-AIIS
Greater trochanter
Lateral epicondyle
Lateral condyle of femur
Lateral condyle of tibia
Head
Neck
Fibula
Lateral malleolus
Calcaneus
Cuboid
Phalanges

Hip bone
Sacrum
Iliopubic eminence
Pubic crest
Body of pubis
Obturator foramen
Lesser trochanter
Femur
Patella
Adductor tubercle
Medial epicondyle
Medial condyle of femur
Medial condyle of tibia
Tibial tuberosity
Tibia
Shin (anterior border of tibia)
Medial malleolus
Talus
Navicular
Cunieforms
Metatarsals

Fig. 24.1: Articulated skeleton showing bones and joints of lower limb

presents a Y-shaped triradiate cartilage (demarcating the three components of the hip bone). The three bones unite by the age of 17 or 18 years.

Obturator Foramen

It is a gap in the lower part of the hip bone located between pubis and ischium. The obturator membrane fills the gap in the living. The membrane also bridges the obturator groove to convert it into obturator canal for the passage of obturator nerve and vessels.

Ilium

The ilium presents following parts:
- Iliac crest or upper end
- Lower end
- Three margins (anterior, posterior and medial)
- Three surfaces (iliac fossa, gluteal surface and sacropelvic surface).

Iliac Crest

It is the subcutaneous curved upper end of ilium extending from the anterior superior iliac spine (ASIS) to the posterior superior iliac spine (PSIS).
- The tubercle of the iliac crest lies about five cm behind the anterior end of the crest on its outer lip. The transtubercular plane passes through the upper margin of L5 vertebra.
- The supracristal plane passes through the highest points of iliac crests (between the spines of third and fourth lumbar vertebrae). This plane is used to determine the site of lumbar puncture.

Segments of iliac crest

The iliac crest is divisible into ventral segment (anterior two third) and dorsal segment (posterior one third).
The ventral segment is further divided into inner lip, intermediate area and outer lip. The dorsal segment is divisible into outer slope and inner slope.

Muscles attached to ventral segment (Fig. 24.2)
- Outer lip of the ventral segment:
  - Origin of tensor fasciae lata in front of iliac tubercle
  - Insertion of external oblique abdominis in its anterior two third
  - Origin of latissimus dorsi in its posterior one third
- Intermediate area gives origin to internal oblique abdominis.
- Inner lip of ventral segment:
  - Origin of transversus abdominis in anterior two-third
  - Origin of quadratus lumborum in posterior one third

Muscles attached to dorsal segment (Fig. 24.3)
- Outer slope gives origin to gluteus maximus
- Inner slope gives origin to erector spinae.

Margins

Anterior margin
- Anterior superior iliac spine gives origin to sartorius and attachment to inguinal ligament
- Anterior inferior iliac spine gives origin to straight head of rectus femoris and attachment to iliofemoral ligament.

Posterior margin

Posterior superior iliac spine lies subjacent to the skin dimple called dimple of Venus (well marked in female) in the upper part of the gluteal region. It corresponds to the spine of second sacral vertebra. This site is used to draw bone marrow from the iliac crest for studying the cells of bone marrow.

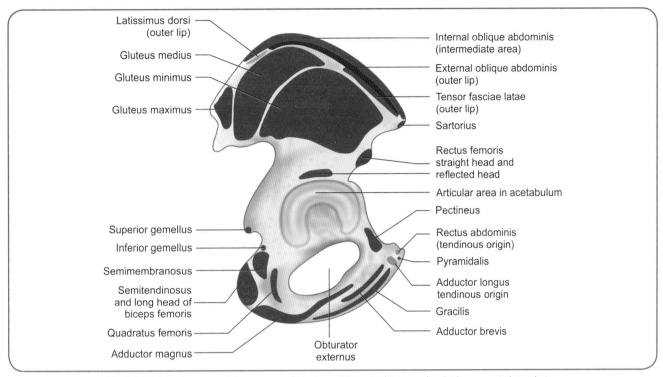

Fig. 24.2: Attachments of three parts of hip bone (ilium, ischium and pubis) as seen in lateral view

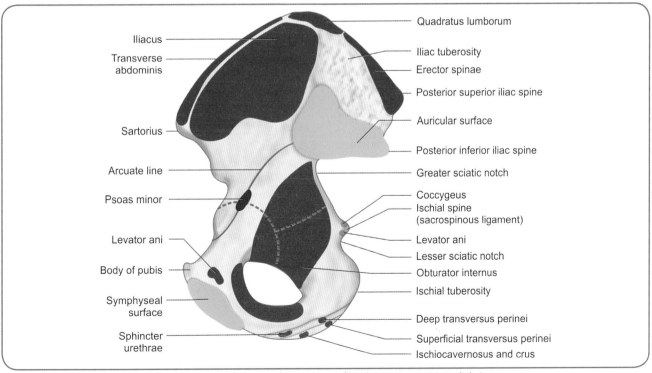

Fig. 24.3: Attachments of three parts of hip bone as seen in medial view

Greater sciatic notch

The greater sciatic notch with the help of sacrotuberous and sacrospinous ligaments forms the greater sciatic foramen, which gives passage to the piriformis muscle, seven nerves (branches of sacral plexus) and three blood vessels.

- Above the Piriformis Muscle
  - Superior gluteal nerve and vessels
- Below the Piriformis
  - Posterior cutaneous nerve of thigh
  - Inferior gluteal nerve and vessels
  - Nerve to quadratus femoris
  - Internal pudendal vessels
  - Pudendal nerve
  - Nerve to obturator internus
  - Sciatic nerve

Medial margin

Its posterior one third is rough; middle third is sharp and anterior third forms an arcuate line, which is continuous with pecten pubis at ilio-pubic eminence.

Linea terminalis

The linea terminalis (lateral boundary of pelvic inlet) is composed of arcuate line, pecten pubis and pubic crest. Some structures cross it to enter the lesser pelvis (internal iliac vessels, ureter, and ovarian vessels in female and vas deferens in male). The round ligament of uterus crosses the linea terminalis to leave the lesser pelvis.

Surfaces

- The iliac fossa is located on the inner aspect of ilium. It is concave and gives origin to iliacus muscle.
- The **sacropelvic surface** is located on inner aspect of ilium behind the medial margin of ilium. It is composed of sacral part dorsally and pelvic part ventrally.
  - The sacral part presents the auricular surface covered with articular cartilage and non-articular area (iliac tuberosity). The auricular surface articulates with sacrum at sacroiliac joint. The iliac tuberosity gives attachment to iliolumbar ligament, dorsal sacroiliac and interosseous sacroiliac ligaments
  - The smooth pelvic surface presents pre-auricular sulcus, which is well marked in female. This sulcus gives attachment to ventral sacroiliac ligament.
- The **gluteal surface** is divided into four areas by posterior, anterior and inferior gluteal lines from before backwards (Fig. 24.2).
  - Gluteus maximus takes origin from the area behind the posterior gluteal line.
  - Gluteus medius takes origin between posterior and anterior gluteal lines
  - Gluteus minimus takes origin between anterior and inferior gluteal lines
  - Reflected head of rectus femoris take origin from the area between inferior gluteal line and margin of acetabulum.

Ischium

Ischium consists of a thick body and a ramus. The body presents two ends (upper and lower), three margins (anterior, posterior and lateral) and three surfaces (femoral, dorsal and pelvic).

- The upper end of the body is united with ilium and pubis at the acetabulum.
- The dorsal part of this area is in direct contact with the sciatic nerve.
- The lower end of the body forms the ischial tuberosity. The ischial ramus arises from the lower end. It joins with the inferior ramus of pubis to form ischiopubic ramus (refer to description of pubis to know details of ischiopubic ramus).

Relations of Ischial Tuberosity

The lower part of the smooth pelvic aspect of the ischial tuberosity is related to the lateral wall of the ischiorectal fossa (pudendal or Alcock's canal). In pudendal nerve block by perineal approach the needle is inserted along the medial side of ischial tuberosity for the depth of about four cm to reach the pudendal canal.

Attachments to ischial tuberosity

- Sacrotuberous ligament is attached to its medial margin
- Quadratus femoris muscle is attached to its lateral margin
- Gluteal surface is divided by a transverse ridge in to upper quadrangular and lower triangular areas.

  The upper quadrangular area is unequally divided by an oblique line in to:
- Superolateral area for origin of semimembranosus
- Superomedial area (placed at lower level) for the origin of semitendinosus and long head of biceps femoris
- The lower triangular area is divided by a vertical line into
- A larger lateral area for origin of ischial part of adductor magnus
- A smaller medial area covered with fibro-fatty tissue since this area comes in contact with the ground in sitting position.

Ischial Spine (Figs 24.2 and 24.3)

The posterior margin of the body presents the ischial spine, which demarcates the greater sciatic foramen from the lesser sciatic foramen.

Relations and attachments of ischial spine

- Sacrospinous ligament is attached to its apex
- Coccygeus and most posterior fibers of levator ani muscle take origin from its pelvic surface. The ureter is related to its pelvic surface
- Internal pudendal vessels and nerve to obturator internus cross its dorsal surface.

CLINICAL CORRELATION

In pudendal nerve block by vaginal approach the ischial spine is the landmark as the pudendal nerve crosses the dorsal aspect of the sacrospinous ligament near the apex of the ischial spine.

Lesser Sciatic Notch

- Superior and inferior gemelli arise from the respective margins of the notch
- Lesser sciatic notch is converted into lesser sciatic foramen by sacrospinous and sacrotuberous ligaments
- Structures passing through Lesser Sciatic Foramen
    - Tendon of obturator internus
    - Nerve to obturator internus
    - Internal pudendal vessels
    - Pudendal nerve

Pubis

The pubis is placed in the anterior part of the hip bone. It consists of the body and superior and inferior rami. The right and left pubic bones articulate at the pubic symphysis.

Body of Pubis

The body of pubis presents pubic crest, pubic tubercle and three surfaces (anterior, posterior and medial).

Pubic crest

Upper palpable margin of the body of pubis is called pubic crest. The conjoint tendon is attached to the pubic crest. The rectus abdominis and pyramidalis take origin from it.

Pubic tubercle

Pubic tubercle is the rounded lateral end of the pubic crest. It is a very important palpable landmark. It is partly covered in male by spermatic cord. The hernia that is superomedial to this tubercle is inguinal hernia and the one that is inferolateral to it is the femoral hernia. The medial end of inguinal ligament is attached to the pubic tubercle.

Surfaces

- The *posterior* or *pelvic surface* is related to urinary bladder. This explains involvement of urinary bladder in fracture of the body of pubis. The posterior surface gives origin to pubococcygeus part of levator ani
- The *medial surface* is known as symphyseal surface because it takes part in pubic symphysis
- The *anterior surface* gives origin to: adductor longus by rounded tendon from the angle between pubic crest and pubic symphysis, gracilis along the lower margin of this surface and adductor brevis above the gracilis.

Superior Ramus

It presents three margins and three surfaces.

Margins

- The *pectineal line* or *pecten pubis* is sharp. It extends from pubic tubercle to the iliopubic eminence and provides attachments to conjoint tendon, lacunar ligament and the pectineus muscle
- The *anterior margin* is called obturator crest. It extends from the pubic tubercle to the acetabular notch
- The *inferior margin* is sharp and takes part in the formation of obturator foramen.

CLINICAL CORRELATION

Shenton's line is a smoothly curved line (with concavity facing down) seen in normal radiographs of hip joint. It is formed by inferior margin of superior ramus of pubis and medial (lower) margin of the femoral neck. Figure 24.4 shows normal Shenton's line and distorted Shenton's line in fracture of neck of femur.

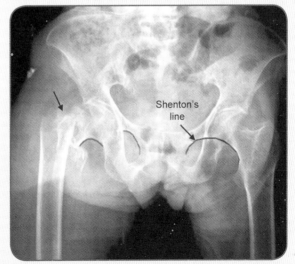

Fig. 24.4: Radiograph of pelvis showing normal Shenton's line on left side and distorted Shenton's line on right side due to fracture of the neck of right femur

Surfaces

- The ***pectineal surface*** is bounded by obturator crest and pectineal line. It gives origin to pectineus muscle
- The ***pelvic surface*** is located between pectineal line and inferior border. It is related to ductus deferens in male and to round ligament of uterus in female
- The ***obturator surface*** is located between obturator crest and inferior border. The obturator groove is present here. The obturator nerve and vessels exit from the pelvis into the medial compartment of thigh through the obturator canal.

Inferior Ramus

It extends from the body of pubis to the ischial ramus, medial to the obturator foramen. The two rami unite to form conjoint ischiopubic ramus. The fusion of the ischial and pubic rami occurs by the age of 6 to 8 years.

Conjoint ischiopubic ramus

It has two margins (superior and inferior) and two surfaces (outer and inner).

Margins of conjoint ramus

- Upper margin gives attachment to obturator membrane
- Lower margin is everted in males. It provides attachment to fascia lata and membranous layer of superficial fascia of perineum (Colles fascia) in both sexes.

Surfaces

- Inner surface is smooth. It forms the lateral limit of the urogenital triangle of the perineum. It is divided into three areas by attachment of superior fascia of urogenital diaphragm and inferior fascia of urogenital diaphragm (perineal membrane)
    - The uppermost area gives origin obturator internus (intrapelvic muscle)
    - The intermediate area gives origin to muscles of deep perineal pouch (sphincter urethrae and deep transverses perinei)
    - The lower area gives attachment to crus of clitoris or penis in front, ischiocavernosus muscle around the crus and superficial transverses perinei muscle behind
- The outer surface gives attachments to adductor magnus, adductor brevis, gracilis and obturator externus.

FEMUR (FIG. 24.5)

The femur is the longest and strongest bone in the body. Its length is one fourth of the height of the individual (approximately 45 cm in a six feet person).

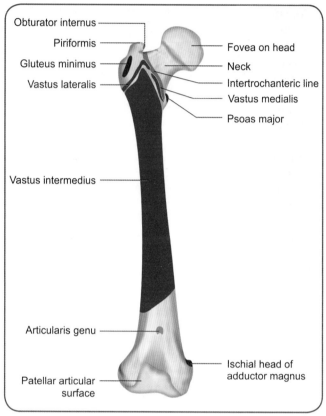

Fig. 24.5: Parts and attachments of femur (thigh bone) in anterior view

Articulations of Femur

The femur articulates with hip bone at hip joint and with patella and tibia at knee joint.

Parts

The femur consists of upper end, shaft and lower end.

Upper End

The upper end presents head, neck, greater trochanter and lesser trochanter.

Head of femur

The head is covered with articular cartilage which articulates with the lunate surface of acetabulum of the hip bone. The ligamentum teres is attached to the fovea capitis, which is a depression by the side of the center of the head.

Neck of femur (Femoral neck)

- A very long and narrow neck connects the head to the shaft. It is obliquely set on the shaft of the femur

- The neck represents the metaphysis of the developing bone and is ossified from the primary center.
- Anteriorly, the intertrochanteric line demarcates the neck from the shaft.
- Posteriorly, the intertrochanteric crest demarcates the neck from the shaft.
- It presents 2 surfaces and 2 margins.
- The anterior surface is fully intracapsular is marked with longitudinal grooves (produced by the retinacular arteries) and numerous vascular foramina.
- The posterior surface is partly intracapsular (as the capsule of hip joint is attached to the posterior surface of the neck as shown in figure 28.8).
- The upper margin is short and concave whereas the lower margin is long, straight and meets the shaft near lesser trochanter.

CLINICAL CORRELATION

Fracture of Femoral Neck

The neck is liable to fractures by slightest trauma in postmenopausal women because of the osteoporotic changes in the bones. The fracture may be intracapsular or extracapsular.

- In intracapsular fracture, the proximal fragment often loses its blood supply due to injuries to retinacular arteries leading to a serious complication called avascular necrosis of head of femur. In extracapsular fracture of the neck the blood supply to the proximal fragment is retained hence there is no avascular necrosis of head.
- In intracapsular fracture of the neck of femur on affected side the limb is shortened and laterally rotated with the toes pointing laterally. The reason for shortening is the upward pull of rectus femoris, hamstring and adductor muscles. The limb is laterally rotated due to lateral rotation of thigh by contraction of gluteus maximus and short lateral rotators of thigh and also the psoas major (due to shift in its axis). The Shenton's line is distorted in fracture of the neck of femur (Fig. 24.4).

Neck Shaft Angle

The neck-shaft angle or angle of inclination is 125°. In coxa vera the angle of inclination is decreased while in coxa valga it is increased.

Greater trochanter

The greater trochanter is a large projection from the lateral aspect of the upper end of femur. It presents upper border and three surfaces (anterior, lateral and medial). The tip or apex of greater trochanter is the postreior part of upper border. It is palpable about a hand's breadth below the midpoint of the iliac crest.

Muscular insertions in greater trochanter

- Apex and adjoining upper margin receive insertion of piriformis muscle.
- Medial surface is divided into upper and lower parts
  - Upper part is for insertion to obturator internus with the two gemelli
  - Lower part is marked by trochanteric fossa for insertion of obturator externus
- Gluteus minimus is inserted into a ridge on the lateral part of anterior surface
- Gluteus medius is inserted on a ridge on the lateral surface.

Lesser trochanter

It is a smaller conical projection from posteromedial part of upper end of femur. It gives insertion to iliopsoas tendon.

Intertrochanteric line

It marks the junction of neck and shaft anteriorly. It gives attachment to the capsule of hip Ejoint in its entire extent and to the bands of iliofemoral ligament to its upper and lower parts. It provides origin to upper most fibers of vasti lateralis and medialis muscles.

Intertrochanteric crest

It connects the two trochanters posteriorly. It shows a rounded quadrate tubercle above its middle part. The quadratus femoris is inserted into quadrate tubercle.

Shaft

The cylindrical shaft of femur is divisible into upper, middle and lower thirds. The shaft is convex forwards because the line of gravity of the body passes behind the hip joints and in front of the knee joints. The weakness caused by the forward convexity of the shaft is compensated by linea aspera (a thickened ridge) on the posterior aspect of the middle third of the shaft (Fig. 24.6).

- The middle third of the shaft presents three margins, medial, lateral and posterior (linea aspera). The linea aspera presents medial and lateral lips (enclosing a narrow intermediate area). There are three surfaces, anterior, medial and lateral
- The upper one third of shaft shows following features. The spiral line is the upwards continuation of medial lip of linea aspera. The gluteal tuberosity is the upward continuation of lateral lip of linea aspera. The spiral line and gluteal tuberosity enclose the posterior surface of the upper one third of the shaft (including the medial, lateral and anterior)
- The lower one third of shaft presents four surfaces like the upper one third. At the lower end of linea aspera the lateral lip continues as lateral supracondylar line

and the medial lip as medial supracondylar line. The supracondylar lines enclose the popliteal surface on the lower one third of the shaft. Thus the lower fourth has 4 surfaces popliteal, anterior, lateral and medial and 4 margins lateral and medial supracondylar lines, medial margins.

Inferiorly, the lateral supracondylar line ends in lateral epicondyle and medial supracondylar line ends in the adductor tubercle.

Attachments of intermuscular septa (Fig. 26.1)

The medial and lateral intermuscular septa (derived from fascia lata) are attached to medial and lateral lips of linea aspera and also to the respective supracondylar lines. The posterior intermuscular septum is attached to the intermediate area on the linea aspera.

Origin of vasti muscles from shaft (Fig. 24.5)

- *Vastus intermedius* (from upper three fourth of anterior and lateral surfaces including lateral lip of linea aspera) and articularis genu (below vastus intermedius).
- *Vastus lateralis* from upper end of intertrochanteric line, adjacent greater trochanter, gluteal tuberosity and upper half of lateral lip of linea aspera.
- *Vastus medialis* from lower end of intertrochanteric line, spiral line, medial lip of linea aspera and upper one fourth of medial supracondylar line

Attachments to posterior aspect of shaft (Fig. 24.6)

- Insertion of deep fibers of gluteus maximus in to gluteal tuberosity.
- Insertion of pectineus from root of lesser trochanter to upper end of linea aspera.
- Linear insertion of adductor brevis starting from the root of lesser trochanter and extending in to the upper half of intermediate area of linea aspera.
- Insertion of adductor longus into middle third of medial lip of linea aspera.
- Linear insertion of adductor magnus (adductor part) from medial margin of gluteal tuberosity, medial lip of linea aspera and medial supracondylar line.
- Insertion of adductor magnus (ischial part) into adductor tubercle.
- Origin of short head of biceps femoris from lateral lip of linea aspera medial to the attachment of lateral intermuscular septum.
- Origins of medial head of gastrocnemius, lateral head of gastrocnemius and plantaris from lower end of the shaft are shown in figure 24.6.

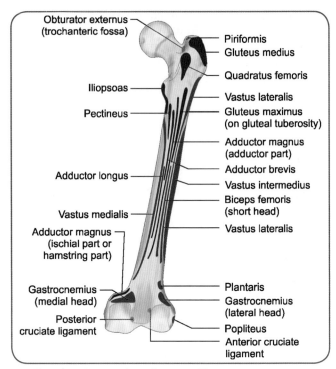

Fig. 24.6: Parts and attachments of femur in posterior view

STUDENT INTEREST

The structures attached to linea aspera are difficult to memorize. The linea aspera gives attachments to 7 muscles and 3 intermuscular septae. To remember the muscles the mnemonic is:

I Like Boys – My Boyfriend Loves Me.

The arrangement of structures from lateral to medial side is: vastus **i**ntermedius, vastus **l**ateralis, lateral intermuscular septum, and short head of **b**iceps femoris, posterior intermuscular septum, adductor **m**agnus, adductor **b**revis, adductor **L**ongus, medial intermuscular septum and vastus **m**edialis).

Lower End

The lower end of the femur bears two large condyles (medial and a lateral), which are separated by an intercondylar notch or fossa on the posterior aspect. The anterior surface of the lower end bears patellar articular area. The anterior, inferior and posterior surfaces of the condyles bear articular areas for articulating with corresponding tibial articular areas.

Medial condyle

- Medial epicondyle is the most prominent point on the medial condyle. The tibial collateral ligament of knee joint is attached to it.
- Above and behind the medial epicondyle it presents adductor tubercle, which is a palpable landmark. The

lower epiphyseal line passes through the adductor tubercle. Any injury to the epiphyseal plate (during childhood) will shorten the limb.
- Its lateral surface forms the medial boundary of intercondylar notch.

Lateral condyle

- Lateral epicondyle is the point of most prominent point on the lateral epicondyle. The fibular collateral ligament of knee joint is attached to it.
- Lateral head of gastrocnemius takes origin from an impression above and behind the lateral epicondyle.
- Popliteus takes origin from the groove below and behind the lateral epicondyle.
- Its medial surface forms the lateral boundary of intercondylar notch.

Intercondylar notch or fossa

It is a deep gap between the inner surfaces of two condyles posteriorly. It presents medial and lateral walls and a floor.
- *Anterior cruciate ligament* is attached to the posterior part of inner surface of lateral condyle.
- *Posterior cruciate ligament* is attached to the anterior part of inner surface of medial condyle.

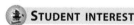 **STUDENT INTEREST**

Mnemonic for cruciate ligaments: **LAMP** (**L**ateral **A**nterior & **M**edial **P**osterior) or **ALPM** (**A**nterior **L**ateral & **P**osterior **M**edial)

Ossification

- Primary center appears for shaft at 8th week of intrauterine life.
- Secondary centers for upper end appear in following order: for head in first year, for greater trochanter at third year and for lesser trochanter at 13th year. These three epiphyses fuse separately with the shaft by 18th year.
- The neck ossifies from primary center.
- Secondary center for the lower end appears just before birth (at 9th month of intrauterine life). The lower epiphysis fuses with the shaft by 20th year.

CLINICAL CORRELATION

The secondary center of ossification at the lower end of femur is unique because unlike secondary centers in other bones it appears just before birth (at 9 months of intrauterine life). It is of medicolegal importance. The presence of this centre is a proof of the viability of the fetus or maturity of the fetus.

Growing End

The lower end is the growing end of femur. The direction of nutrient foramen is towards the upper end. The nutrient artery is usually derived from the second perforating branch of profunda femoris artery.

PATELLA (KNEE-CAP)

The patella is the largest sesamoid bone in the body. It develops in the tendon of quadriceps femoris. The patella is located in front of the lower end of femur (with which it articulates).

The patella functions as both the lever and pulley. As a lever, the patella magnifies the force exerted by quadriceps femoris during extension of knee. As a pulley, the patella alters the direction of the pull of quadriceps femoris for the joint during extension movement. However, in flexion movement the patella straddles the knee joint and is in contact with both condyles of femur.

Parts

The patella is triangular in shape. It presents base (pointing upwards), apex (pointing downwards), two margins (lateral and medial) and two surfaces (anterior and posterior).
- The anterior surface is subcutaneous and rough (Fig. 24.7A). It gives insertion to quadriceps femoris tendon and ligamentum patellae is attached to its apex.
- The posterior surface (Fig. 24.7B) bears a large articular area above and a smaller nonarticular area below. A vertical ridge divides the articular area into larger lateral area and smaller medial area. The medial articular area is separated from a very narrow medial vertical facet. The medial area comes in contact with medial femoral condyle in extension whereas the vertical facet comes in contact in full flexion of knee joint.

Attachments

- Rectus femoris and vastus intermedius are inserted into the base.
- Lateral patellar retinaculum (expansion from vastus lateralis) is attached to lateral margin.
- Medial patellar retinaculum and the lower fleshy fibers of vastus medialis (called vastus medialis oblique) are attached to medial margin.
- Ligamentum patellae is attached to the apex.

Relations

- Subcutaneous prepatellar bursa is related to the anterior surface of patella.

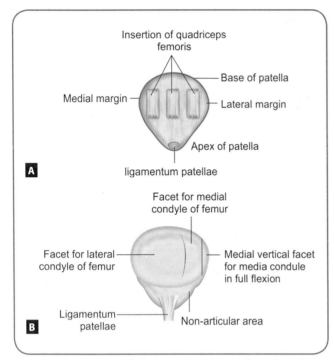

Figs 24.7A and B: A. Features of anterior surface of patella
B. Features of posterior surface of fibula

- Infrapatellar pad of fat is related to the lower nonarticular part of posterior surface.

Ossification

Patella ossifies from several centers that develop in quadriceps tendon during 3 to 6 years. Ossification is complete at puberty.

ADDED INFORMATION

Prevention of Lateral Dislocation of Patella

The patella has a natural tendency to dislocate laterally. The quadriceps femoris is obliquely placed compared to the femur but the ligamentum patellae is in line with the tibial tuberosity. As a result of this inclination, whenever quadriceps femoris contracts it pulls the patella upwards and laterally (rectus femoris is attached to anterior inferior iliac spine, which is laterally placed compared to patella). This inherent tendency of the factors that counter the tendency of patella to dislocate laterally

- Forward projection of lateral condyle of femur (compared to medial condyle)
- Stronger medial pull of vastus medialis oblique (Fig. 26.16)
- Stronger medial pull by medial patellar retinaculum

CLINICAL CORRELATION

- Recurrent dislocation of patella on extension of knee may occur if the factors, which keep its position are diseased, for example, weakness of quadriceps muscle, traumatic rupture of medial patellar retinaculum, congenitally underdeveloped lateral condyle of femur or greater Q angle due to patella alta or genu valgum.
- Patella may be fractured by direct trauma or by sudden and forceful contraction of quadriceps femoris.

TIBIA (SHIN BONE)

The tibia is the medial bone of the leg. It is a strong bone as it is a weight bearing bone in standing position.

Parts

The tibia consists of:
- Broad upper end
- Shaft
- Narrow lower end

The medial malleolus is a bony projection arising from the medial side of the lower end. It is a palpable landmark at the medial aspect of ankle.

Articulations

- Knee joint
- Superior tibiofibular joint
- Middle tibiofibular joint
- Inferior tibiofibular joint
- Ankle joint

Upper End

The upper end of tibia presents lateral and medial condyles, and intercondylar area on the superior aspect. It presents tibial tuberosity on the anterior aspect.

Medial Condyle

- The superior surface of medial condyle shows oval articular surface for articulation with medial condyle of femur and for the medial meniscus.
- Its posterior surface presents a deep groove for the insertion of semimembranosus.

Lateral Condyle

- The superior surface of lateral condyle shows circular articular area for articulation with lateral condyle of femur and lateral meniscus.

- The inferolateral part of posterior surface of lateral condyle shows a rounded facet for articulation with head of fibula at superior tibiofibular joint
- The anterior surface of lateral condyle presents a facet (Gerdy's tubercle) for attachment of iliotibial tract.

Intercondylar Area (Fig. 24.8)

An intercondylar non-articular area is present between the two articular surfaces on the superior surfaces the two condyles. There is an elevation in the middle part of this area which is called intercondylar eminence or tubercle. Three structures are attached in front of the tubercle and three behind the tubercle.

Intra-articular Structures Attached to Intercondylar Area (in Anteroposterior Order):
- Anterior horn of medial meniscus
- Anterior cruciate ligament
- Anterior horn of lateral meniscus
- Posterior horn of lateral meniscus
- Posterior horn of medial meniscus
- Posterior cruciate ligament.

> **STUDENT INTEREST**
>
> Mnemonic for structures at intercondylar area: MAL-LMP (anterior horn of Medial meniscus, Anterior cruciate ligament, anterior horn of Lateral meniscus, posterior horn of Lateral meniscus, posterior horn of Medial meniscus, Posterior cruciate ligament)
> Additional Mnemonic: Mobile And Laptop- Laptop Mobile Pen-drive

Tibial Tuberosity

It is an elevation on the anterior surface of upper end of tibia. The ligamentum patellae is attached to its upper smooth part and the subcutaneous infrapatellar bursa is related to its lower rough part.

> **CLINICAL CORRELATION**
>
> In Osgood Schlatter disease in young growing athletes (mostly boys), stress of repeated contraction of quadriceps femoris is transmitted to tibial tuberosity. This leads to strain on secondary center of ossification in tibial tuberosity, which may cause multiple avulsion fractures. There is excess bone growth in tibial tuberosity producing a painful swelling.

Shaft

The shaft presents three borders (anterior lateral and medial) and three surfaces (lateral, medial and posterior).

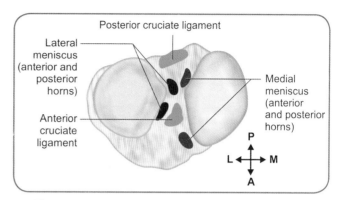

Fig. 24.8: Structures attached to intercondylar area of tibia

- **Anterior border** or shin is sharp and entirely subcutaneous. It begins at the lower end of tibial tuberosity o the anterior border of medial malleolus
- **Medial border** extends from medial condyle to posterior border of medial malleolus
- **Lateral** or **interosseous border** extends from lateral condyle to anterior margin of fibular notch on the lower end of tibia. It gives attachment to interosseous membrane.

Surfaces

Medial surface

It is a subcutaneous surface. It lies between anterior and medial borders.

Insertion on medial surface

Its upper end receives insertion of sartorius, gracilis and semitendinosus from before backwards. The pattern created by linear insertions of their tendons on the tibia resembles the foot of a goose, which in Greek is pes anserinus (Fig. 24.9). Therefore these three muscles are called anserine muscles and the bursa between them and tibial collateral ligament attached deep to the tendons is known as anserine bursa.

> **STUDENT INTEREST**
>
> ***Mnemonic for three anserine muscles:*** Gracy between Surgeon and Sister

> **CLINICAL CORRELATION**
>
> - Anserine bursa provides a cushion for the motion between the knee joint and the three tendons. Overuse of muscles especially in athletes may cause inflammation of the bursa leading to pes anserine bursitis.
> - Long saphenous vein (accompanied by saphenous nerve) crosses the lower third of the medial surface. It is often cannulated in front of the medial malleolus.

Contd...

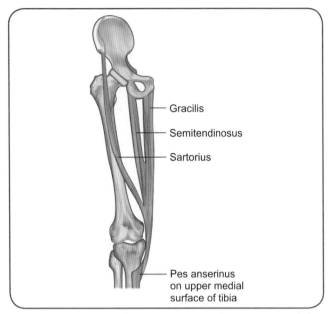

Fig. 24.9: Insertion of pes anserinus muscles on upper medial surface of tibia

Contd...

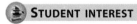 **CLINICAL CORRELATION**

- For purpose of bone grafting, pieces from medial surface and the shin are used
- Upper part of medial surface is the favored site for marrow puncture and intra-osseous infusion in very small children.

Lateral surface (Fig. 24.10)

It is between anterior and interosseous margins. It forms the lateral boundary of anterior compartment of leg (Fig. 30.1).

- Its upper two third gives origin to tibialis anterior muscle.
- Its lower third is related to the tendons of tibialis anterior and extensor hallucis longus, anterior tibial artery, deep peroneal nerve, tendons of extensor digitorum longus and peroneus tertius (from medial to lateral as shown in Fig. 24.11).

STUDENT INTEREST

Mnemonic for order of structures at lower third of lateral surface of tibia: The Hostels Are Not Dirty Places.

Posterior surface

It is between medial and lateral borders.

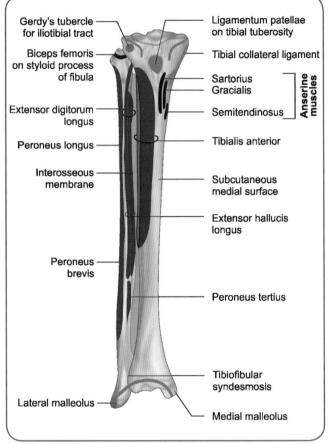

Fig. 24.10: Attachments of tibia and fibula as seen from anterior aspect

- Soleal line is a roughened oblique ridge, which gives attachment to fascia covering popliteus and origin of soleus.
- A triangular area above the soleal line receives insertion of popliteus.
- The posterior surface below soleal line is divided into medial and lateral areas by a vertical line. A nutrient foramen is located at the upper end of vertical line. The nutrient canal is directed downwards.
- The medial area below the soleal line provides origin to flexor digitorum longus.
- The lateral area below the soleal line provides origin to tibialis posterior.
- ***The lower fourth of the posterior surface is related from medial to lateral to:*** Tibialis posterior, flexor digitorum longus, posterior tibial artery, tibial nerve and flexor hallucis longus (Fig. 24.12).

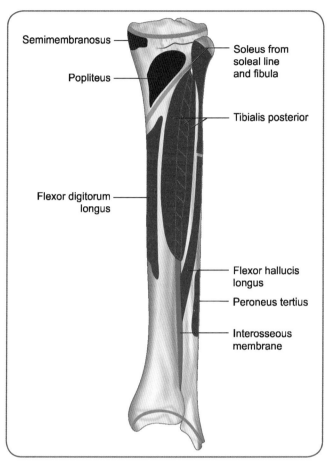

Fig. 24.11: Attachments of tibia and fibula as seen from posterior aspect

Lower End

The lower end of the tibia is smaller than its upper end. It presents 5 surfaces (anterior, posterior medial, lateral and inferior) and a projection called medial malleolus from the medial surface.

- The anterior surface is crossed by structures in the anterior compartment of leg (same as lateral surface described above).
- The posterior surface is related to structures that enter the sole from the posterior compartment of leg (same as relations of lower fourth of posterior surface of shaft).
- Laterally it presents fibular notch for articulation with fibula to form inferior tibiofibular syndesmosis.
- The inferior surface has articular facet for articulating with facet on the superior surface of talus at ankle joint.

Medial Malleolus

The lower end projects medially as medial malleolus, which is subcutaneous. The posterior surface of medial malleolus is grooved by tendon of tibialis posterior (Fig. 24.12). The lateral surface of medial malleolus bears a comma shaped articular facet for articulating with malleolar facet on medial surface of talus. The apex of the medial malleolus gives attachment to deltoid ligament of ankle joint.

Growing End

The upper end of tibia is its growing end. The nutrient foramen points inferiorly. The nutrient artery is derived from posterior tibial artery and is the largest nutrient artery.

Blood Supply

- Nutrient artery arises from posterior tibial artery. Tibial nutrient artery is the largest nutrient artery in the body. It enters the bone distal to the soleal line and runs downwards in the nutrient canal to enter the medullary cavity where it divides in to 3 ascending branches and 1 descending branch.
- Periosteal arteries arise from muscular branches of anterior and posterior tibial arteries. Since lower one third of the shaft of tibia is devoid of muscular attachments it lacks supply from periosteal arteries.

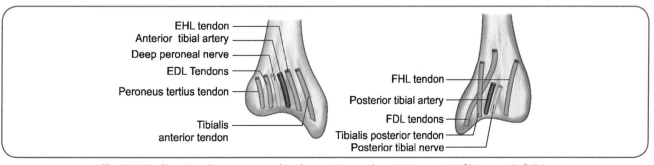

Fig. 24.12: Showing the structures related to anterior and posterior aspects of lower end of tibia

The vascularity of lower one third of tibia is relatively poor hence fractures at lower one third take longer time to heal or do not heal.

FIBULA

The fibula is the lateral bone of the leg. It is very thin because it does not transmit weight. In shape it resembles a brooch, which means fibula in Greek.

Articulations

- Superior tibiofibular joint
- Middle tibiofibular joint
- Inferior tibiofibular joint
- Ankle joint

Features

The fibula consists of upper end, shaft and lower end.

Upper End

The upper end presents head, neck and styloid process.
- The head of fibula bears a rounded facet superiorly for articulating with reciprocal facet on lateral condyle of tibia at superior tibiofibular joint.
- The styloid process is an upward projection from the posterolateral aspect of head. The fibular collateral ligament is attached to it and the biceps femoris muscle is inserted into it.
- The neck of fibula is palpable. The common peroneal nerve can be rolled against the posterolateral surface of the neck.

Shaft (Fig. 24.13)

The shaft of fibula presents three margins, anterior, posterior and medial or interosseous (which give attachment to anterior intermuscular septum, posterior intermuscular septum and the interosseous membrane of the leg respectively). There are three surface of fibula called medial, lateral and posterior.

Surfaces

- **Medial** or **extensor surface** is narrow. It gives origin to extensor digitorum longus, extensor hallucis longus and peroneus tertius.
- **Lateral** or **peroneal surface** gives origin to peroneus longus and peroneus brevis.
- **Posterior** or **flexor surface** presents peroneal crest or medial crest that divides the posterior surface into medial and lateral areas. The medial area gives origin to tibialis posterior and lateral area to flexor hallucis longus. The peroneal artery is closely related to the medial crest. The nutrient foramen is located near the medial crest. It is directed downwards.

🦫 STUDENT INTEREST

Peroneal artery is closely related to medial crest (which divides the posterior surface of fibula in to lateral and medial areas).

⌀ CLINICAL CORRELATION

The fibula is an ideal bone for taking pieces for bone grafting. The bone graft is taken from the site of nutrient foramen so that the graft will have its own artery in the new location.

Lower End (Lateral Malleolus)

The lower end of fibula is expanded to form lateral malleolus, which is half cm lower than the medial malleolus. The lateral malleolus presents four surfaces as follows:
- Medial surface (Fig. 24.14) bears anteriorly a triangular articular facet and a malleolar fossa posteriorly. The

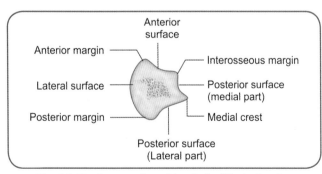

Fig. 24.13: Cross-section of the shaft of fibula showing borders and surfaces

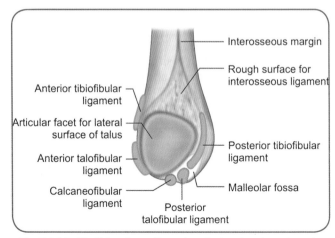

Fig. 24.14: Medial surface of lateral malleolus showing triangular articular facet anteriorly and rough malleolar fossa posteriorly

upper part of this fossa gives attachment to posterior tibiofibular ligament and the lower part to posterior talofibular ligament.

- Lateral surface is subcutaneous.
- Anterior surface provides attachment to anterior tibiofibular and talofibular ligaments.
- Posterior surface presents a groove for tendons of peroneus brevis and peroneus longus. The peroneus brevis is deeper to the peroneus longus.

🏊 STUDENT INTEREST

To identify the side of fibula (Fig. 24.15): First identify the malleolar fossa on the lower end of fibula. Hold the lower end between your thumb and index finger by putting the thumb in to the malleolar fossa and index finger on the lateral surface. You will be able to hold in this fashion only right fibula in your right hand and left fibula in your left hand.

Growing End

The upper end of fibula is its growing end. The direction of nutrient foramen is towards the ankle and nutrient artery is a branch of peroneal artery.

Ossification

Fibula ossifies from one primary center for shaft and two secondary centers for two ends. The secondary center for lower end appears by 1 – 2 years and fuses with the shaft by 18 years. The secondary center for upper end of fibula appears by 3 – 4 years and fuses with the shaft by 20 years.

The rule of ossification states that the secondary center that appears first fuses with the shaft last. Therefore the lower end of fibula breaks the rule of ossification. The explanation for this unusual feature is as follows:

As per the rule, pressure epiphysis appears before traction epiphysis. The center for lower end of fibula (pressure epiphysis) appears first but the upper epiphysis fuses last because it is the growing end of the fibula.

⌀ CLINICAL CORRELATION

Fractures of Bones of Leg

- The common site of fracture of tibia is at the junction upper two third and lower third of the shaft. The junction is the narrowest part of tibia.
- Tibia is the most common long bone to fracture and most commonly it is the compound or open fracture (due to its exposed position).
- Tibial shaft fractures have the highest rate of nonunion among the long bones of the body. This is due to relatively poor blood supply of lower third of tibia. Absence of muscle attachments in the distal third adds to its poor vascularity (periosteal supply is deficient). When there is fracture of shaft involving the nutrient artery chances of nonunion or delayed union are more.
- Fracture of neck of fibula is likely to injure common peroneal nerve.
- Pott's fracture occurs if the foot is trapped in a rabbit hole in the ground. There is fracture of lateral malleolus, medial malleolus and posterior margin of lower end of tibia in succession.

SKELETON OF FOOT (FIG. 24.16)

The foot consists of 28 bones (7 tarsal, 5 metatarsal, 14 phalanges and 2 sesamoid bones (in the tendons of insertion of flexor hallucis brevis).

Tarsal Bones

There are seven small irregular tarsal bones, which articulate with each other and with the metatarsal bones to form segmented levers in the foot.

Rows of Tarsal Bones

- Proximal row: Calcaneus below and talus above it
- Distal row: Cuneiform bones (lateral cuneiform, intermediate cuneiform and medial cuneiform) and the cuboid bone

Talus (Figs 24.17A, B and C)

The talus is located on the upper surface of calcaneus. ***One peculiar feature of talus is that it has no muscular attachments.***

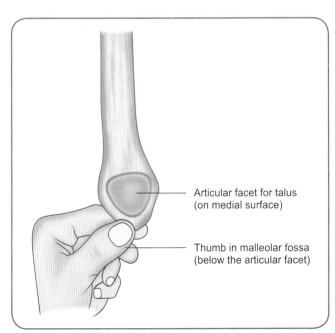

Articular facet for talus (on medial surface)

Thumb in malleolar fossa (below the articular facet)

Fig. 24.15: Showing the method to hold the lower end of fibula between thumb and index finger to assign side to the bone

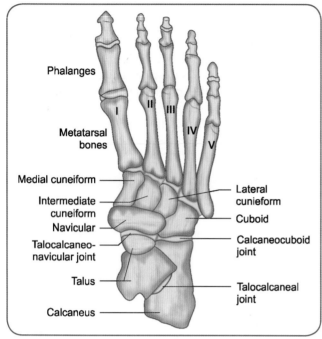

Fig. 24.16: Showing bones and joints of the articulated foot

Articulations of talus

- Ankle joint
- Subtalar or posterior talocalcanean joint
- Talocalcaneonavicular joint

Features

The talus is shaped like a tortoise with a body, neck and head.

Head of talus

- Its oval distal surface articulates with the navicular bone.
- Its plantar surface bears three facets as follow:
  - Posterior facet articulates with sustentaculum tali of calcaneus.
  - Anterolateral to the above facet, there is a facet for calcaneus.
  - On medial side there is a third facet, which comes in contact with fibrocartilaginous upper surface of spring ligament.

Neck of talus

The neck is present between the head and body. It has dorsal and plantar surfaces.

- The narrow medial end of the planter surface is called sulcus tali, which takes part in the formation of sinus tarsi along with reciprocal sulcus calcanei.

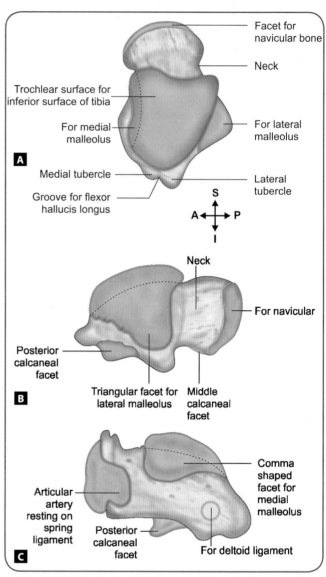

Figs 24.17A to C: Articular facets on right talus **A.** as seen in superior view; **B.** as seen in lateral view and **C.** as seen in medial view (Note the articular facet by which the head of talus rests on the spring ligament)

- The plantar surface provides attachment to interosseous talocalcaneal and cervical ligaments, which are the contents of sinus tarsi (Fig. 24.18).

Body of talus

The body presents five surfaces, superior, inferior, lateral, medial and posterior.

- Superior surface bears trochlear articular surface, which articulates with articular surface of lower end of tibia.

- Inferior surface bears articular facet for articulating with posterior facet of calcaneus to form subtalar joint.
- Medial surface has a comma shaped articular surface for articulation with a corresponding facet on lateral surface of medial malleolus of tibia. The deltoid ligament of ankle joint is attached to the non-articular part of the medial surface.
- Lateral surface has a triangular articular facet for articulating with similar facet on medial surface of lateral malleolus of fibula.
- Posterior surface is grooved by tendon of flexor hallucis longus. This groove is flanked by medial and lateral tubercles. When the lateral tubercle is a separate bone, it is called os trigonum (an example of atavistic epiphysis).

Calcaneus or Heel Bone (Figs 24.18A and B)

The calcaneus is the largest and strongest bone of the foot. It forms the heel of the foot. It is the first tarsal bone to ossify. It presents six surfaces, anterior, posterior, medial, lateral, superior and inferior. Its narrow anterior surface bears facet, medial surface presents shelf like projection called sustentaculum tali and inferior surface is rough (this information is sufficient to assign side to the bone).

Articulations of calcaneus

- Subtalar joints
- Talocalcaneonavicular joint
- Calcaneocuboid joint (Fig. 24.18B)

Surfaces

- The anterior surface presents a concavo-convex articular facet for cuboid.
- The posterior surface is divisible into three areas from above downwards. The upper part is smooth as it is related to a synovial bursa. The middle part receives insertion of tendocalcaneus and plantaris. The lower part is in contact with fibrofatty tissue.
- The superior or dorsal surface is divisible into three areas. The posterior one third is rough and covered with fibrofatty tissue. The middle one third bears the posterior facet for talus. The anterior one third is divided into anteromedial articular area and non-articular area. The anteromedial area shows middle and anterior facets for talus. The middle facet is located on sustentaculum tali. The non-articular area is further divided into narrow medial part and wider lateral part. The narrow medial part is called sulcus calcanei, which gives attachment to interosseous talocalcaneal ligament and cervical ligament. The lateral area provides origin to extensor digitorum brevis and gives

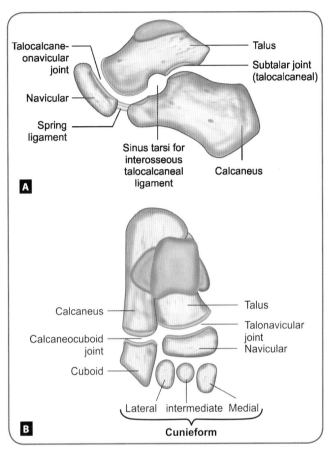

Figs 24.18A and B: A. Showing sinus tarsi (which contains interosseous talocalcaneal ligament and cervical ligament); **B.** Showing talonavicular (part of talocalcaneonavicular joint) and calcaneocuboid joint

attachment to stem of Y shaped inferior extensor retinaculum.

- The inferior or plantar surface is characterized by anterior tubercle anteriorly. The short plantar ligament is attached to it. Posteriorly this surface is marked by tuber calcanei or calcaneal tuberosity, which is subdivided into lateral and medial processes. The long plantar ligament is attached to the area between anterior tubercle and calcaneal tuberosity.
- The lateral surface is subcutaneous. Its anterior part is marked by a small elevation called peroneal trochlea or tubercle. The inferior extensor retinaculum is attached to it and the tendons of peroneus brevis (above) and of peroneus longus (below) are closely related to it.
- The medial surface is marked by a shelf like projection called sustentaculum tali from its upper anterior part. A middle articular facet for the head of talus is present on the superior aspect of the projection. The tendon of flexor hallucis longus grooves the inferior surface

of the sustentaculum tali whereas the tendon of flexor digitorum longus is related to its medial surface. The medial surface of sustentaculum tali gives attachment to spring ligament, superficial fibers of deltoid ligament and a slip from the tibialis posterior muscle.

Navicular Bone

The name navicular (in Latin) is derived from its resemblance to a small ship. The navicular bone lies along the medial margin of the foot in front of the head of talus. It presents 6 surfaces.
- The anterior surface has three facets for articulation with the three cuneiform bones.
- The posterior surface is deeply concave. It articulates with the head of talus.
- The medial surface presents navicular tuberosity, which receives the main insertion of tibialis posterior. The tuberosity is directed downwards. It is separated from plantar surface by an inferiorly directed groove (occupied by tendon of tibialis posterior).
- The lateral surface may present a facet for cuboid bone.
- The plantar surface provides attachment to plantar calcaneonavicular ligament.
- The dorsal or superior surface gives attachment to talonavicular ligament.

Cuboid Bone (Fig. 24.18B)

It is roughly cubical in shape. It is the lateral bone of the distal row of tarsal bones lying in front of the calcaneus. It presents 6 surfaces.
- Its anterior surface bears facets for articulation with bases of fourth and fifth metatarsals.
- Its posterior surface bears concavo-convex facet to articulate with reciprocal facet of anterior surface of calcaneus.
- The plantar surface is marked by a deep groove (anteriorly) for lodging the tendon of peroneus longus. The plantar surface gives attachment to long and short plantar ligaments. It also receives a slip of insertion of tibialis posterior.
- The dorsal surface is rough.
- The medial surface has articular facet for articulation with lateral cuneiform.
- The lateral surface is narrow and notched by tendon of peroneus longus.

Cuneiform Bones

The medial, intermediate and lateral cuneiform bones are wedge-shaped and are part of the medial longitudinal arch.

Articulations
- The posterior surfaces of the three cuneiforms articulate with navicular bone.
- The distal surface of medial cuneiform articulates with the base of first metatarsal, that of intermediate cuneiform with base of second metatarsal and that of lateral cuneiform with the base of third metatarsal.
- The lateral surface of lateral cuneiform articulates with cuboid and base of fourth metatarsal bone.

Attachments

Medial cuneiform receives insertion of tibialis posterior (on plantar surface), peroneus longus (on lateral side of plantar surface) and tibialis anterior (on medial and plantar surfaces).

Ossification Centers of Tarsal Bones (Table 24.1)

Ossification centers in lower limb at birth

The radiograph of knee and foot in full term newborn usually shows five ossification centers, two around the knee (lower end of femur and upper end of tibia) and three in the foot, (calcaneus, talus and cuboid).

Metatarsal Bones

There are five metatarsal bones, which are numbered from medial to lateral side.
- The first metatarsal is short and stout for weight bearing. The head of the first metatarsal bone makes pressure contact with the ground at the beginning of taking a step. The sesamoid bones in the tendons of flexor hallucis brevis articulate directly with the plantar surface of this bone.
- The second metatarsal is the longest and least mobile.
- The fifth metatarsal has a tuberosity at its base, which can be palpated along the lateral margin of foot. The tuberosity receives insertion of peroneus brevis. Sometimes the pull of contraction of this muscle may fracture the tuberosity. Sometimes the tuberosity may

TABLE 24.1: Ossification centers of tarsal bones

Tarsal bone	Time of appearance
Calcaneus	3rd month of IUL
Talus	6th month of IUL
Cuboid	Just before birth
Lateral cuneiform	In first year
Medial cuneiform	In second year
Intermediate cuneiform and Navicular	In third year

ossify by separate center and remain separate from the base, in which case it is known as os Vesalius.

The metatarsal bones and phalanges of the foot provide insertion to a large number of long muscles of the leg and to the short muscles of the foot.

⚕ CLINICAL CORRELATION

Fractures of Bones of Foot

- The fractures of talus and calcaneus are not common. But they may be crushed in landing on the calcaneus from a height.
- Though fracture of talus is rare, forceful dorsiflexion of foot may fracture the neck of talus (for example in on forceful pressure on brake during head on collusion of the car). Arteries supplying the talus enter through its neck and course backwards in the body. They are injured in fracture of the neck. Avascular necrosis of the body of talus is the complication of this fracture (compare this with fracture of scaphoid in hand).
- The tuberosity of the fifth metatarsal bone may be avulsed by trivial twisting injuries of the forefoot.
- Fatigue fractures (march fractures) are common in metatarsal bones. This is due to repeated small bending stresses to the bones. The second metatarsal bone is the most frequently fractured bone in young adults.

Sesamoid Bones in Lower Limb

- Patella in tendon of quadriceps femoris
- Fabella in lateral head of gastrocnemius
- Rider's bone in tendon of adductor longus
- Os peroneum in tendon of peroneus longus where it winds round to enter the canal in the cuboid.
- Two sesamoid bones in the tendons of insertion of flexor hallucis brevis (also known as hallux sesamoids).

Accessory Bones in Skeleton of Foot

- Os trigonum (separate ossification center for lateral tubercle of talus).
- Os Vesalius or Vesalianum (tuberosity of 5th metatarsal ossifies from separate center).
- Os naviculare secundarium or accessory navicular bone is an extra navicular bone seen from birth.

25

Surface Features, Cutaneous Nerves, Venous and Lymphatic Drainage of Lower Limb

Chapter Contents

INTRODUCTION

The lower limb is subdivided into the following regions:
- Gluteal region
- Thigh,
- Popliteal fossa
- Leg
- Ankle
- Foot

SURFACE FEATURES

- The iliac crest, which is palpable in its entire extent, forms the superior limit of the gluteal region. The highest point of the iliac crest is at the level of the space between the spines of L3 and L4 vertebrae.
- The anterior superior iliac spine is easy to palpate in thin individuals.
- The tubercle of the iliac crest is located 5 cm behind the anterior superior iliac spine. The plane passing through it is known as transtubercular plane and it corresponds to the spine of L5 vertebra.
- The posterior superior iliac spine is indicated by a skin dimple, which is located four cm lateral to the spine of second sacral vertebra. One can palpate the sacroiliac joint at this site.
- The pubic symphysis is felt at the lowest limit of abdominal wall in the median plane. The pubic crest, which is the superior margin of the pubis and its lateral end, called pubic tubercle are palpable parts of the pubic bone.
- The ischial tuberosity is easily palpable in sitting position. The weight of the body is supported by the ischial tuberosities in this position.
- The greater trochanter of femur can be felt a hand's breadth below the midpoint of the iliac crest.
- The condyles of femur are subcutaneous hence easily palpable, when the knee is flexed or extended.
- The adductor tubercle is felt above and behind the medial epicondyle of femur. It is continuous with the lower end of medial supracondylar line. The lower epiphyseal line of femur passes through the adductor tubercle.
- The patella or kneecap moves during flexion and extension of knee joint. Its lateral and medial margins are felt, when the knee is flexed.
- The tibial tuberosity is felt five cm below the apex of patella. The tibial condyles form visible and palpable landmarks at the medial and lateral sides of ligamentum patellae.
- The anterior border of tibia (called shin) is sharp and palpable in its entire extent.
- The medial subcutaneous surface of tibia lies medial to the shin.
- The medial malleolus at the lower end of tibia is subcutaneous and the great saphenous vein runs along its anterior margin.

- The head of fibula is subcutaneous at the posterolateral aspect of the knee and is palpable at the level of the superior margin of tibial tuberosity. The neck of the fibula is palpable distal to the head. The lower end of shaft of fibula is subcutaneous.
- The lateral malleolus is subcutaneous. Its tip extends further distally than that of medial malleolus.
- The posterior, lateral and medial surfaces of calcaneus are palpable. The sustentaculum tali is usually felt as a small prominence about a fingerbreadth below the tip of medial malleolus.
- The peroneal trochlea is felt as a small tubercle on the lateral aspect of the calcaneus, two cm distal to the tip of lateral malleolus. The tendon of peroneus brevis passes above and the tendon of peroneus longus passes below the peroneal trochlea.
- The head of talus is palpable anterior to the medial malleolus if the foot is everted and anteromedial to the lateral malleolus if the foot is inverted.

- The head of the first metatarsal bone is a prominent landmark on the medial aspect of distal foot. The tuberosity of the fifth metatarsal bone is palpable at the midpoint of the lateral margin of foot. The shafts of metatarsals and phalanges are palpable on the dorsum of foot.

CUTANEOUS INNERVATION OF LOWER LIMB (FIGS 25.1A AND 25.1B)

The cutaneous nerves of the lower limb are derived from five sources, subcostal nerve (T12), branches of lumbar plexus, branches of sacral plexus and the dorsal rami of lumbar and sacral nerves.

Gluteal Region

The gluteal region is the only part of the lower limb that receives sensory supply from dorsal as well as ventral rami.

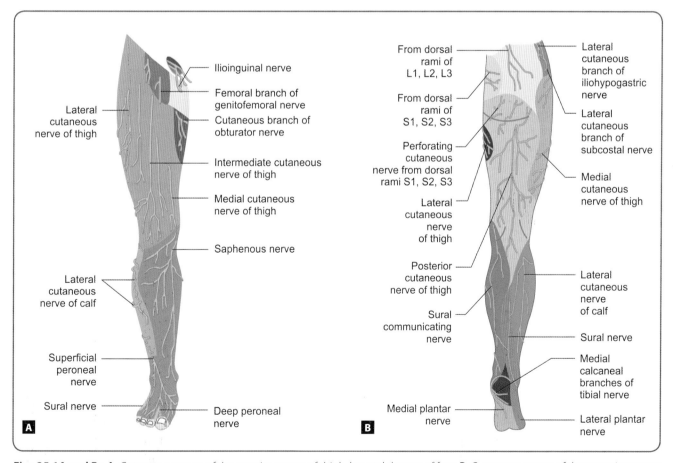

Figs 25.1A and B: A. Cutaneous nerves of the anterior aspect of thigh, leg and dorsum of foot; **B.** Cutaneous nerves of the posterior aspect of thigh, leg and sole

The region may be divided into four unequal areas, which receive cutaneous nerves from different sources.

- Superolateral area receives twigs from the lateral cutaneous branch of subcostal nerve (T12) and of iliohypogastric nerve (L1). These branches pass anterior and posterior to the iliac tubercle to reach the level of greater trochanter.
- Inferolateral area receives branches from lateral cutaneous nerve of thigh (L2, L3), which is a branch of lumbar plexus.
- Superomedial area receives branches from the dorsal rami of L1, L2, L3 nerves and of S1, S2, S3 nerves.
- Inferomedial area receives twigs from the gluteal branches of posterior cutaneous nerve of thigh (S1, S2, S3) and a few twigs from perforating cutaneous nerve (S2, S3), both branches of sacral plexus. The last named cutaneous nerve perforates the sacrotuberous ligament as well as the gluteus maximus muscle.

Front of Thigh

Six cutaneous nerves supply the skin of the front of thigh.
- Direct sensory branches of the lumbar plexus are:
  - Ilioinguinal nerve
  - Femoral branch of genitofemoral nerve
  - Lateral cutaneous nerve of thigh
- Branches of femoral nerve are:
  - Medial femoral cutaneous nerve
  - Intermediate femoral cutaneous nerve
  - Saphenous nerve.

Additionally, the obturator nerve supplies skin of the medial side through its contribution to the subsartorial plexus.

Back of Thigh

Cutaneous nerves of the back of thigh are:
- Posterior cutaneous nerve of thigh.
- Lateral cutaneous nerve of thigh.
- Medial anterior femoral cutaneous nerve of thigh.

Popliteal Fossa

Posterior cutaneous nerve of thigh and medial femoral cutaneous nerve.

Front of Leg

- Saphenous nerve (branch of femoral nerve).
- Lateral cutaneous nerve of calf (branch of common peroneal nerve in popliteal fossa).
- Superficial peroneal nerve (terminal branch of common peroneal nerve).

Back of Leg

- Sural nerve (a branch of tibial nerve in the popliteal fossa).
- Sural communicating nerve (branch of common peroneal nerve in the popliteal fossa).
- A few twigs from posterior cutaneous nerve of thigh and from medial femoral cutaneous nerve of thigh.

Dorsum of Foot

- Superficial peroneal nerve supplies the larger intermediate area.
- Sural nerve supplies the lateral margin.
- Saphenous nerve supplies the medial side up to the base of great toe.

Dorsum of Toes

A total of five nerves supply the dorsal aspects of the toes:
- Sural nerve supplies the lateral side of the little toe.
- Deep peroneal nerve supplies the adjacent sides of first and second toes (first inter-digital cleft).
- Superficial peroneal nerve supplies the remaining toes.
- Medial plantar nerve supplies the nail beds of medial three and half toes.
- Lateral plantar nerve supplies the nail beds of lateral one and half of toes.

Sole of Foot

- Medial calcanean nerve (branch of tibial nerve) supplies the heel.
- Cutaneous branches of medial plantar nerve.
- Cutaneous branches of l lateral plantar nerve.

💡 **ADDED INFORMATION**

Dermatomes of Lower Limb (Figs 25.2A and B)

The ventral rami of lumbar and sacral nerves pleat together to form lumbar and sacral plexuses through which the cutaneous supply of the lower limb is derived. The gluteal region is the only exception that receives sensory nerves additionally from the dorsal rami of L1 to S3 spinal nerves (Fig. 25.1B). In the case of the limbs, dermatome is the area of skin supplied by one ventral ramus through its various cutaneous branches. Therefore, S1 dermatome receives S1 fibers from the cutaneous branches of several peripheral nerves carrying S1 fibers. Only if the sensory rootlets of first sacral nerve are damaged will there be complete anesthesia in S1 dermatome. In injury to the peripheral nerve, the nerve fibers belonging to more than one segment of the spinal cord will be involved and hence the sensory effects will not coincide with any one dermatome.

Contd…

Contd...

 ADDED INFORMATION

The embryonic development of the lower limb helps to understand its dermatomal map. When the lower limb bud elongates it drags down the nerves arising from L1 to S3 segments of spinal cord. Due to the medial rotation of the lower limb bud, the pre-axial digit of the lower limb comes to occupy medial side of the limb bud whereas the postaxial digit moves on the lateral side of the limb bud. The dorsal or extensor surface except the gluteal region comes to lie anteriorly while the ventral or flexor surface faces posteriorly. The pre-axial border starts near the midpoint of thigh and descends to the knee. It then curves medially to descend to the medial malleolus and reach the great toe along the medial margin of foot. In broad terms, the lumbar dermatomes lie in succession from L1 to L5 on the front of the limb. L4 and L5 lie side by side in the front of leg and L5 dermatome occupies the middle of the dorsum of the foot. L5 dermatome includes the great toe and S1 includes the little toe and lateral side of sole and dorsum of foot as of the sole of the foot. S1 dermatome ascends on the back of the leg to be followed by the S2 dermatome up to the gluteal fold and S3 dermatome above it in the gluteal region.

 CLINICAL CORRELATION

The skin on the S1 dermatome on the lateral side of sole is scratched while eliciting Babinski sign.

VENOUS DRAINAGE OF LOWER LIMB

It is essential to know the anatomy of the veins of the lower limb to understand the pathogenesis, diagnosis and surgical treatment of the varicosity of the veins of lower limb. Varicosity is a condition in which the superficial veins of lower limb become tortuous and dilated.

Subdivisions

The veins of the lower limb are divided into the following three groups:
1. Superficial or subcutaneous veins in the superficial fascia
2. Deep veins accompanying the arteries located deep to the deep fascia
3. Perforating veins (passing through the deep fascia) to connect the superficial and deep veins

Long Superficial Veins

- Great or long saphenous vein
- Small or short saphenous vein

The above two veins originate in dorsal venous arch on the dorsum of foot.

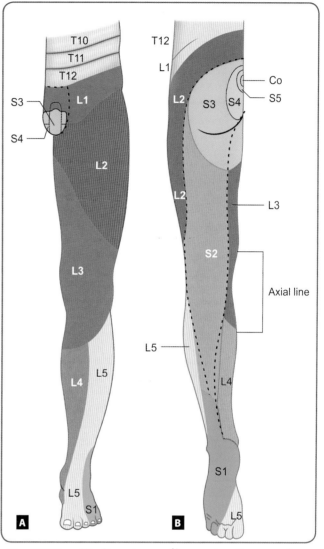

Figs 25.2A and B: Dermatomes of lower extremity as seen from A. Anterior aspect; and B. Posterior aspect

Dorsal venous arch

The dorsal venous arch is located on the distal parts of the metatarsal bones. It receives the dorsal digital and dorsal metatarsal veins and communicates with proximally located dorsal venous network. Along the sides of foot there are medial and lateral marginal veins, which drain both the dorsal and plantar aspects of the respective sides in to the dorsal venous arch.

Great saphenous vein (Fig. 25.3)

The word 'saphenous', which is Greek in origin, means easily seen. Since the saphenous vein lies in the superficial fascia it is easily seen. The great saphenous vein is the longest vein in the body. It is thick-walled and contains numerous valves, which allow the blood to flow towards

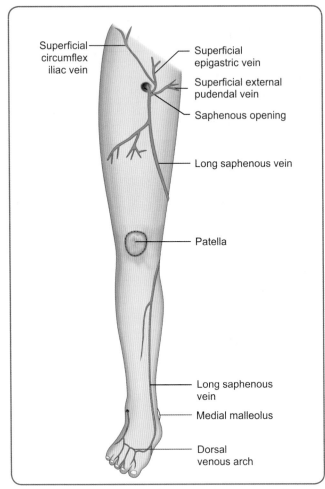

Superficial circumflex iliac vein

Superficial epigastric vein

Superficial external pudendal vein

Saphenous opening

Long saphenous vein

Patella

Long saphenous vein

Medial malleolus

Dorsal venous arch

Fig. 25.3: Origin, course, tributaries and termination of long saphenous vein

heart. The valves divide the long column of blood in short segments so as to reduce the pressure on the distal part of the vein during prolonged standing.

Formation

The formation of great saphenous vein is described in two ways.

1. The medial end of venous arch and medial marginal vein of the foot continue as great saphenous vein.
2. The union of dorsal digital vein of the medial side of big toe and the medial end of dorsal venous arch form the great saphenous vein.

Course and relations

- At the ankle, the great saphenous vein enters the leg at a very constant point. It ascends in the interval between the anterior aspect of the medial malleolus and the tendon of tibialis anterior muscle. Then it remains in contact for a short distance with the distal third of medial subcutaneous surface of the tibia. In

this part of its course it is accompanied by saphenous nerve. Further, it ascends along the medial border of tibia to reach the posterior aspect of the medial side of the knee.

- At the back of the knee, it is about a hands breadth behind the medial border of patella.
- In the thigh, the vein ascends along the medial aspect of the front of the thigh until it reaches the saphenous opening in the fascia lata. A few branches of medial cutaneous nerve of thigh are closely related to it here.
- The great saphenous vein pierces the cribriform fascia at the saphenous opening along with the three superficial branches of the femoral artery (superficial circumflex iliac, superficial epigastric and superficial external pudendal arteries) and lymph vessels.
- It terminates into the femoral vein after piercing the anterior wall of the femoral sheath. A valve guarding the saphenofemoral junction is located at a point about 3.5 to 4 cm inferolateral to the pubic tubercle.

Tributaries

- At the ankle, it receives blood from the sole and the dorsum of foot.
- In the leg, it receives anterior vein of the leg and posterior arch vein, which is formed on the medial malleolus and ascends on the medial aspect of the calf to join the great saphenous vein. The posterior arch vein is connected to the posterior tibial venae comitantes (deep veins) by three ankle perforators. Some surgeons refer the posterior arch vein as vein of Leonardo da Vinci.
- In the thigh, the great saphenous vein receives the anterolateral vein of thigh and posteromedial vein of thigh. Before it passes through the saphenous opening it receives three tributaries, namely, superficial epigastric vein, superficial external pudendal vein and superficial circumflex iliac vein (Fig. 25.3).
- After passing through the saphenous opening but before piercing the femoral sheath it receives deep external pudendal vein (last tributary).

Surface marking of great saphenous vein

Though one can see the long saphenous vein in thin people in its course in the foot and leg it is necessary to know its surface marking in the entire extent because this vein is used for venous cut downs and for coronary artery bypass graft.

- At the ankle the vein passes upwards about 2.5 cm anterior to the medial malleolus.
- In the leg it ascends crossing the medial surface and the medial border of tibia to reach the posteromedial aspect of the knee.

- At the knee it lies about a hand's-breadth posterior to the medial margin of patella.
- In the thigh it ascends along the medial aspect of the front of thigh to enter the saphenous opening.
- Termination of the vein is indicated by centre of the saphenous opening, which is roughly four cm below and lateral to the pubic tubercle.

One should know the surface marking of the termination of saphenous vein while performing various tests to assess saphenofemoral valve competency.

Small saphenous vein

It begins as the continuation of lateral marginal vein of foot or is formed by the union of dorsal digital vein of lateral side of the little toe and lateral end of dorsal venous arch. The short saphenous vein has numerous valves.

Course and relations (Fig. 25.4)

- At first the short saphenous vein ascends posterior to the lateral malleolus and then on the lateral side of the tendocalcaneus.
- It passes along the middle of the calf and pierces the deep fascia in the lower part of the popliteal fossa to open into the popliteal vein above the level of the back of the knee joint (the termination may show variations. It may join the great saphenous vein in the proximal thigh, or it may bifurcate, one branch joining the great saphenous vein and the other joining the popliteal vein).
- In the leg the short saphenous vein is accompanied by sural nerve.

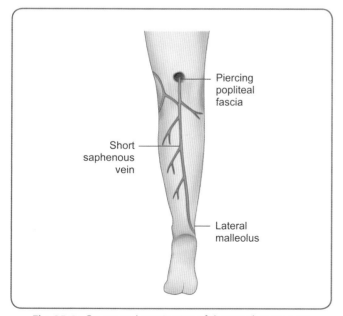

Fig. 25.4: Course and termination of short saphenous vein

Tributaries

At the ankle it receives veins from the sole and dorsum of foot. It receives several cutaneous tributaries of the leg and communications from the great saphenous vein. The perforating vein may connect it to the deep veins of the calf.

Deep Veins of Lower Limb

The deep veins accompany the arteries. The contractions of the muscles (soleus and gastronomies) propel the venous blood upward. Valves are more in deep veins compared to the superficial veins. The deep veins receive blood from superficial veins through perforators (Fig. 25.5).

Major deep veins of lower limb

- Deep veins of the sole (medial and lateral plantar veins)
- Venae comitantes accompanying the dorsalis pedis, posterior tibial and anterior tibial arteries
- Popliteal vein
- Femoral vein.

Factors facilitating venous return

In the standing position the venous blood has to flow against gravity.

The following factors help the venous return:

- The deep veins of the leg lie in the tight fascial compartment along with the arteries. When the muscles of the calf contract there is rise in the pressure inside the compartment, which compresses the deep veins. The valves open up and blood is propelled in upward direction.
- The soleus contains venous sinuses filled with blood and on contraction it squeezes the blood out into the deep veins. For this reason the soleus is regarded as the peripheral heart and the calf muscles collectively work as a venous pump.
- During relaxed state of the muscles the blood is sucked from the superficial to the deep veins through the perforators.
- The pulsations of accompanying arteries help in propelling the blood in the veins.
- The valves in superficial and deep sets of veins allow the blood to flow in upward direction only.
- The negative pressure in the thoracic cavity sucks the blood in the venous system towards heart in standing or recumbent positions.

Perforating Veins or Perforators (Fig. 25.5)

There are about five perforating veins, which connect the great saphenous vein to the deep veins of leg and thigh. These veins are called perforators because they perforate

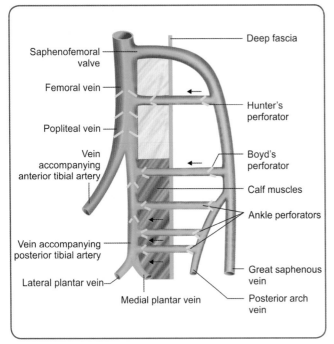

Fig. 25.5: Perforating veins connecting great saphenous vein to the deep veins of leg and thigh (arrows indicate the direction of flow of blood from superficial to deep veins)

the deep fascia. Their unique feature is that they contain unidirectional valves, which allow the blood to flow only from the superficial veins to the deep veins. In this way the perforating veins minimize the load of the superficial veins. The incompetence of the valves of the perforators is one of the causes of dilatation of superficial veins of lower limb.

Position of perforating veins

- Between the medial malleolus and mid-calf there are three ankle perforators of Cockett connecting the posterior arch vein to the venae comitantes of posterior tibial artery. So, these perforators indirectly connect the great saphenous vein to the deep veins of leg.
- At the upper end of the calf there is tibial tubercle perforator or Boyd's perforator that connects the venae comitantes of the posterior tibial artery to the great saphenous vein.
- In the intermediate third of thigh one vein called Hunterian perforator or perforator of Dodd connects the great saphenous vein to the femoral vein in the subsartorial canal. This perforator passes through the fascial roof of the canal.

CLINICAL CORRELATION

- Great saphenous vein is often chosen for a venous cut down in an emergency, when the superficial veins elsewhere are collapsed and invisible. A small skin incision is placed just in front of the medial malleolus (taking care not to injure the accompanying saphenous nerve) to expose the vein for giving intravenous fluids.
- Great saphenous vein is suited for coronary arterial graft as it is a muscular vein. A segment of the patient's great saphenous vein in the thigh is removed to prepare venous graft which is sutured bypassing the blocked coronary artery (Fig. 41.9).
- In varicosity of lower limb, the superficial veins are dilated and tortuous (Figs 25.6 and 25.7). This is common in people, whose jobs require prolonged standing (bus conductors, traffic police, nurses, etc.). Incompetence of valves in perforating veins and incompetence in saphenofemoral valve are major causes of varicosity.
- Trendelenburg test is performed to find out whether the saphenofemoral valve is incompetent or the valves in the perforators are incompetent. The patient lies down in supine position and then asked to raise the leg to empty the superficial veins. The saphenofemoral junction is closed by thumb and the patient is asked to stand up. Immediate filling of the great saphenous vein from above after release of the pressure indicates the incompetence of saphenofemoral valve. This is positive Trendelenburg test. Slow filling from below without releasing the pressure indicates the incompetent valves in the perforating vein or veins. This is also a positive test. The positive tests are indications for operative treatment.

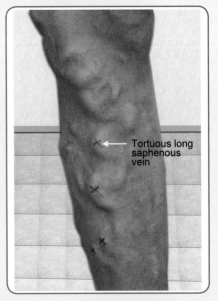

Fig. 25.6: Unilateral varicosity in the leg of a patient (arrow showing)

Contd…

Contd...

CLINICAL CORRELATION

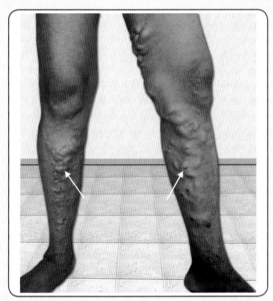

Fig. 25.7: Bilateral varicose veins in the legs of the patient (arrow showing)

- Sometimes, a varicose ulcer (Fig. 25.8) develops in the skin near the medial malleolus. This is due to venous stasis reducing oxygen supply to the skin. Initially the skin becomes dry and discolored and later sloughs producing ulcer.
- Deep vein thrombosis (DVT) or phlebothrombosis in deep veins of the calf (Fig. 25.9) is the most feared complication after major surgical operation. During postoperative convalescence there is minimum activity of the legs, which favors venous stasis and thrombosis. The emboli from the thrombus enter venous circulation to reach the right side of heart and from there enter the pulmonary arteries. Blockage of pulmonary arteries or artery by embolus culminates in life threatening pulmonary embolism.

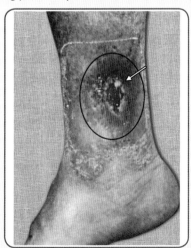

Fig. 25.8: Varicose ulcer just above the medial malleolus

Contd...

Contd...

CLINICAL CORRELATION

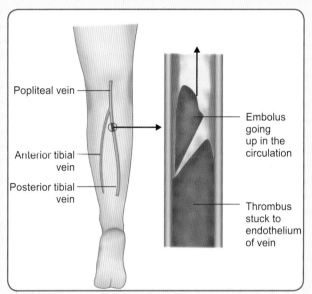

Fig. 25.9: Showing deep vein thrombosis (DVT) in deep vein of calf (posterior tibial vein) and the detached embolus released into the circulation

LYMPHATIC DRAINAGE OF LOWER LIMB

The lymph nodes and lymph vessels of the lower limb are divided into superficial and deep groups.

Superficial Group (Figs 25.10A and B)

The superficial inguinal lymph nodes are located in the superficial fascia of the inguinal region and are normally palpable. They are arranged into two groups or sets (resembling the alphabet T).

1. Horizontally disposed lymph nodes parallel to and just below the inguinal ligament.
2. Vertically disposed lymph nodes along the terminal part of great saphenous vein.

Areas of Drainage

Medial inguinal lymph nodes of horizontal group

- External genitalia in both sexes except the glans penis or clitoris
- Lower end of vagina in female
- Terminal part of male urethra
- Lower part of anal canal
- Medial half of the anterior abdominal wall below the umbilicus
- Part of fundus of uterus (tubo-uterine junction) in female

Lateral inguinal lymph nodes of horizontal group

- Gluteal region
- Lateral half of anterior abdominal wall below the umbilicus
- Entire lower limb except lateral part of foot, heel and lateral part of back of leg

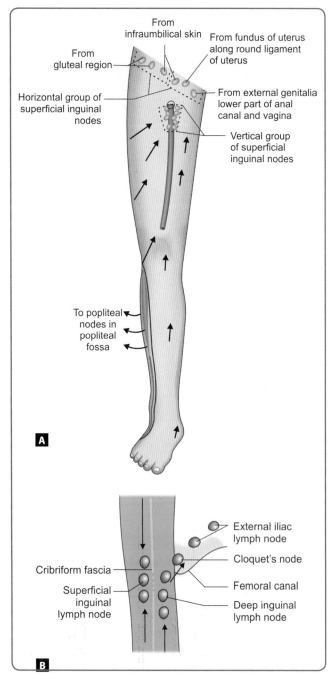

A

B

Figs 25.10A and B: A. Superficial lymph vessels of lower limb; **B.** Direction of lymph flow in superficial and deep inguinal lymph nodes.

Deep Group (Fig. 25.11)

The deep lymph nodes are located deep to the deep fascia.

- Deep inguinal lymph nodes
- Popliteal nodes

Deep Inguinal Lymph Nodes

They are located in the femoral triangle in relation to femoral vessels They receive lymph from the deeper tissues of the thigh, the popliteal lymph nodes and from the superficial inguinal lymph nodes. The efferent vessels from the deep group drain into the external iliac nodes. One member of the deep group called Cloquet node, is located in the femoral canal. It receives lymph from the glans penis in male and clitoris in female.

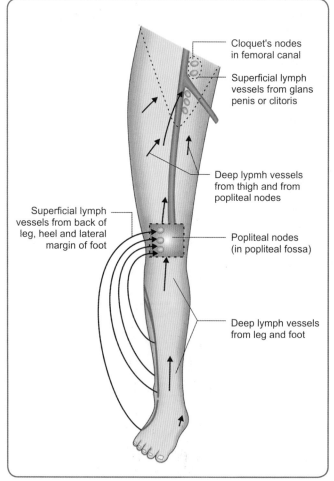

Fig. 25.11: Showing areas of drainage of popliteal and deep inguinal lymph nodes

Popliteal Lymph Nodes (Fig. 29.23)

The popliteal lymph nodes are embedded in the fat in the popliteal fossa. They are about three to six in number and are disposed in three sets.

1. Superficial or posterior lymph node at sapheno-popliteal venous junction.
2. Deepest or anterior lymph node between knee joint and popliteal artery.
3. Intermediate lymph nodes on either side of the popliteal vessels.
   The popliteal lymph nodes are unique because they are the only deep lymph nodes that receive both superficial and deep lymph vessels.
4. Superficial lymph node receives superficial vessels from lateral side of foot, the heel and the lateral half of the back of the leg because these lymph vessels travel with small saphenous vein, which opens into popliteal vein.
5. Intermediate lymph nodes receive deep lymph vessels accompanying the deep blood vessels (anterior and posterior tibial) from the entire leg and foot.
6. The most anterior node receives lymph from the knee joint.

The efferent vessels from the popliteal nodes reach the deep inguinal lymph nodes.

CLINICAL CORRELATION

- The lesion of prepuce, penis, labia majora, scrotum, lower part of vagina, uterotubal junction (part of fundus of uterus), lower part of anal canal will cause enlargement of horizontal chain of superficial inguinal lymph nodes. A boil or abscess in the gluteal region will cause inflammation and swelling of lateral nodes of horizontal group.
- Enlargement of popliteal lymph nodes occurs in inflammatory lesions of heel, lateral side of the foot and back of leg.

Contd…

Contd…

CLINICAL CORRELATION

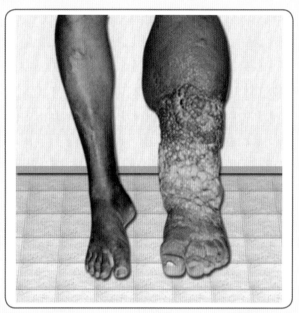

Fig. 25.12: Photo of a patient showing elephantiasis of lower limb due to blockage of lymph vessels of lower limb

- The lymphatic vessels of the lower limb may be blocked by micro-filarial parasites (Wuchereria Bancrofti). This usually manifests as massive edema of the lower limb (elephantiasis as seen in a patient (Fig. 25.12).
- In inflammatory lesions of the lower limb, the inguinal lymph nodes in vertical chain are enlarged and painful.
- The melanoma originates from the melanocytes of the skin. The common site of this tumor is on any one of the medial toes. Since this cancer spreads by lymphatics, there is enlargement of inguinal nodes. Therefore, the affected toe is amputated along with complete removal of the inguinal lymph nodes.

26

Front of Thigh

Chapter Contents

INTRODUCTION

The thigh extends from the hip to the knee. The proximal extent of the thigh is bounded by the inguinal region or groin anteriorly, perineum medially and the gluteal fold posteriorly. Distally, the thigh extends anteriorly to the front of the knee and posteriorly to the popliteal fossa. The thigh is divided into three osteofascial compartments by intermuscular septa, which pass from the fascia lata to the linea aspera of femur.

OSTEOFASCIAL COMPARTMENTS (FIG. 26.1)

- Anterior or extensor compartment containing extensor muscles supplied by femoral nerve.
- Posterior or flexor compartment containing hamstring muscles supplied by sciatic nerve.
- Medial or adductor compartment containing adductor muscles supplied by obturator nerve.

Superficial Fascia of Thigh

In the upper part of the front of thigh, the superficial fascia consists of two layers (superficial fatty layer and deep membranous layer). These two layers are continuous in front of the inguinal ligament with corresponding layers of anterior abdominal wall. The membranous layer is fused with the deep fascia of thigh along a horizontal line starting from the pubic tubercle and passing for about eight cm laterally. This line is referred to as Holden's line (Fig. 26.2). This line of fascial fusion seals the space between the membranous layer of superficial fascia and the external oblique aponeuroses in the infraumbilical abdominal wall. This explains why the extravasated urine (in rupture of urethra in perineum) deep to the membranous layer of superficial fascia in the anterior abdominal wall does not descend in to the thigh below this line.

Deep Fascia of Thigh (Fascia Lata)

The deep fascia of the thigh encircles the thigh like a stocking. It has a wide attachment superiorly. It is attached to all the bony prominences at the knee inferiorly.

Upper Attachment

- *Anteriorly:* To inguinal ligament
- *Laterally:* To iliac crest
- *Medially:* To body and inferior ramus of pubis and ramus and tuberosity of ischium
- *Posteriorly:* To sacrotuberous ligament, sacrum and coccyx

In the gluteal region it splits to enclose the gluteus maximus muscle.

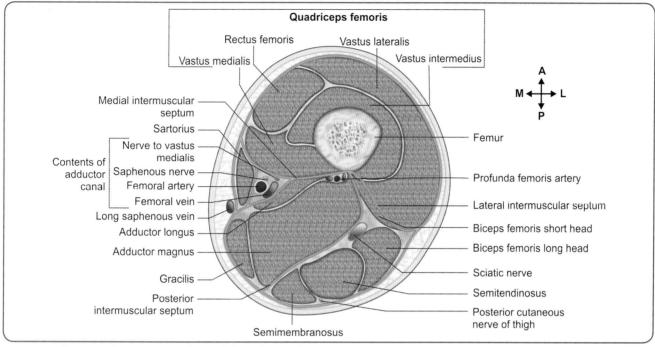

Fig. 26.1: Cross-section at the level of midthigh to depict the osteofascial compartments of thigh with their contents

Inferior Attachment

- Anteriorly to patella, condyles of femur and tibia and head of fibula.

  (Patella is held to the tibial condyles by lateral and medial patellar retinacula which are thickened bands of deep fascia and through which lateral and medial vasti are inserted into respective margins of patella).
- Posteriorly, the fascia lata continues as the popliteal fascia.

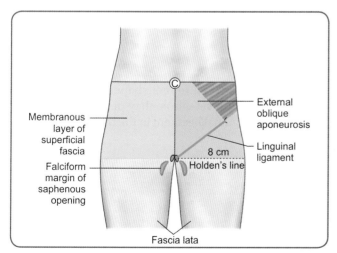

Fig. 26.2: Showing Holden's line below the inguinal ligament (it is a line of fusion of membranous layer of superficial fascia with fascia lata)

Special features of fascia lata

- Saphenous opening is the deficiency in deep fascia. It is covered by cribriform fascia, which is pierced by multiple structures giving it a sieve like appearance.
- Iliotibial tract is the thickened part of deep fascia laterally extending like a band from the iliac crest to lateral tibial condyle. It splits superiorly to enclose the tensor fascia latae.
- The intermuscular septa arising from the deep fascia course internally towards the linea aspera of the femur. The lateral, medial and posterior intermuscular septa divide the thigh in to anterior, posterior and medial compartments.

Saphenous opening (Fig. 26.3)

This is an oval aperture in the deep fascia of the thigh or fascia lata. It is about 3cm long and 1.5 cm wide. The center of the opening lies about 3 to 4 cm infero-lateral to the pubic tubercle. It has a sharp falciform margin, which bounds it on superior, lateral and inferior aspects. The medial margin however is smooth and sloping and merges with fascia covering the anterior surface of pectineus. It must be appreciated that the falciform margin, which is at a superficial plane forms the anterior relation of the femoral sheath while the medial margin, which is at a deeper plane passes posterior to the sheath. The two margins of

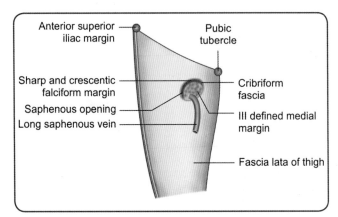

Fig. 26.3: Showing position of saphenous opening and its falciform margin

the opening are connected by the cribriform fascia, which is so called because of its sieve-like appearance. The long saphenous vein, lymph vessels and superficial external pudendal, superficial epigastric and superficial circumflex iliac arteries (branches of the femoral artery) pierce the cribriform fascia.

📖 STUDENT INTEREST

Saphenous opening is very important surgically. Therefore its surface marking is a must know.

Iliotibial tract or band (Fig. 26.4)

It is a thickened part of fascia lata on the lateral aspect of thigh.

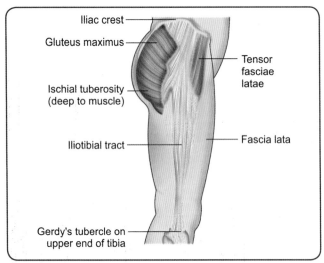

Fig. 26.4: Showing iliotibial tract on lateral side of thigh and gluteal region

Attachments
- ***Superiorly:*** To the anterior part of iliac crest.
- ***Inferiorly:*** To the anterior surface of lateral condyle of tibia on a circumscribed area (Gerdy's tubercle).

Functional Importance
- The iliotibial tract provides insertion to tensor fasciae latae and gluteus maximus muscles. The tract extends their insertion to the tibia.
- It plays a crucial role to stabilize in extended position (especially during running).

✒ CLINICAL CORRELATION

Iliotibial Tract (Band) Syndrome

This syndrome is characterized by stinging sensation just lateral to the knee joint or along the entire extent of iliotibial tract. The cause is the continuous rubbing of the tract on lateral condyle of tibia during running or cycling producing inflammation in the area of contact. The surgical sectioning of the tract relieves the symptoms (if cortisone injection at the site of contact is not effective).

ANTERIOR COMPARTMENT OF THIGH

The main contents of anterior or extensor compartment of thigh are:
- Large mass of quadriceps femoris muscle
- Sartorius
- Tensor fasciae latae
  (Apart from muscles in the floor of femoral triangle)
- Femoral nerve
- Femoral artery
- Femoral vein
  (The femoral vessels in their initial course in the femoral triangle are wrapped up in the femoral sheath).

Femoral Sheath

The femoral sheath is a funnel-shaped fascial envelope around the femoral vessels as they descend behind the medial half of inguinal ligament in the thigh.

Formation

The fascia transversalis forms the anterior wall of the sheath and the fascia iliaca forms the posterior wall. The lateral wall of the sheath is straight while its medial wall is sloping. The femoral sheath closes inferiorly because of

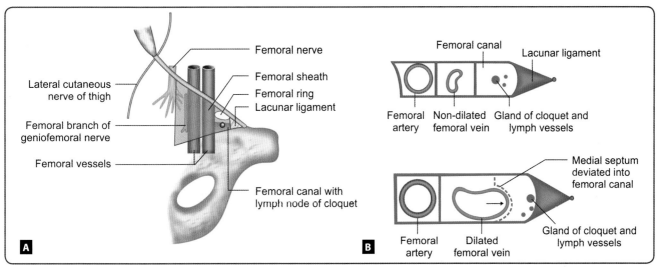

Figs 26.5A and B: **A.** Femoral sheath showing its compartments with their contents (Note that femoral nerve is outside the femoral sheath); **B.** Simplified diagram to depict use of femoral canal as a dead space for expansion of femoral vein during times of increased venous return from the lower limb (arrow showing)

the blending of its anterior and posterior walls with the tunica adventitia of femoral vessels.

Three Compartments of Femoral Sheath (Fig. 26.5A)

The femoral sheath is divided in the following three compartments by two anteroposterior septa:
1. Femoral canal is medial compartment.
2. Intermediate compartment contains the femoral vein
3. Lateral compartment contains femoral artery and femoral branch of genitofemoral nerve.

Femoral canal

The femoral canal is about two cm long. It contains the lymph node of Cloquet and fibro-fatty tissue. The canal provides dead space for the expansion of femoral vein during times of increased venous return (Fig. 26.5B).

Femoral ring is the upper opening of the femoral canal. It is directed towards the abdomen. It can admit the tip of a little finger. It is wider in females due to wider pelvis. The femoral ring is closed by femoral septum, which is made of the extraperitoneal fatty tissue. The boundaries of the femoral ring are of surgical importance. The lateral margin is formed by femoral vein, anterior margin by inguinal ligament, posterior by pectineus muscle and the medial margin by the base of lacunar ligament. If the abnormal obturator artery is present, it lies on the base of the lacunar ligament (medial boundary of femoral ring).

CLINICAL CORRELATION

- The femoral ring is the weak area in the lower part of the abdominal wall. The protrusion of abdominal contents covered by parietal peritoneum through the femoral ring in the femoral canal is called the femoral hernia. It is more common in females due to the greater width of the femoral ring. The femoral hernia presents as a globular swelling in the groin. Its distinguishing features are its relations to the pubic tubercle and inguinal ligament. It is situated inferolateral to the pubic tubercle and inferior to the inguinal ligament as against the inguinal hernia, which is supero-medial to the pubic tubercle.

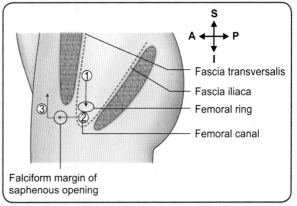

Fig. 26.6: Schematic diagram to show the path of femoral hernia (**1.** downward, **2.** forward and **3.** upward)

- The path of the femoral hernia is at first downward, then anterior and then upward (Fig. 26.6). First it enters the femoral canal and then passes through its anterior wall in to

Contd...

Contd...

⚕ CLINICAL CORRELATION

the saphenous opening, where it turns upwards around the sharp falciform margin of saphenous opening. It is useful for the surgeon to know the path of the hernia in order to reverse the path while manually reducing the hernia.

- The femoral hernia is prone to strangulation because of the compression of the neck of the hernial sac at the narrow femoral ring. The strangulation endangers the blood supply of the herniated intestinal loop. The relief of the strangulated loop is obtained by cutting the lacunar ligament so as to enlarge the femoral ring. The surgeon must be familiar with the anatomical relations of the abnormal obturator artery to the femoral ring while incising the lacunar ligament to enlarge the femoral ring. If the abnormal obturator artery (Fig. 26.7) is in lateral relation to the ring it is its safe position. If it is in medial relation to the ring (in contact with lacunar ligament) it is prone to inadvertent injury and bleeding during enlargement of femoral ring by cutting the lacunar ligament.

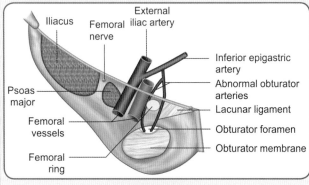

Fig. 26.7: Relations of abnormal obturator artery to femoral ring (it is a safe relation when the artery is in lateral relation to the ring and it is an unsafe when the artery is in medial relation to the ring)

 STUDENT INTEREST

Femoral canal is the medial and very short compartment of femoral sheath. It contains lymph node of Cloquet and provides passage for lymph vessels. It opens in to the abdominal cavity by femoral ring, which is closed by fibrofatty tissue (femoral septum). The medial margin of femoral ring is the lacunar ligament. Femoral canal is important on three accounts: (1) provides room for lymph node of Cloquet and is the only path for lymph vessels of lower limb to join the external iliac lymph nodes (2) provides space for expansion of femoral vein during increase in venous return (3) is the site of femoral hernia.

Femoral Triangle

The femoral triangle (Scarpa's triangle) is a triangular space in the upper third of the thigh below the inguinal ligament and medial to the sartorius muscle.

Boundaries (Fig. 26.8A)

- *Base:* Inguinal ligament.
- *Medial:* Medial border of adductor longus muscle.
- *Lateral:* Medial border of sartorius.
- *Apex:* Meeting of the medial borders of adductor longus and sartorius muscles.
  At the apex, the femoral triangle is continuous with the subsartorial canal.
- *Gutter-shaped floor:* By four muscles (medial to lateral), adductor longus, pectineus, psoas major and iliacus (Fig. 26.8B).
- *Roof:* Fascia lata with some features like saphenous opening and cribriform fascia.

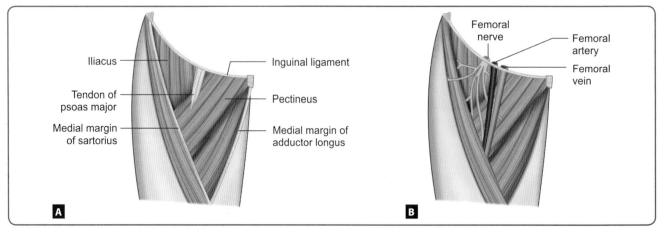

Figs 26.8A and B: A. Showing boundaries and floor of the femoral triangle; **B.** Showing the main contents of femoral triangle

Contents (Fig. 26.8B)

The main contents of the femoral triangle are as follows:
- Femoral nerve and its branches.
- Femoral artery and its branches.
- Femoral vein with its tributaries.
- Lateral cutaneous nerve of thigh.
- Femoral branch of genitofemoral nerve.
- Deep inguinal lymph nodes.

Brief Description of the Main Neurovascular Structures

- The femoral nerve breaks up in the femoral triangle in to a bunch of three sensory and six muscular branches. The sensory branches are, intermediate and medial femoral cutaneous nerves and the saphenous nerve. The muscular branches supply the sartorius, pectineus and separate branches to the four heads of quadriceps femoris.
- The femoral artery enters the base of the triangle at midinguinal point. Its upper part, along with femoral vein is enclosed in the femoral sheath. The femoral artery gives three superficial branches (superficial epigastric, superficial circumflex iliac and superficial external pudendal), deep external pudendal and profunda femoris artery. Two branches of the profunda femoris artery (lateral and medial circumflex femoral) originate in the femoral triangle.
- The femoral vein receives the long saphenous vein besides smaller tributaries.

Exit of Contents from Femoral Triangle (Fig. 26.9)

- The femoral vessels leave through the apex to enter the subsartorial canal.
- The profunda femoris vessels leave through the floor, via a gap between pectineus and adductor longus muscles.
- The medial circumflex femoral vessels pass through the gap between psoas major and pectineus muscles.
- The lateral circumflex femoral vessels pass behind the sartorius.
- The superficial branches of the femoral artery pierce the cribriform fascia.
- The saphenous nerve and nerve to vastus medialis leave through the apex. The other muscular branches enter the respective muscles in the triangle itself while the other cutaneous nerves pierce the deep fascia of the triangle.

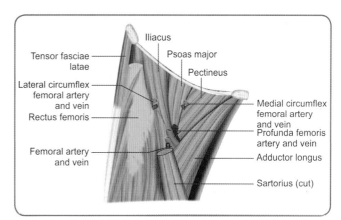

Fig. 26.9: Sites of exit of the vessels through femoral triangle (Note that a stab wound at the apex of the triangle is likely to injure four large-sized blood vessels—femoral artery, femoral vein, profunda vein and profunda artery in anteroposterior order)

Relations at Apex of Femoral Triangle (Fig. 26.9)

At the apex of the triangle four vessels and two nerves come in close relation. The femoral vessels passing through the apex are separated by the adductor longus from the profunda vessels. These large sized four vessels are arranged from anterior to posterior order as follows: femoral artery, femoral vein, profunda vein, and profunda artery. All these vessels are involved in a stab injury or bullet injury at the apex.

CLINICAL CORRELATION

A number of anatomical structures give rise to swelling in the groin or upper part of femoral triangle. Therefore while examining a case of lump in the groin a clinician thinks of various anatomical structures in the femoral triangle, which may be involved.
- The subcutaneous fatty tissue may form a lipoma.
- The femoral and inguinal herniae present as swelling. The relation to pubic tubercle helps in distinguishing the swelling of femoral hernia from that of inguinal hernia. The femoral hernia is inferolateral to the pubic tubercle whereas inguinal hernia is superomedial to it.
- The dilatation or aneurysm of femoral artery forms a pulsatile swelling.
- Hematoma due to injury to the femoral vein (for example during venipuncture).
- Dilatation of terminal part of great saphenous vein.
- Neuroma arising from femoral nerve.
- Psoas abscess in psoas sheath.
- Swollen inguinal lymph nodes due to inflammatory lesions or malignancy.
- Ectopic testis in the femoral triangle.

Subsartorial Canal or Adductor Canal

The subsartorial canal (Hunter's canal) is located in the middle third of the medial side of the thigh. It is triangular on cross section.

Extent

It extends from the apex of femoral triangle to the tendinous opening in adductor magnus through it opens in to the popliteal fossa.

Boundaries (Fig. 26.10)

The subsartorial canal has anterolateral, anteromedial (roof) and posterior boundaries.
- ***Anterolateral boundary:*** Vastus medialis
- ***Anteromedial boundary or fibrous roof:*** Overlapped by sartorius
- ***Posterior boundary or floor:*** Adductor longus above and adductor magnus below.

Main Contents

- Femoral artery
- Femoral vein
- Saphenous nerve
- Nerve to vastus medialis

Note: A vascular branch of the anterior division of obturator nerve, a genicular branch of posterior division of obturator nerve and descending genicular artery from lower part of femoral artery are inside the canal for a brief course)

Exit of Contents

- The femoral artery and vein leave through the posterior wall at the tendinous opening in the adductor magnus.
- The saphenous nerve leaves by piercing the roof.
- The nerve to vastus medialis leaves by entering the vastus medialis.

    Relations of major contents of the subsartorial canal are described with 'Femoral Artery' in ensuing text.

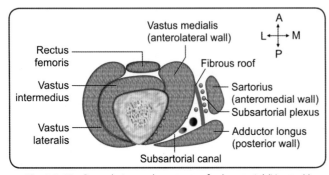

Fig. 26.10: Boundaries and contents of subsartorial (Hunter's) canal on left side

 ADDED INFORMATION

The subsartorial plexus of nerves supplies the skin of the medial side of thigh. It is located between the fibrous roof and the sartorius. It is formed by twigs from the saphenous nerve, medial cutaneous femoral nerve and anterior division of obturator nerve.

CLINICAL CORRELATION

- In the treatment of aneurysm of popliteal artery, the surgeon ligates the femoral artery in subsartorial canal. The principle of this procedure depends on the presence of anastomotic channels around the knee through which blood reaches the popliteal artery despite ligation of femoral artery.
- For surgical approach to the femoral artery in the subsartorial canal, a skin incision is placed along the line of anterior border of middle third of sartorius. The superficial and deep fasciae are divided and the sartorius is retracted. The fibrous roof of the canal is incised to expose the femoral artery. John Hunter was the first to describe the exposure and ligation of the femoral artery in subsartorial canal in treating the aneurysm of popliteal artery. That is why this canal is named after Hunter.

Femoral Nerve

The femoral nerve is a branch of lumbar plexus, which is housed in the substance of the psoas major muscle located on the posterior abdominal wall. The dorsal branches of the ventral rami of second, third and fourth lumbar spinal nerves join to form the femoral nerve (root value- L2, L3, L4).

Course (Fig. 26.11)

Abdominal course

The femoral nerve emerges from the lateral margin of psoas major muscle and descends to reach the iliac fossa, where it located between the iliacus and psoas major muscles. It supplies branches to iliacus at this level.

Short course in femoral triangle in the thigh

It enters the femoral triangle behind the inguinal ligament lying outside the femoral sheath. It is related laterally to the femoral artery (which is inside the femoral sheath). It is located in the groove between psoas and iliacus.

Termination

The femoral nerve terminates into anterior and posterior divisions just below the inguinal ligament. Hence, it has a very short trunk in the femoral triangle.

Branches in femoral triangle

The branches are divided according their origin from the trunk, anterior division and posterior division of femoral nerve.

Muscular branches

- From the trunk to pectineus
- From anterior division to sartorius
- From posterior division to four parts of quadriceps femoris.

Cutaneous branches

- From anterior division—medial and intermediate femoral cutaneous nerves of thigh
- From posterior division-saphenous nerve.

🔖 CLINICAL CORRELATION

- The femoral nerve may be compressed or injured at the base of the triangle, where it lies in the groove between the iliacus and psoas muscles due to psoas abscess. Injury to the femoral nerve results in atrophy of extensor muscles of thigh with inability to extend the leg at the knee joint and loss of knee jerk.
- The femoral nerve block can be easily achieved in the femoral triangle by injecting the anesthetic solution at a point one-finger breadth lateral to the point of femoral pulse, which is just below the midinguinal point.

Saphenous Nerve

It is a branch of the posterior division of femoral nerve. It is the longest cutaneous nerve in the body.

Course (Fig. 26.11)

The saphenous nerve leaves the femoral triangle along with femoral vessels through the apex to enter the subsartorial canal. It lies anterior to the femoral vessels at the apex of femoral triangle. During its course through the subsartorial canal, it crosses in front of the femoral artery from lateral to medial side. It leaves the subsartorial canal along with saphenous branch of descending genicular artery by piercing the fibrous roof at the lower end of the canal. In its further course it descends vertically along the medial side of knee lying behind the sartorius. The saphenous nerve pierces the deep fascia of leg between the tendons of sartorius and gracilis to become superficial. In the leg it descends with the great saphenous vein along the medial side, passes in front of the medial malleolus to enter the dorsum of the foot, where it reaches up to the base of big toe.

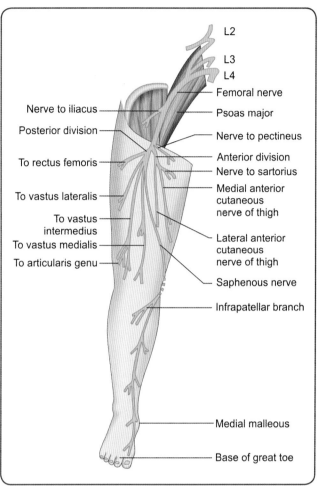

Fig. 26.11: Origin, course and branches of femoral nerve (Note that the saphenous nerve, the longest cutaneous branch of femoral nerve, reaches up to the base of great toe)

Branches

- In the thigh, the saphenous nerve gives a twig to the subsartorial plexus. Its infrapatellar branch contributes to the patellar plexus along with medial, intermediate and lateral femoral cutaneous nerves of thigh.
- In the leg, it supplies the skin of medial side of front of leg and the medial side of ankle.
- In the foot, it supplies the skin of the medial side of the dorsum of foot up to the base of big toe.

🔖 CLINICAL CORRELATION

Saphenous Nerve Graft

The superficially located saphenous nerve is favored for nerve grafting.

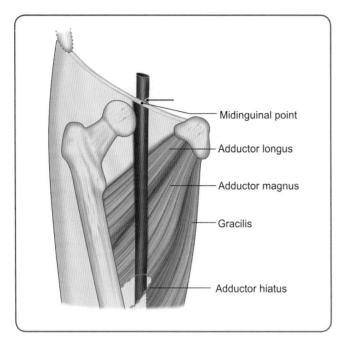

Fig. 26.12: Showing the extent of the femoral artery (the arrow indicates the site of compression of femoral artery against the head of femur)

Femoral Pulse (Fig. 26.13)

The clinicians feel the femoral artery in the femoral triangle just below the midinguinal point (a point half way between the anterior superior iliac spine and pubic symphysis) by palpating against the head of femur (Fig. 26.12). Bilateral weak femoral pulse compared to the radial pulse is indicative of coarctation (narrowing) of arch of aorta. The femoral pulse may be reduced or obliterated by atherosclerotic changes or emboli in proximal arteries).

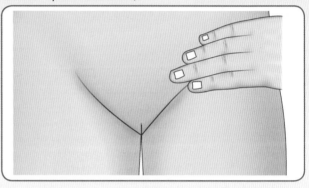

Fig. 26.13: Site of palpation of femoral pulse

Femoral Artery

The femoral artery is the chief artery of the lower limb.

Extent (Fig. 26.12)

It begins as the continuation of the external iliac artery at the midinguinal point. After coursing through the femoral triangle and subsartorial canal it leaves the thigh through adductor hiatus or tendinous opening in the adductor magnus muscle, where it enters the popliteal fossa to continue as popliteal artery.

Surface Marking

To draw the femoral artery on the surface, the thigh is kept in a position of slight flexion, abduction and lateral rotation. The upper two-third of a line drawn from the midinguinal point to the adductor tubercle represents the femoral artery in the thigh. The upper one third of this line represents the femoral artery in femoral triangle while the middle third represents the femoral artery in the subsartorial canal.

Relations in Femoral Triangle

Anterior relations from superficial to deep are the skin, superficial fascia with inguinal lymph nodes, fascia lata and anterior wall of femoral sheath. The posterior relations are the posterior wall of the femoral sheath, nerve to pectineus and tendon of psoas major muscle. This tendon separates the artery from the capsule of hip joint. At this site the artery can be compressed against the head of the femur through the skin. The femoral nerve and its branches form the lateral relation. The femoral vein lies medial to the artery (Fig. 26.9) except at the apex, where it lies posterior to the artery.

Branches in Femoral Triangle (Fig. 26.14)

Superficial and deep branches originate in femoral triangle.
- Three superficial branches are superficial epigastric, superficial external pudendal and superficial circumflex iliac arteries.
- The deep branches are deep external pudendal, profunda femoris and muscular branches.

Relations in Subsartorial Canal

- Saphenous nerve crosses the femoral artery anteriorly from lateral to medial side.
- Nerve to vastus medialis is lateral to the femoral artery and leaves the canal by entering the vastus medialis in the upper part of the canal.
- Femoral vein, which is posterior to the artery in the upper part of the canal, becomes its lateral relation distally.
- Adductor longus above and magnus below are related posteriorly.

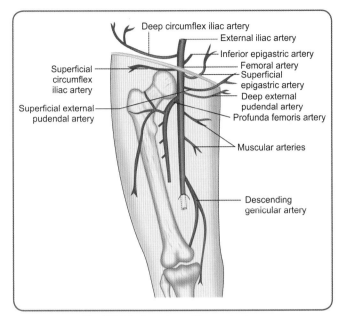

Fig. 26.14: Branches of femoral artery

Branches in Subsartorial Canal (Fig. 26.14)

- Muscular branches.
- Descending genicular artery leaves the canal by descending in the substance of the vastus medialis. It divides in to an articular and a saphenous branch. The latter accompanies the saphenous nerve as it emerges through the roof of the subsartorial canal.

CLINICAL CORRELATION

- Since the femoral artery is relatively superficial in position in the thigh; it is easy to approach the artery for various procedures. To inject radio-opaque dye in the arteries of abdomen (aortic angiography, celiac artery angiography, superior and inferior mesenteric angiography etc) the catheter is introduced through the femoral artery. It is also a favored vessel for coronary angiography or for coronary angioplasty (retrograde catheterization). The route of the catheter for reaching coronary ostia is as follows – femoral artery → external iliac artery → common iliac artery → abdominal aorta → thoracic aorta → arch of aorta → ascending aorta → coronary ostia.
- The femoral angiography (Fig. 26.15) is performed to visualize the femoral artery and its branches in suspected cases of femoral artery occlusion.
- Sudden occlusion in the femoral artery usually occurs due to emboli from the heart (myocardial infarction or thrombi in the left atrium in mitral stenosis). It presents as five "P"s- pain, pallor, paraesthesia (altered sensations), paralysis and pulselessness. The serious complication of acute occlusion is gangrene of the lower limb.

Contd...

Contd...

CLINICAL CORRELATION

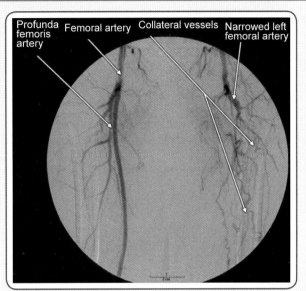

Fig. 26.15: Femoral angiogram showing normal right femoral artery and narrowed left femoral artery (arrow showing)

- In gradual narrowing of the femoral artery as a result of atherosclerosis, the circulation to lower limb is maintained through collateral channels.

Femoral Vein

The femoral vein begins at the tendinous opening in the adductor magnus as the continuation of popliteal vein. It ascends in the subsartorial canal and then enters the femoral triangle. After traversing the intermediate compartment of the femoral sheath the femoral vein continues upward as the external iliac vein just medial to the midinguinal point.

Relations

The femoral vein has changing relation to the femoral artery in its course at various levels.

- At the tendinous opening, the femoral vein is lateral to the femoral artery.
- In the subsartorial canal, the vein gradually crosses posterior to the artery so that at the apex of the femoral triangle it lies posterior to the femoral artery.
- At the base of the femoral triangle the femoral vein lies medial to the femoral artery.

Valves in Femoral Vein

The femoral vein contains four to five valves, the most constant being the saphenofemoral valve (competency of this valve is tested by Trendelenburg test).

Tributaries

- Great saphenous vein
- Profunda femoris vein
- Lateral circumflex femoral vein
- Medial circumflex femoral vein

Muscles of Anterior Compartment

The psoas major and iliacus muscles are described with posterior abdominal wall (Chapter 53). The pectineus muscle is described with medial compartment of thigh (Chapter 27).

Tensor Fasciae Latae

This muscle is located at the junction of the front of thigh and gluteal region at the lateral side (Fig. 26.3). It is enclosed between two layers of fascia lata.
- **Origin:** From the outer lip of the anterior part of the iliac crest and the lateral surface of anterior superior iliac spine.
- **Insertion:** Into the iliotibial tract through which it gains attachment to the lateral condyle of tibia.
- **Nerve supply:** Superior gluteal nerve.

Actions

- Tensor fasciae latae assists the gluteus medius and minimus muscles in abduction and medial rotation of the thigh.
- It stabilizes the knee joint in standing position and helps in extension of the knee joint through the iliotibial tract.

⚖ STUDENT INTEREST

Tensor fasciae latae muscle shares its insertion with gluteus maximus but shares its nerve supply with gluteus medius and minimus.

Sartorius (Fig. 24.9)

The word **sartorius** is derived from the Latin word sartor meaning tailor. Hence sartorius is called the tailor's muscle. The sartorius is the longest muscle in the body.
- **Origin:** From anterior superior iliac spine.
- **Insertion:** Into the upper part of subcutaneous medial surface of the shaft of tibia anterior to the insertion of gracilis and semitendinosus muscles.
- **Nerve supply:** The femoral nerve in the femoral triangle

Course and relations

The sartorius courses obliquely in latero-medial direction in the thigh from its origin to insertion. It forms the lateral boundary of the femoral triangle and covers the fibrous roof of the subsartorial canal. On its way to insertion it passes close to the medial boundary of the popliteal fossa.

Actions

- Sartorius is the only muscle that flexes both hip and knee joints.
- It helps in adduction and lateral rotation of thigh (while sitting cross-legged on the ground).

Quadriceps Femoris (Fig. 26.16)

Quadriceps femoris is a very bulky muscle, which almost fills the anterior compartment of thigh. It has four components having separate names (rectus femoris, vastus lateralis, vastus medialis and vastus intermedius). Each component has a separate origin but a common insertion. It crosses the hip and knee joints.

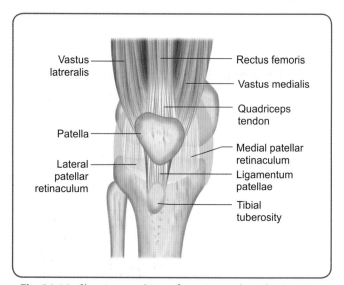

Fig. 26.16: Showing quadriceps femoris muscle and its insertion

Rectus femoris (Kicking muscle)

Rectus femoris is a straight muscle. Its superficial fibers are bipennate and deep fibers are parallel.
- ***Origin (double origin from ilium)***
  - Straight head from the anterior inferior iliac spine.
  - Reflected head from a groove above the acetabulum.
- ***Insertion:*** The two heads unite to form a fusiform belly, which passes vertically downwards superficial to the other components to end in a common tendon for insertion in to patella.

Vastus lateralis

It is the largest component of quadriceps femoris.

Origin: From the upper part of intertrochanteric line, anterior border of greater trochanter, lateral lip of gluteal tuberosity and upper part of lateral lip of linea aspera.

Vastus medialis

- ***Origin:*** From lower part of intertrochanteric line, spiral line of femur, entire length of medial lip of linea aspera and upper one fourth of medial supracondylar line
- ***Insertion:*** Into patella by common tendon

Vastus intermedius

- ***Origin:*** From lateral and anterior surfaces of the femoral shaft.
- ***Insertion:*** By common tendon in to patella

Articularis genu

It is a small slip of muscle that is detached from lowest part of vastus intermedius.
- ***Origin:*** From the front of the lower part of shaft of femur
- ***Insertion:*** In to suprapatellar synovial bursa of knee joint

Common insertion (Fig. 26.16)

The four parts of quadriceps femoris unite to form a common tendon (quadriceps tendon), which is inserted into the margins of patella. The insertion is prolonged over the front of patella as the strong ligamentum patellae to the tuberosity of tibia.

Actions

- The quadriceps femoris muscle is a powerful extensor of the knee joint. It straightens the lower limb (extends)

 ADDED INFORMATION

Details of Insertion
- The rectus femoris and vastus intermedius are inserted into the upper margin of patella.
- The lower fleshy fibers of vastus medialis insert in to the medial margin of patella (this part of vastus medialis is known as vastus medialis oblique as against its remaining part, which is known as vastus medialis longus).
  Note that the attachment of vastus medialis to medial margin of patella extends longer than that of vastus lateralis to the lateral margin of patella.
- The medial and lateral patellar retinacula are the expansions from the sides of patella to the respective condyles of tibia.
- The combination of quadriceps tendon, patella and ligamentum patellae is known as patello-femoral complex.

during the act of standing from sitting position. The tone of the quadriceps muscle is very important to the stability of the knee joint.
- The tendinous expansions of medial and lateral vasti form the patellar retinacula, which blend with the capsule of knee joint to reinforce it.
- The rectus femoris alone acts on the hip joint. It is the flexor of hip joint.
- The articularis genu retracts the synovial membrane superiorly during extension of the knee joint in order to prevent injury.

Nerve supply

All parts of quadriceps femoris are separately innervated by postreior division of femoral nerve. The articularis genu receives a twig from the nerve to vastus intermedius.

Testing function of quadriceps femoris

The quadriceps femoris is tested with the subject lying on the back with knee joint partially flexed. When the subject is asked to extend the knee against resistance the normal quadriceps muscle can be seen and felt easily.

 STUDENT INTEREST

Rectus femoris is the only component of quadriceps femoris that crosses both hip and knee joints. It is the flexor of hip joint and extensor of knee joint (actions which are used while kicking).

CLINICAL CORRELATION

- Vastus lateralis is a bulky muscle hence preferred for intramuscular injection.
- Patellar tendon reflex is elicited by tapping ligamentum patellae with a knee hammer. The positive response consists of extension of the leg at knee joint. The reflex consists of afferent limb (femoral nerve), efferent limb (femoral nerve) and the spinal center (L2, L3 and L4 segments). The reflex is lost in injury to femoral nerve or injury to spinal reflex center.
- The disuse atrophy of quadriceps femoris results due to immobilization of knee joint on account of any cause (arthritis or plaster cast). Reduction in size of the quadriceps femoris due to atrophy is found out by measuring the circumference of each thigh. For preventing the disuse atrophy active exercises (physiotherapy) are started as early as possible in patients in whom lower limbs are immobilized.

ADDED INFORMATION

Normally, between the oblique line of quadriceps muscle and the straight line of patellar ligament there is valgus angle opening on lateral side. The supplement of the valgus angle is called the quadriceps angle or Q angle (normal value is around 10 to 12°). In fact it is the Q angle that is responsible for the natural tendency of patella to dislocate laterally. To counteract this tendency the vastus medialis oblique muscle pulls the patella medially in addition to the bony factors. If the value of Q angle is greater than 15° there is lateral pull on patella. This causes the patella to rub against the lateral condyle of femur resulting in patellar pain initially and later its dislocation laterally.

27

Gluteal Region, Posterior Compartment of Thigh and Sciatic Nerve

Chapter Contents

GLUTEAL REGION

The gluteal region or buttock is a prominent bulge (on each side) produced by the subcutaneous fat and the bulky gluteus maximus muscle on the back of the pelvis.

Boundaries (Fig. 27.1)

The gluteal region is bounded superiorly by the iliac crest and superomedially by the sacrum. Inferiorly the gluteal sulcus separates it from the thigh. Medially there is an inter-gluteal or natal cleft. A line joining the anterior superior iliac spine to the front of the greater trochanter of femur limits the region laterally.

Communications

- The gluteal region communicates with the pelvic cavity through the greater sciatic foramen (gateway to gluteal region).
- It communicates with the ischiorectal fossa through the lesser sciatic foramen.
- Inferiorly, it is continuous with the posterior compartment of thigh.

Surface Landmarks (Fig. 27.1)

- Fold of the buttock is a transverse skin crease indicating the lower limit of gluteal region.

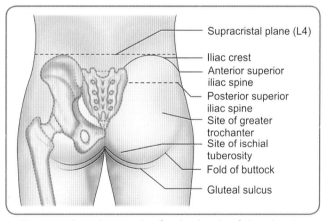

Fig. 27.1: Boundaries and surface landmarks of gluteal region

- Gluteal sulcus is a groove beneath the gluteal fold. It corresponds to lower margin of gluteus maximus muscle.
- Iliac crest is felt along its entire extent. It is the upper limit of gluteal region.
- Anterior superior iliac spine, iliac tubercle and posterior superior iliac spine.
- Ischial tuberosity is bony prominence felt deep to the lower margin of gluteus maximus about 5cm above the gluteal fold and from the median plane. It can be felt by pressing the fingers upwards in to the medial part of gluteal fold.

- Tip of greater trochanter of femur lies about one hand's breadth below the iliac tubercle.
- Sacrum lies between the two hip bones. Upper 3 sacral spines are palpable in the midline.
- Natal or inter-gluteal cleft is between the buttocks in the midline beginning at level of S3 vertebra.
- Coccyx lies behind the anus in the posterior end of the natal cleft.

Superficial Fascia

The superficial fascia of the gluteal region is thick and filled with fat. A number of cutaneous nerves are present in the superficial fascia (Fig. 27.2).

Cutaneous Nerves (Fig. 27.2)

The cutaneous nerves of gluteal region are derived from both posterior (dorsal) and anterior (ventral) rami of spinal nerves as follows:

Upper Posterior Quadrant

Posterior or dorsal rami of L1, L2, L3 and S1, S2, S3 spinal nerves

Lower Posterior Quadrant

- Branches of posterior cutaneous nerve of thigh (S1, S2, S3 -from sacral plexus).
- Perforating cutaneous nerve (S2, S3- from sacral plexus).

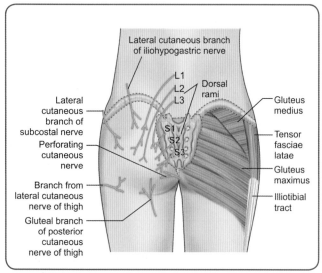

Fig. 27.2: Cutaneous nerves of gluteal region shown on left side and gluteus maximus, gluteus medius and tensor fasciae latae are shown on the right side

Upper Anterior Quadrant

- Lateral cutaneous branch of subcostal nerve (T12).
- Lateral cutaneous branch of iliohypogastric nerve (L1—from lumbar plexus).

Lower Anterior Quadrant

Branches of lateral cutaneous nerve of thigh (L2, L3—lumbar plexus).

Deep Fascia

The deep fascia of gluteal region is attached above to the iliac crest and behind to the sacrum. Along the iliac crest it splits twice to enclose tensor fasciae latae and gluteus maximus. The unsplit fascia between the two muscles forms the gluteal aponeurosis that covers the gluteus medius. On the lateral aspect, the deep fascia is thickened to form iliotibial tract.

Gluteus Maximus

The gluteus maximus (Fig. 27.2) is the largest and the most superficial muscle of the gluteal region. It has a coarse texture due to a large number of fibrous septa in its substance.

Origin

- Outer slope of the dorsal segment of iliac crest.
- Outer surface of ilium behind the posterior gluteal line.
- Aponeurosis of erector spinae.
- Posterior surface of adjacent sacrum and coccyx.
- Sacrotuberous ligament.

Insertion (Figs 27.2 and 24.6)

- Three-fourth of the muscle is inserted by tendinous fibers into the iliotibial tract.
- One fourth of the muscle is inserted into the gluteal tuberosity of femur.
  Nerve Supply: Inferior gluteal nerve

Actions

- The gluteus maximus is a powerful extensor of thigh on the trunk or of trunk on the thigh at the hip joint in such activities as running, climbing steps and rising from sitting position.
- It is the lateral rotator of thigh.
- Acting from its insertion, it can straighten the trunk after stooping by rotating the pelvis backward on the head of femur (this action is in association with hamstring muscles).

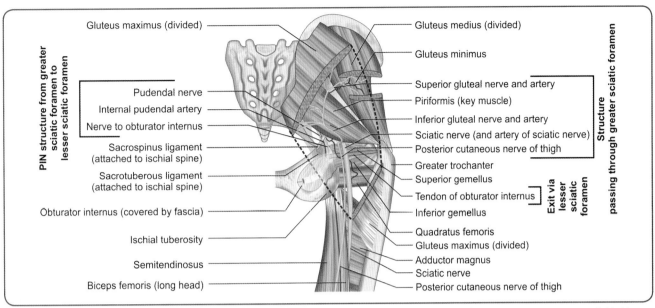

Fig. 27.3: Structures under cover of gluteus maximus (Note the continuity of gluteal region with posterior compartment of thigh)

- It maintains the upright position of trunk by preventing the pelvis from rotating forward on the head of femur (thus retaining the center of gravity behind the hip joint).
- It stabilizes the knee joint through iliotibial tract.

Testing Function of Gluteus Maximus

The subject lying in prone position is asked to raise the thigh against resistance. Inability to do so indicates weakness of the muscle.

Structures Under Cover of Gluteus Maximus (Figs 27.3 and 27.4)

Bony structures

- Ischial spine
- Ischial tuberosity
- Greater and lesser sciatic foramina
- Greater trochanter

Ligaments

- The sacrotuberous ligament extends from the ischial tuberosity to the lower lateral part of sacrum and coccyx and both posterior inferior and posterior superior iliac spines. The perforating cutaneous nerve from the sacral plexus pierces this ligament to enter the gluteal region.
- The sacrospinous ligament extends from the tip of ischial spine to the lower lateral part of sacrum and coccyx. It lies deep to sacrotuberous ligament. The pudendal nerve passes over the apex of the ligament to enter the lesser sciatic foramen.

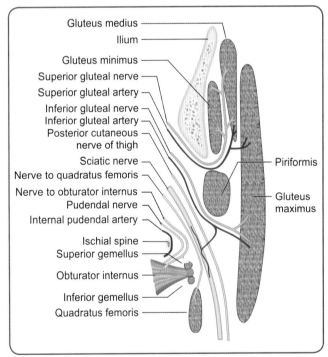

Fig. 27.4: Schematic diagram to depict structures under cover of gluteus maximus

Morphology

- Sacrotuberous ligament is regarded as the continuation of biceps femoris muscle.
- Sacrospinous ligament is regarded as aponeurotic part of coccygeus muscle.

Bursae

- A large trochanteric bursa separates the gluteus maximus from the greater trochanter.
- The gluteofemoral bursa is present between the tendon of gluteus maximus and origin of vastus lateralis.
- The ischial bursa lies between the gluteus maximus and the lower medial part of ischial tuberosity. This bursa may become inflamed due to excessive friction producing ischial bursitis (weaver's bottom).

Muscles

- Gluteus medius and deep to it the gluteus minimus.
- Piriformis.
- Tendon of obturator internus with fleshy bellies of gemelli muscles.
- Quadratus femoris and the tendon of obturator externus deep to it.
- Origin of hamstring muscles from the ischial tuberosity.

Gluteus Medius

Origin

From outer surface of ilium between anterior and posterior gluteal lines

Insertion

Into the lateral aspect of greater trochanter along an oblique ridge.

Gluteus Minimus

Origin

From outer surface of ilium between anterior and inferior gluteal lines

Insertion

In to greater trochanter on the anterolateral ridge.

Nerve Supply

Both gluteus medius and minimus muscles are supplied by superior gluteal nerve.

Actions

- The gluteus medius and minimus muscles abduct the thigh at the hip joint, when the limb is free to move.
- Their anterior fibers bring about medial rotation and flexion of thigh.
- Their important function is to support the pelvis in walking. When a person stands on one foot and the foot of the opposite side is raised from the ground to take a step, the contraction of the glutei medius and minimus muscles of the supported side raises the contralateral pelvis a little (Fig. 27.5). In this way the contraction of the muscles on one side prevents the pelvis of the opposite side from sinking down, when the foot on that side is off the ground. These actions on the right and left sides of pelvis occur alternately during walking and depend on the integrity of three factors, namely, the normal glutei medius and minimus, normal hip joint and intact femoral neck.

Testing Function

- The subject lies prone with knee flexed at 900. The subject is asked to push the foot outward against resistance. Inability to do so means weakness of gluteus medius and minimus muscles.
- The subject lies prone or supine with thighs adducted at hip. The thighs are abducted against resistance.

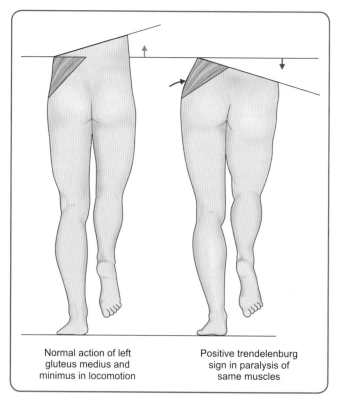

| Normal action of left gluteus medius and minimus in locomotion | Positive trendelenburg sign in paralysis of same muscles |

Fig. 27.5: Showing the action of the normal gluteus medius and minimus muscles on the pelvis of opposite side during locomotion and the effect of paralyzed gluteus medius and minimus muscles on the pelvis of opposite side during locomotion (green arrow shows the normal action and red arrow indicates dipping of the opposite pelvis when the muscle is paralyzed as shown by indigo arrow)

Paralysis of Gluteal Muscles

- In paralysis of gluteus maximus muscle (for example due to poliomyelitis or due to injury to inferior gluteal nerve), the gait of the person has a typical backward lurch during every step forward. This is explained by the fact that due to non-action of the muscle the center of gravity is retained by tilting the hip backward.
- In paralysis of glutei medius and minimus the pelvis of the unsupported (normal side) side sinks, when the patient tries to stand on the limb of affected side. This is known as positive Trendelenburg's sign (Fig. 27.5). In an attempt to raise the opposite foot the centre of gravity is shifted lateral to the hip joint of supported side by flexing the trunk to that side. This produces a characteristic dipping or lurching gait (also known as abductor lurch).

Short Lateral Rotators of Thigh

There are four muscles, which fall in this category, piriformis, and obturator internus with gemelli, obturator externus and quadratus femoris. These short muscles are collectively called the short lateral rotators of thigh at the hip joint. However, their main function is to act as ligaments, which retain the head of femur in the acetabulum.

Piriformis (Fig. 55.2B and 27.6)

It is located partly in the pelvis and partly in the gluteal region.

Origin

Is inverted E-shaped from the pelvic surface of the sacrum.

Insertion

Into the apex and adjoining upper margin of greater trochanter of femur.

Course and relations

- Inside the pelvis its important anterior relations are rectum, sacral plexus and branches of internal iliac artery. From its origin it turns laterally towards the greater sciatic foramen, through which it enters the gluteal region.
- The piriformis almost fills the greater sciatic foramen. It is regarded as the key muscle of the gluteal region because the nerves and blood vessels entering the gluteal region are arranged in relation to it at the greater sciatic foramen as shown in Fig. 27.3.

Nerve supply

The intrapelvic part of the piriformis receives direct branches from the ventral rami of the fifth lumbar and upper two sacral nerves.

Actions

It laterally rotates the extended thigh and abducts the flexed thigh.

In piriformis syndrome the sciatic nerve is compressed due to spasm or hypertrophy of the piriformis muscle at the greater sciatic foramen.

Obturator Internus (Fig. 55.2A)

The obturator internus muscle is partly in the pelvis and partly in the gluteal region. Its intrapelvic part is described with muscles of the pelvis in Chapter 55.

Origin

From the inner surface of obturator membrane and the surrounding bones (ischium, ilium and pubis).

Insertion

Common tendon of triceps coxae (obturator internus with gemelli) on upper part of medial surface of greater trochanter.

Relations

The tendon of the obturator internus muscle enters the gluteal region through the lesser sciatic foramen. The tendon provides the insertion for the superior gemellus and for the inferior gemellus. The obturator internus tendon and the two gemelli together constitute triceps coxae. They are related anteriorly to the sciatic nerve.

Nerve supply

Nerve to obturator internus, a branch of sacral plexus.

Action

Helps in lateral rotation of the extended thigh.

Gemelli

There are two gemelli, superior gemellus and inferior gemellus.

Origin

Superior gemellus from posterior aspect of ischial spine and inferior gemellus from the uppermost part of ischial tuberosity.

Insertion

Both gemelli insert into the tendon of obturator internus and their insertion is extended along with obturator internus to the medial surface of greater trochanter.

Nerve supply

The superior gemellus is supplied by nerve to obturator internus and the inferior gemellus is supplied by nerve to quadratus femoris.

Actions

The gemelli laterally rotate the extended thigh and abduct the flexed thigh.

Quadratus Femoris

This is a small quadrilateral muscle lying between the inferior gemellus and superior margin of adductor magnus.

Origin

From the lateral border of ischial tuberosity.

Insertion

Into the quadrate tubercle located on intertrochanteric crest of femur.

Nerve supply

Nerve to quadratus femoris, a branch of sacral plexus.

Action

Lateral rotator of thigh.

Obturator Externus

This muscle is described along with muscles of the medial compartment of thigh in chapter 28. Only its tendon appears in the gluteal region in close contact with the back of the neck of femur on its way to insertion in to the trochanteric fossa.

Nerves

The following seven branches of the sacral plexus (inside the pelvic cavity) enter the gluteal region via the greater sciatic foramen.
- Sciatic nerve
- Posterior cutaneous nerve of thigh
- Superior gluteal nerve
- Inferior gluteal nerve
- Nerve to obturator internus
- Nerve to quadratus femoris
- Pudendal nerve

Arteries

The following arteries are seen in the gluteal region:
- The superior and inferior gluteal arteries (accompanying the corresponding nerves) and internal pudendal artery are the branches of internal pudendal artery.
- The medial circumflex femoral artery, which is the branch of profunda femoris artery, enters from the thigh.

Nerves in Gluteal Region

- The superior gluteal nerve (L4, L5, and S1) arises from sacral plexus in the pelvis and enters the gluteal region via the greater sciatic foramen above the piriformis. It is accompanied by superior gluteal vessels. Lying in the interval between gluteus medius and minimus it supplies the gluteus medius, gluteus minimus and tensor fasciae latae. An inadvertent intramuscular injection in the superomedial quadrant of the gluteal region may injure the superior gluteal nerve.
- The inferior gluteal nerve (L5, S1, S2) arises from the sacral plexus and enters the gluteal region through the greater sciatic foramen below the piriformis along with the inferior gluteal vessels. It supplies the gluteus maximus muscle only.
- The nerve to quadratus femoris (L4, L5, S1) is a branch of sacral plexus. It enters the gluteal region through the greater sciatic foramen by passing below the piriformis. It descends initially behind the dorsal surface of ischium and in front of sciatic nerve, and then in front of the superior gemellus and tendon of obturator internus muscle. It supplies gemellus inferior and quadratus femoris. It may also give an articular twig to the hip joint.
- The nerve to obturator internus (L5, S1, S2) is a branch of sacral plexus. It enters the gluteal region through the greater sciatic foramen along with pudendal nerve and internal pudendal vessels. It supplies a branch to the superior gemellus. It crosses the dorsal surface of the base of ischial spine and enters the lesser sciatic foramen to supply branches to the pelvic surface of obturator internus muscle.
- The pudendal nerve (S2, S3, S4) is a branch of the sacral plexus. It has a very short course in the gluteal region. It crosses the sacrospinous ligament to enter

the lesser sciatic foramen. The internal pudendal artery accompanies the pudendal nerve. The internal pudendal artery is sandwiched between the nerve to obturator internus laterally and pudendal nerve medially (PIN relation as shown in Fig. 27.6). The pudendal nerve and the internal pudendal artery are described in detail in Chapter 58.

- The posterior cutaneous nerve of thigh (S1, S2, and S3) or posterior femoral cutaneous nerve arises from the sacral plexus. It enters the gluteal region by passing below the piriformis. It courses through four regions namely, gluteal, posterior compartment of thigh, popliteal fossa and back of leg.
  - In the gluteal region, it lies on the superficial aspect (posterior) of the sciatic nerve immediately deep to the gluteus maximus.
  - In the postreior compartment of thigh, it descends lying superficial to the long head of biceps femoris and deep to the deep fascia of thigh.
  - It enters the popliteal fossa and pierces the deep fascia. It descends in the superficial fascia to the level of middle of the calf along with short saphenous vein.
  - It supplies a few cutaneous twigs to the inferolateral part of gluteal region. Its perineal branch pierces the fascia lata and fascia of Colles to enter the superficial perineal pouch and supplies the skin of the posterior aspect of scrotum or labia majora. The cutaneous twigs are distributed to the skin of the

back of thigh, popliteal fossa and the upper half of the back of leg.

 STUDENT INTEREST

Posterior cutaneous nerve of thigh lies deep to the deep fascia until it pierces the popliteal fascia.

- The sciatic nerve enters the gluteal region via the greater sciatic foramen. A detailed account of sciatic nerve follows later.
- The perforating cutaneous nerve (S2, S3) is a branch of sacral plexus. It enters the gluteal region by perforating the sacrotuberous ligament and supplies the skin of the postero-inferior area of gluteal region (Fig. 27.2).

Arteries of Gluteal Region (Fig. 27.6)

The following branches of internal iliac artery enter the gluteal region:

- The superior gluteal artery is a branch of the posterior division of internal iliac artery. It enters the gluteal region along with the corresponding nerve above the piriformis. It divides into superficial and deep branches. The superficial branch supplies the gluteus maximus. The deep branch divides into upper and lower branches. The upper or ascending branch anastomoses with superficial and deep circumflex iliac and ascending branch of lateral circumflex and iliolumbar arteries near the anterior superior iliac spine. The lower or descending branch takes part in trochanteric anastomosis.
- The inferior gluteal artery is a branch of anterior division of internal iliac artery. Along with inferior gluteal nerve it enters the gluteal region below the piriformis. The inferior gluteal artery gives muscular branches mainly to gluteus maximus muscle and anastomotic branches that take part in trochanteric and cruciate anastomosis. Its most important branch is an artery to sciatic nerve or the companion artery of sciatic nerve, which sinks into the substance of the sciatic nerve. Artery to sciatic nerve is a remnant of axis artery of lower limb.
- Internal pudendal artery is a branch of anterior division of internal iliac artery. It enters the gluteal region via greater sciatic foramen below the piriformis muscle in company with pudendal nerve and nerve to obturator internus. It crosses the ischial spine to enter the lesser sciatic foramen to enter the lateral wall of ischiorectal fossa.

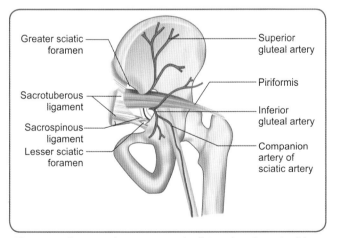

Fig. 27.6: Showing the superior and inferior gluteal arteries (Note the branch of inferior gluteal artery accompanying the sciatic nerve)

ADDED INFORMATION

Trochanteric Anastomosis

It is located in the trochanteric fossa of femur and following four arteries take part into its formation.
- Descending branch of the superior gluteal artery.
- A branch from inferior gluteal artery.
- Ascending branch of lateral circumflex femoral artery.
- Ascending branch of medial circumflex femoral artery.

The trochanteric anastomosis provides the chief source of blood supply to the head of femur.

Cruciate Anastomosis

The cruciate anastomosis is located in the interval between the upper margin of adductor magnus and lower margin of quadratus femoris. The following four arteries take part in this anastomosis.
- Transverse branch of medial circumflex femoral artery.
- Transverse branch of lateral circumflex femoral artery.
- Descending branch of inferior gluteal artery.
- Ascending branch of first perforating artery.

Since this anastomosis is the link between the internal iliac artery and profunda femoris artery, it provides collateral circulation to fill the femoral artery (if it is blocked proximal to the origin of profunda femoris artery).

POSTERIOR COMPARTMENT OF THIGH

Contents of Posterior Compartment

- Hamstring muscles.
  - Long head of biceps femoris.
  - Semitendinosus.
  - Semimembranosus.
  - Ischial part of adductor magnus).
- Short head of biceps femoris.
- Sciatic nerve.
- Posterior cutaneous nerve of thigh.

There is no major artery in the back of thigh as the hamstrings and short head of biceps femoris are supplied by perforating branches of profunda femoris artery.

Hamstring Muscles

The posterior compartment of thigh contains a group of muscles called hamstrings. The tendons of these muscles are found in the region of ham (poples) in the lower part of the back of the thigh (popliteal region).

Characteristics of Hamstring Muscles

To be called a hamstring the muscle must have the following four features:
- Origin from ischial tuberosity (Fig. 27.7).

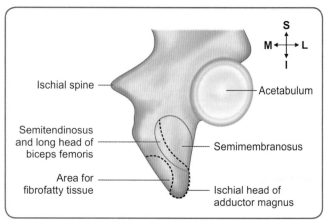

Fig. 27.7: Origin of hamstring muscles from the posteroinferior aspect of ischial tuberosity

- Insertion into either tibia or fibula.
- Nerve supply by tibial part of sciatic nerve.
- Extensor of hip joint and flexor of knee joint.

Biceps femoris

This muscle has two heads. The long head is a true hamstring muscle while the short head is not.
- ***Origin of long head:*** From the muscular impression on the superomedial area of the ischial tuberosity along with semitendinosus (Fig. 27.8).
- ***Origin of short head:*** From the lateral lip of linea aspera of femur.
- ***Insertion:*** By a common tendon into the head of fibula
- ***Nerve supply:*** Long head by tibial part of sciatic nerve high up in the thigh and short head by common peroneal part of sciatic nerve in the thigh.
- ***Actions:*** Long head produces extension of hip joint and flexion of knee joint but the short head produces only flexion of knee joint.

Semitendinosus

This muscle is so named because it has a very long tendon that begins in midthigh.
- ***Origin:*** From the muscular impression on the supero-medial area of ischial tuberosity, in common with long head of biceps femoris.
- ***Insertion:*** Into the medial surface of tibial shaft between sartorius and gracilis.
- ***Nerve supply:*** Tibial part of the sciatic nerve.

Semimembranosus

The muscle is so called because it splits into membranous slips at its insertion.
- ***Origin:*** From the supero-lateral area of ischial tuberosity by a broad flat tendon.

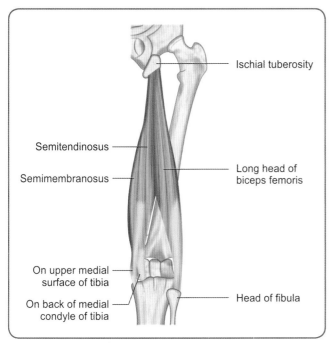

Fig. 27.8: Attachments of long head of biceps femoris, semitendinosus and semimembranosus

- **Insertion:** Mainly into a groove at the back of the medial condyle of tibia.

Extensions from the insertion of semimembranosus (Fig. 27.9)

- Oblique popliteal ligament of knee joint
- Fascia covering the popliteus muscle
- A series of slips to the medial margin of tibia

Nerve Supply: Tibial part of the sciatic nerve.

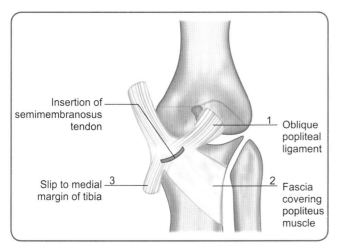

Fig. 27.9: Depicting three extensions (1, 2, 3) from insertion of semimembranosus on the back of medial condyle of tibia

Adductor magnus

The ischial part of adductor magnus is described along with adductor group of muscles in chapter 28.

Actions of hamstrings

- The hamstring muscles extend the thigh at the hip joint and flex the leg at the knee joint.
- With knee semiflexed, biceps femoris acts as lateral rotator of knee.
- With knee semiflexed, semitendinosus and semimembranosus act as medial rotators of knee joint.

Testing function of hamstrings

In prone position with knee extended, the subject is asked to flex the knee against resistance.

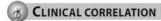

CLINICAL CORRELATION

Pulled Hamstrings is a painful condition in which the attachment of hamstrings to the ischial tuberosity is torn. It is more common in professional runners as extension of hip and flexion of knee is essential for running.

Sciatic nerve

The sciatic nerve is the thickest nerve in the body. It is about 1.5 to 2 cm wide. The sciatic nerve begins from the sacral plexus in the pelvis and terminates at the upper angle of popliteal fossa in to tibial nerve and common peroneal (common fibular) nerve. The sciatic nerve supplies the muscles of the posterior compartment of the thigh and through its terminal branches it supplies all the muscles of the leg and foot. It has a wide sensory supply, which includes the entire leg and foot except the area supplied by the saphenous (a branch of femoral nerve) and posterior cutaneous nerve of thigh.

High division of sciatic nerve

Occasionally, the sciatic nerve divides into terminal branches high up inside the pelvis or in the gluteal region or in the upper thigh. The mode of exit from greater sciatic foramen may be different as shown in Figs 27.10A and B.

Root value

The sciatic nerve is the largest branch of the sacral plexus (L4, L5, S1, S2, S3), which is located in the pelvis in front of the piriformis muscle.

Components

The sciatic nerve has two components which are enclosed in a common connective tissue sheath.

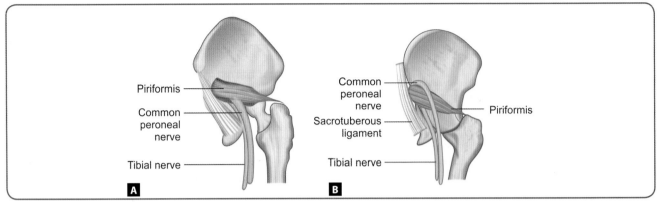

Figs 27.10A and B: Showing intrapelvic division of sciatic nerve and the mode of exit of its terminal branches in to the gluteal region. **A.** Common peroneal nerve pierces piriformis muscle; **B.** Common peroneal nerve emerges above the piriformis

- Tibial component is medial. It consists of ventral divisions of L4, L5, S1, S2, and S3 ventral rami.
- Common peroneal component is lateral. It consists of dorsal divisions of L4, L5, S1 and S2 ventral rami of spinal nerves.

Exit from pelvis

- Normally, the sciatic nerve exits from pelvis to enter the gluteal region through the greater sciatic foramen below the piriformis (Fig. 27.3). It is the most lateral structure below the piriformis.
- In intra-pelvic division of sciatic nerve, the common peroneal component either pierces the piriformis or passes above it and the tibial component passes below the piriformis (Figs 27.10A and B).

Course and relations in gluteal region

From the lower margin of the piriformis the sciatic nerve descends to enter the posterior compartment of thigh. It passes downwards through the inferomedial quadrant of the gluteal region.

Medial relations

Inferior gluteal vessels and posterior cutaneous nerve of thigh

Anterior relations or bed of sciatic nerve (Fig. 27.11)

From above downwards, the sciatic nerve is related to:
- Posterior surface of body of ischium
- Superior gemellus, tendon of obturator internus and inferior gemellus
- Quadratus femoris
- Upper part of adductor magnus

Posterior relation

The sciatic nerve is covered by the gluteus maximus muscle.

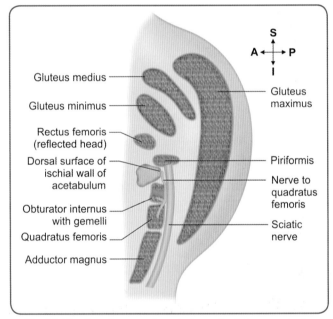

Fig. 27.11: Showing anterior relations of sciatic nerve in the gluteal region

Course and relations in posterior compartment of thigh

- In the back of the thigh, the sciatic nerve descends vertically lying between the adductor magnus anteriorly and long head of biceps femoris posteriorly.
- The long head of the biceps femoris crosses the sciatic nerve from medial to lateral side as it goes from ischial tuberosity (origin) to the head of fibula (insertion).
- The sciatic nerve gives a branch to the short head of biceps femoris from its lateral side (common peroneal component).
- It usually terminates at the upper angle of popliteal fossa by dividing into tibial and common peroneal nerves.

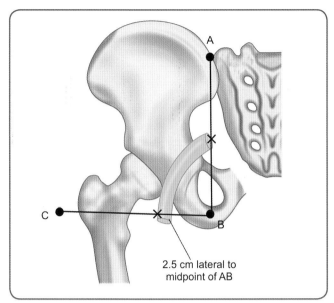

2.5 cm lateral to midpoint of AB

Fig. 27.12: Surface marking of sciatic nerve in the gluteal region. A-Posterior superior iliac spine, B-Ischial tuberosity, C-Greater trochanter

Surface marking

- To represent the gluteal course of the sciatic nerve (Fig. 27.12) two points are marked. The upper point corresponds to a point about 2 to 2.5 cm lateral to the midpoint of a line joining the posterior superior iliac spine and the ischial tuberosity. The lower point is marked midway between the greater trochanter and ischial tuberosity. A thick curved line (with outward convexity) joining the two points represents the nerve.
- To represent the sciatic nerve in the thigh, a straight line is drawn from the lower point (mentioned above) to the upper angle of popliteal fossa.

Arterial supply (Fig. 27.6)

The sciatic nerve receives a special artery called companion artery of sciatic nerve (arteria Nervi ischiadici), a branch of inferior gluteal artery. This artery enters the substance of the sciatic nerve. When the sciatic nerve is cut in above knee amputation (AKA), the companion artery is secured and ligated to avoid profuse bleeding. Its embryological importance is that it is an example of the axis artery of lower limb.

Branches in the gluteal region

Articular branches to the hip joint

Branches in the thigh

- Muscular branches arise from its medial side (tibial part) for long head of biceps femoris, semitendinosus, semimembranosus and ischial part of adductor magnus.
- Muscular branch arises from its lateral side (common peroneal part) to short head of biceps femoris.

Therefore, the medial side of sciatic nerve is considered its side of danger and lateral side its safe side.

⊘ CLINICAL CORRELATION

- Sciatica is caused by compression of the lower lumbar and upper sacral nerve roots or by pressure on the sacral plexus. The patient experiences radiating pain down the posterior aspect of thigh, posterior and lateral sides of leg and lateral part of foot. On doing straight leg raising test the pain was aggravated. In this test the patient lies supine and is asked to extend both leg and thigh on the affected side. The extended lower limb is raised by holding the foot. This causes pain in the leg due to strain on the sciatic nerve.
- Seeping foot is due to temporary compression of the sciatic nerve against femur, at the lower border of gluteus maximus muscle, when a person sits on the hard edge of a chair for a long time.
- For anesthetic block of sciatic nerve, the site chosen for injection is a few cm inferior to the midpoint of the line joining posterior superior iliac spine and apex of greater trochanter.

Effects of Injury to Complete Sciatic Nerve (for example in posterior dislocation of hip joint)

- Paralysis of the muscles of posterior compartment of thigh and of posterior compartment of leg and of foot.
- Sensory loss below the knee with sparing of the skin supplied by saphenous nerve and postreior cutaneous nerve of thigh.

Effects of Injury to Tibial Component Only (of sciatic nerve)

- Paralysis of all the muscles of posterior compartment of leg and of sole of the foot leading to inability to stand on the toes (due to loss of plantarflexion of foot).
- Loss of Achilles tendon reflex.
- Sensory loss on the sole of the foot, which may lead to trophic ulcers on the sole.

Effects of Injury to Common Peroneal Component Only (of sciatic nerve)

- Paralysis of the muscles of anterior and lateral compartments of leg resulting in inability to stand on heel (foot drop due to involvement of deep peroneal nerve) and inability to evert foot (due to involvement of superficial peroneal nerve).

Contd...

Contd…

Contd…

CLINICAL CORRELATION

- Sensory loss on the anterolateral side of leg and dorsum of foot except for the area supplied by saphenous nerve (medial side of lower part of leg and medial border of foot as far as the root of great toe).

Intragluteal Injections

The intramuscular injections in gluteal region (Fig. 27.13) are commonly used for administration of antibiotics or iron etc. The gluteal muscles provide a large surface area for absorption of drugs. Injecting in the superomedial quadrant endangers the superior gluteal nerve and vessels. Injecting in inferomedial quadrant endangers the sciatic nerve and inferior gluteal nerve and vessels. Sometimes only the lateral part of the sciatic nerve may be injured causing effects of common peroneal nerve injury like foot drop. Therefore, superolateral quadrant is a safe site for intramuscular injection in the gluteus medius muscle. The point of injection is just posteroinferior to the anterior superior iliac spine.

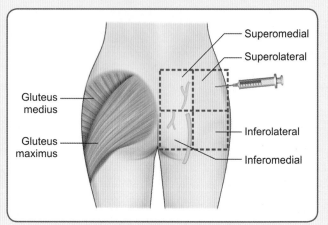

Fig. 27.13: Safe quadrant in gluteal region for intramuscular injection

28

Adductor or Medial Compartment of Thigh and Hip Joint

Chapter Contents

ADDUCTOR COMPARTMENT OF THIGH

The adductor compartment of thigh contains six muscles, obturator nerve, obturator vessels and the profunda femoris vessels. The muscles in the adductor compartment are obturator externus, pectineus, gracilis and adductor magnus, longus and brevis muscles. The obturator externus is functionally not the adductor muscle but the remaining five muscles are adductors. The adductor muscles collectively are called the rider's muscles.

Arrangement of Adductor Muscles (Fig. 28.1)

The muscles are arranged in three strata:
- **Superficial stratum:** Pectineus, adductor longus and gracilis.
- **Intermediate stratum:** Obturator externus and adductor brevis.
- **Deep stratum:** Adductor magnus.

Muscles in Superficial Stratum

Pectineus (Fig. 28.2)

The pectineus is a composite (or hybrid) muscle that belongs to medial and anterior compartments of thigh. It is located in the medial part of the floor of femoral triangle.
- **Origin:** From the pecten pubis of the superior ramus of pubis.

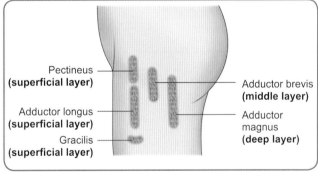

Fig. 28.1: Showing arrangement of adductor muscles in adductor compartments in schematic format

- **Insertion:** Into the posterior aspect of femur on a line extending from the lesser trochanter to the linea aspera.

Relations
- **Anteriorly:** To the posterior wall of femoral sheath and the femoral vessels contained inside it.
- **Posteriorly:** To the capsule of the hip joint, obturator externus and the adductor brevis from above downward. The anterior division of obturator nerve descends between the posterior surface of the pectineus and the obturator externus and adductor brevis muscles.
- **Medially:** To adductor longus and the profunda femoris vessels enter the gap between the two.

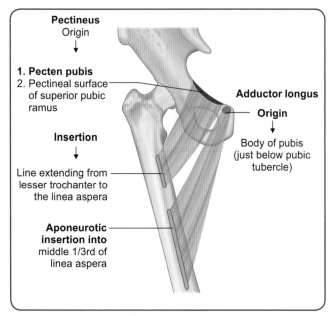

Fig. 28.2: Attachments of pectineus and adductor longus muscles

- *Laterally:* To psoas major and the medial circumflex, femoral vessels enter the gap between the pectineus and psoas major muscles.

Nerve supply

- A branch from the femoral nerve supplies from its anterior aspect.
- A branch from anterior division of obturator nerve (or by accessory obturator nerve when present) supplies from its posterior aspect.

Actions

Pectineus is a flexor of the thigh and assists in adduction of the thigh.

Adductor Longus (Fig. 28.2)

- *Origin:* From the front of the body of pubis (just below the pubic tubercle) by a narrow tendon (rider's bone is a sesamoid bone in the tendinous origin).
- *Insertion:* By a wide aponeurosis into the linea aspera of the back of femur.

Relations

- The medial margin of adductor longus forms the medial boundary of the femoral triangle. It forms the most medial part of the floor of femoral triangle, where its lateral margin lies edge to edge with pectineus.
- Anteriorly (near the origin), it is crossed by spermatic cord in male and in the femoral triangle and subsartorial canal, it is related to femoral vessels (Fig. 26.12).

- Posteriorly, it is related to profunda femoris vessels, anterior branch of obturator nerve and adductor brevis muscle.

Nerve supply: Anterior division of obturator nerve.

Actions

It is the adductor and medial rotator of thigh at the hip joint.

Gracilis

This muscle derives its name from the Latin word *gracilis* meaning *slender*. The gracilis is a thin and flat muscle. It is the most superficial of the adductor muscles.

- *Origin:* From the medial margin of the lower half of the body of pubis and the lower part of conjoint ischiopubic ramus. It descends vertically to become tendinous at the level of medial condyle of femur.
- *Insertion:* By a narrow, flattened tendon into the upper part of medial surface of tibia between the insertions of sartorius and semitendinosus (Fig. 24.8).
- *Nerve Supply:* Anterior division of obturator nerve.

Actions

- It is an adductor and medial rotator of thigh at the hip joint.
- It is an accessory flexor of leg at the knee joint.

> ### ✎ CLINICAL CORRELATION
>
> **Gracilis Graft**
> Being easily accessible and functionally a weak muscle, the gracilis is suitable for muscle graft to replace the damaged muscle in some other part of the body. To include the nerve and blood vessels inside the graft, it is important to know that the entry point of the neurovascular bundle of gracilis is at its upper end.

Muscles in Intermediate Stratum

Obturator externus

This muscle is a content of the adductor compartment and is innervated by obturator nerve but it does not function like other five muscles of this compartment.

- *Origin:* From the external surface of the obturator membrane and the bony margins of the obturator foramen.
- *Insertion:* Into the trochanteric fossa of femur.
- *Nerve Supply:* Posterior division of obturator nerve.

Actions

- The obturator externus is a lateral rotator of thigh.

- Its tendon spirals round the back of neck of femur. This enables it to act like a ligament steadying the head of femur in the acetabulum.

Adductor brevis

- *Origin:* From the external aspect of body and inferior ramus of pubis.
- *Insertion:* Into a line extending from the base of the lesser trochanter to upper part of linea aspera.

Relations

- The adductor brevis lies between the pectineus and adductor longus in front and the adductor magnus behind.
- It is sandwiched between the anterior and posterior divisions of the obturator nerve.

Vascular relations

- Medial circumflex femoral artery runs between the adductor brevis (below) and obturator externus (above).
- First to third perforating arteries (branches of profunda artery) arise in relation to the adductor brevis muscle, first at the level of its upper border, the second in front of it and the third at its lower border.

Nerve supply

It is usually supplied by anterior division of obturator nerve but may receive a branch from the posterior division as well.

Action: Adductor of thigh

Muscle in Deep Stratum

Adductor magnus (Fig. 28.3)

This is a large composite or hybrid muscle, which has two parts (adductor part and ischial or hamstring), which differ in origin, insertion, nerve supply and actions.

Adductor part of adductor magnus

- *Origin:* From the ischiopubic ramus.
- *Insertion:* Horizontal fibers into gluteal tuberosity and middle oblique fibers into the linea aspera and proximal part of medial supracondylar line.

Osseoaponeurotic openings at insertion of adductor part

The long insertion of the adductor part is interrupted by five osseo-aponeurotic openings, bridged by tendinous arches attached to the linea aspera.

- Upper four openings are small and transmit four perforating branches of profunda femoris artery.
- Lowest opening is large and called *adductor* or *tendinous hiatus*. It transmits the femoral vessels into

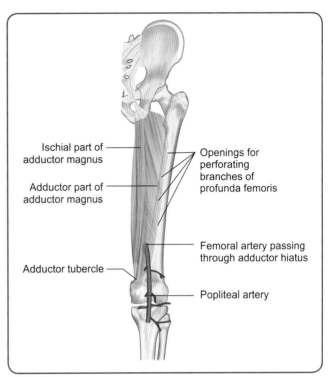

Fig. 28.3: Showing the adductor magnus muscle and the osseo-aponeurotic openings at its insertion

the popliteal fossa. This opening lies on the medial supracondylar line of femur at the junction of the middle and lower thirds of thigh.

Ischial part of adductor magnus

The ischial part is located posterior to the adductor part.

- *Origin:* From the inferolateral quadrant of the ischial tuberosity.
- *Insertion:* By a rounded tendon into the adductor tubercle of femur.

Relations of adductor magnus

- *Anteriorly:* Related to pectineus, adductor brevis and adductor longus muscles from above downwards and to the posterior division of obturator nerve, profunda vessels and the femoral vessels in the lower part of adductor canal.
- *Posteriorly:* Related to the sciatic nerve and the hamstring muscles.

Nerve supply

- *Adductor part:* By posterior division of the obturator nerve.
- *Ischial part:* By tibial component of the sciatic nerve.

Actions

- Adductor part adducts and medially rotates the thigh.
- Ischial part extends the hip joint and flexes the knee joint.

Obturator Nerve (Fig. 28.4)

The obturator nerve is a branch of the lumbar plexus, located on posterior abdominal wall. Its root value is L2, L3 and L4 (ventral divisions of ventral rami of spinal nerves). It emerges from the medial margin of the psoas major muscle and crosses the pelvic brim anterior to the sacroiliac joint to enter the pelvic cavity.

Course inside Pelvis

- The obturator nerve courses forward on the lateral pelvic wall along the upper margin of obturator internus muscle. In a female, it is related to lateral surface of the ovary.
- The obturator artery (a branch of anterior division of internal iliac artery) accompanies the obturator nerve. The neurovascular bundle thus formed enters the obturator canal.
- The obturator nerve terminates into anterior and posterior divisions in the obturator canal.
- The anterior and posterior divisions leave via the obturator foramen to enter the medial compartment of thigh along with the obturator artery.

Course and Distribution of Anterior Division

The anterior division of the obturator nerve descends at first, in front of the obturator externus muscle and then in front of adductor brevis. It passes behind the pectineus and adductor longus muscles.

Branches

- Articular branch to the hip joint.
- Muscular branches to pectineus, adductor longus, adductor brevis and gracilis.
- Vascular filament to the femoral artery.
- A cutaneous branch to communicate with branches of medial femoral cutaneous nerve and saphenous nerve to form subsartorial plexus (which supplies the skin of medial side of the thigh).

Course and Distribution of Posterior Division

The posterior division of the obturator nerve passes through the obturator externus muscle and descends on the anterior surface of adductor magnus lying behind the adductor brevis. Distal to the lower limit of the adductor magnus the posterior division continues in the popliteal fossa as the slender genicular branch.

Branches

- Muscular branches to obturator externus, adductor brevis (if it does not receive supply from anterior division) and the adductor part of adductor magnus.
- Genicular branch passes through the lower part of adductor magnus to enter popliteal fossa. It supplies the articular capsule of the knee joint and after piercing the oblique popliteal ligament supplies the interior of the knee joint.

CLINICAL CORRELATION

- Bilateral obturator neurectomy (cutting the nerve) is performed to relieve severe adductor spasm. Because the thighs are held in adducted position in adductor spasm, the lower limbs cross each other like the scissors. This is seen in some neurological disorders.
- The pain due to disease of hip joint may be referred to knee joint and to the medial side of the thigh. This is because of the common nerve supply of the joints through the articular branches of obturator nerve and of cutaneous supply to the medial side of thigh (through its contribution to subsartorial plexus).

Blood Vessels in Adductor Compartment

The following three blood vessels enter the adductor compartment of thigh:

- The obturator artery enters through the obturator foramen from the pelvis.

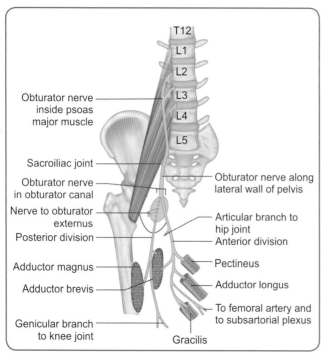

Fig. 28.4: Course and distribution of obturator nerve

- The profunda femoris artery enters through the gap between the pectineus and adductor longus muscles from the femoral triangle.
- The medial circumflex femoral branch of the profunda femoris artery enters through the gap between the pectineus and the psoas major muscle from the femoral triangle.

Obturator Artery

The obturator artery is a branch of anterior division of internal iliac artery. It accompanies the obturator nerve in the pelvis (lying below the obturator nerve). Immediately after its emergence from the obturator canal, it divides into anterior and posterior branches.

Note: The pelvic course of obturator artery is described in chapter 55 along with branches of internal iliac artery

Branches in thigh

- Muscular branches to the muscles in the medial compartment of thigh from both anterior and posterior divisions of obturator artery.
- Acetabular branch to the hip joint arises from the posterior division of obturator artery and enters the hip joint via acetabular notch to travel along the ligamentum teres to the head of the femur.
- The terminal branch of posterior terminal branch of obturator artery enters the hip joint through the acetabular notch and then passes along the ligament of head to the head to supply the head of femur.

Profunda Femoris Artery (Deep Femoral Artery)

This is the main artery providing blood to all the muscles of thigh. Though it originates in the front of thigh in the femoral triangle, its main course is in the adductor compartment. Its branches, however, enter all the compartments and take part in the chain of arterial anastomoses in the back of thigh.

Origin of profunda femoris (Fig. 28.5)

The profunda femoris artery arises from the lateral aspect of the femoral artery in the femoral triangle about 3.5 to 4 cm below the inguinal ligament. However, the point of origin may be variable.

Course in femoral triangle

- From its origin the profunda femoris gradually turns medially to pass posterior to the femoral vessels. In this course it lies on the anterior aspect of pectineus muscle.

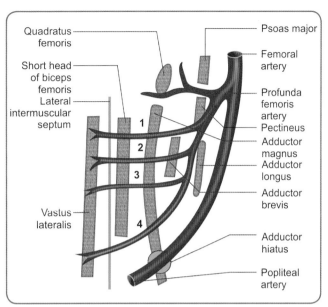

Fig. 28.5: Profunda femoris artery and its perforating branches (numbered 1 to 4)

- It leaves the femoral triangle through the gap between the pectineus and adductor longus to enter the adductor compartment.

Branches in femoral triangle

- Medial circumflex femoral artery
- Lateral circumflex femoral artery
- Muscular branches

Course and branches in medial compartment

- At the level of the apex of femoral triangle, the profunda femoris artery and accompanying vein are separated from the femoral vessels by adductor longus. The gunshot or stab injury at this level may injure all the four blood vessels.
- In its further descent the profunda femoris lies at first between the adductor longus in front and adductor brevis behind. Beyond the lower limit of adductor brevis it lies between the adductor longus in front and adductor magnus behind.
- At the level of midthigh it enters the adductor magnus to continue as the fourth perforating artery.

Branches in thigh

- First perforating artery
- Second perforating artery
- Third perforating artery
- Fourth perforating artery (continuation of profunda femoris artery).

Medial Circumflex Femoral Artery (MCFA)

This artery usually arises from the posteromedial aspect of the profunda femoris artery in the femoral triangle.

Course

The medial circumflex femoral artery takes a circuitous route as it passes through three regions, femoral triangle and medial compartment of thigh and gluteal region. It leaves the femoral triangle by passing between the psoas major and pectineus muscles. It travels in posterior direction between the obturator externus and adductor brevis and then enters the gluteal region, where it passes between the quadratus femoris and upper margin of adductor magnus (Fig. 28.5).

Branches

- Transverse branch takes part in cruciate anastomosis.
- Ascending branch passes up in the gluteal region on the tendon of the obturator externus and takes part in trochanteric anastomosis.

 STUDENT INTEREST

> The ascending branch of MCFA forms a vascular ring around the femoral neck by anastomozing with ascending branch of LCFA. The posterior retinacular branches from this vascular ring provide blood to the head and neck of the femur. The medial circumflex femoral artery is thus the chief arterial supply to the head of femur.

- Acetabular artery enters the acetabulum along with a similar branch from obturator artery to supply the femoral head.

Lateral Circumflex Femoral Artery (LCFA)

This is a lateral and larger branch arising near the root of profunda femoris artery. It turns laterally between the anterior and posterior divisions of femoral nerve and leaves the femoral triangle by passing deep to the sartorius. After passing deep to the rectus femoris it divides in to ascending, transverse and descending branches.

- Ascending branch runs along the intertrochanteric line lateral to the hip joint and forms an anastomotic ring around the femoral neck with ascending branches of medial circumflex femoral artery and takes part in trochanteric anastomosis in the gluteal region.
- Transverse branch passes laterally anterior to the vastus intermedius and pierces the vastus lateralis to reach the posterior aspect for taking part in cruciate anastomosis.
- Descending branch runs down along the anterior border of vastus lateralis. It supplies the vastus lateralis and its one long branch descends in the substance of

vastus lateralis to anastomose with lateral superior genicular branch of popliteal artery to take part in anastomosis around the knee joint.

Perforating Arteries (Fig. 28.6)

Out of the four perforating arteries upper three are the branches of profunda femoris artery and the fourth one is the continuation of the profunda femoris artery.

The upper three perforating arteries pierce the insertion of adductor magnus (lying very close to the femur) to reach the flexor compartment. In the flexor compartment they supply the hamstring muscles and communicate with each other by anastomotic branches. They pierce the origin of short head of biceps femoris and the lateral intermuscular septum to terminate in the vastus lateralis in the extensor compartment. Additionally the first perforator takes part in cruciate anastomosis. The second perforator gives a nutrient branch to the femur and the fourth perforator anastomoses with the superior muscular branches of the popliteal artery.

💡 **ADDED INFORMATION**

> **Anastomoses of Profunda Femoris Artery**
> - Spinous anastomosis at anterior superior iliac spine.
> - Trochanteric anastomosis in the gluteal region.
> - Cruciate anastomosis in the upper part of thigh at the level of lesser trochanter.
> - Vertical anastomotic chains between branches of perforating arteries in the middle of thigh.
> - In the lower part of thigh the branches of popliteal artery anastomose with fourth perforating and lateral circumflex femoral arteries.

🔖 **CLINICAL CORRELATION**

> - The deeply located profunda femoris artery is in close proximity to the femoral shaft. Hence it is prone to injury in fracture of femoral shaft. It may also be injured due blunt injury to the thigh without fracture of the femur. The artery is also liable to injury in surgical procedures like fixing metallic screws in the femur.
> - Rupture of the profunda femoris artery causes severe bleeding inside the thigh muscles, which may result in thigh compartment syndrome.
> - The preferred site of femoral artery ligation is proximal to the origin of profunda femoris. This ensures the arterial supply to lower limb via the anastomoses between branches of profunda and branches of internal and external iliac arteries.
> - In blockage of femoral artery beyond the origin of profunda femoris, the arterial supply to the lower limb is maintained via the anastomoses of branches of profunda femoris with those of popliteal artery.

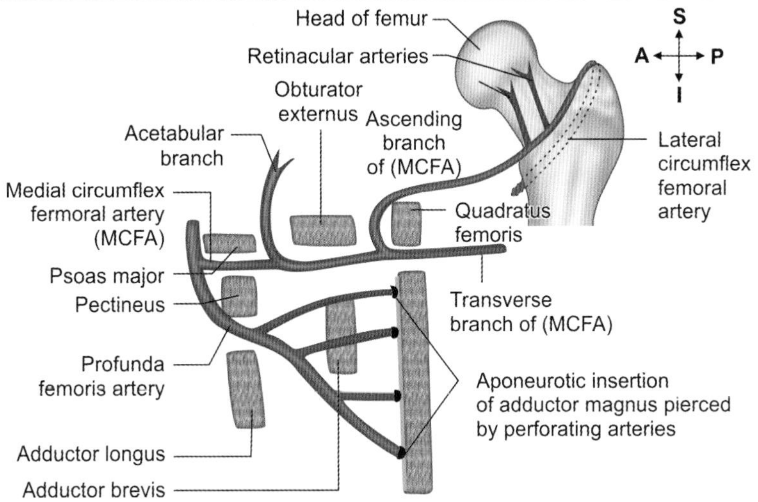

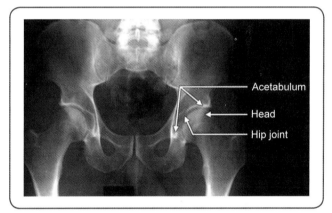

Fig. 28.6: Origin, course and distribution of three branches of medial circumflex femoral artery (MCFA)

HIP JOINT OR COXAL JOINT

The hip joint is an example of multiaxial ball and socket type of synovial joint. Its primary functions are to support the body weight in standing position and to transmit the forces during movements of trunk upon the femur like walking and running. The range of movements in all directions is possible in this joint because the long and narrow neck of the femur makes an angle with the shaft called **neck shaft angle** or **angle of inclination**.

Articular Surfaces

The bones taking part in the hip joint are the head of femur and the acetabulum of the hip bone. Figure 28.7 shows the radiological appearance of the bones taking part in the hip joint.

Acetabulum

The **acetabulum** (in Latin means **cup**) is a cup-shaped cavity formed by the union of ilium, ischium and pubis of the hip bone.
- The rim of the acetabulum presents a notch in its lower part. This notch gives attachment to the transverse acetabular ligament and to the ligament of head of femur.
- The fibrocartilaginous labrum acetabulare deepens the acetabulum. The labrum, which is attached to the rim of acetabulum and to the transverse acetabular ligament, forms a tight fit around the neck of femur.
- The horseshoe-shaped articular surface (lunate surface) of acetabulum is covered with articular cartilage. It is thickest and widest superiorly, where the maximum body weight is transmitted to the femur.

Fig. 28.7: Anteroposterior radiograph of adult male showing bones taking part in hip joint

- The nonarticular part of acetabulum is known as **acetabular fossa**. It is filled with Haversian pad of fat, which is intracapsular but extrasynovial.

Head of Femur

The spherical femoral head is covered by hyaline articular cartilage, except for a rough pit where the ligament of the head of femur is attached. The articular cartilage is thickest in the center and thins out towards the periphery.

Fibrous Capsule

The capsule is very strong and surrounds the joint tightly.

Medial attachment to acetabulum

The capsule is attached to the margins of the acetabulum, labrum acetabulare and transverse acetabular ligament.

Lateral attachment to upper end of femur

Anteriorly, it is attached to the intertrochanteric line of upper end of femur. Thus the entire anterior surface of neck is intracapsular and posteriorly, it is attached to the posterior surface of the neck at a short distance (about a cm) medial to the intertrochanteric crest. Thus the posterior surface of the neck is partly intracapsular.

Special Parts of Capsule

- Zona orbicularis is the inner part of the capsule consisting of circularly arranged fibers. It forms a tight collar for the neck of the femur.
- Retinacula are the longitudinal fibers on the outer part of the capsule (very well developed anteriorly). Many of these longitudinal fibers originate from the capsule at the site of its attachment to the intertrochanteric line and turn sharply towards the femoral head in close contact with the anterior surface of the neck of femur. These longitudinal bundles are called *retinacula*, which produce grooves on the femoral neck. Their main function is to support the retinacular arteries running towards the head.

Ligaments (Fig. 28.8)

The fibrous capsule covers the joint. The capsule is strengthened in three places to form the iliofemoral, pubofemoral and ischiofemoral ligaments.

Iliofemoral ligament (Ligament of Bigelow)

The iliofemoral ligament is anteriorly placed. It is the thickest and a very powerful ligament. Its shape is like inverted Y.

Attachments:
- Superiorly, to anterior inferior iliac spine
- Inferiorly, to the intertrochanteric line of femur by medial and lateral bands and intervening thin part (Fig. 28.8).

The iliofemoral ligament prevents the natural tendency of the body to fall backward (overextension of hip joint). The tendency to fall backward is on account of the fact that the line passing through the center of gravity of the body lies slightly behind the hip joints.

Pubofemoral ligament (Fig. 28.8)

It is triangular in shape. It is attached to the iliopubic eminence, superior pubic ramus and obturator crest by base. It blends with the capsule and deep surface of the medial band of iliofemoral ligament inferiorly. It limits abduction and lateral rotation of thigh.

Ischiofemoral ligament (Fig. 28.8)

The ischiofemoral ligament reinforces the posterior side of the capsule. It is attached to the ischium below the lower

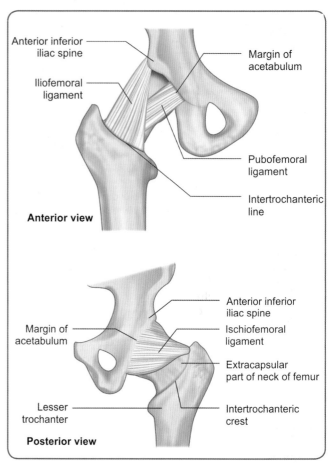

Fig. 28.8: Ligaments of hip joint (iliofemoral, pubofemoral and ischiofemoral)

margin of acetabulum. From this attachment the fibers spiral superolaterally to merge with the fibrous capsule. The ischiofemoral ligament limits the medial rotation of hip joint.

Transverse acetabular ligament

It converts the acetabular notch into acetabular foramen through which pass acetabular branch of obturator artery, acetabular branch of medial circumflex femoral artery and articular branch of anterior division of obturator nerve.

Ligament of head of femur

This ligament extends from the acetabular notch to the fovea on the head of femur. It carries the articular vessels and nerves to the head of the femur.

Synovial membrane (Fig. 28.9)

The synovial membrane lines the inner surface of the fibrous capsule. It covers the intracapsular part of the neck as far as the articular margin of the head of femur. It also covers the acetabular labrum, ligament of the head of

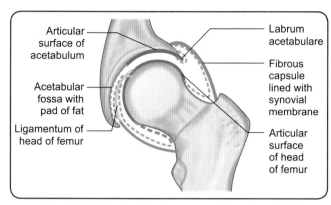

Fig. 28.9: Showing the fibrous capsule and synovial membrane of hip joint

femur and Haversian pad of fat inside the acetabular fossa. The synovial fold surrounding the ligament of the head of femur carries the blood vessels and nerves entering the joint through the acetabular foramen. The synovial membrane lining the intracapsular part of the neck is raised into folds by the retinacular fibers. Occasionally, the synovial membrane may protrude through as opening in the anterior part of capsule between iliofemoral and ischiofemoral ligaments to become continuous with psoas bursa.

Relations of Joint (Fig. 28.10)

The joint is surrounded by muscles as follows:

Anterior (from medial to lateral)

- Lateral part of pectineus separates the femoral vein from the hip joint.
- Tendon of psoas separates the femoral artery from the joint and the femoral nerve is in the gap between psoas tendon and iliacus (a bursa intervenes between the joint and iliopsoas tendon).
- Straight head of rectus femoris and deep layer of iliotibial tract (which blends with the capsule of the joint)

Superior

Reflected head of rectus femoris medially and gluteus minimus, gluteus laterally.

Inferior

Lateral part of pectineus and obturator externus muscle along with medial circumflex femoral artery.

Posterior (Most Important Relations)

From below upwards the relations are the tendon of obturator externus (separating the capsule from quadratus femoris), tendon of obturator internus with the gemelli (separating the capsule from sciatic nerve) and piriformis. Superficial to the above mentioned close relations is the gluteus maximus muscle.

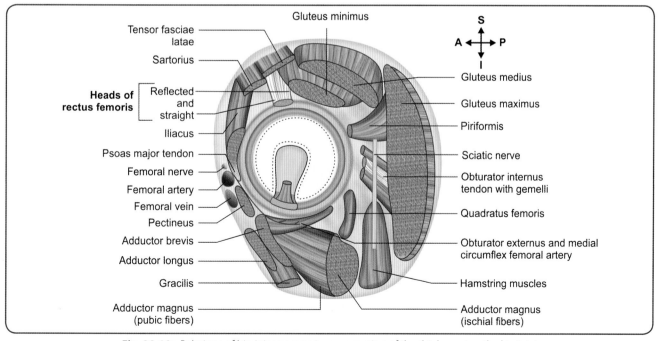

Fig. 28.10: Relations of hip joint as seen in cross-section of the thigh passing the hip joint

Arterial Supply (Fig. 28.11)

- The area of femoral head around the fovea is supplied by acetabular branch of obturator artery and acetabular branch of medial circumflex femoral artery. This source is of little significance.
- Major parts of the head and neck receive blood from arterial circle around the capsular attachment, in which the medial circumflex femoral artery is the chief source. The retinacular arteries arise from this vascular ring, pierce the capsule and run along the neck of femur to supply it and the head. The retinacular arteries are the sole supply of head and neck. Their rupture due to intracapsular fracture of the femoral neck results in avascular necrosis of the head of femur.
- The nutrient artery of the femur is an additional source.

Nerve Supply

The joint receives articular twigs from femoral nerve via a branch to rectus femoris, nerve to quadratus femoris, anterior division of obturator nerve and from superior gluteal nerve.

Movements

The movements of hip joint take place around three axes, transverse, anteroposterior and vertical.

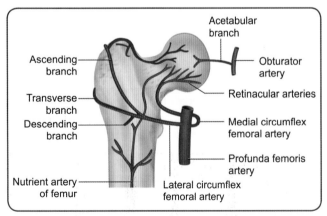

Fig. 28.11: Arterial supply of head and neck of femur (MFCA is the chief source)

TABLE 28.1: Muscles Responsible for Movements of Hip Joint

Movement	Main muscles	Accessory muscles
Flexion	Iliopsoas	Pectineus, sartorius, rectus femoris
Extension	Gluteus maximus	Hamstring muscles
Adduction	Adductors—longus, brevis and magnus	Pectineus and gracilis
Abduction	Gluteus—medius and minimus	Tensor fasciae latae
Medial rotation	Gluteus—medius and minimus	Tensor fasciae latae and adductor muscles
Lateral rotation	Obturator externus and internus, gemelli, quadratus femoris	Piriformis, gluteus maximus, sartorius
Circumduction	Sequential contraction of all muscles responsible for above movements	

Flexion and Extension

These movements occur around transverse axis. The range of flexion is greater. The flexion is limited when the anterior surface of thigh touches the anterior abdominal wall. The extension is limited when the thigh and trunk are in the same vertical line.

Adduction and Abduction

These movements occur around anteroposterior axis. Adduction is limited by contact with the opposite thigh. In abduction, the thigh moves laterally. Abduction is very crucial during walking. The abduction movement in the supported hip joint enables the pelvis on the opposite side to lift up (in preparation of taking a step).

Medial and Lateral Rotation

Rotation takes place around vertical axis. The axis of rotation does not pass through the shaft of femur because of the presence of neck-shaft angle. It passes through the head and the lateral condyle of the femur when the limb is on the ground. During medial rotation, the medial condyle of femur turns backwards with concomitant forward movement of the greater trochanter. In lateral rotation, the lateral condyle of femur moves backwards with concomitant backward movement of the greater trochanter.

ADDED INFORMATION

Palpation of Bony Landmarks in Clinical Examination of Hip Joint
- Anterior superior iliac spine
- Greater trochanter, and the
- Ischial tuberosity

Greater Trochanter

The greater trochanter is located at a hand's breadth below the tubercle of iliac crest. Upward displacement of greater trochanter indicates shortening of the limb due to fracture dislocations in hip region.

Methods to Palpate Greater Trochanter
- Nelaton's line is drawn with the patient lying on the normal side, from the anterior superior iliac spine to the most prominent part of ischial tuberosity. Normally the tip of greater trochanter is at or just below this line.
- Schoemaker's line is a straight line that extends from the tip of greater trochanter to the anterior superior iliac spine and upwards over the anterior abdominal wall to reach the umbilicus. If the greater trochanter is elevated the line reaches below the umbilicus.

CLINICAL CORRELATION

- Fracture of the neck of femur may be intracapsular or extracapsular (Figs 28.12A and B). Intracapsular fracture includes subcapital, transcervical and basal. The subcapital fracture is more common in postmenopausal women (thinning of cortical bone due to deficiency of estrogen) and is produced by a minor trip. In this type of fracture the retinacular arteries are injured leading to delay in healing or nonunion of fracture. Its serious complication is avascular necrosis of head of the femur with resultant loss of function of the hip joint. Extracapsular fracture of the neck (for example, intertrochanteric fracture) is relatively less serious as the retinacular arteries are saved (Fig. 28.12B).
- The characteristic feature of intracapsular fracture of the neck of femur is shortening of the affected limb. The length of entire lower limb is measured from anterior superior iliac spine to the medial malleolus and of thigh from anterior superior iliac spine to the adductor tubercle. The limb is held in laterally

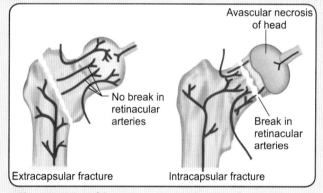

Figs 28.12A and B: A. Extracapsular fracture of neck of femur (no break in retinacular arteries); **B.** Intracapsular fracture of neck of femur (break in retinacular arteries and resultant avascular necrosis of the femoral head)

Contd...

Contd…

rotated position with toes pointing laterally (Fig. 28.13). The shortening of the lower limb occurs due to powerful upward pull of rectus femoris and adductor and hamstring muscles. The lateral rotation of the lower limb is explained as follows. The head of femur separates from the shaft (carrying the trochanter) in intracapsular fracture. So the shaft of femur can rotate independent of the head. The gluteus maximus and short lateral rotator muscles rotate the femur laterally. The psoas major becomes a lateral rotator after fracture due to shift in the axis of its action.

- The neck- shaft angle is also known as angle of inclination (Fig. 28.14A to C)). The normal neck-shaft angle is 125° in adult and 160° in children. When there is increase in the angle, it is called ***coxa valga***. It is found in congenital dislocation of hip joint. Coxa valga limits the adduction movement of the hip joint. If the angle is reduced, it is called ***coxa vara***. It limits the abduction at the hip joint
- Fig. 28.15 depicts the radiograph of a patient with dislocation of prosthetic hip joint on right side. In hip replacement the diseased head of the femur is replaced by a metallic head fixed to the patient's femoral shaft by bone cement and a plastic socket replaces the patient's acetabulum.
- Pain arising in hip joint is referred to knee joint due to common innervation of the two joints through branches of sciatic, femoral and obturator nerves.
- In posterior dislocation of hip joint, the head of femur dislocates in the gluteal region, where it may compress the sciatic nerve.
- Congenital dislocation in hip joint is more common than any other joint in the body. In this, the head dislocates into the gluteal region due to congenitally deficient upper margin of acetabulum. This causes lurching gait and positive Trendelenburg sign.

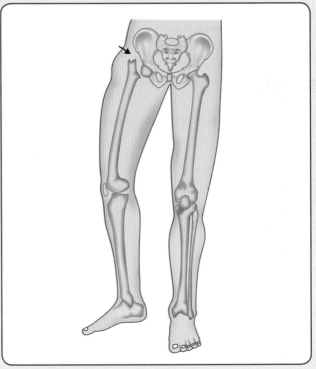

Fig. 28.13: Fracture of neck of right femur resulting in upward and posterior displacement of greater trochanter (indicated by arrow) and the limb is held in laterally rotated position

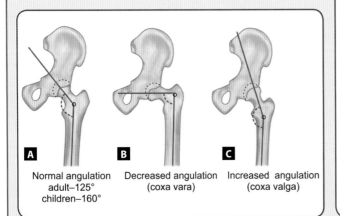

A Normal angulation adult–125° children–160° **B** Decreased angulation (coxa vara) **C** Increased angulation (coxa valga)

Figs 28.14A to C: Clinical importance of neck shaft angle (angle between long axis of neck of femur and long axis of shaft of femur)

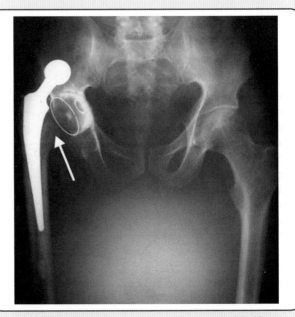

Fig. 28.15: Radiograph showing dislocation of head of femur in prosthetic hip joint (arrow showing)

29

Popliteal Fossa and Knee Joint

Chapter Contents

POPLITEAL FOSSA

The popliteal fossa is a diamond-shaped hollow situated behind the knee joint. It is an important region because it gives passage to the main vessels and nerves from the thigh to the leg.

Boundaries (Fig. 29.1)

The tendons of hamstring muscles form the superolateral and superomedial boundaries. The fleshy origins of the flexor muscles of the leg form the inferolateral and inferomedial boundaries.
- ***Superolaterally:*** Tendons of biceps femoris.
- ***Superomedially:*** Tendons of semitendinosus and semimembranosus.
- ***Inferolaterally:*** Lateral head of gastrocnemius and plantaris.
- ***Inferomedially:*** Medial head of gastrocnemius.
- Roof or the posterior wall is the deep fascia (popliteal fascia), which is pierced by small saphenous vein, superficial lymphatics, and posterior cutaneous nerve of thigh.
- Floor or anterior wall is divisible into three parts (Fig. 29.2)
  1. Upper part by the popliteal surface of femur.
  2. Intermediate part by capsule of the knee joint (oblique popliteal ligament).
  3. Lower part by fascia covering the popliteus muscle.

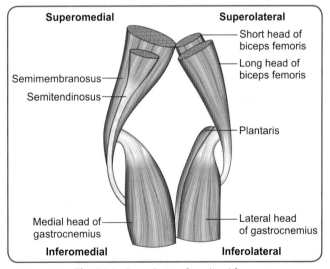

Fig. 29.1: Boundaries of popliteal fossa

Contents

- Popliteal artery and its branches (Fig. 29.3)
- Popliteal vein and its tributaries
- Tibial nerve and its branches
- Common peroneal nerve and its branches
- Posterior cutaneous nerve of thigh
- Descending genicular branch of posterior division of obturator nerve

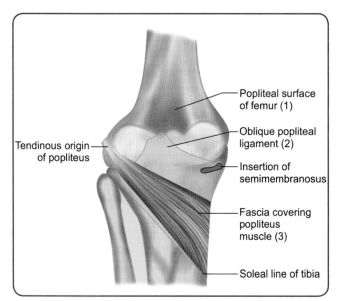

Fig. 29.2: Three parts (numbered 1 to 3 from above downwards) of the floor of popliteal fossa

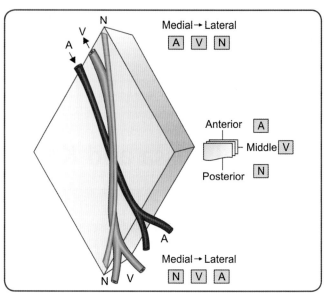

Fig. 29.4: Neurovascular relations in right popliteal fossa (A) Popliteal artery, (V) Popliteal vein, (N) Tibial nerve

- In the upper part, the relation is A-V-N from medial to lateral.
- In the middle part, the relation is A- V - N in anteroposterior order.
- In the lower part the relation is N – V- A from medial to lateral.

Note: Common peroneal nerve is also an important content. But it is not part of the main neurovascular bundle as it inclines in lateral direction from the superior angle of the fossa and leaves the fossa following the tendon of biceps femoris (Fig. 29.6).

Popliteal Artery (Fig. 29.3)

The popliteal artery is the continuation of femoral artery at the level of tendinous opening (hiatus magnus) in adductor magnus muscle. It is the deepest structure in the popliteal fossa as it is located in close contact with the floor of the fossa. The popliteal artery runs obliquely across the fossa with a lateral inclination to reach the distal border of the popliteus muscle, where it terminates in to anterior and posterior tibial arteries.

Surface Marking

The popliteal artery is marked on the popliteal fossa by joining the following three points:
1. Upper point is 2.5 cm medial to the midline at the junction of middle and lower thirds of thigh.
2. Middle point is at the level of knee joint in the midline.
3. Lower point is in the midline on the back of leg at the level of tibial tuberosity.

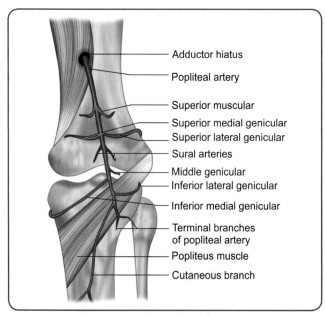

Fig. 29.3: Extent and branches of popliteal artery

- Popliteal lymph nodes in close proximity to the popliteal vessels.
- Popliteal fat.

Main Neurovascular Bundle (Fig. 29.4)

The main neurovascular bundle containing tibial nerve, popliteal artery and popliteal vein displays triple relations as follows:

Relations

Anterior or deep

The popliteal artery is related to the floor of fossa (popliteal surface of femur, capsule of knee joint and fascia covering the popliteus). This relationship endangers the popliteal artery in supracondylar fracture of femur and in posterior dislocation of knee joint.

Posterior or superficial

- Proximally, semimembranosus muscle.
- Distally, gastrocnemius and plantaris.
- At intermediate level: popliteal artery is separated from skin and fasciae by fat and crossed by tibial nerve and popliteal vein from medial to lateral side (popliteal vein being sandwiched between popliteal artery and tibial nerve).

Relation of Popliteal Artery to Popliteal Lymph Nodes

One popliteal lymph node lies between the popliteal artery and the capsule of the knee joint and a few lymph nodes surround the popliteal vessels.

 STUDENT INTEREST

Remember that popliteal artery is a very close relation of the popliteal surface of femur and back of the knee joint. In the middle part of the popliteal fossa, it is crossed by tibial nerve and popliteal vein from medial to lateral side. It terminates at the distal margin of popliteus muscle into anterior tibial and posterior tibial arteries.

Branches (Fig. 29.3)

- Superior muscular branches supply the muscles in the thigh (hamstrings).
- Sural arteries supply the soleus, gastrocnemius and plantaris muscles.
- Lateral and medial superior genicular arteries, lateral and medial inferior genicular arteries and middle genicular artery supply the knee joint.

CLINICAL CORRELATION

- The popliteal pulse is the most difficult to feel among the peripheral pulses. The best position of the knee joint for this purpose is 120° flexion. The clinician puts fingertips of both hands in the popliteal fossa (to feel the artery in the lower part of fossa where it is resting on popliteus) and the thumbs on patient's patella (Figs 29.5A and B).
- The popliteal artery is used for measuring blood pressure in lower limb; for example, in patients suffering from coarctation of aorta. The BP cuff is tied around the patient's thigh and Korotkoff sounds are heard by keeping the diaphragm of the stethoscope on the popliteal fossa.

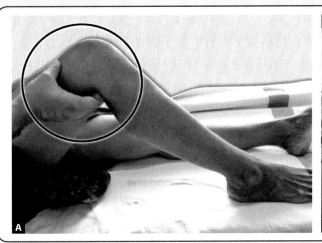 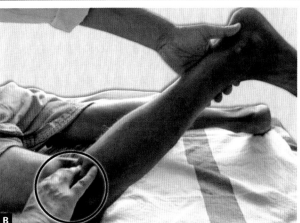

Figs 29.5A and B: Methods of palpation of popliteal pulse. **A.** Supine position of the patient; **B.** Prone position of the patient

Genicular Anastomosis

The arterial anastomosis around the knee joint is called the genicular anastomosis. It maintains adequate blood flow during flexion of knee joint when the popliteal artery is compressed. The following branches of popliteal, anterior and posterior tibial, femoral and profunda femoris arteries take part in the anastomosis.

- The superior medial genicular artery anastomoses with inferior medial genicular artery and with descending genicular branch of femoral artery, and
- The inferior medial genicular artery anastomoses with superior medial genicular and with saphenous branch of descending genicular artery.
- The superior lateral genicular artery anastomoses with inferior lateral genicular artery and with descending branch of lateral circumflex femoral artery.
- The inferior lateral genicular artery passes deep to the fibular collateral ligament to anastomose with superior lateral genicular artery, anterior and posterior tibial recurrent branches of anterior tibial artery and circumflex fibular branch of posterior tibial artery.

Popliteal Vein

Formation

The popliteal vein begins at the distal margin of the popliteus muscle by the union of venae comitantes accompanying the anterior and posterior tibial arteries.

Relations

The popliteal vein has triple relation to the popliteal artery. The vein lies medially in the lower part, it crosses superficially (posteriorly) in the middle part (between the two heads of gastrocnemius) and lies laterally at the upper part.

Termination

The popliteal vein continues as the femoral vein at the adductor hiatus.

Tributaries

- Small saphenous vein
- Veins accompanying the branches of the popliteal artery.

The swellings in the popliteal fossa originate not only from structures in the fossa but also from structures inside the knee joint (as the knee joint is a very close anterior relation of popliteal fossa). This is the reason why knee joint is examined in a case of popliteal swelling and popliteal fossa is examined in the case of the joint disorder.

- The popliteal aneurysm due to dilatation of popliteal artery presents as a pulsatile midline swelling in the popliteal fossa. This may cause edema of leg due to compression of popliteal vein. The stasis of blood in the aneurysm may favor formation of thrombosis and emboli, which may enter the distal arteries causing pain and ulceration and gangrene in the toes. The operative treatment of popliteal aneurysm consists of exposing and clamping the popliteal artery. Another method of treatment is to use saphenous vein graft to replace the dilated part of the popliteal artery. Yet another time-honored method pioneered by John Hunter is to ligate the femoral artery in the subsartorial canal. This method is based on the anatomical fact that arteries taking part in genicular anastomosis enlarge to provide collateral arterial supply to the leg (when femoral artery is ligated).
- Popliteal abscess is a painful swelling that presents as a red swelling in the popliteal fossa. It usually arises from the inflammation of popliteal lymph nodes.
- Varicosity of the terminal part of the small saphenous vein may present as swelling.
- A cystic swelling in the popliteal fossa is usually due to inflammation of the bursae around the knee joint or due to protrusion of the synovial membrane through the fibrous capsule of knee joint. Examples of cystic swelling are, Baker's cyst and semimembranosus bursitis (refer to semimembranosus bursa of knee joint).

Tibial Nerve in Popliteal Fossa

Root Value-ventral divisions of ventral rami of L4, L5, S1, S2, S3.

The tibial nerve is the larger terminal branch of the sciatic nerve. It enters the popliteal fossa through the upper angle. It bears triple relation to the popliteal vessels. In the upper part it lies lateral to the vessels. In the middle of the fossa it crosses the vessels superficially (posteriorly) and in the distal part it lies medial to the vessels.

Termination

At the distal margin of popliteus muscle it continues in the posterior compartment of leg as the tibial nerve in company with posterior tibial vessels.

Genicular, Cutaneous and Muscular Branches (Fig. 29.6)

- Three genicular nerves for the supply of knee joint are:
    1. Superior medial genicular nerve
    2. Middle genicular nerve
    3. Inferior medial genicular nerve

Note: The middle genicular nerve pierces the oblique popliteal ligament (middle part of the floor of the fossa) to enter the knee joint.

- The only cutaneous branch is the sural nerve. It descends between the heads of gastrocnemius and after leaving the fossa pierces the deep fascia of leg to become superficial. It supplies the posterior part of leg and lateral border of foot including the lateral margin of little toe. Since it is easily accessible it is favored for nerve grafting.
- The muscular branches (five in number) arise in the distal part of fossa.
- Branches that arise from the lateral side of tibial nerve supply following muscles:
    1. Lateral head of gastrocnemius
    2. Plantaris
    3. Soleus
    4. Popliteus
- A branch arising from the medial side supplies:
    5. Medial head of gastrocnemius

Note: Nerve to popliteus has peculiar course. It descends on the posterior surface of the popliteus muscle and winds round its distal margin to supply the popliteus from its anterior or deep aspect. It supplies not just popliteus muscle but also tibialis posterior muscle, all three tibiofibular joints and tibia.

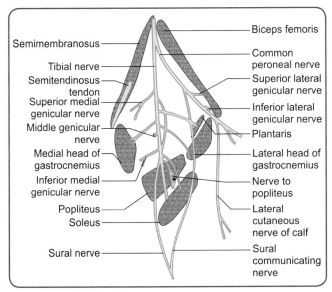

Fig. 29.6: Distribution of tibial and common peroneal nerves in popliteal fossa

Surface Marking

It is represented by a vertical line starting from the upper angle of popliteal fossa to a point in the midline at the level of tibial tuberosity.

CLINICAL CORRELATION

Effects of Injury to Tibial Nerve in Popliteal Fossa

The tibial nerve is rarely injured in popliteal fossa because of its relatively protected position in the fossa. However, if injured, all the muscles of calf and intrinsic muscles of foot are paralyzed. This results in talipes calcaneovalgus deformity of foot (foot is everted and dorsiflexed). The patient walks on the heel. The sensory loss mainly affects the sole including plantar aspects of toes and nail beds.

Common Peroneal Nerve

Root Value-dorsal divisions of ventral rami of L4, L5, S1, S2.

The common peroneal nerve is the smaller terminal branch of the sciatic nerve. It enters the popliteal fossa through the upper angle and lies medial to the biceps femoris tendon. It follows this tendon to the back of the head of the fibula. It then curves forward lying in close contact with the lateral side of the neck of fibula, where it divides in to its terminal branches deep to the peroneus longus muscle.

Palpation of Common Peroneal Nerve

It is palpated by rolling it against the neck of fibula.

Branches in Popliteal Fossa (Fig. 29.6)

The common peroneal nerve has no muscular branches but gives two articular and two cutaneous branches in the popliteal fossa.

- Two genicular branches are:
    1. Superior lateral genicular nerve
    2. Inferior lateral genicular nerve
- Two cutaneous branches are:
    1. Lateral cutaneous nerve of leg
    2. Sural (peroneal) communicating nerve

Branches at the Neck of Fibula

- Recurrent genicular nerve arises just before its termination (Fig. 30.2). It passes through the tibialis anterior muscle along with anterior tibial recurrent artery, supplies a twig to the muscle and reaches the knee joint.
- The terminal branches of common peroneal nerve are the superficial peroneal nerve and deep peroneal

nerve. The superficial peroneal nerve enters the peroneal compartment of leg while the deep peroneal nerve enters the anterior compartment of leg.

Surface Marking

The common peroneal nerve is indicated on the surface by a line starting from the upper angle of the popliteal fossa along the tendon of biceps femoris to the back of the head of fibula.

 CLINICAL CORRELATION

Effects of Injury to Common Peroneal Nerve

- The common peroneal nerve is superficial hence it is unprotected compared to the tibial nerve. It is a commonly injured nerve in the lower limb. It may be injured in fracture of the neck of fibula or due to direct pressure of a tightly applied plaster cast. It is affected in Hensen's disease and becomes tender and thickened.
- Injury to common peroneal nerve leads to paralysis of dorsiflexors of the ankle joint and evertors of foot supplied through its deep peroneal and superficial peroneal branches respectively. The paralysis of the above muscles results in foot drop deformity (inverted and plantarflexed foot). The patient walks on the toes.
- There is sensory loss on the dorsum of foot and toes excluding the medial and lateral margins of the foot and the lateral side of little toe.

Popliteal Lymph Nodes

The popliteal nodes belong to the deep group of lymph nodes. They are usually five to six in number. They are embedded in the fat of popliteal fossa.

- One lymph node is present at the sapheno-popliteal junction. This node receives superficial lymph vessels draining the lateral side of the foot including the little toe, lateral side of heel and lateral side of the back of leg.

Note: This is one example where deep lymph nodes receive superficial lymph vessels.

- One lymph node is present between the popliteal artery and the capsule of knee joint. It receives lymph from the joint.
- The remaining nodes are grouped around the popliteal vessels. They receive lymph vessels draining all the deep structures below the knee.

The efferent vessels from the popliteal nodes travel with the popliteal vessels and so pass through the adductor hiatus. Then they accompany the femoral vessels to reach the deep inguinal nodes.

 CLINICAL CORRELATION

Palpation of Popliteal Lymph Nodes

The popliteal lymph nodes are enlarged in injury to deeper tissues of the foot. Palpation of popliteal lymph nodes is as follows. The deep fascia of the popliteal fossa can be relaxed by passively flexing the knee. The examiner holds the knee with hands and explores the fossa for enlarged lymph nodes with the fingers of both hands.

KNEE JOINT

The knee joint is the largest and the most complicated synovial joint in the body. It is classified as a modified hinge joint with a mobile transverse axis. In addition to flexion and extension it allows a small degree of rotation. The knee joint is composed of three articulations, right and left condylar joints between the tibial and femoral condyles and a saddle joint between the patella and the patellar surface of the femur. The knee joint is a major weight-bearing joint. Its stability depends on its ligaments and quadriceps mechanism (extensor apparatus).

Articular Surfaces

There are three articular surfaces covered with articular cartilage. They are not congruent with each other.

1. Proximal articular surfaces on the lower end of femur
2. Distal articular surfaces on the upper end of tibia
3. Patellar articular surfaces

Proximal or Femoral Articular Surfaces

The articular surface covers the posterior, inferior and anterior surfaces of the medial and lateral condyles of femur. The articular surfaces of the two condyles are continuous with each other anteriorly but are separated by intercondylar notch posteriorly. The proximal articular surface is divisible into three parts.

1. *Patellar articular surface* or trochlear surface is present on the anterior aspect. It is subdivided into larger lateral and smaller medial areas by a vertical groove. The larger lateral articular surface is elevated (compared to the medial). A small semilunar area of the articular surface on the medial condyle adjoining the anterior margin of intercondylar fossa comes in contact with the medial articular facet of patella in full flexion.
2. *Tibial articular surface* on the medial femoral condyle is longer in antero-posterior axis and is obliquely set compared to the articular surface on the lateral femoral condyle.

3. ***Tibial articular surface*** on the lateral femoral condyle is straight, less curved and smaller by about two cm than the corresponding surface on the medial condyle.

Distal or Tibial Articular Surfaces (Figs 29.7A and B)

The distal articular surfaces are present on the upper surfaces of the condyles of tibia as the lateral and medial condylar surfaces separated by a rough non-articular area. They are slightly concave centrally but flat peripherally, where they come in contact with the corresponding menisci.

- Articular surface on medial tibial condyle is oval and its anteroposterior diameter is greater than the transverse diameter
- Articular surface on lateral tibial condyle is circular and its posterior part extends on the posterior aspect of lateral condyle, where the tendon of popliteus glides.

Patellar Articular Surface

The posterior surface of patella bears a large articular area, which is divided by a vertical groove in to larger lateral and smaller medial areas. Near the medial margin of the patella there is a narrow semilunar strip for contact with medial condyle of femur in full flexion. The rest of the lateral and medial areas are divided into three facets on each side. These facets come in contact with femur one by one as the knee passes from the position of full extension to that of flexion.

Fibrous Capsule

The unique feature of the capsule of the knee joint is that it is deficient in the anterior part of the joint. The strong quadriceps femoris tendon, patella and ligamentum patellae take the place of the deficient capsule.

Upper Attachment of Capsule to Femur (Figs 29.7A and B)

The capsule is attached about half to one cm beyond the articular margins of femoral condyles with the exception that it is deficient anteriorly (where it is pierced by suprapatellar bursa), is attached to the intercondylar line posteriorly and encloses the tendinous origin of popliteus laterally.

Lower Attachment of Capsule to Tibia

The capsule is attached to tibia about half to one cm beyond the articular margins of tibial condyles except anteriorly where it descends from the margins of condyles

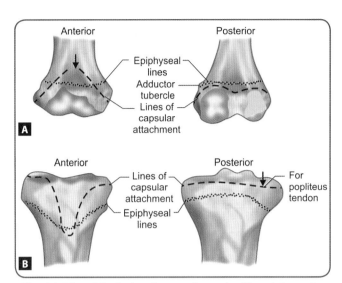

Figs 29.7A and B: A. Attachment of capsule of knee joint to the lower end of femur; **B.** Attachment of capsule of knee joint to tibia (Arrows indicate the gaps in the capsule)

along tibial tuberosity where the capsule is deficient due to ligamentum patellae and posteriorly it presents a gap behind the lateral condyle for the exit of the tendon of popliteus.

Ligaments

There are five important ligaments, ligamentum patellae, oblique popliteal ligament, arcuate popliteal ligament, tibial collateral ligament and fibular collateral ligament.

Ligamentum Patellae or Patellar Ligament

The ligamentum patellae is the continuation of the central part of the tendon of quadriceps femoris. It is attached to the lateral and medial patellar retinacula on either side.

It extends from the apex of the patella to the upper margin of tibial tuberosity. Posteriorly, its upper part is related to a large infrapatellar pad of fat (Fig. 29.23) and lower part to the deep infrapatellar bursa (Fig. 29.21). Anteriorly, the lower part is related to subcutaneous infrapatellar bursa (Fig. 29.21).

> **⌀ CLINICAL CORRELATION**
>
> Ligamentum patellae is used for eliciting patellar reflex or knee jerk by tapping it with a knee hammer.

Tibial Collateral Ligament (TCL) (Fig. 29.8)

This ligament is the thickening of the medial part of the capsule. It forms a very strong flat band, about eight to nine cm long.

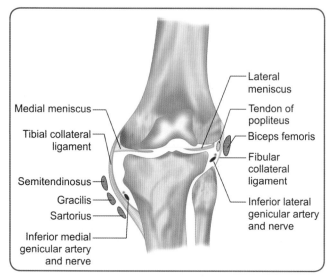

Fig. 29.8: Attachments and relations of tibial and fibular collateral ligaments

Attachments

It is attached superiorly to the medial epicondyle of femur. Inferiorly, it is divided into a long superficial part and a short deep part.

The superficial part is attached to the medial surface of tibia between the medial margin of tibia and the insertions of sartorius, gracilis and semitendinosus.

The deep layer is fused with the capsule and is attached to the articular margin of media condyle of tibia (Fig. 29.9).

Relations

Superficial part is related medially to inferior genicular nerve and vessels. Its lower end is covered by tendons of sartorius, gracilis and semitendinosus.

Deep part merges with fibrous capsule and with the peripheral margin of medial meniscus (this is a very important relation).

Morphology

TCL represents the lower part of the ischial component of adductor magnus muscle.

Fibular Collateral Ligament (FCL)

The fibular collateral ligament is rounded, cord like and short.

Attachments (Fig. 29.10)

The fibular collateral ligament extends from the lateral epicondyle of femur to the lateral surface of the head of fibula.

Relations

Superficially the tendon of biceps femoris (which is split by the ligament) overlaps the ligament.

Its deep relations are the tendon of popliteus (which separates it from the lateral meniscus) and the inferior lateral genicular nerve and vessels (Fig. 29.10).

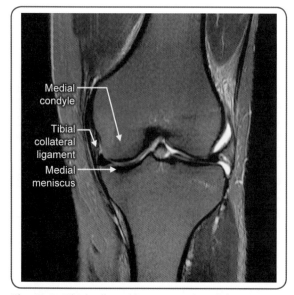

Fig. 29.9: Tibial collateral ligament and medial meniscus in MRI of knee joint

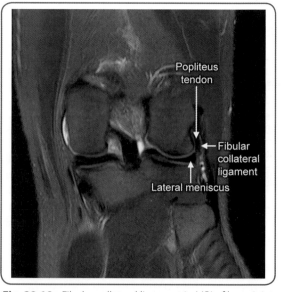

Fig. 29.10: Fibular collateral ligament in MRI of knee joint

Morphology

The fibular collateral ligament represents the upper part of peroneus longus muscle.

 CLINICAL CORRELATION

Testing Integrity of Collateral Ligaments

The patient is seated on a high stool with legs hanging down but not touching the ground. The lower end of femur is grasped firmly with one hand. The tibia is moved in lateral and medial direction. Excessive lateral movement of tibia suggests rupture of tibial collateral ligament while excessive medial movement of tibia suggests rupture of fibular collateral ligament.

Oblique Popliteal Ligament

The oblique popliteal ligament is a broad band, which strengthens the capsule posteriorly. It is an expansion from the tendon of insertion of semimembranosus (Fig. 27.9). It extends from the posterior aspect of the medial condyle of tibia to the lateral part of intercondylar line and lateral condyle of femur.

The popliteal artery is in close contact with this ligament. It is pierced by three structures, middle genicular artery, middle genicular nerve and genicular branch of the posterior division of obturator nerve.

Arcuate Popliteal Ligament

This is Y-shaped ligament. Its stem is attached to the styloid process of head of fibula. Its posterior limb is attached to posterior end of the intercondylar area of tibia and the anterior limb attaches to the lateral condyle of femur passing deep to the fibular collateral ligament.

Intra-articular Structures (Figs 29.11 and 29.12)

The following structures are present inside the knee joint.
- Cruciate ligaments
- Semilunar cartilages or menisci
- Ligaments of Wrisberg and Humphrey
- Infrapatellar pad of fat
- Transverse ligament and coronary ligaments
- Synovial membrane
- Tendon of popliteus.

Cruciate Ligaments

The anterior and posterior cruciate ligaments cross each other like a letter X. They are named anterior and posterior depending on their attachment to the tibia. They provide strong connection between tibia and femur. Since the ligaments invaginate the synovial membrane from behind their anterior aspect only are covered with synovial membrane hence they are described as intracapsular but extrasynovial.

Anterior cruciate ligament (ACL)

Its tibial end is attached to the anterior part of intercondylar area of tibia and the femoral end is attached to the posterior part of the medial surface of lateral condyle in the intercondylar notch (Fig. 29.11). ACL runs from its tibial superiorly, posteriorly and laterally to reach its femoral end. It is supplied by middle genicular artery (Fig. 29.13).

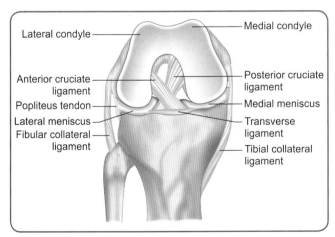

Fig. 29.11: Intra-articular structures of knee joint as seen from anterior aspect of flexed knee joint

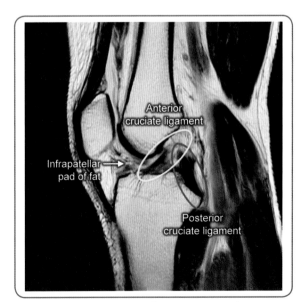

Fig. 29.12: MRI appearance of some intra-articular structures [yellow circle shows ACL (anterior cruciate ligament) and red circle shows PCL (posterior cruciate ligament)]

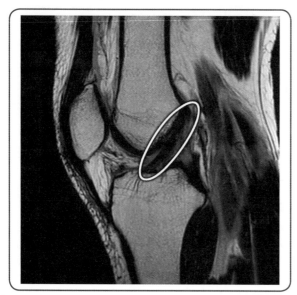

Fig. 29.13: MRI appearance of anterior cruciate ligament in sagittal plane (circle is showing the attachment of anterior cruciate ligament)

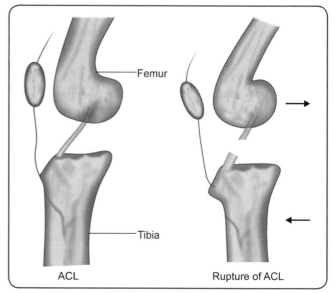

Fig. 29.14: Positive anterior drawer sign in rupture of anterior cruciate ligament (ACL)

Function

It prevents posterior dislocation of femur on tibia and anterior dislocation of tibia on femur. It becomes taut in extension along with all the other ligaments.

> 🔟 **CLINICAL CORRELATION**
>
> **Drawer Test for Integrity of ACL (Fig. 29.14)**
>
> The patient lies in the supine position with the hip and knee joints flexed. With ankle joint (of the same side) firmly held in hand, the tibia is pulled forward. If there is excessive forward movement of tibia, it is anterior drawer sign, which is indicative of injury to ACL.
>
> **Rupture of ACL**
>
> Isolated rupture of anterior cruciate ligament may occur if the knee is forcibly hyperextended. The patient presents with acute pain and swelling of the knee joint. The anterior drawer sign is positive. Hemarthrosis (blood inside the joint) of knee joint is often present.

Posterior cruciate ligament (PCL)

Its tibial end is attached to the posterior part of the intercondylar area of tibia and the femoral end is attached to the anterior part of the lateral surface of the medial condyle in the intercondylar notch (Fig. 29.11). PCL is directed from its tibial end superiorly, anteriorly and medially to reach femoral end. It is supplied by middle genicular artery (Fig. 29.15).

Function

It prevents anterior dislocation of femur on tibia and posterior dislocation of tibia on femur. It becomes taut during flexion along with anterior cruciate ligament.

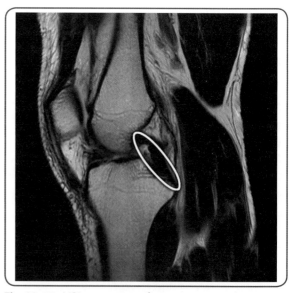

Fig. 29.15: MRI appearance of posterior cruciate ligament in sagittal plane

Drawer Test for Integrity of PCL (Fig. 29.16)

The patient lies in supine position with the knee and hip kept flexed. With ankle joint (of same side) firmly held by hand the examiner pushes the tibia posteriorly. If the tibia moves excessively in posterior direction it is called posterior drawer sign. This sign is indicative of injury to posterior cruciate ligament.

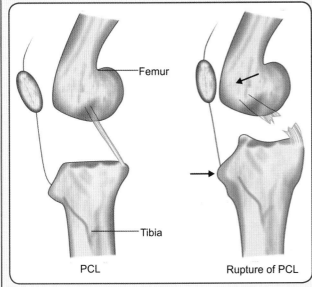

Fig. 29.16: Positive posterior drawer sign in rupture of posterior cruciate ligament

Menisci or Semilunar Cartilages (Fig. 29.17)

The lateral and medial menisci are plates of fibrocartilage placed on the articular surface of respective tibial condyle. The menisci divide the joint cavity in to two chambers in each half, meniscofemoral above and meniscotibial below.

The menisci are wedge- shaped plates with thick peripheral and thin inner margins. The peripheral margin is attached to the fibrous capsule and to tibial condyles by the coronary ligaments. The menisci deepen the shallow articular surfaces of tibial condyles.

Parts of menisci

Each meniscus presents:
- Anterior and posterior horns or ends (attached to tibia)
- Superior concave surface and inferior surfaces.

The transverse ligament connects the anterior horns of the two menisci to each other.

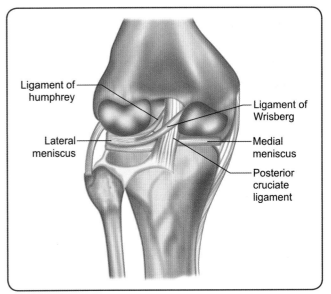

Fig. 29.17: Showing the position of lateral and medial menisci (also seen are the ligaments arising from posterior horn of lateral meniscus embracing posterior cruciate ligament)

Medial meniscus

It is a C-shaped cartilage. The two ends of the C represent the two horns of the meniscus, which are attached to the intercondylar area of tibia. Its periphery is fused with the fibrous capsule in the region of tibial collateral ligament. This close proximity of the medial meniscus and the tibial collateral ligament makes the medial meniscus less mobile and more prone to tears.

Lateral meniscus

It is circular in shape. The points of attachments of the anterior and posterior horns of the lateral meniscus to the intercondylar area are very close to each other (within the points of attachments of the two horns of medial meniscus). The intracapsular tendon of popliteus intervenes between the lateral meniscus and the fibrous capsule. The peripheral attachment of the lateral meniscus to the capsule is lax hence the lateral meniscus is more mobile compared to medial. The popliteus protects the lateral meniscus from injuries (on account of the fact that a few fibers of popliteus attached to its posterior horn keep meniscus out of harm's way).

Meniscofemoral ligaments of Humphrey and Wrisberg

The posterior horn of lateral meniscus sends two slips, one in front and one behind the posterior cruciate ligament to gain attachment to the medial condyle of femur. These

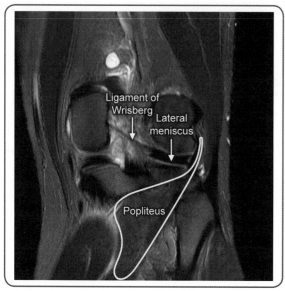

Fig. 29.18: MRI of knee joint showing some intra-articular structures including the ligament of Wrisberg (posterior meniscofemoral ligament)

slips are referred to as anterior meniscofemoral ligament of Humphrey and posterior meniscofemoral ligament of Wrisberg (Fig. 29.18).

Nutrition of menisci

- The peripheral thick part is vascular and supplied by the capsular blood vessels
- The inner thin part is avascular and nourished by synovial fluid.

Functions of menisci

- The menisci make the tibial articular surface more concave and congruent with the femoral condylar surface
- They act as shock absorber
- They help in evenly spreading the synovial fluid on the articular surfaces
- The menisci divide the joint cavity in to two chambers for independent movements. The flexion and extension takes place in meniscofemoral compartment while the rotation occurs in the meniscotibial compartment.

CLINICAL CORRELATION

- The internal derangement of the knee joint causes serious interference with the joint function. The collateral ligaments, cruciate ligaments and the menisci are the structures that are injured. The injury to any of these structures is associated with traumatic synovitis. A combination of injury to the tibial collateral ligament, medial meniscus and anterior cruciate ligament is called 'unhappy triad' of knee joint (Fig. 29.19)

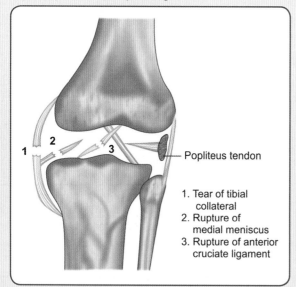

1. Tear of tibial collateral
2. Rupture of medial meniscus
3. Rupture of anterior cruciate ligament

Fig. 29.19: Unhappy triad of knee joint

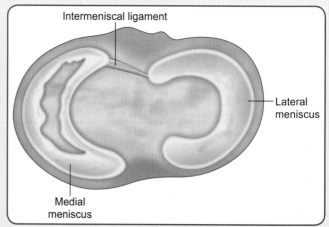

Fig. 29.20: Bucket-handle tear of medial meniscus of right knee joint

- The medial meniscus injuries are more common than that of lateral meniscus because it is less mobile. A sudden blow on the lateral side of a flexed weight-bearing knee can cause rupture of the tibial collateral ligament with a concomitant tear in the medial meniscus. The bucket handle rupture (Fig. 29.20) of the medial meniscus is common in football players. On rupture of the meniscus the patient feels sudden pain in the knee. The knee gets locked in the flexed position and swollen due to synovitis. The chances of the knee getting struck on the medial side are far less in sports hence the injury to fibular collateral ligament is much less. The protective factors of the lateral meniscus are its mobility and the role of popliteus.

Synovial Membrane (Fig. 29.21)

The knee joint has the most extensive synovial membrane.

The synovial membrane lines the inner surface of the capsule and covers the nonarticular parts of tibial and femoral condyles inside the joint and is attached to the margins of patella.

- *Above the patella*, the synovial membrane extends upward deep to the tendon of quadriceps femoris for a short distance in the lower thigh as suprapatellar bursa. The articularis genu attached to this bursa holds it in position. From the margins of patella the synovial membrane covers the inner aspects of lateral and medial patellar retinacula. Below the patella it extends deep to ligamentum patellae from which it is separated by infrapatellar pad of fat.
- *Anteriorly*, the synovial membrane extends from the deep surface of the ligamentum patellae in the posterior direction This layer of synovial membrane forms the right and left alar folds on either side and an infrapatellar fold in the midline. The infrapatellar fold is attached to the most anterior point of the intercondylar notch of the femur.
- *Posteriorly*, the synovial membrane lines the posterior part of fibrous capsule and the posterior edges of the menisci. It extends anteriorly as a fold inside the intercondylar notch to cover the anterior and lateral aspects of both cruciate ligaments and anterior aspect of ACL. This fold is attached to the margins of intercondylar area of tibia and forms a partial partition between the two halves of the joint.

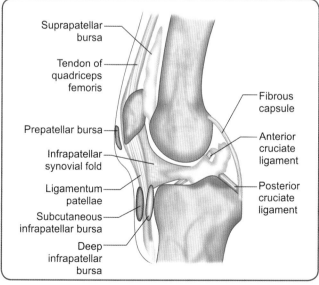

Fig. 29.21: Bucket-handle tear of medial meniscus of right knee joint

To understand synovial membrane, intra-articular ligaments and menisci and relations of knee joint it is essential to practice diagram of cross section of the knee joint.

Bursae in Relation to Knee Joint

Several bursae are found around the knee joint, of which four are in communication with the joint cavity. The bursae are divided into three groups according to their location.

1. *Anterior Group* (Fig. 29.22A and B)
- Subcutaneous prepatellar bursa is present between the lower part of patella and the skin.
- Subcutaneous infrapatellar bursa occupies the space between the ligamentum patellae and the skin.
- Deep infrapatellar bursa lies between the ligamentum patellae and tibial tuberosity.
- Suprapatellar bursa is the extension of joint cavity superiorly behind the tendon of quadriceps femoris. Effusion in the knee joint distends this bursa, which is described as water on the knee. On physical examination the patella appears to float over the femur.

2. *Lateral Group*
- Bursa between the lateral head of gastrocnemius and the joint capsule.
- Bursa between the tendon of biceps femoris and fibular collateral ligament.
- Bursa between the tendon of popliteus and the fibular collateral ligament.
- Popliteus bursa between the lateral condyle of tibia and the tendon of popliteus communicates with the joint cavity.

3. *Medial Group*
- A bursa between the medial head of gastrocnemius and the fibrous capsule is known as Brodie's bursa. It communicates with the joint cavity.
- A bursa between the tibial collateral ligament and the tendons of sartorius, gracilis and semitendinosus is called bursa anserine. The term pes anserinus is derived from the foot of the goose appearance of insertion of these three tendons on the medial surface of tibia. This bursa is in communication with joint cavity.
- Bursa between the superficial and deep parts of tibial collateral ligament.
- Bursa between the insertion of semimembranosus and medial condyle of tibia may communicate with the knee joint.

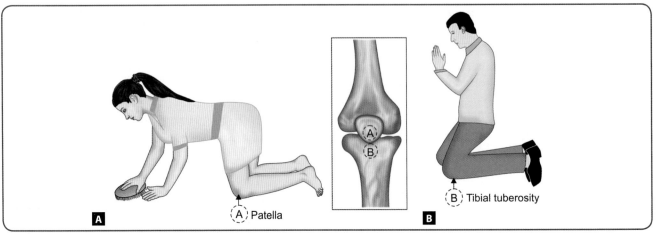

Figs 29.22A and B: Anatomical basis of: **A.** Housemaid's knee (prepatellar bursitis); **B.** Clergyman's knee (inflammation of subcutaneous infrapatellar bursa) due to frequent adoption of specific body posturis

- Prepatellar bursitis or housemaid's knee (Fig. 29.22A) results due to inflammation of subcutaneous prepatellar bursa
- Clergyman's knee (Fig. 29.22B) results due to inflammation of subcutaneous infrapatellar bursa
- Semimembranosus bursitis is a chronic inflammation of the bursa related to insertion of semimembranosus muscle. It may present as a cystic swelling in the medial part of the popliteal fossa. Baker's cyst is a fluctuant swelling in the popliteal fossa either due to inflammation of the same bursa or due to projection of synovial membrane from a diseased joint.

Relations of Knee Joint (Fig. 29.23)

- **Anteriorly:** Tendon of quadriceps femoris, patella and ligamentum patellae.
- **Anteromedially:** Medial patellar retinaculum.
- **Anterolaterally:** Lateral patellar retinaculum.
- **Posteromedially:** Tendons of semimembranosus, sartorius, semitendinosus and gracilis.
- **Posterolaterally:** Tendon of biceps femoris and common peroneal nerve above the joint and tendon of popliteus inside the joint.
- **Posteriorly:** Popliteal artery (Fig. 29.24), popliteal vein and tibial nerve.

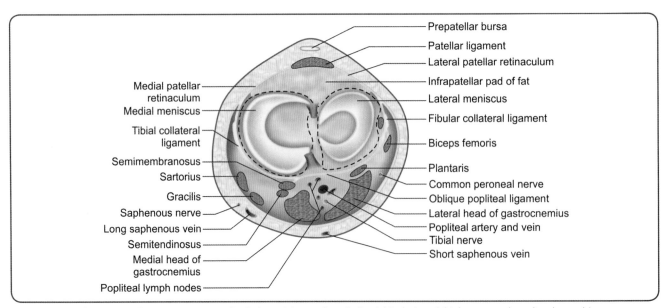

Fig. 29.23: Transverse section of right knee joint to show its "at risk" relations (tibial nerve and popliteal vessels)

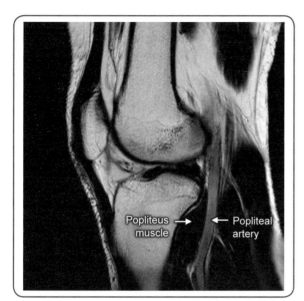

Fig. 29.24: MRI of knee joint showing close relation of popliteal artery to the back of knee joint

Nerve Supply

- Femoral nerve through its branches to vasti
- Posterior division of the obturator nerve via descending genicular branch
- Tibial and common peroneal nerves via genicular branches in popliteal fossa
- Common peroneal nerve via recurrent genicular branch outside the fossa

Arterial Supply

Knee joint is richly supplied through an arterial anastomosis in which following arteries take part:

- Four genicular branches of popliteal artery in popliteal fossa
- Descending branch of lateral circumflex femoral artery and descending genicular branch of femoral artery
- Circumflex fibular branch of posterior tibial artery and anterior and posterior tibial recurrent branches from the anterior tibial artery.

Note: Middle genicular branch of popliteal artery does not take part in the anastomosis since it enters the knee joint by piercing the oblique popliteal ligament

Movements of Knee Joint

The knee joint permits flexion, extension, lateral rotation and medial rotation.

- The flexion-extension occurs on a mobile transverse axis, which shifts forward during extension and backward during flexion. In this movement the femoral condyles move on the tibia and the menisci in the meniscofemoral compartment
- The rotation occurs around a vertical axis in the meniscotibial compartment. There are two types of rotation in the knee joint. The conjunct rotation (about 20-30°) is part of locking-unlocking mechanism. The adjunct rotation (about 50-70°) occurs in the semiflexed knee. Active muscle contraction is necessary for adjunct rotation.

Extension

During the last 20 to 30° of extension of knee there is conjunct or automatic medial rotation of femur on the tibia (when the foot is on the ground) or lateral rotation of tibia on the femur (if the foot is off the ground). This 20 to 30° of rotation at the final stage of extension is part and parcel of the movement of extension. It is described as a screw home movement or locking. In the locked position the knee joint is maximally congruent and the ligaments are taut. A person is able to stand for hours together without strain to the quadriceps femoris in locked position.

The muscles responsible for extension are quadriceps femoris and tensor fasciae latae.

Flexion

From the fully extended knee, the flexion begins by the unlocking movement. Unlocking consists of lateral rotation of femur or medial rotation of tibia (depending on whether the foot is on or off the ground). This rotation at the beginning of flexion is conjunct but requires contraction of popliteus muscle (key of knee joint).

After the joint id unlocked further flexion is carried out by hamstring muscles assisted by gracilis, sartorius and popliteus. In a stationary foot gastrocnemius is active.

Rotation in Semiflexed Knee

In the semiflexed knee about 50 to 700 of adjunct rotation is possible with the help of active contraction of muscles.

- ***Medial rotation:*** By popliteus, semitendinosus and semimembranosus
- ***Lateral rotation:*** By biceps femoris

 STUDENT INTEREST

Locking is defined as medial rotation of femur on the tibia during last stage of extension of knee joint, when the foot is on the ground. Unlocking is defined as lateral rotation of femur on tibia at the beginning of flexion of locked knee, when the foot is on the ground. Unlocking needs active contraction of popliteus hence popliteus is called 'key of knee joint'.

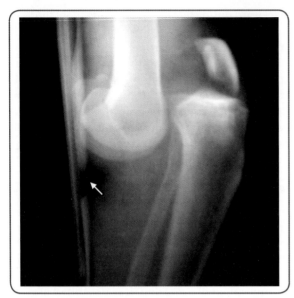

Fig. 29.25: Radiograph showing posterior dislocation of knee joint and lower end of femur compressing the popliteal artery (arrow showing)

Radiological Anatomy

- The tibial and femoral condyles are visualized with the shadow of patella overlying the femur. The intercondylar tubercles of tibia are seen projecting in the joint space. The shadow of the infrapatellar fat pad is visible inside the joint.
- Fabella (a sesamoid bone in lateral head of gastrocnemius at its origin) and patella are best visible in the lateral view.
- MRI and ultrasound are very useful to study intra-articular structures (Fig. 29.25).

CLINICAL CORRELATION

- Knee joint replacement is performed when joint function is totally lost due to degenerative disease
- Runner's knee or patellofemoral pain syndrome manifests as pain near the patella after sitting for a long stretch with knees flexed
- In posterior dislocation of knee joint the popliteal artery is in danger of injury (Fig. 29.24).

30

Compartments of Leg and Retinacula Around Ankle

Chapter Contents

ANTERIOR COMPARTMENT OF LEG

The leg is that part of the lower limb between the knee and ankle. It is divided into three osteofascial compartments by bones of the leg (tibia and fibula) and the intermuscular septae (Fig. 30.1). The compartments are named anterior or extensor, lateral or peroneal and posterior or flexor.

Superficial Fascia

The surface landmarks, cutaneous nerves and superficial veins are dealt in chapter 25.

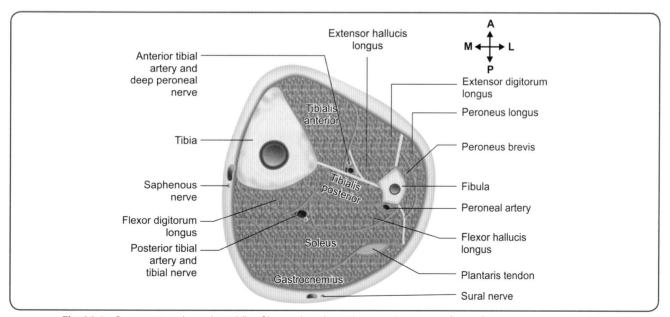

Fig. 30.1: Cross-section through middle of leg to show boundaries and contents of osteofascial compartments of leg

Deep Fascia of Leg

- The deep fascia of the leg is continuous above with the fascia lata. It is strengthened in the region of knee by expansions from the tendons of sartorius, gracilis and semitendinosus medially and biceps femoris laterally. The deep fascia is attached to the condyles of tibia, head of fibula, tibial tuberosity and patella. The patella is attached to the tibial condyles by the medial and lateral patellar retinacula, which are thickened bands of deep fascia, reinforced by tendons of vastus medialis and lateralis respectively.
- At the anterior and medial borders of tibia the deep fascia becomes continuous with the periosteum covering the subcutaneous medial surface of the tibia.
- Two intermuscular septa pass from the deep aspect of the deep fascia towards the fibula. The anterior intermuscular septum, which intervenes between the lateral and anterior compartments, is attached to the anterior border of fibula. The posterior intermuscular septum, which intervenes between the lateral and posterior compartments, is attached to the posterior border of fibula.
- At the ankle, the deep fascia is modified to form flexor, extensor and peroneal retinacula, which help in strapping down the tendons at the ankle.

Boundaries (Fig. 30.1)

- **Lateral boundary:** Anterior intermuscular septum.
- **Medial boundary:** Lateral surface of tibia.
- **Postreior boundary:** Interosseous membrane and the narrow medial surface of fibula.
- **Anterior boundary:** Deep fascia of leg.

Contents (Fig. 30.2)

- Four muscles of the anterior compartment are tibialis anterior, extensor hallucis longus, and extensor digitorum longus and peroneus tertius.
- Anterior tibial artery and accompanying veins (the main vessels).
- Deep peroneal nerve
- A perforating branch of peroneal artery (which enters the anterior compartment from the posterior compartment by piercing the interosseous membrane.

Tibialis Anterior (TA)

- **Origin:** From the lateral condyle of tibia, upper two thirds of its lateral surface and adjacent interosseous membrane.

- **Insertion:** Into medial surface of medial cuneiform and base of first metatarsal bone.
  The anterior tibial recurrent artery (a branch of anterior tibial artery) and recurrent genicular nerve (a branch of common peroneal nerve at its bifurcation) pass through the upper part of tibialis anterior.
- **Nerve supply:** By deep peroneal nerve and recurrent genicular nerve.
- **Actions**
  - Dorsiflexion of foot at the ankle joint.
  - Inversion of the foot at the midtarsal and subtalar joints.
  - Providing support to medial longitudinal arch of the foot.

Testing function

The subject is asked to dorsiflex the foot against resistance of examiner's hand placed across the dorsum of the foot.

Extensor Hallucis Longus (EHL)

- **Origin:** Middle two fourth of the medial surface of fibula and adjacent interosseous membrane.
- **Insertion:** Into the base of terminal phalanx of the great toe.
- **Nerve supply:** By deep peroneal nerve.
- **Actions**
  - Dorsiflexion of foot at the ankle.
  - Dorsiflexion of the great toe.
  - Support of medial longitudinal arch.

Testing function of EHL

The subject attempts to dorsiflex the great toe against resistance.

Extensor Digitorum Longus (EDL)

- **Origin:** Upper three fourth of the medial surface of the fibula, adjacent interosseous membrane and anterior intermuscular septum. The extensor digitorum longus divides in to four tendons on the dorsum of foot.
- **Insertion:** Tendons of second to fourth toes are joined by the tendons of extensor digitorum brevis. Each of the 4 tendons is inserted in to the base of middle phalanx and into the base of terminal phalanx through dorsal digital expansion.
- **Nerve supply:** By deep peroneal nerve.
- **Actions**
  - Dorsiflexion of foot
  - Extension of lateral four toes

Testing function

The subject is asked to dorsiflex the toes against resistance.

Peroneus Tertius

- *Origin:* From lower part of medial surface of fibula (in continuation with the extensor digitorum longus).
- *Insertion:* Into the dorsal surface of the base of fifth metatarsal bone.
- *Nerve supply:* By deep peroneal nerve.
- *Actions*
  - Dorsiflexion of foot.
  - Weak evertor of foot.

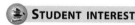 **STUDENT INTEREST**

Note that extensor hallucis longus, extensor digitorum longus and peroneus tertius take origin from fibula and tibialis anterior alone takes origin from tibia. Deep peroneal nerve supplies these 4 extensor muscles which are dorsiflexors of foot at ankle joint.

Anterior Tibial Artery (Fig. 30.2)

The anterior tibial artery is the smaller terminal branch of the popliteal artery in the back of the leg at the distal margin of the popliteus (in the back of leg).

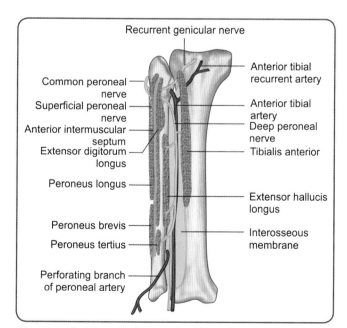

Fig. 30.2: Structures in the anterior compartment of leg (Peroneus longus and brevis are seen in the lateral compartment separated by anterior intermuscular septum from the anterior compartment)

Entry into anterior compartment

The anterior tibial artery enters the anterior compartment by passing through an opening in the upper part of the interosseous membrane.

Course in anterior compartment

It descends in contact with the anterior surface of the interosseous membrane and is flanked by venae comitantes. The artery is deeply placed in the upper two thirds of the leg but becomes superficial in the lower third.

Termination

The anterior tibial artery ends at a point midway between lateral and medial malleoli, where it continues as the dorsalis pedis artery of the foot.

Relations

- Posteriorly the proximal two-third of the artery rests directly on the interosseous membrane but its lower third is in contact with the lateral surface of tibia and front of ankle joint.
- The upper one third of the artery is flanked by tibialis anterior (medially) and extensor digitorum longus (laterally), middle one third is flanked by tibialis anterior and extensor hallucis longus and lower one third is flanked by tendon of extensor hallucis longus medially) and tendons extensor digitorum longus laterally.

Note: That the changed relation to EHL is due to crossing of EHL tendon in front of the anterior tibial artery at the junction of middle and lower third of the artery.

Changing relation to deep peroneal nerve

In the upper part, the nerve is laterally placed in relation to the artery as they descend on the anterior aspect of the interosseous membrane. Gradually the nerve comes to lie anterior to the artery but at the lower part it goes back once again to its lateral position.

Branches

- Anterior and posterior recurrent genicular branches take part in knee anastomosis.

Note: Origin of posterior tibial recurrent artery is in the back of leg and anterior tibial recurrent artery ascends through the tibialis anterior muscle.

- Muscular branches to muscles in anterior compartment.
- Anterior medial and anterior lateral malleolar arteries take part in medial and lateral malleolar network around ankle joint.

Anterior Tibial Pulse

The anterior tibial pulse is felt at the midpoint of the front of the ankle.

Deep Peroneal Nerve (Fig. 30.3)

The deep peroneal nerve is one of the terminal branches of the common peroneal nerve. It begins in the lateral compartment of leg at the lateral side of the neck of fibula under cover of upper fibers of peroneus longus muscle.

Entry into anterior compartment

The deep peroneal nerve enters the anterior compartment by piercing the anterior intermuscular septum, which intervenes between the lateral and anterior compartments.

Course in anterior compartment

- Initially, the deep peroneal nerve courses medially lying deep to the extensor digitorum longus. It joins the anterior tibial vessels from the lateral side and the neurovascular bundle thus formed travels down on the anterior surface of the interosseous membrane between the extensor digitorum longus and extensor hallucis longus on the lateral side and tibialis anterior on the medial side.

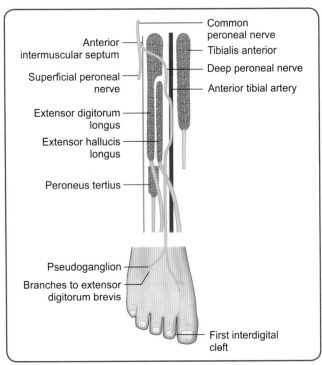

Fig. 30.3: Origin, course and termination of deep peroneal nerve

- In the lower part of the leg, the tendon of extensor hallucis longus crosses the neurovascular bundle from lateral to medial side.
- The deep peroneal nerve is called the nervus hesitans due to its changing relations to the anterior tibial artery. At first it is lateral to anterior tibial artery and then it gradually comes in front of the artery but at the lower level again goes back in lateral position (as if the nerve hesitates to cross the artery). For this reason the deep peroneal nerve is called nervous hesitans.

Branches in Anterior Compartment

- Muscular branches to the four muscles of the compartment.
- Articular branch to the ankle joint.

Course and Branches on Dorsum of Foot

On entering the dorsum of foot, the deep peroneal nerve terminates by dividing into lateral and medial branches (Fig. 30.4).

The medial terminal branch travels distally deep to deep fascia to reach the first interdigital cleft, where it becomes cutaneous. Before becoming cutaneous it supplies first dorsal interosseous muscle and metatarsophalangeal joint of big toe. After piercing the deep fascia it supplies cutaneous branches to adjacent sides of first and second toes.

The lateral terminal branch passes laterally deep to extensor digitorum brevis, where enlarges in to a pseudoganglion. The branches of the pseudoganglion supply the extensor digitorum brevis and tarsal and metatarsophalangeal joints of middle three toes.

Extensor Retinacula of Ankle (Fig. 30.4)

There are two thickened bands in front of the ankle called superior and inferior extensor retinacula. The function of these bands is to hold the extensor tendons strapped to the ankle joint. In the absence of the retinacula the tendons will jump forward during dorsiflexion.

Superior Extensor Retinaculum

Attachments

- *Laterally:* To the lower part of subcutaneous anterior surface of fibula.
- *Medially:* To the anterior margin of tibia above the medial malleolus.
- *Superficial relations* (from medial to lateral side).

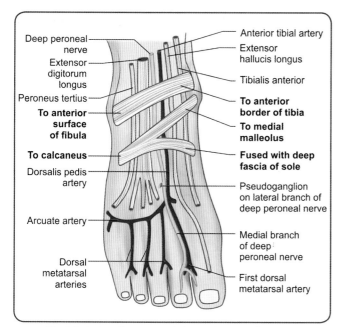

Fig. 30.4: Attachments and deep relations of extensor retinacula of foot

Saphenous nerve, great saphenous vein, medial and lateral terminal branches of the superficial peroneal nerve

- **Deep Relations** (from medial to lateral).
  Tibialis anterior, extensor hallucis longus, anterior tibial artery, deep peroneal nerve, extensor digitorum longus and peroneus tertius.

🏅 STUDENT INTEREST

Mnemonic
The Himalayas Are Never Dry Places

- **Synovial sheaths:** The extensor tendons as they pass deep to the superior extensor retinaculum acquire synovial sheaths. The function of the synovial sheath is to permit frictionless movements of the tendons. Inflammation of the tendon synovial sheath is called tenosynovitis.

Inferior Extensor Retinaculum

It is a Y-shaped retinaculum on the dorsum of foot as it has a stem and two bands (upper and lower). The stem of the Y points laterally and the two limbs medially.

Attachments

Laterally: The stem is attached to the upper surface of the anterior part of calcaneus.
Medially: Its upper band is attached to anterior border of tibia above the medial malleolus and the lower band

passes to the medial side of the foot to fuse with the deep fascia of the sole.

Note: As the extensor tendons pass deep to the extensor retinacula, they are surrounded by synovial sheaths (which permit frictionless movements of the tendons)

⌀ CLINICAL CORRELATION

- Injury to deep peroneal nerve produces motor and sensory effects as follows:
  - Paralysis of extensors (dorsiflexors) of ankle joint (muscles of anterior compartment) leads to a deformity called foot drop in which the ankle is held in plantarflexed position.
  - Sensory loss in the first interdigital cleft.
- Anterior compartment syndrome develops as a result of sudden strenuous exercise to muscles in anterior compartment. This causes swelling of the muscles within an unyielding space and symptoms due to pressure on anterior tibial artery and deep peroneal nerve. To relieve the compression, the deep fascia of the leg is surgically incised (fasciotomy) along the whole length of the compartment.

🏅 STUDENT INTEREST

- It is observed that anterior compartment syndrome (fresher's syndrome) occurs in freshers in the colleges and in new recruits in defense services and police forces, who are subjected to undergo rigorous exercises (to which they are not accustomed).
- If a medical student in the ward observes a physician pinching the skin between 1st toe and 2nd toe of right foot of the patient, with the knowledge of sensory innervation of dorsum, the student should instantly understand that the physician is testing the deep peroneal nerve of right side.

PERONEAL COMPARTMENT

The peroneal or the lateral compartment of the leg is the smallest compartment.

Boundaries (Fig. 30.1)

- **Anteriorly:** By anterior intermuscular septum.
- **Posteriorly:** By posterior intermuscular septum.
- **Medially:** By lateral surface of the fibula.
- **Laterally:** By deep fascia of the leg.

Contents

- Peroneus longus and brevis muscles.
- Termination of common peroneal nerve at the neck of fibula.

- Deep peroneal nerve in upper part of the compartment.
- Superficial peroneal nerve is the nerve of lateral compartment.
- Recurrent genicular branch of common peroneal nerve (Fig. 30.2).

The lateral compartment does not have its own artery.

Peroneus Longus (Fig. 30.5)

The peroneus longus muscle is superficial to the peroneus brevis.

- **Origin:** From the head of fibula and upper two thirds of lateral surface of fibula (Between these two sites of origin, there is a gap through which the common peroneal nerve passes).
- **Insertion:** Peroneus longus becomes tendinous in the lower part of the leg. Its long tendon changes direction around the lateral malleolus, where it is lodged in groove along with peroneus brevis. On the lateral side of the calcaneus, it courses forwards in the foot below

the peroneal trochlea to reach the lateral margin of foot, where it changes direction to pass through the groove on the plantar surface of cuboid. Then it crosses the so obliquely from lateral to medial side to reach its insertion on lateral aspect of medial cuneiform and base of first metatarsal bone.

- **Nerve supply:** superficial peroneal nerve.
- **Actions:** Evertor of foot and support to lateral longitudinal arch.

Special features of peroneus longus

- It has a very long tendon, which changes direction at twice.
- Its tendon crosses across the sole obliquely from lateral to medial side deeply grooving the plantar surface of cuboid bone.
- Common peroneal, deep peroneal and superficial peroneal nerves lie deep to it at the neck of fibula. The superficial peroneal nerve passes through the peroneus longus for a short distance.

Peroneus Brevis

The peroneus brevis lies deep to the peroneus longus muscle.

- **Origin:** From lower two thirds of the lateral surface of fibula.
- **Insertion:** The tendon of peroneus brevis grooves the lateral malleolus and courses forwards above the peroneal trochlea to insert in to the lateral aspect of the tuberosity of the base of the fifth metatarsal bone.
- Nerve supply and actions are similar to peroneus longus muscle.

> 💡 **ADDED INFORMATION**
>
> **Synovial Sheath of Peroneal Tendons**
>
> The tendons of peroneus longus and brevis are very close to each other as they pass deep to the peroneal retinacula. They are covered with a common synovial sheath from the lateral malleolus to peroneal trochlea. Beyond this point there is a separate synovial sheath for each tendon up to its insertion. The reason for two synovial sheaths is that separate osteofascial spaces are formed by a septum from extending from inferior peroneal retinaculum to the peroneal trochlea.

Peroneal Retinacula (Fig. 30.6)

The peroneal retinacula are the thickened bands of deep fascia on the lateral side of the ankle. The tendons of peroneus longus and brevis muscles pass deep to them. The small saphenous vein and sural nerve pass superficial to the superior peroneal retinaculum.

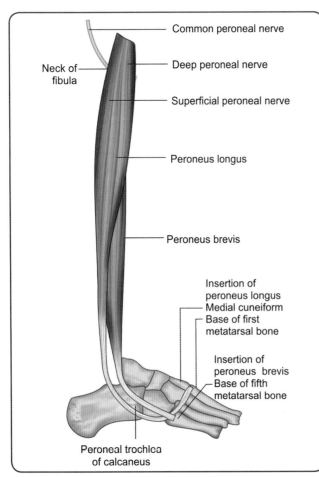

Fig. 30.5: Muscles of lateral or peroneal compartment of leg

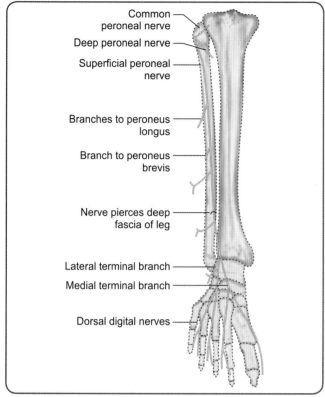

Fig. 30.6: Origin, course, branches and termination of superficial peroneal nerve

- Superior peroneal retinaculum is attached to the back of lateral malleolus above and to the lateral surface of calcaneus below.
- Inferior peroneal retinaculum is attached to the lateral surface of calcaneus posteriorly and to the stem of the inferior extensor retinaculum anteriorly. Some of the fibers of the retinaculum are attached to the periosteum of peroneal trochlea as it crosses the trochlea. This gives rise to two osteofascial canals for the tendons of peroneus longus and brevis. This explains why the originally common synovial sheath of the peroneal tendons becomes double distally (Fig. 30.7).

Superficial Peroneal Nerve (Fig. 30.6)

The superficial peroneal nerve is one of the terminal branches of the common peroneal nerve deep to the peroneus longus muscle at the lateral side of the neck of fibula. It is the nerve of lateral compartment of leg as it supplies the two peroneal muscles in this compartment.

From its beginning at the neck of fibula, it travels downwards in the intermuscular plane between the peroneus longus and peroneus brevis muscles. At the junction of upper two-thirds and lower one third of the leg it pierces the deep fascia of the leg to enter the superficial fascia.

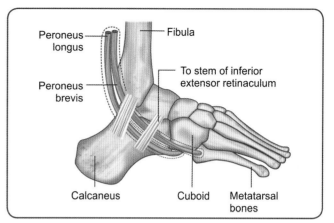

Fig. 30.7: Attachments and deep relations of peroneal retinacula

The superficial peroneal nerve divides into medial and lateral branches in the lower part of leg. Both the terminal branches cross in front of the extensor retinaculum to enter the dorsum of foot.

Branches in Leg

- Muscular branches to peroneus longus and peroneus brevis muscles
- Cutaneous branches to lateral part of leg

Distribution on Dorsum of Foot

The medial and lateral terminal branches supply the skin of the larger intermediate area of the dorsum. The medial terminal branch divides into two dorsal digital nerves, which supply the medial side of great toe and adjacent sides of second and third toes.

The lateral terminal branch divides into two dorsal digital branches for the adjacent sides of third and fourth and fourth and fifth toes.

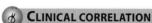

CLINICAL CORRELATION

Injury to Superficial Peroneal Nerve

- Weakness of eversion of the foot (due to paralysis of erectors of foot, namely peroneus longus and brevis).
- Sensory loss on the lateral aspect of leg extending on the intermediate area on dorsum of foot.
- Sensory loss on dorsum of all toes except the first interdigital cleft and lateral side of fifth toe.

POSTERIOR COMPARTMENT OF LEG

The posterior compartment is the largest osteofascial compartment of leg. Superiorly it is continuous with the popliteal fossa. And inferiorly it is continuous with the sole of foot deep to the flexor retinaculum.

Boundaries (Fig. 30.1)

- *Anterior boundary:* By posterior surfaces of tibia and fibula and the interosseous membrane, posterior surface of fibula and posterior intermuscular septum.
- *Posterior boundary:* By deep fascia of the leg.
- *Lateral boundary:* Posterior intermuscular septum.
- *Medial boundary:* Attachment of deep fascia of leg of the medial border of tibia.

Subdivisions

The posterior compartment is subdivided into three parts (superficial, middle and deep) by two fascial septa.

1. The transverse fascial septum intervenes between superficial division (containing gastrocnemius, soleus and plantaris) and middle subdivision (flexor digitorum longus and flexor hallucis longus and popliteus). It is attached above to the soleal line of tibia, medially to medial border of tibia, laterally to posterior border of fibula and is continuous with the flexor retinaculum below.
2. The deep fascial layer intervenes between the middle subdivision and deep subdivision (containing tibialis posterior). It is attached medially to the vertical ridge on the posterior surface of tibia and laterally to the medial crest on the posterior surface of fibula.

Superficial Muscles of the Back of Leg (Fig. 30.8)

Gastrocnemius, plantaris and soleus form a massive muscular mass in the calf. They are strong muscles because they support and propel the body. Together the two headed gastrocnemius and soleus form a three headed triceps surae.

Gastrocnemius

The gastrocnemius is a bulky muscle with two heads.
- *Origin of lateral head:* From lateral aspect of lateral condyle of femur by a tendon. (Occasionally a sesamoid bone, called fabella develops in the tendon of lateral head).
- *Origin of medial head:* From upper and posterior part of medial condyle behind the adductor tubercle and adjacent part of the popliteal surface of femur just above the medial condyle. The tendinous origin of medial head is separated from the capsule of knee joint by a bursa.
- *Insertion:* Tendon of gastrocnemius muscle joins tendons of plantaris and soleus to form tendocalcaneus by which it is inserted into the middle one third of the posterior surface of calcaneus.

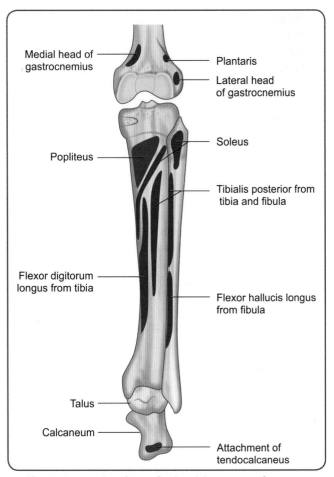

Fig. 30.8: Muscles of superficial and deep strata of posterior compartment of leg

- *Nerve supply:* Medial and lateral heads receive separate branches from the tibial nerve in the popliteal fossa.

Actions
- Gastrocnemius is the plantar flexor of ankle joint in flexed position of knee.
- It is the flexor of knee joint.
- It is active during running and jumping.

⚕ CLINICAL CORRELATION

Tennis leg is a painful calf injury in which there is a tear of medial belly of gastrocnemius at its musculotendinous junction due to overstretching.

Plantaris

It is a fusiform muscle with small belly and long tendon, lying under cover of the lateral head of gastrocnemius. The plantaris is a vestigial muscle and plantar aponeurosis is considered to be its degenerated part.

- *Origin:* From the lower third of lateral supracondylar ridge of femur.
- *Insertion:* Into calcaneus through the tendocalcaneus

Nerve Supply

A branch from tibial nerve in the popliteal fossa innervates it.

 CLINICAL CORRELATION

> The plantaris tendon is used for tendon grafting in the repair of ruptured long tendons in the hand (palmaris longus tendon serves similar purpose).

Soleus

It is given the name soleus from its resemblance to the sole (flat fish). It is a very powerful and massive muscle situated deep to gastrocnemius. It is a multipennate muscle

- *Horse shoe shaped origin:* From the upper one third of the posterior surface of fibula, soleal line of tibia, middle third of the medial border of tibia and the tendinous arch of soleus posterior to the neurovascular structures of the compartment.
- *Insertion:* By tendocalcaneus in to the middle one third of posterior surface of calcaneus.
- *Nerve supply:* Branches of tibial nerve in the popliteal fossa.

Actions

- Soleus is a powerful plantar flexor of ankle joint (though relatively slower).
- It is a postural muscle.
- It is active during normal walking.

 STUDENT INTEREST

> You stroll with the help of soleus but win long jumps and running races with the help of gastrocnemius.

Calf muscle pump

Gastrocnemius and soleus together constitute a calf muscle pump for facilitating venous return from the lower limb. The soleus is regarded as the peripheral heart because it houses large venous sinuses, which are connected to the superficial veins by perforating veins. These veins pass through soleus. Thus contraction of soleus helps in sucking the blood from the superficial veins in to the perforating veins and propelling it towards the deep veins of the posterior compartment.

Tendocalcaneus (Achilles tendon)

The tendocalcaneus is the thickest and strongest tendon in the body (length 15 cm). It begins in the middle of the calf

though its anterior aspect receives muscle fibers of soleus almost to its lower end. About four cm above the calcaneus it becomes flattened and is inserted into the middle third of the posterior surface of calcaneus. This tendon is very important in conserving the energy and releasing it in the next stage in gait cycle. Unlike the other long tendons at the ankle the tendocalcaneus is not enveloped in the synovial sheath. It is related to two bursae. The calcaneal bursa, between the calcaneus and the tendocalcaneus is prone to inflammation in long distance runners. There is a bursa between the tendon and the skin (adventitious bursa).

Testing function of gastrocnemius and soleus

On asking the subject to stand on toe, the tendocalcaneus and triceps surae become visible and palpable (if contracting normally).

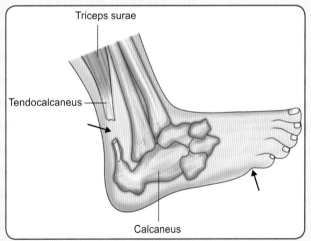 **CLINICAL CORRELATION**

> - Sprain and rupture of tendocalcaneus (Fig. 30.9) are common injuries. The rupture causes sudden pain in the calf. Due to retraction of the muscle bellies of gastrocnemius proximally, a gap can be felt in the tendon. There is loss of plantarflexion of the foot. The ruptured tendon can be sutured and strengthened using fascia lata.
> - Ankle jerk or Achilles tendon reflex is elicited as follows. On tapping the tendon with knee hammer there is reflex contraction of triceps surae with resultant plantarflexion of the foot. The nerve responsible for this is the tibial nerve and the spinal center is S1 segment. So in paralysis of triceps surae the patient will not be able to stand on the toes and there will be loss of ankle jerk.
>
> **Fig. 30.9:** Rupture of tendocalcaneus resulting in dorsiflexed foot (arrow showing)

Posterior tibial artery

The posterior tibial artery is one of the terminal branches of the popliteal artery at the lower margin of the popliteus muscle (deep to gastrocnemius). The venae comitantes and the tibial nerve closely associated with it form a neurovascular bundle that enters the posterior compartment by passing under the tendinous arch of soleus.

Course and relations (Fig. 30.10)

The posterior tibial artery passes vertically downwards and slightly medially to reach the posteromedial side of ankle and terminates into lateral and medial plantar arteries deep to the flexor retinaculum.

Superficial relations

In the upper two thirds of leg, it is separated by the superficial transverse septum from the superficial calf muscles.

In the lower third of the leg, it covered with skin and fasciae.

At the ankle, it is covered by flexor retinaculum and abductor hallucis.

Deep relations

In the upper three fourth of leg, it rests on the posterior surfaces of tibialis posterior.

In the lower one third of leg, it rests on flexor digitorum longus muscle and on posterior aspect of tibia.

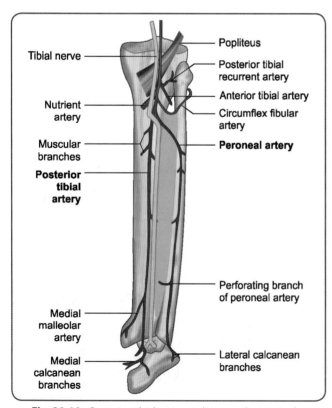

Fig. 30.10: Posterior tibial artery and peroneal artery in the posterior compartment of leg

At the ankle, it directly rests on the capsule of the ankle joint.

Relation to tibial nerve

The tibial nerve crosses the posterior tibial artery as follows. It is at first medial to the posterior tibial artery but gradually changes to posterior position and in the lower part it lies lateral to the artery.

Surface marking

The posterior tibial artery corresponds to a line from the midline on the back of the leg at the level of the neck of fibula to a point midway between the tendocalcaneus and medial malleolus.

> **CLINICAL CORRELATION**
>
> The posterior tibial pulse (Fig. 30.11) is palpated against the calcaneus about 2 cm below and behind the medial malleolus. This is a peripheral pulse like dorsalis pedis pulse in the distal part of lower limb. This pulse is diminished in cases of arterial insufficiency due to narrowing of arteries on account of atherosclerosis (Fig. 32.5).
>
>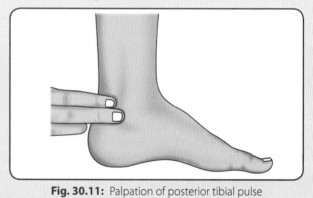
>
> **Fig. 30.11:** Palpation of posterior tibial pulse

Branches

- Circumflex fibular artery passes through the substance of the soleus and winds round the lateral side of the neck of fibula. It takes part in genicular anastomosis.
- Nutrient artery of the tibia arises near the origin of posterior tibial artery and enters the nutrient foramen just below the soleal line.
- Muscular branches are for muscles of the back of leg.
- Communicating branch joins with the similar branch of peroneal artery.
- Medial malleolar branch takes part in medial malleolar network.
- Medial calcanean branches pierce the flexor retinaculum and supply the skin of the heel.
- Peroneal artery (Fig. 30.10) is the largest branch that arises about 2.5 cm to the below the distal margin of popliteus. It supplies the muscles of posterior and

lateral compartments. It travels the entire length of the posterior compartment lying in close contact with the medial crest of the fibula in a fibrous tunnel between the tibialis posterior and flexor hallucis longus muscles. It terminates on the lateral aspect as the lateral calcanean branches, which take part in the lateral malleolar network.

The branches of the peroneal artery are as follows:
- Muscular to the peroneal muscles.
- Nutrient artery to the fibula.
- Communicating branch to join with communicating branch of posterior tibial artery.
- Perforating branch passes through lower part of interosseous membrane to enter the anterior compartment.

  The perforating artery after reaching anterior aspect of the leg anastomoses with the lateral malleolar branch of anterior tibial artery and with the lateral tarsal artery (a branch of dorsalis pedis) to form lateral malleolar network. The perforating branch is sometimes enlarged in which case it may replace the dorsalis pedis artery
- Lateral calcanean artery is the continuation of peroneal artery.

Note: Peroneal artery is an example of axis artery of lower limb

CLINICAL CORRELATION

Arterial insufficiency in the leg is characterized by intermittent claudication in which there is pain in the calf muscles on walking but the pain disappears after resting. On walking, when the demand for more blood is not met, the muscle ischemia causes pain. This is due to narrowing of the arteries. The causes of narrowing of the arteries are atherosclerosis, diabetes and hypertension. In young men habituated to smoking a condition called thrombo-angitis obliterans (TAO) affects the arteries of the leg. The serious complication of arterial insufficiency is gangrene of the toes or foot or the leg (Fig. 32.4).

Posterior tibial veins

The veins accompanying the posterior tibial artery (venae comitantes) are the posterior tibial veins. These veins begin deep to the flexor retinaculum by the union of veins accompanying the lateral and medial plantar arteries. The tributaries of the posterior tibial veins are the veins from the muscles of posterior compartment, especially the venous plexus in the soleus and peroneal veins. The perforating veins connecting these veins to the great saphenous vein are provided with unidirectional valves so that blood flows from the superficial to the deep veins. The venae comitantes of the posterior and anterior tibial arteries unite at the lower margin of popliteus muscle to form popliteal vein.

CLINICAL CORRELATION

Deep Vein Thrombosis (DVT)
The deep veins of the leg are clinically very important because they are prone to thrombosis if there is prolonged immobilization of lower limb for any reason (plaster cast on leg or postoperative period). If the thrombus is detached, it enters the venous circulation and reaches the pulmonary arteries via right side of heart causing fatal pulmonary embolism.

Tibial nerve

The tibial nerve in the popliteal fossa continues as the tibial nerve of posterior compartment of leg at the distal border of popliteus muscle. It enters the posterior compartment along with posterior tibial vessels deep to the tendinous arch of the soleus.

Course and relations

The relations of tibial nerve are similar to those of the posterior tibial artery.
- The tibial nerve is closely applied to the anterior surface of the deep transverse septum throughout its course.
- It lies medial to the posterior tibial vessels deep to the tendinous arch of soleus.
- Below this level the tibial nerve crosses the accompanying vessels posteriorly from medial to lateral direction.
- At the ankle, the tibial nerve is lateral to the posterior tibial artery.
- The tibial nerve divides deep to the flexor retinaculum into lateral and medial plantar nerves.

Branches
- Muscular branches to tibialis posterior, flexor digitorum longus and flexor hallucis longus. The soleus may also receive a branch in the leg.
- Articular branches supply the ankle joint.
- Medial calcanean branches pierce the flexor retinaculum to supply the skin over the heel.

CLINICAL CORRELATION

Effects of Injury to Tibial Nerve
Being deep in location injury to tibial nerve is less common in both popliteal fossa and posterior compartment of leg. When injured it shows following effects.
- Paralysis of all the muscles of the posterior compartment of leg and all the intrinsic muscles of the foot (because of which foot is held in calcaneovalgus position due to unresisted action of dorsiflexors and evertors).
- Sensory loss on the sole (due to which trophic ulcers may develop on sole).

Popliteus (Fig. 29.2)

The popliteus is located in the lower part of the floor of popliteal fossa. This muscle is important in unlocking a locked knee joint. So it is referred to as the key of the knee joint.

- *Origin:* From anterior end of the popliteal groove on the lateral condyle of femur(Fig. 30.8).
  Its origin is tendinous and is located inside the capsule of knee joint (a few of its fibers arise from the back of lateral meniscus).
- *Insertion:* Popliteus tendon expands in a triangular fleshy belly, which is inserted into the posterior surface of tibia above the soleal line.

Relations of intracapsular tendon

The intracapsular tendon of popliteus intervenes between the lateral meniscus and the fibular collateral ligament. The long tendon enclosed in synovial sheath pierces the posterior part of fibrous capsule, below the arcuate popliteal ligament.

Relations of fleshy part of popliteus in popliteal fossa

- Posterior surface is covered with a strong fascia, which is an extension from the insertion of semimembranosus muscle. This surface is related to the popliteal vessels and tibial nerve.
- Anterior surface is in contact with the posterior surface of tibia above soleal line.

Relations at distal margin of popliteus

- The popliteal artery terminates into anterior and posterior tibial arteries.
- The popliteal vein is formed by union of anterior and posterior tibial veins (venae comitantes).
- The tibial nerve enters into the posterior compartment of leg.
- The nerve to popliteus winds round this margin to reach the anterior surface of the muscle.

Nerve supply

- Nerve to popliteus is a branch of the tibial nerve in the popliteal fossa. This nerve reaches the lower (distal) margin of the muscle to wind round it to reach and enter its anterior surface.
- The nerve to popliteus also supplies a few twig to tibialis posterior muscle, articular branches to tibiofibular joints and tibia.

Actions

- Unlocking the locked knee at the beginning of flexion of knee joint.
- Flexion of knee joint and lateral rotation of semiflexed knee.
- Protection to lateral meniscus from injury.

Flexor digitorum longus (FDL)

This deep muscle of the leg is the long flexor of lateral four digits.

- *Origin:* From posterior surface of tibia (Fig. 30.12) below the soleal line and medial to the tibial origin of tibialis posterior.

Course

The tendon of flexor digitorum longus crosses superficial to the tendon of tibialis posterior in the distal part of the leg. At the ankle, it passes behind the flexor retinaculum and then enters the sole. In the sole, the tendon turns laterally to cross superficial the tendon of flexor hallucis longus.

William Turner's slip

The common tendon of flexor digitorum longus receives some fibers (called *William Turner's slip*) from the tendon of flexor hallucis longus during the crossing. This intertendinous connection serves to strengthen the action of flexor digitorum longus.

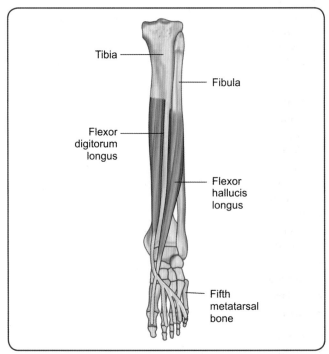

Fig. 30.12: Origin of flexor digitorum longus from tibia and flexor hallucis longus from fibula and insertion of Flexor digitorum longus (FDL) in lateral four toes and Flexor hallucis longus (FHL) in great toe (Note the crossing of FDL and FHL tendons in the second layer of sole)

Insertion of flexor digitorum accessories into the tendon of FDL

The common tendon of flexor digitorum longus receives the insertion of flexor digitorum accessorius on its lateral side. This connection serves to straighten the pull of action of flexor digitorum longus on the toes.

- **Insertion of FDL:** The common tendon splits into four digital tendons for four lateral toes. Each digital tendon gives origin to the lumbrical muscle of the foot. Finally the digital tendon enters the fibrous flexor sheath, pierces the tendon of flexor digitorum brevis and is inserted into the plantar surface of the bases of terminal phalanges of lateral four toes.
- *Nerve supply:* Tibial nerve in the posterior compartment of the leg

Actions

- Plantarflexion of lateral four toes and of foot.
- Support to the arches of foot.

Note: That FDL in the leg is comparable to flexor digitorum profundus of forearm in the pattern of insertion and in giving origin to lumbricals.

Flexor hallucis longus (FHL)

This muscle is much larger than the flexor digitorum longus.

Origin: From posterior surface of the fibula (Fig. 30.8) below the origin of soleus, from fascia covering tibialis posterior and from lower part of interosseous membrane

Course

- In the leg, the tendon of flexor hallucis longus passes obliquely downward and medially and lies in a groove on the lower end of tibia, and then passes deep to the flexor retinaculum.
- After entering the sole, it grooves the posterior surface of the talus and then the sustentaculum tali of the calcaneus.
- It crosses the tendon of flexor digitorum longus in the second layer of sole and in doing so, gives a fibrous slip (William Turner's slip) to the digitorum tendon.
- **Insertion:** into the base of the distal phalanx of the great toe
- *Nerve supply:* Tibial nerve in the leg

Actions

- Plantarflexion of great toe and of the ankle joint.
- Support to the medial longitudinal arch of foot.

Tibialis posterior

The tibialis posterior is the most anterior or deeply placed muscle in the posterior compartment of leg. It is overlapped by the larger flexor hallucis longus on lateral side and relatively smaller flexor digitorum longus on medial side.

Origin: from upper two-thirds of posterior aspect of interosseous membrane and adjacent parts of posterior surfaces of tibia and fibula.

Course

In the distal part of the leg, its tendon passes deep to the tendon of flexor digitorum longus. Then it passes in a groove behind the medial malleolus enclosed in a synovial sheath and passes deep to the flexor retinaculum to reach the sole. In the sole, it lies inferior to the plantar calcaneonavicular ligament (spring ligament).

- **Insertion:** Main insertion on the tuberosity of the navicular bone and by slips to the all tarsal bones (except talus) and to bases of second to fourth metatarsal bones.
- **Nerve supply:** Tibial nerve in postreior compartment and nerve to popliteus

Actions

- Chief invertor of foot.
- Weak plantarflexion of the foot.
- Main support to medial longitudinal arch.

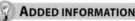 **ADDED INFORMATION**

Synovial Sheaths of Flexor Tendons

- Synovial sheath for tibialis posterior starts four cm above the medial malleolus and ends just proximal to its insertion into the navicular bone.
- Synovial sheath for flexor hallucis longus starts at the malleolar level proximally and to the base of first metatarsal bone distally.
- Synovial sheath for the flexor digitorum longus begins just above the medial malleolus and reaches the level of navicular bone.

Inflammation of the synovial sheaths around the tendons gives rise to tenosynovitis.

Segmental Innervation of Muscles of Lower Limb

Iliopsoas	L2, L3
Sartorius	L2, L3
Adductor muscles	L2, L3, L4
Quadriceps femoris	L2, L3,L4
Tibialis anterior and posterior	L4, L5,
Gluteus minimus and medius	L4, L5 ,S1
Gluteus maximus	L4, L5, S1, S2
Hamstrings	L4, L5, S1, S2
Gastrocnemius	L4, L5, S1, S2
Soleus	L5, S1, S2
Flexor hallucis and FDL	S1, S2
Extensor hallucis longus	L5, S1

Flexor retinaculum (Fig. 30.13)

It is a thick band of deep fascia on the medial aspect of and behind and below the medial malleolus. From its upper attachment it is directed inferiorly, posteriorly and laterally.

Attachments

- *Medially or above:* To the medial malleolus.
- *Laterally or below:* To the medial process of the tubercle of calcaneus.

Its distal border gives origin to the abductor hallucis muscle.

The medial calcaneal nerve (a branch of tibial nerve) and the medial calcaneal artery (a branch of posterior tibial artery) pierce the retinaculum.

Deep relations

From above downwards (or medio-laterally) are: Tibialis posterior tendon, flexor Digitorum longus tendon, posterior tibial Artery, tibial Nerve and flexor Hallucis longus tendon (Fig. 30.13).

 STUDENT INTEREST

Mnemonic
Tom Dick AN Harry

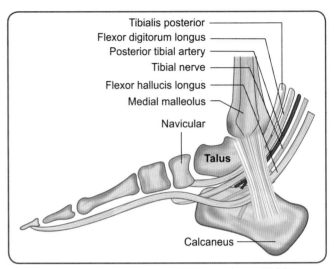

Fig. 30.13: Attachments and deep relations of flexor retinaculum of foot

🎼 **CLINICAL CORRELATION**

In tarsal tunnel syndrome the tibial nerve is compressed in the osseofibrous tunnel behind the medial malleolus deep to flexor retinaculum. The symptoms are, burning, tingling and pain in the sole of the foot. Surgical division of the flexor retinaculum relieves the severe and persistent pain.

Tibiofibular Joints and the Ankle Joint

TIBIOFIBULAR JOINTS

There are three joints between tibia and fibula as mentioned below (Fig. 31.1):

1. Proximal (or superior) tibiofibular joint
2. Middle tibiofibular joint
3. Distal (inferior) tibiofibular joint.

- **Superior or proximal tibiofibular joint:** This is a plane type of synovial joint between the lateral condyle of tibia and the head of the fibula. The joint capsule is thick anteriorly and posteriorly. The fibular collateral ligament and the tendon of biceps femoris are related to the superolateral aspect of the joint. The tendon of the popliteus enclosed in the synovial sheath passes across the posteromedial aspect of the joint. In 10% of people the synovial sheath of the popliteus may communicate with the synovial cavity of the joint. A slight amount of gliding movement is permitted in the joint. The nerve to popliteus and the recurrent genicular nerve (a branch of common peroneal nerve) innervate the joint.

- **Middle tibiofibular joint:** This is a fibrous joint between the shafts of tibia and fibula connected by interosseous membrane.
  - **Interosseous membrane of leg:** This is a fibrous membrane that stretches between the interosseous borders of tibia and fibula thus, intervening between the anterior and the posterior compartments of the leg. The direction of fibers in the membrane is downward and laterally from the tibia to the fibula.

At the lower end, the interosseous membrane is in continuity with the interosseous ligament of distal tibiofibular joint.

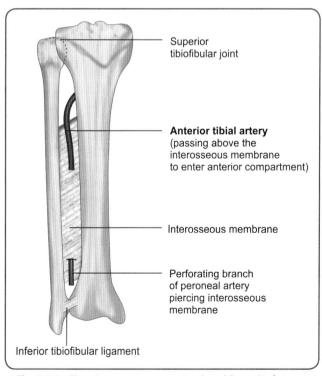

Labels: Superior tibiofibular joint; **Anterior tibial artery** (passing above the interosseous membrane to enter anterior compartment); Interosseous membrane; Perforating branch of peroneal artery piercing interosseous membrane; Inferior tibiofibular ligament

Fig. 31.1: Showing superior or proximal, middle and inferior or distal tibiofibular joints

The anterior tibial artery enters the anterior compartment of leg through a large oval opening above the superior margin of the membrane. The perforating branch of peroneal artery pierces the membrane (Fig. 31.1) near its lower margin to enter the anterior compartment of leg. The nerve to popliteus supplies the membrane.

- ***Functions of interosseous membrane are as follows:***
  - The anterior surface of the membrane provides partial origin to all the four muscles of anterior compartment of leg. The posterior surface of the membrane gives partial origin to the tibialis posterior and flexor hallucis longus
  - It holds tibia and fibula together
  - It partitions the flexor and extensor compartments of the leg with the help of the bones of leg.
- ***Inferior or distal tibiofibular joint:*** This is a syndesmosis type of fibrous joint and the strongest among the tibiofibular articulations. The interosseous ligament is the connecting bond between the medial convex surface of the distal end of fibula and the rough fibular notch of the lateral surface of the distal end of tibia. The inferior tibiofibular syndesmosis receives twigs from the nerve to popliteus and from deep peroneal nerve.

Accessory Ligaments

- Interosseous ligament is the strongest bond between the lower ends of tibia and fibula. It is continuous above with the interosseous membrane of the leg. It connects the medial rough surface of the distal end of fibula and the rough lateral surface of the lower end of tibia.
- Anteriortibiofibular ligament covers the interosseous ligament anteriorly.
- Stronger posterior tibiofibular ligament covers the posterior aspect of the interosseous ligament. Its lower and deep part is called inferior transverse tibiofibular ligament. It is composed of yellow elastic fibers which pass transversely from malleolar fossa of fibula to the posterior margin of articular surface of tibia almost of the medial malleolus. It helps in deepening the socket of ankle joint.
- Inferior transverse tibiofibular ligament is the inferior part of posterior tibiofibular ligament containing yellow elastic fibers. It extends beyond the lower limits of tibia and fibula as it stretches from the proximal end of malleolar fossa to the posterior border of the tibial articular surface. It deepens the socket of ankle joint.

ANKLE OR TALOCRURAL JOINT

The ankle joint is a strong weight-bearing joint of the lower limb. It is a synovial joint of hinge variety.

Articulating Bones

It is a compound articulation between the lower end of tibia, lower end of fibula and the talus (Figs 31.2A and 31.2B).

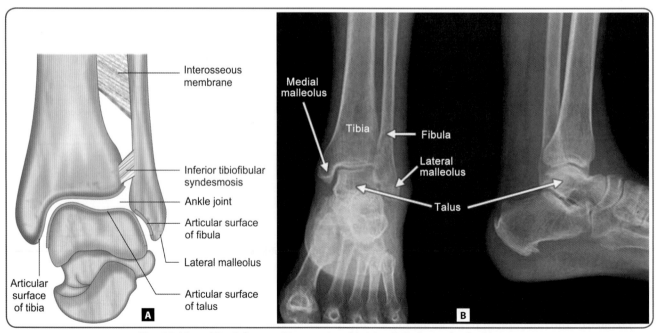

Figs 31.2A and B: A. Bones taking part in ankle joint; **B.** Radiograph of ankle joint

Articular Surfaces

Proximal Articular Surface

The articular facets on the lower end of tibia including on the medial malleolus, articular facet of lateral malleolus of fibula and inferior transverse tibiofibular ligament together form the tibiofibular socket.

Distal Articular Surface

The articular facets are present on the superior, lateral and medial surfaces of the talus. These facets form a continuous articular area.

- *Comma-shaped facet* on the medial aspect of the talus articulates with the facet on the medial malleolus.
- *Triangular facet* on the lateral aspect of talus articulates with the corresponding facet on lateral malleolus.
- *Trochlea on the superior aspect* of talus is for articulation with inferior surface of lower end of tibia.

    The trochlea is wider in front than behind. During dorsiflexion of the foot the grip of the malleoli on the talus is strongest because this movement forces the anterior wider part of trochlea posteriorly between the malleoli. The ankle joint is relatively unstable during plantarflexion because the narrower posterior part of the trochlea does not fill the tibiofibular socket. Therefore, injuries to ankle occur mostly during plantarflexion and inversion.

Fibrous Capsule

The capsule is attached superiorly to the margins of articular surfaces of the tibia and the malleoli. It is attached inferiorly to the margins of articular surfaces of the talus.

Synovial Membrane

The synovial membrane lines the fibrous capsule except the anterior and posterior aspects of the capsule where fatty pads intervene between the capsule and the synovial membrane. It is attached to the margins of the articular surfaces. There is an extension of synovial membrane between the tibia and fibula just below the interosseous ligament of the distal tibiofibular joint.

Ligaments of Ankle Joint

Deltoid Ligament or Medial Ligament of Ankle Joint

The deltoid ligament is large and very strong. Because it is triangular in shape it gains its name *'deltoid'* (Fig. 31.3).

- *Upper attachment of deltoid ligament* is to the apex and margins of medial malleolus.
- *Lower attachment of superficial part of deltoid ligament* from before backwards, is to navicular bone

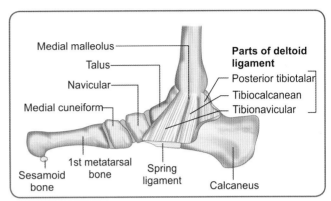

Fig. 31.3: Attachments of deltoid ligament of ankle joint (note that anterior tibiotalar part of deltoid ligament is not shown in this view)

spring ligament, to sustentaculum tali and to medial tubercle and adjacent medial surface of talus.

According to the lower attachments, the superior part of deltoid ligament is divisible into tibionavicular ligament, tibiocalcanean ligament and posterior tibiotalar ligament.

- *Lower attachment of deep part of deltoid ligament*, is to the anterior part of medial surface of talus. The deep part is called *anterior tibiotalar ligament*.

Lateral Ligament of Ankle Joint (Fig. 31.4)

This ligament is divided in to three discrete parts, namely, anterior talofibular, posterior talofibular and calcaneofibular.

- Anterior talofibular ligament extends from the anterior border of lateral malleolus to the lateral aspect of the neck of talus.
- Posterior talofibular ligament runs from the distal part of malleolar fossa of lower end of fibula to the posterior tubercle of talus.

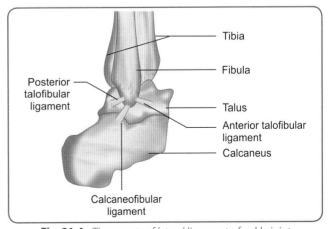

Fig. 31.4: Three parts of lateral ligament of ankle joint

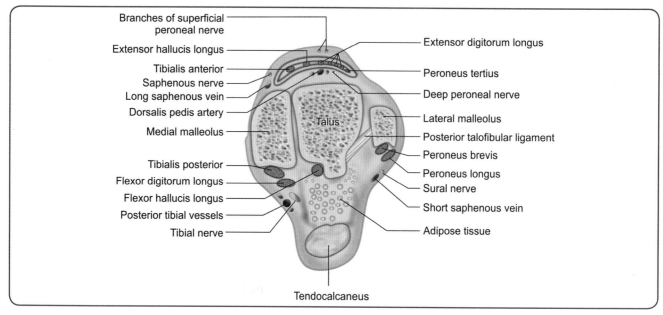

Fig. 31.5: Horizontal section through ankle joint depicting the structures surrounding it

- Calcaneofibular ligament is cord like and extends from the distal end of lateral malleolus to the lateral surface of calcaneus.

Relations (Fig. 31.5)

- **Anteriorly:** Tibialis anterior, extensor hallucis longus, anterior tibial artery, deep peroneal nerve, extensor digitorum longus and peroneus tertius
- **Posteromedially:** Tibialis posterior, flexor digitorum longus, posterior tibial artery, tibial nerve and flexor hallucis longus
- **Posterolaterally:** Tendons of peroneus longus and brevis
- **Posteriorly:** Tendocalcaneus separated from the joint by fibrofatty tissue

Arterial Supply

Through rich arterial anastomoses around the ankle.

Nerve Supply

By articular branches of deep peroneal and tibial nerves.

Movements

The movements permitted at the ankle joint are dorsiflexion and plantarflexion.

- In **dorsiflexion** the dorsum of the foot moves toward the anterior surface of leg and thus the angle between the foot and the leg is reduced. This enables one to strike the ground with the heel during walking.
- In **plantarflexion** the dorsum moves away from the anterior surface of leg. This enables one to raise the heel from the ground and touch the toes to the ground as in running.

Muscles Producing Dorsiflexion

Tibialis anterior, extensor digitorum longus, extensor hallucis longus and peroneus tertius.

Muscles Producing Plantarflexion

Gastrocnemius, soleus, tibialis posterior, flexor hallucis longus and flexor digitorum longus.

Radiology

Radiological anatomy of ankle joint is well shown in anteroposterior view of plain radiograph. The tip of the lateral malleolus is at a lower level than that of the medial. The joint cavity is of uniform size on all sides. Occasionally an accessory bone (os trigonum) may be seen at the back of talus (not be mistaken for fracture of talus).

CLINICAL CORRELATION

- Ankle joint is the most frequently injured joint. The ankle injuries occur in plantarflexed position of the foot. The lateral ligament in more often injured compared to the medial. A sprained ankle results due to tear of anterior talofibular and calcaneofibular ligaments when the foot is twisted in lateral direction (inversion injury). In forcible eversion of foot the deltoid ligament may be torn. At times the deltoid ligament pulls the medial malleolus thereby causing avulsion fracture of the medial malleolus.
- Pott's Fracture (fracture- dislocation of the ankle) occurs when the foot is caught in the rabbit hole in the ground and the foot is forcibly everted. In this condition at first there is an oblique fracture of the shaft and lateral malleolus of fibula.
- The strong eversion pull on the deltoid ligament causes transverse fracture of the medial malleolus. If the tibia is carried anteriorly the posterior margin of the distal end of tibia is also broken by the talus producing tri-malleolar fracture (because in this situation the broken distal end of tibia is considered the third malleolus).

The Foot

Chapter Contents

INTRODUCTION

The foot consists of upper surface or dorsum of the foot and lower surface or sole.

DORSUM OF FOOT

The dorsum contains the dorsal venous arch, tendons, extensor digitorum brevis muscle, nerves and the dorsalis pedis artery.

Sensory Nerve Supply (Fig. 32.1)

- *Saphenous nerve:* Along medial margin of dorsum upto the base of big toe.
- *Sural nerve:* Along lateral side of dorsum and lateral side of little toe.
- *Superficial peroneal nerve:* Supplies the larger intermediate area of dorsum, medial side of big toe and all other toes (except the first interdigital cleft and the lateral side of fifth toe).
- *Deep peroneal nerve:* Supplies first interdigital cleft.
- *Medial plantar nerve:* Nail beds of medial three and half toes.
- *Lateral plantar nerve:* Nail beds of lateral one and half toes.

Dorsal Venous Arch

The dorsal venous arch drains the dorsum of the foot and toes via the dorsal metatarsal veins. The small saphenous

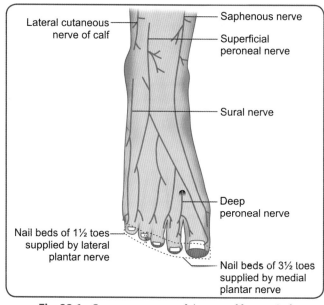

Fig. 32.1: Cutaneous nerves of dorsum of foot and of dorsum of toes

vein begins at the lateral end of dorsal venous arch and the great saphenous vein on the medial end.

DEEP PERONEAL NERVE ON DORSUM (FIGS 30.3 AND 30.4)

Tendons and Muscle on Dorsum (Fig. 30.4)

The tendons of the four muscles of the anterior compartment pass on the dorsum to reach their respective distal attachments. If the foot is dorsiflexed the tendon of tibialis anterior becomes visible and can be felt on the medial side of foot. The tendon of extensor hallucis longus can be felt just lateral to tibialis anterior tendon, when the big toe is dorsiflexed. The four tendons of extensor digitorum longus are visible in the distal part of dorsum on dorsiflexion of lateral four toes. The tendon of peroneus tertius is not distinctly visible.

Extensor Digitorum Brevis (Fig. 32.2)

The extensor digitorum brevis is the only muscle on the dorsum of the foot. It is felt in living as a small fleshy elevation anterior to the lateral malleolus on the dorsum.
- ***Origin:*** From anterior part of upper surface of calcaneus.
- ***Insertion:*** By four tendons to 1st, 2nd, 3rd and 4th toes.
  The tendons for 2nd, 3rd and 4th toes end in to corresponding tendons of extensor digitorum longus and

insert via dorsal expansion in to middle and terminal phalanx.

The tendon of most medial part of extensor digitorum brevis (called extensor hallucis brevis) is inserted in to the base of proximal phalanx of big toe.

Actions
- Extensor digitorum muscle extends the metatarso-phalangeal and interphalangeal joints of middle three toes.
- Extensor hallucis brevis extends proximal phalanx only of big toe.

Nerve supply

The extensor digitorum brevis is supplied by lateral terminal branch of deep peroneal nerve through the pseudoganglion.

Dorsalis Pedis Artery (Fig. 32.3)

The dorsalis pedis artery (dorsal artery of foot) is the direct continuation of anterior tibial artery midway between the malleoli. It courses downwards and medially on the dorsum of the foot to reach the proximal end of the first intermetatarsal space, where it turns downwards between the two heads of the first dorsal interosseous muscle. It enters the sole and ends by completing the plantar arch medially.

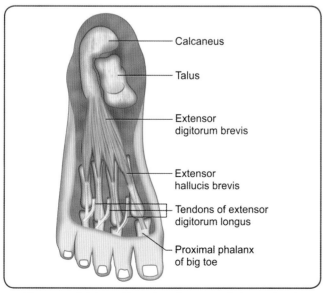

Fig. 32.2: Origin and insertion of extensor digitorum brevis

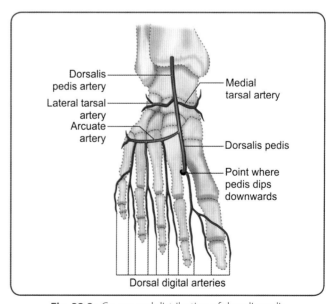

Fig. 32.3: Course and distribution of dorsalis pedis artery on the foot

---

- Palpation of dorsalis pedis pulse (Fig. 32.4) is very easy because of the superficial location of the artery. It is felt just lateral to the extensor hallucis longus tendon against the tarsal bones. A diminished or absent dorsalis pedis pulse indicates arterial insufficiency of the lower limb caused by block in any one of the proximal arteries (cause may be thrombosis, embolism or arteriosclerosis in femoral, popliteal or anterior tibial arteries). Figure 32.5 shows the gangrene of the foot due to vascular insufficiency.
- Diabetic foot is a complication of uncontrolled diabetes. There is gangrene formation in the foot. Gangrene means death of tissues with purification due to three factors, high blood glucose, arterial insufficiency and neuritis (diabetic neuropathy due to high sugar). The treatment of diabetic foot is amputation through ankle.

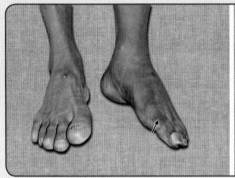
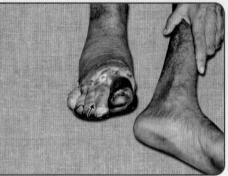

Fig. 32.4: Palpation of dorsalis pedis pulse

Fig. 32.5: Gangrene of the foot and toes due to arterial insufficiency (arrow showing)

Surface marking

A line starting from the midpoint between the malleoli to the proximal end of first intermetatarsal space represents the dorsalis pedis artery.

Relations (Fig. 32.3)

- On the deep (inferior) aspect, dorsalis pedis artery lies successively on the capsule of ankle joint, talus, navicular and intermediate cuneiform bones.
- On the superficial or superior aspect, the skin, fasciae, and inferior extensor retinaculum cover it and distally the extensor hallucis brevis crosses it.
- Medially, it is related to the tendon of extensor hallucis longus.
- Laterally, it is related to medial tendon of extensor digitorum longus and medial terminal branch of deep peroneal nerve.

Branches

There are four named branches of dorsalis pedis artery:
1. Lateral tarsal artery
2. Medial tarsal artery
3. Arcuate artery
4. First dorsal metatarsal artery

Arcuate artery (Fig. 32.3)

The arcuate artery has the shape of the arch with forward convexity. It passes laterally across the bases of metatarsal bones deep to the extensor tendons. It terminates by taking part in the lateral malleolar network.

Dorsal metatarsal arteries

The dorsal metatarsal arteries are four.
- The first dorsal metatarsal artery is the direct branch of dorsalis pedis artery, at the point where it dips into the first intermetatarsal space.
- The second, third and fourth dorsal metatarsal arteries arise from the convexity of the arcuate artery.

At the interdigital cleft each dorsal metatarsal artery divides in two dorsal digital arteries for the adjacent sides of first and second, second and third, third and fourth, and fourth and fifth digits. The first dorsal metatarsal artery (a direct branch of dorsalis pedis artery) gives a twig to the medial side of the big toe while the fourth artery gives a twig to the lateral side of little toe.

Each dorsal metatarsal artery is connected to the arteries of sole by two sets of perforating arteries.

The proximal set consists of perforating arteries for the second to fourth spaces, which connect the dorsal metacarpal arteries to the plantar arch.

The distal set of perforating arteries connects each dorsal metatarsal artery to the corresponding plantar metatarsal arteries.

SOLE OF FOOT

The sole of the foot bears the weight of the body and is subjected to the maximum wear and tear. Hence it is covered by thick skin with keratinized layer of epidermis. The subcutaneous fat is divided into small loculi by fibrous septa, which anchor the skin to the deep fascia. The fibrofatty tissue is particularly well developed at three sites, which come in contact with the ground, namely, the heel and heads of the metatarsals and pulp of terminal digits.

Sensory Nerve Supply (Fig. 32.6)

- The medial calcanean branches of tibial nerve supply the skin over the heel.
- The cutaneous branches of medial plantar nerve supply the skin of the medial half of the sole and the plantar digital branches of the same nerve supply the plantar aspect of the great, second, third and medial half of fourth toes.
- The cutaneous branches of lateral plantar nerve supply the lateral half of sole and the plantar digital branches of the same nerve supply the plantar aspect of lateral half of fourth toe and the entire fifth toe.

Arterial Supply of Heel

The heel receives blood from two sources as follows:

1. Medial aspect of heel from medial calcanean branches of the posterior tibial artery.
2. Lateral aspect of heel from lateral calcanean branch of peroneal artery.

Deep Fascia of Sole

The deep fascia of sole is called plantar fascia. The central part of the plantar fascia is much thicker than its lateral and medial parts.

Plantar Aponeurosis (Fig. 32.7)

The thick central part of the plantar fascia is triangular in shape. It is known as the plantar aponeurosis. It is regarded as the degenerated tendon of plantaris muscle.

Parts

It presents an apex proximally and a base distally. The base splits in to five processes.

Attachments

- The apex is attached to the medial tubercle of calcaneus.
- Its base splits into five slips (one for each toe) proximal to the metatarsal heads. Each slip divides into a superficial and a deep stratum. The superficial stratum is connected to the superficial transverse metatarsal ligament. The deep stratum of each slip divides into two parts, which pass on either side of flexor tendons and fuse with the deep transverse metatarsal ligaments, plantar ligaments of metatarsophalangeal joints and fibrous flexor sheath at the base of each proximal phalanx.

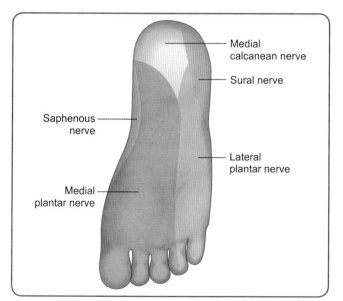

Fig. 32.6: Sensory nerve supply of the sole

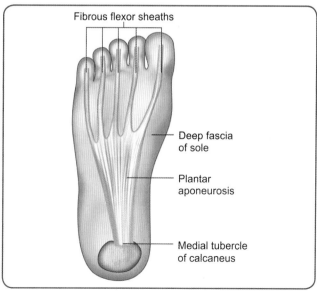

Fig. 32.7: Plantar aponeurosis and its five slips distally

- Laterally the plantar aponeurosis is continuous with the plantar fascia covering the abductor digiti minimi.
- Medially the plantar aponeurosis is continuous with the plantar fascia covering the abductor hallucis.
- A lateral intermuscular septum projects from the lateral margin of plantar aponeurosis. It is attached to the fibrous sheath of peroneus longus tendon and the fifth metatarsal bone.
- A medial intermuscular septum projects from the medial margin of the plantar aponeurosis. It is attached to a large number of ligaments, tarsal bones and fascia over the muscles and tendons.

Function

The plantar aponeurosis gives protection to the plantar nerves and blood vessels.

It provides support to the arches of foot.

> **CLINICAL CORRELATION**
>
> - Chronic inflammation of the posterior bony attachment of the plantar aponeurosis (at its apex) is called plantar fasciitis. This causes pain in the heel. This condition is common in people, who have to stand for long stretches
> - Plantar fascia may tear at its apex. This is more common in policemen hence called policeman's heel
> - Ossification at the apex of the aponeurosis leads to formation of calcanean spur.

Fibrous Flexor Sheath

The deep fascia over the toes is modified to form a fibrous flexor sheath, which along with the phalanx gives rise to an osseofibrous tunnel for the flexor tendons in each digit.

Proximally, the fibrous sheath is continuous with the fibrous slips of plantar aponeurosis. It is attached to the margins of the phalanges and to the base of terminal phalanx. The sheath contains long and short flexor tendons surrounded by synovial sheath in each of the lateral four toes. In the sheath of great toe there is only one tendon of flexor hallucis longus lined by synovial sheath.

The function of the fibrous flexor sheath is to restrain the flexor tendons during movements of the toes.

Muscles of the Sole

The intrinsic muscles of the sole (total 18) and tendons of muscles of leg (total 4) passing through the sole are arranged into four layers from superficial to the deep aspect of the sole. The nerves and vessels travel through two neurovascular planes in the sole. The first neurovascular plane lies between the first and second layers of muscles

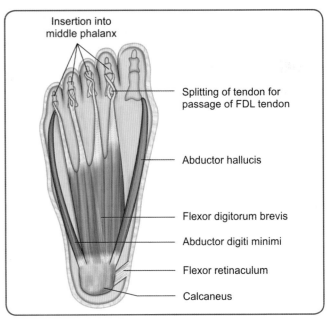

Fig. 32.8: Muscles in the first layer of sole

while the second neurovascular plane lies between the third and fourth layers.

Muscles in First Layer (Fig. 32.8)

There are three muscles in the first layer:
1. Abductor hallucis
2. Flexor digitorum brevis
3. Abductor digiti minimi

Abductor hallucis

This muscle lies along the medial margin of the foot.
- **Origin:** From medial tubercle of calcaneus and flexor retinaculum.
- **Insertion:** Into plantar surface and partly in to the medial surface of the base of the proximal phalanx of big toe after fusing with lateral tendon of insertion of flexor hallucis brevis.
- **Nerve Supply:** By a twig from trunk of medial plantar nerve.
- **Action:** Abduction of big toe (to move it away from second toe) and flexion of big toe.

Flexor digitorum brevis

The flexor digitorum brevis lies immediately deep to the plantar aponeurosis.
- **Tendinous origin:** From medial tubercle of calcaneus and from plantar aponeurosis.
- **Insertion:** Distally it divides into four tendons for the lateral four toes. Each tendon enters the fibrous flexor

sheath along with the tendon of flexor digitorum longus. At the base of proximal phalanx the tendon of flexor digitorum longus perforates the tendon of flexor digitorum brevis, which divides again to get inserted in to both sides of the plantar surface of the middle phalanx.

Note: The mode of insertion of the flexor digitorum brevis is similar to that of flexor digitorum superficialis of the hand.

- *Nerve Supply:* By a twig from the trunk of the medial plantar nerve
- *Action:* Flexion of lateral four toes.

Abductor digiti minimi

This muscle lies along the lateral margin of the foot.
- *Origin:* From the lateral and medial tubercles of calcaneus and from plantar aponeurosis.
- *Insertion:* In to the lateral side of proximal phalanx of little toe.
- *Nerve Supply:* By a twig from the lateral plantar nerve.
- *Actions:* Flexion and abduction of little toe.

Long Flexor Tendons and Muscles in Second Layer

1. The tendons of flexor hallucis longus and of flexor digitorum longus.
2. Lumbrical muscles and flexor digitorum accessorius (Fig. 32.9).

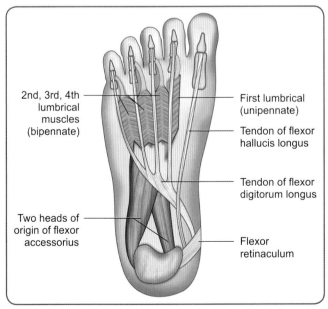

Fig. 32.9: Muscles and tendons in the second layer of sole

Labels:
2nd, 3rd, 4th lumbrical muscles (bipennate)
First lumbrical (unipennate)
Tendon of flexor hallucis longus
Tendon of flexor digitorum longus
Two heads of origin of flexor accessorius
Flexor retinaculum

Long flexor tendons

There is a crossing of the tendons of flexor digitorum longus and flexor hallucis longus in the second layer, during which the long flexor tendon of flexor hallucis longus gives few fibers through the William Turner's slip to the common tendon of flexor digitorum longus.

The common tendon of flexor digitorum longus receives insertion of the flexor digitorum accessorius.

The four tendons of flexor digitorum longus give origin to four lumbrical muscles.

Flexor digitorum accessorius

- *Origin by two heads:* Fleshy medial head from medial surface of calcaneus and tendinous lateral head from the lateral tubercle of calcaneus.
- *Insertion:* Into lateral side of the common tendon of FDL.
- *Nerve supply:* A branch from the trunk of lateral plantar nerve.
- *Actions:* Flexor digitorum accessorius straightens the oblique pull of action of the flexor digitorum longus on the lateral four toes. It assists in the plantarflexion of the same toes.

Lumbrical muscles

There are four lumbrical muscles, which are numbered from medial to lateral side. The first lumbrical is unipennate whereas the remaining three are bipennate muscles.
- *Origin:* From the tendon of flexor digitorum longus (Fig. 32.9).
- *Insertion:* Each lumbrical ends in a tiny tendon, which curves round the medial side of the corresponding metatarsophalangeal joint and is inserted into the extensor expansion and through it into the base of middle and terminal phalanges of lateral four toes. In this way, the first lumbrical is inserted into the extensor expansion of second toe, the second into third toe, the third into fourth toe and the fourth into the fifth toe.
- *Nerve Supply:* first lumbrical by medial plantar nerve and the other three by deep branch of lateral plantar nerve.
- *Actions:* Flexion at metatarsophalangeal joint and extension of inter-phalangeal joints.

Muscles in the Third Layer (Fig. 32.10)

The third layer consists of three muscles, flexor hallucis brevis, adductor hallucis, and flexor digiti minimi brevis.

Flexor hallucis brevis

- *Origin by two heads:* From medial part of the plantar surface of cuboid bone and from the lateral cuneiform bone.

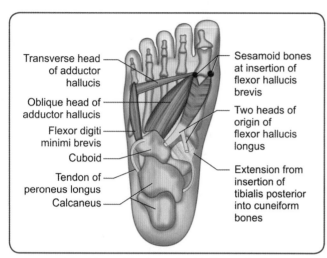

Fig. 32.10: Muscles in the third layer of sole

- **Insertion:** Distally the common muscle belly ends into two tendons, which are inserted into the respective side of the base of proximal phalanx of big toe.

A well-developed sesamoid bone occurs in each tendon near its insertion.

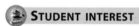 **STUDENT INTEREST**

This muscle has two heads of origin and two tendons of insertion of which medial tendon blends with abductor hallucis and lateral tendon with adductor hallucis and its tendons of insertion contain two sesamoid bones.

- **Nerve Supply:** A branch of medial plantar nerve
- **Actions:** Flexion of proximal phalanx of big toe.

Adductor hallucis

- **Origin by two head:** Smaller transverse head from plantar aspect of the metatarsophalangeal joints of third, fourth and fifth toes and larger oblique head from the plantar aspect of the bases of second, third and fourth metatarsal bones.
- **Insertion:** By common tendon in to the lateral part of the base of proximal phalanx of big toe after fusing with lateral tendon of insertion of flexor hallucis brevis.
- **Nerve Supply:** A branch from deep branch of lateral plantar nerve.
- **Action:** Adduction of big toe.

Flexor digiti minimi brevis

- **Origin:** From medial part of plantar aspect of the base of fifth metatarsal bone.
- **Insertion:** Into lateral side of the base of the proximal phalanx of little toe.

- **Nerve Supply:** By superficial branch of lateral plantar nerve.
- **Action:** Flexion of proximal phalanx of little toe.

Muscles and Tendons in Fourth Layer

The fourth layer contains four dorsal interossei (which are bipennate) and three palmar interossei (which are unipennate) in addition to the tendons of peroneus longus and tibialis posterior muscles.

Interossei muscles of foot

The interossei muscles are located between the metatarsal bones. They are numbered from medial to lateral side.

Plantar interossei (Fig. 32.11A)

- **Origin:** From medial sides of the shafts of 3rd to 5th metatarsal bones.
- **Insertion:** Into medial side of the base of the proximal phalanx of its own digit and partly into the extensor expansion.

Dorsal interossei (Fig. 32.11B)

- **Origin:** From the adjacent sides of shafts of 1 to 5 metatarsal bones.
- **Insertion:** Each dorsal interosseous muscle ends in a tendon, which is inserted into the proximal phalanx and the extensor expansion as follows.

1st on medial side of proximal phalanx of second toe, 2nd, 3rd and 4th on lateral sides of proximal phalanges of 2nd, 3rd and 4th toes

Nerve supply of interossei

All interossei of foot are supplied by lateral plantar nerve as follows:

- Superficial branch of lateral plantar nerve supplies the interossei of the fourth space (third plantar and fourth dorsal).
- Deep branch of lateral plantar nerve supplies the remaining interossei.

Dorsal interossei of first and second spaces receive additional twigs from the deep peroneal nerve.

Actions

The action of the interossei takes place around an axis passing through the second toe.

- The plantar interossei adduct the toes toward the second toe.
- The dorsal interossei abduct the toes away from the second toe.
- In the case of the second toe either the lateral or medial movement is abduction.
- The interossei and the lumbricals bring about the extension of interphalangeal joints and the flexion of metatarsophalangeal joints.

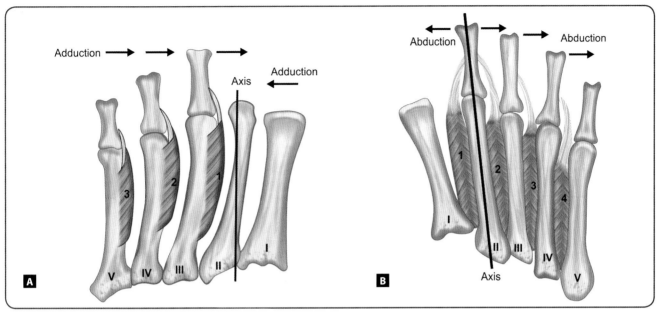

Figs 32.11A and B: A. Plantar interossei (Unipennate) and **B.** Dorsal interossei (Bipennate)

ARTERIES OF SOLE (FIG. 32.12)

The medial plantar artery, lateral plantar artery and the plantar arch supply the structures in the sole.

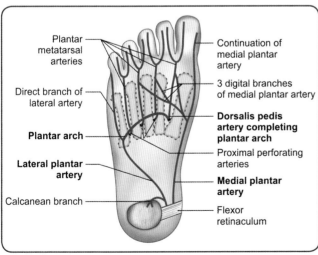

Fig. 32.12: Lateral and medial plantar arteries and plantar arterial arch

Medial Plantar Artery

This is the smaller terminal branch of the posterior tibial artery. It begins deep to the flexor retinaculum and enters the sole under cover of the abductor hallucis along with the medial plantar nerve. It courses forward lying in the interval between the abductor hallucis and flexor digitorum brevis.

Branches

- Cutaneous branches to the skin of the medial side of sole.
- Muscular branches.
- One superficial digital branch arises from the lateral side of medial plantar artery and trifurcates in to three digital branches, which join the first, second and third plantar metatarsal arteries (branches of plantar arch).

  The medial plantar artery (diminished in caliber after giving off muscular and superficial digital branch) continues along the medial side of big toe to anastomose with the digital branch of the first plantar metatarsal artery to the medial side of big toe.

Lateral Plantar Artery

This is the larger terminal branch of the posterior tibial artery. It begins deep to the flexor retinaculum. It enters the sole under cover of the abductor hallucis muscle along with the lateral plantar nerve.

Parts of Lateral Plantar Artery

- First part is the lateral plantar artery proper coursing between the first and second layers of sole
- Second part takes major share in the formation of plantar arch, coursing between the third and fourth layers of sole.

Course and relations of first part

The lateral plantar artery (with the accompanying nerve) runs in lateral and oblique direction lying between the flexor digitorum brevis (the muscle of first layer of sole) and the flexor accessorius (the muscle of the second layer of sole). It reaches the base of the fifth metatarsal bone on the lateral margin of the foot, where the first part ends.

Branches of first part

- Muscular branches
- Cutaneous branches to the lateral half of the sole
- Anastomotic branches, which join the lateral malleolar network
- Fifth plantar metatarsal artery.

Plantar Arch (Second Part of Lateral Plantar Artery)

The lateral plantar artery turns deep (superior) and runs in the medial direction across the sole lying plantar (inferior) to the bases of the metatarsal bones. This part of the artery is called the plantar arch. It ends by joining the termination of dorsalis pedis artery (in the first intermetatarsal space).

The plantar arch thus, extends from the base of the fifth metatarsal bone to the proximal end of the first intermetatarsal space and travelling between the muscles of the third and fourth layers. The plantar arch presents a concavity proximally and convexity distally. The deep branch of the lateral plantar nerve lies in the concavity of the plantar arch.

Branches of plantar arch (Fig. 32.12)

- Three proximal perforating arteries ascend through proximal parts of 2nd, 3rd and 4th inter-metatarsal spaces and join the corresponding dorsal metatarsal arteries.
- 1st, 2nd, 3rd and 4th plantar metatarsal arteries are called the common plantar digital arteries after uniting with the digital branches of medial plantar artery. The distal perforating arteries take origin from distal part of each plantar metatarsal artery. It joins to the distal part of the dorsal metatarsal artery.
- The proper plantar digital arteries are formed by division of common plantar arteries for the supply of

adjacent sides of 1st and 2nd toes, 2nd and 3rd toes, 3rd and 4th toes and 4th and 5th toes.

Note: The first plantar metatarsal artery sends a proper plantar digital artery to the medial side of the big toe (which anastomoses with continuation of medial plantar artery). The lateral side of the little toe receives a proper plantar digital branch directly from the lateral plantar artery.

> ### CLINICAL CORRELATION
>
> **Bleeding Wounds of Plantar Arch**
>
> It is difficult to control the bleeding from the plantar arch by direct ligature due to its deep location. The immediate treatment consists of compression of the femoral artery. The compression of anterior tibial alone or posterior tibial alone or of both the tibial arteries may not be effective due to presence of anastomoses around the ankle, in which the peroneal artery also takes part.

VEINS OF SOLE

The veins in the sole accompany the arterial trunks and their branches. The venae comitantes accompanying the lateral and medial plantar arteries unite deep to the flexor retinaculum to form the venae comitantes accompanying the posterior tibial artery.

NERVES OF SOLE

The sole of the foot contains the lateral and medial plantar nerves, which are the terminal branches of the tibial nerve. They begin deep to the flexor retinaculum. They enter the sole with the lateral and medial plantar arteries under cover of the abductor hallucis.

Medial Plantar Nerve (Fig. 32.13)

This is the larger terminal branch of the tibial nerve. At first it passes deep to the abductor hallucis along the medial margin of the foot and then appears between abductor hallucis and flexor digitorum brevis. It ends by dividing in to proper digital branch to big toe and three common digital plantar branches. It gives cutaneous, muscular and articular branches.

Branches from the Trunk of Medial Plantar Nerve

- Cutaneous branches to the skin of medial half of sole
- Muscular branches to abductor hallucis and flexor digitorum brevis.

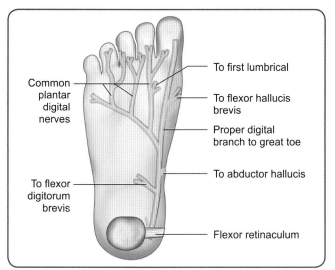

Fig. 32.13: Course and distribution of medial plantar nerve

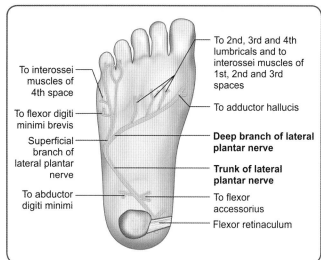

Fig. 32.14: Course and distribution of medial plantar nerve

Branches and Distribution of Terminal Branches

- Proper digital branch to big toe supplies a muscular branch to the flexor hallucis brevis and the skin of medial side of big toe
- Three common plantar digital nerves supply the adjacent sides of 1st and 2nd, 2nd and 3rd and 3rd and 4th toes. The first common plantar digital nerve supplies a muscular branch to the first lumbrical.

  All proper digital nerves supply the skin of the plantar aspect of the toes and also the nail bed on the dorsal aspect of the toes.

- Articular branches arise from the trunk and digital nerves for the supply joints.

 STUDENT INTEREST

Sensory distribution of toes by medial plantar nerve (medial three and half toes) is similar to that of median nerve in the hand except that median nerve supplies lateral three and half fingers)

CLINICAL CORRELATION

- Morton's metatarsalgia is a condition in which a neurofibroma occurs on the digital nerve supplying the adjacent sides of third and fourth toes. The pressure of the tight fitting shoe may be the cause of this condition, which causes severe pain in the third and fourth toes
- Medial plantar nerve may be compressed at flexor retinaculum(tarsal tunnel syndrome) or under the abductor hallucis muscle.

Lateral Plantar Nerve (Fig. 32.14)

The lateral plantar nerve is the smaller terminal branch of the tibial nerve. It begins deep to the flexor retinaculum. It enters the sole under cover of abductor hallucis and then passes forward and laterally across the sole in oblique direction to reach the tuberosity of the fifth metatarsal bone, where it divides into superficial and deep branches. During its oblique course it lies between the flexor accessorius muscle of the second layer and the flexor digitorum brevis muscle of the first layer. At its termination, the lateral plantar nerve lies between the flexor digitorum brevis and the abductor digiti minimi. It gives cutaneous and muscular branches.

Branches of the Trunk of Lateral Plantar Nerve

- Muscular branches to flexor digitorum accessorius and abductor digiti minimi
- Cutaneous branches to the lateral part of the sole.

Superficial Branch of Lateral Plantar Nerve

The superficial branch runs distally along the lateral border of sole and divides into two common plantar digital nerves. It is a mixed nerve.

- Lateral common plantar digital nerve supplies three muscles, namely, flexor digiti minimi brevis, fourth dorsal interosseous and third plantar interosseous and skin of lateral side of little toe
- Medial common plantar digital nerve often connects with the third common plantar digital branch of the medial plantar nerve. It divides in to proper plantar digital nerves for the adjacent sides of the fourth and fifth toes.

Deep Branch of Lateral Plantar Nerve

The deep branch turns medially from the base of fifth metatarsal bone and travels across the sole between the muscles of the third and fourth layers of sole to terminate into the adductor hallucis muscle.

Branches and Distribution

The deep branch of lateral plantar nerve is purely motor. It supplies a nine muscles of sole listed below:

1. Lateral three lumbricals
2. First, second and third dorsal interossei
3. First and second plantar interossei
4. Adductor hallucis.

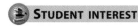 **STUDENT INTEREST**

> The distribution of lateral plantar nerve is comparable to ulnar nerve in the hand. Through its superficial and deep branches it supplies 12 muscles in foot and sensory supply via superficial branch to lateral one and half toes)

JOINTS OF FOOT

There are numerous joints between the tarsal, metatarsal and phalangeal bones of the foot (Fig. 32.15). They include inter-phalangeal, metatarsophalangeal, tarsometatarsal, intermetatarsal and intertarsal joints.

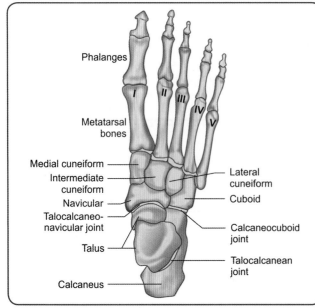

Fig. 32.15: Skeleton of the foot

Intertarsal Joints

The intertarsal joints are divided into two subtypes as follows:

Major Intertarsal Joints

- Subtalar or posterior talocalcanean joint
- Talocalcaneonavicular joint
- Calcaneocuboid joint.

Note: Talocalcaneonavicular and calcaneocuboid joints together form midtarsal or transverse tarsal joint.

The major intertarsal joints allow movements of inversion and eversion of foot.

Small Intertarsal Joints

- Cuneonavicular joint
- Cuboideonavicular joint
- Cuneocuboid joint
- Intercuneiform joints

The small joints of the foot provide certain amount of resilience to the tarsus but the amount of movement is very small.

Subtalar joint

The subtalar joint is the posterior talocalcanean joint belonging to the plane variety of synovial joint. It is an articulation between the concave posterior facet on the inferior surface of the body of talus and the convex posterior facet on the superior surface of calcaneus. The joint is surrounded by fibrous capsule.

Ligaments

- Lateral and medial talocalcanean ligaments strengthen the joint on each side.
- Interosseous talocalcanean ligament is a bilaminar band, which occupies the sinus tarsi (tarsal canal). It descends obliquely from the sulcus tali to sulcus calcanei and separates the talocalcaneonavicular and posterior talocalcanlean joints
- Cervical ligament is lateral to the sinus tarsi and extends from the upper surface of calcaneus to the inferolateral tubercle of the neck of talus.

Talocalcaneonavicular joint

The talocalcaneonavicular joint is a compound joint consisting of anterior talocalcanean and talonavicular articulations. It is a ball and socket type of synovial joint.

The articular surface of the rounded head of the talus fits in to the socket formed by the posterior surface of navicular bone and the middle and anterior talar facets on the calcaneus along with the superior surface of the spring ligament.

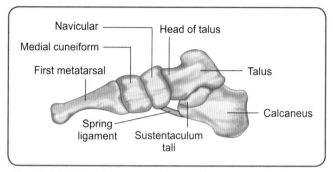

Fig. 32.16: Spring ligament or plantar calcaneonavicular ligament

A fibrous capsule surrounds the articulating bones. The synovial cavity of this joint is separate from the other joints.

Ligaments

- Plantar calcaneonavicular spring ligament (Fig. 32.16)
- Calcaneonavicular part of bifurcate ligament (connecting the calcaneus to the navicular bone).

Spring ligament (Plantar calcaneonavicular ligament)

The spring ligament is a powerful ligament.

Attachments

- **Anteriorly:** To plantar surface of navicular bone
- **Posteriorly:** To anterior margin of sustentaculum tali
- **Upper surface:** Bears a fibrocartilaginous facet, which supports the infero-medial part of the head of talus
- **Lower surface:** Is supported by tendon of tibialis posterior muscle
- **Medial margin:** Gives attachment to the deltoid ligament of the ankle joint.

The spring ligament is the most important ligament in the foot as it maintains the medial longitudinal arch by supporting the head of talus. It provides resilience to the medial longitudinal arch.

Bifurcate ligament

The bifurcate ligament is Y shaped with a stem and two limbs. The stem is attached to anterior part of upper surface of calcaneus. The medial limb is called calcaneonavicular ligament and lateral limb is called calcaneocuboid ligament. The former supports the talocalcaneonavicular joint and the latter supports the calcaneocuboid joint.

Calcaneocuboid joint

The calcaneocuboid joint is a saddle variety of synovial joint having independent synovial cavity. The bones taking part in this joint are the anterior surface of calcaneus and the posterior surface of cuboid. The joint lies along the lateral side of foot.

Ligaments

- Long plantar ligament is the longest ligament, which extends from the plantar surface of calcaneus to the plantar surface of cuboid and beyond it to the bases of the three metatarsal bones (second to fourth). It converts the groove on the plantar surface of cuboid in a tunnel for the tendon of peroneus longus
- Short plantar ligament is called the plantar calcaneocuboid ligament. It lies superior to the long plantar ligament. It stretches from the anterior tubercle of the calcaneus to the adjoining part of cuboid
- Calcaneocuboid part of bifurcate ligament extends from the stem of the bifurcate ligament to the dorsal aspect of cuboid.

MOVEMENTS OF THE FOOT

Inversion and Eversion

The inversion and eversion are the movements of the foot, which take place at the subtalar and midtarsal (talocalcaneonavicular and calcaneocuboid) joints. These movements occur along an oblique axis and are basically rotation movements of the foot on the talus.

Definition

- Inversion is defined as a movement in which the medial border of the foot is raised and the sole faces medially. Inversion is accompanied by plantarflexion and adduction of forefoot
- Eversion is defined as a movement in which the lateral border of the foot is raised and the sole faces laterally. Eversion id accompanied by dorsiflexion and abduction of forefoot.

💡 **ADDED INFORMATION**

Movements when the Foot is off the Ground

The degree of inversion is greater when the foot is off the ground. Inversion is a combination of adduction of forefoot, lateral rotation or supination of forefoot and plantarflexion at ankle. Similarly the degree of eversion is also greater when the foot is off the ground. Eversion is a combination of abduction of the forefoot, medial rotation or pronation of forefoot and dorsiflexion at the ankle.

Movements when the Foot is on the Ground

When the foot is on the ground it is bearing the weight of the body. Therefore inversion and eversion are more restricted. They consist of only one movement and that is lateral rotation or supination of the forefoot in inversion and medial rotation or pronation of the forefoot in eversion. Pronation raises the heads of lateral metatarsals and supination raises the heads of medial one or two metatarsals. This type of rotation allows us to stand upright on a sloping ground.

Functional Importance

The movements of inversion and eversion are necessary while walking on uneven and sloping ground. They enable the body to move sideways over the foot while the foot is fixed. It is not possible to reproduce the movements of inversion and eversion in an artificial limb. Therefore, an amputee wearing an artificial limb finds difficulty in walking on uneven ground.

Muscles Producing Inversion

They pass medial to the axis of rotation. Tibialis anterior and tibialis posterior are the main invertors of the foot (assisted by flexor digitorum longus and flexor hallucis longus).

Muscles Producing Eversion

They pass lateral to the axis of rotation. The peroneus longus, brevis are the main evertors of the foot (assisted by peroneus tertius).

ARCHES OF FOOT

The human foot is aptly described as an architectural marvel. Its construction is the best example of the structural adaptation to function. The foot has two major functions. It supports the body weight during standing and progression and it acts as a lever to propel the body forwards during walking, running and jumping. To fulfill the first function the foot must be pliable to withstand the stresses and to fulfill its second function it must be transformable into a lever. A segmented arched lever converts the foot in to a spring to make it ideally suited for its functions. The bones of the foot are arranged in the form of longitudinal and transverse arches (Figs 32.17A and B).

The arches of the foot are present from birth. Due to the presence of subcutaneous fat the arching is not apparent during infancy and childhood. Gradually the plantar surface acquires the concave appearance and the characteristic footprint with weight bearing points on sole is evolved.

Functions of Arches

The medial longitudinal arch functions as a propulsive force during locomotion being more elastic and dynamic. The lateral longitudinal arch functions as a static organ of support and weight transmission. Besides this the arches act as shock absorbers. The concavity of the arches provides protection to the deeply located nerves and vessels of the sole.

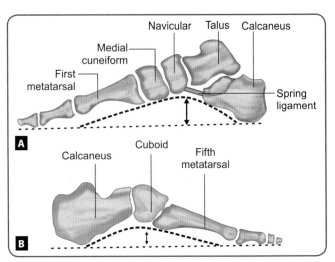

Figs 32.17A and B: A. Medial view of medial longitudinal arch **B.** Lateral view of lateral longitudinal arch

Types of Arches

- Longitudinal arches are medial and lateral
- Transverse arch is present as half arch per foot. Only when the two feet are held close to each other the transverse arch becomes complete.

Parts of Longitudinal Arches

The longitudinal arches have anterior and posterior pillars, summit and joints. The supports of the arches are more or less similar to the mechanical supports of the overhead bridges.

Medial longitudinal arch (Fig. 32.17A)

The bones of the medial longitudinal arch from behind forward are calcaneus, talus, navicular, cuneiform bones and medial three metatarsal bones including the two sesamoid bones under the head of the first metatarsal bone.

- **Posterior pillar:** Short and sturdy calcaneus.
- **Summit:** Head of the talus (keystone of medial longitudinal arch).
- **Anterior pillar:** Heads of medial three metatarsal bones and the sesamoid bones in the tendons of flexor hallucis brevis.

The medial longitudinal arch is taller than the lateral. It is more dynamic and pliant due to the presence of joints in this arch (such as talocalcaneonavicular and subtalar joints).

Supports of medial arch (Fig. 32.18)

- The summit of the arch (head of the talus) transfers the body weight to the other bones of the foot. Therefore,

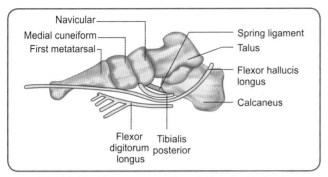

Fig. 32.18: Main supports of medial longitudinal arch

support to the talus is very important. The head of the talus is held in a socket provided by the navicular, sustentaculum tali and the spring ligament. The combination of the spring ligament and the underlying tibialis posterior tendon forms a dynamic support to the head. Additionally, flexor hallucis longus and flexor digitorum longus assist

- The anterior and posterior pillars of the medial arch are held together by the plantar aponeurosis, abductor hallucis and flexor hallucis brevis. These structures act as tie beams of the arch

- The combined action of the tendon of tibialis anterior and deltoid ligament of the ankle joint is to exert a sling action from above. The slips of insertion of the tibialis posterior in all the tarsal bones (except the talus) provide the support from below.

Lateral longitudinal arch (Fig. 32.17B)

The bones forming the lateral longitudinal arch from behind forwards are calcaneus, cuboid and lateral two metatarsals. This arch being very short almost touches the ground. The heads of lateral two metatarsal bones form the anterior pillar while the posterior pillar is the calcaneus. The calcaneocuboid joint is the important joint in this arch. The lateral arch being lower and less mobile than the medial is adapted to transmit weight and thrusts.

Supports of lateral arch

The long plantar and short plantar (plantar calcaneocuboid) ligaments are the main ligamentous supports of this arch. The plantar aponeurosis and the intrinsic muscles of little toe function as tie beam of this arch. The tendons of peroneus brevis and tertius, which are inserted in to the base of the fifth metatarsal bone act as slings from above. The tendon of peroneus longus, which grooves the cuboid and courses transversely across the sole, provides the support to the cuboid bone (and the calcaneocuboid joint) from above, through its pulley like action (Fig. 32.19).

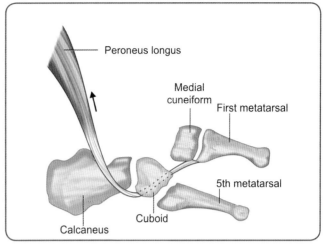

Fig. 32.19: Support provided by peroneus longus tendon to the lateral longitudinal arch

Transverse arch

Each foot is composed of a series of transverse arches. The bony components of the transverse arch are the bases of the metatarsals and the cuboid and the three cuneiform bones. The factors that maintain the transverse arch are the interosseous ligaments and the dorsal interossei muscles. The tendon of peroneus longus and the adductor hallucis muscle play a major role in support to this arch.

📖 STUDENT INTEREST

Arches of foot is an essay or short answer question in theory paper. The important joints and ligaments of the foot must be understood to know the arches of foot. Learn definitions of inversion and eversion and do not confuse the movements of ankle joint (dorsiflexion and plantar flexion) and movement of subtalar and midtarsal joints (inversion and eversion).

🔖 CLINICAL CORRELATION

Deformities of Foot

- Pes planus or flat foot is due to collapse of medial longitudinal arch. The support to the head of the talus is lost hence it is pushed downward between the calcaneus and navicular bones. During long periods of standing, the plantar aponeurosis and other plantar ligaments including the spring ligament are overstretched, which may gradually result in flattening of the medial longitudinal arch with lateral deviation of foot. A person with flat foot has clumsy gait with susceptibility to trauma. The nerves and vessels of sole are compressed, which produces pain and swelling of foot

Contd...

Contd…

Contd…

🎼 CLINICAL CORRELATION

- Pes cavus means highly arched foot. It is associated with claw foot in which there is dorsiflexion of metatarsophalangeal joints and plantarflexion of interphalangeal joints.
- Rocker bottom feet are the ones in which there is plantar convexity. This is found in babies born with trisomy 18 (Edward syndrome).
- The hallux valgus refers to the deformity in which the big toe passes transversely under the second toe (Fig. 32.20) and there is abnormal prominence of head of first metatarsal bone on the medial side of the foot, just behind the big toe. There is collapse of the transverse arch due to varus position of first metatarsal bone. The exposed and prominent head of first metatarsal tends to rub on the shoe, giving rise to an adventitious bursa called bunion. The patient experiences pain and fatigue in the foot during routine walking.
- Talipes is a Latin word meaning clubfoot. There are different types of talipes. In talipes equinus, the foot is plantarflexed and the person walks on toes(like a horse). In talipes calcaneus, the foot is dorsiflexed and the person walks on heel. In talipes varus the foot is inverted and the person walks on lateral margin of foot. In talipes valgus, the foot is everted and the person walks on medial margin of foot.
- In talipes equinovarus deformity, the foot is held in plantarflexed and inverted position due to paralysis of dorsiflexors and evertors (for example due to injury to common peroneal nerve).
- The hammertoe deformity is produced due to paralysis of lumbricals and interossei. There is hyperextension at the metatarsophalangeal joints, hyperflexion of proximal interphalangeal joints and extension at the distal interphalangeal joints in lateral four toes.

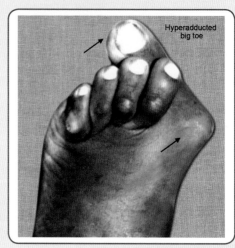

Fig. 32.20: Hallux valgus deformity of big toe and adventitious bursa or bunion on the head of first metatarsal bone

💡 ADDED INFORMATION

Development of Arteries of Lower Limb

The fifth lumbar segmental artery enters the embryonic lower limb bud and its remnants are the following arteries of definitive stage.
- Inferior gluteal artery
- Companion artery of sciatic nerve (branch of inferior gluteal artery)
- Popliteal artery
- Peroneal artery
- Plantar arch.

33

Clinicoanatomical Problems and Solutions

CASE 1

A patient with 4 gm hemoglobin was given intramuscular injections of iron in the gluteal region. After a few weeks, the patient complained of difficulty while stepping on the right foot while walking. Clinical examination revealed sensory loss in the intermediate area of the dorsum of right foot and dorsum of all toes except lateral side of little toe and first interdigital cleft. The patient experienced difficulty in dorsiflexing and everting the right foot.

Questions and Solutions

1. Name the nerve that is injured by the injection needle in the gluteal region.

Ans. Sciatic nerve is injured due to inadvertent injection.

2. Name the two components of this nerve giving the root value of each.

Ans. i. Tibial or medial part (L4, L5, S1, S2, S3)
ii. Common peroneal or lateral part (L4, L5, S1, S2)

3. Which component is injured in the above patient based on the symptoms and signs?

Ans. Common peroneal component is injured.

4. Explain sensory and motor loss in the above patient.

Ans. When the common peroneal component of sciatic nerve is injured it amounts to loss of function of its terminal branches (deep peroneal and superficial peroneal nerves). The sensory loss experienced by the patient is typical of injury to superficial peroneal nerve. Difficulty in eversion is due to loss of motor supply of peroneus longus and brevis (supplied by superficial peroneal nerve). Difficulty in dorsiflexion of foot is due to loss of motor supply of tibialis anterior, extensor hallucis longus and extensor digitorum longus muscles in the extensor compartment of leg (supplied by deep peroneal nerve).

CASE 2

A 55-year-old policeman with a history of chronic dull ache in both legs came to the hospital, when he noticed dilated and tortuous veins on the medial side of his both legs. The skin on the medial malleolus was found to be discolored, dry and scaly.

Questions and Solutions

1. Name the clinical condition mentioning the vein involved.

Ans. Bilateral varicose veins (varicosity) of lower limb due to dilatation of long saphenous veins.

2. What is the relation of this vein to medial malleolus?

Ans. It ascends 2.5 cm in front of medial malleolus.

3. Name the closely related cutaneous nerve to this vein in this location.

Ans. Saphenous nerve

4. Name the veins that connect it to the deep veins of lower limb.

Ans. Perforating veins connect the superficial and deep veins in leg and thigh.

5. What is the direction of flow of blood in the connecting veins?

Ans. From superficial veins to deep veins

6. What is the sharp margin of saphenous opening called?

Ans. Falciform margin

CASE 3

A 78-year-old woman was not able to move her right lower limb after a minor fall. On examination it was noted that the toes of her right foot were pointing laterally. On measuring the length, the right limb was found to be shorter. X-ray showed intra-capsular fracture of femoral neck and general osteoporosis.

Questions and Solutions

1. What is the reason for shortening of right lower limb in this patient?

Ans. Contraction of hamstrings, rectus femoris and adductor muscles pulls the shaft of femur upwards.

2. What is the reason for the characteristic position of the right foot?

Ans. The thigh is laterally rotated by contraction of gluteus maximus and short lateral rotators of thigh. In fracture of neck of femur, the psoas major muscle also becomes lateral rotator due to shift in its axis.

3. What is the serious complication of this type of fracture?

Ans. Avascular necrosis of femur occurs due to rupture of the retinacular arteries that pass along the neck of femur.

CASE 4

A football player, on receiving a blow on the lateral side of the right knee, felt a sharp pain in the knee. The knee was swollen especially above the patella. The drawer signs were negative. Radiological examination did not show any fracture.

Questions and Solutions

1. Which intra-articular structure is torn in this patient?

Ans. Medial meniscus

2. Name the type of tear that usually occurs in it in the sports injury.

Ans. Bucket handle tear

3. What are components of the 'unhappy triad' of knee joint?

Ans. i. Rupture of anterior cruciate ligament
ii. Tear of medial meniscus
iii. Injury to tibial collateral ligament

4. What is suprapatellar bursa? Which muscle is inserted into it?

Ans. Suprapatellar bursa is an extension of the synovial cavity above the patella and behind the quadriceps tendon in the thigh. Articularis genu is inserted into it.

5. What is housemaid's knee?

Ans. Inflammation of prepatellar bursa is called housemaid's knee.

CASE 5

A 50 year old woman came to the hospital, when she noticed a lemon sized swelling in the upper thigh. On examination, the swelling was found to be inferior and lateral to the pubic tubercle and it was seen to push in to the saphenous opening.

Questions and Solutions

1. Which hernia gives rise to swelling below and lateral to pubic tubercle?

Ans. Femoral hernia

2. Name the passage through which the hernia enters the thigh.

Ans. Femoral canal

3. Give the name and the boundaries of the upper opening of the passage.

Ans. The femoral ring is the name of the upper opening of the passage. Its boundaries are: in front—inguinal ligament, medially—lacunar ligament, laterally—femoral vein the middle compartment of femoral sheath, posteriorly—pectineus and fascia.

4. Describe the direction of the hernia and the importance of this knowledge to the surgeon.

Ans. The femoral hernia at first comes downwards in the femoral canal then it goes anteriorly into the saphenous opening and finally turns upwards against the falciform margin of the saphenous opening. In manual reduction of the hernia the surgeon reverses the order by pushing the hernia, downwards, posteriorly and upwards.

CASE 6

A 20-year-old tennis player twisted his right foot while playing. He could not move his foot due to severe pain. On examination there was swelling of right ankle, black and blue discoloration on lateral side of ankle and restricted and painful movements. Radiographs of the right ankle showed no fracture of lower end of tibia, fibula and talus.

Questions and Solutions

1. Which ligament of ankle joint is commonly sprained?

Ans. Lateral collateral ligament of ankle joint

2. What are the parts of this ligament?

Ans. i. Anterior tibiofibular
ii. Posterior tibiofibular
iii. Calcaneofibular

3. Name the bones taking part in the ankle joint.

Ans. The bones, which take part in this articulation are—the lower end of tibia, lower end of fibula and the talus.

4. Name the ligament of inferior tibiofibular joint that deepens the tibiofibular socket of ankle joint.

Ans. Inferior transverse tibiofibular ligament

5. Explain foot drop.

Ans. Foot drop or drop foot is the deformity of foot in which the foot looks floppy (drooping downwards) causing difficulty in walking. There is loss of ability to raise the foot at the ankle joint (loss of dorsiflexion). The muscles in the anterior (extensor) compartment of leg (tibialis anterior, extensor digitorum longus and extensor hallucis longus are paralyzed due to injury to deep peroneal nerve (the nerve of anterior compartment of leg). Foot drop can also occur if common peroneal nerve is damaged at fibular neck or if sciatic nerve is injured in gluteal region.

SINGLE BEST RESPONSE TYPE MULTIPLE CHOICE QUESTIONS

1. Which of the following is not attached to fibula?
   a. Tibialis anterior
   b. Extensor hallucis longus
   c. Extensor digitorum longus
   d. Peroneus tertius

2. Which muscle is used for intramuscular injection in gluteal region?
   a. Gluteus maximus
   b. Gluteus medius
   c. Gluteus minimus
   d. Piriformis

3. Profunda femoris artery leaves the femoral triangle through:
   a. Apex
   b. Behind sartorius
   c. Between psoas major and pectineus
   d. Between pectineus and adductor longus

4. Which bursa is affected in Clergyman's knee?
   a. Prepatellar
   b. Suprapatellar
   c. Subcutaneous infrapatellar
   d. Deep infrapatellar bursa

5. Which is not a branch of common peroneal nerve?
   a. Lateral inferior genicular
   b. Recurrent genicular
   c. Sural
   d. Sural communicating

6. Femoral branch of genitofemoral nerve is located in:
   a. Femoral canal
   b. Inguinal canal
   c. Middle compartment of femoral sheath
   d. Lateral compartment of femoral sheath

7. Skin of the medial side of big toe is supplied by:
   a. Deep peroneal nerve
   b. Saphenous nerve
   c. Superficial peroneal nerve
   d. Sural nerve

8. Lateral cutaneous branches of the following pair of nerves enter the gluteal region:
   a. Subcostal and iliohypogastric
   b. 11th intercostal and subcostal
   c. Perforating cutaneous and ilioinguinal
   d. Iliohypogastric and ilioinguinal

9. Muscles of which of the following pair are supplied by same nerve?
   a. First lumbrical and second lumbrical of foot
   b. Popliteus and plantaris
   c. Superior gemellus and inferior gemellus
   d. Obturator externus and obturator internus

10. The structure that comes out of the lesser sciatic foramen is:
    a. Tendon of obturator internus
    b. Pudendal nerve
    c. Internal pudendal artery
    d. Nerve to obturator internus

11. Bucket handle tear usually occurs in:
    a. Lateral meniscus
    b. Anterior cruciate ligament
    c. Medial meniscus
    d. Posterior cruciate ligament

12. Ankle joint is most stable in following position:
    a. Fully dorsiflexed
    b. Partially dorsiflexed
    c. Fully plantarflexed
    d. Partially plantarflexed

13. Meniscofemoral ligaments are attached to which horn of the following meniscus?
    a. Anterior horn of lateral meniscus
    b. Posterior horn of lateral meniscus
    c. Anterior horn of medial meniscus
    d. Posterior horn of medial meniscus

14. Pes anserinus is the term used for insertion of the following muscles except:
    a. Semitendinosus
    b. Sartorius
    c. Semimembranosus
    d. Gracilis

15. Obturator artery is a branch of:
    a. External iliac artery
    b. Common iliac artery
    c. Posterior division of internal iliac artery
    d. Anterior division of internal iliac artery

16. Violent inversion of foot leads to avulsion of a tendon that is inserted into tuberosity of the fifth metatarsal bone. Identify the tendon that is avulsed:
    a. Peroneus brevis   b. Peroneus longus
    c. Peroneus tertius   d. Tibialis posterior

17. Which dermatome is located over the little toe?
   a. L4
   b. L5
   c. S1
   d. S2

18. Which of the following arteries would be compressed in posterior compartment syndrome of leg?
   a. Posterior tibial artery and anterior tibial artery
   b. Medial and lateral plantar arteries
   c. Popliteal artery and perforating branch of peroneal artery
   d. Posterior tibial and peroneal arteries

19. The surface marking of saphenous opening is:
   a. Superomedial to pubic tubercle
   b. Superolateral to pubic tubercle
   c. Three to four cm inferolateral to pubic tubercle
   d. Three to four cm lateral to pubic tubercle

20. Which nerve is tested by the lady medical student when she pinches the skin of a diabetic patient between big toe and second toe?
   a. Superficial peroneal
   b. Deep peroneal
   c. Sural
   d. Saphenous

KEY TO MCQ

1. a	**2.** b	**3.** d	**4.** c	**5.** c	**6.** d	**7.** c	**8.** a
9. b	**10.** a	**11.** c	**12.** c	**13.** b	**14.** c	**15.** d	**16.** a
17. c	**18.** d	**19.** c	**20.** b				

Section 5

THORAX

Bones of Thoracic Cage

Chapter Contents

INTRODUCTION

The thoracic cage is otherwise known as the skeleton of thorax. It is an osseocartilaginous cage that permits increase and decrease in capacity of thorax during respiratory movements.

BOUNDARIES OF THORACIC CAGE (FIG. 35.1)

- **Anteriorly:** Sternum
- **Posteriorly:** Anterior surfaces of the bodies of the twelve thoracic vertebrae and the intervening intervertebral discs.
- **On each side:** Twelve pairs of ribs with their costal cartilages.

All the ribs articulate posteriorly with vertebrae by costovertebral and costotransverse joints. Their anterior attachments are, however, different. The costal cartilages of upper seven ribs articulate with the sternum by sternocostal or chondrosternal joints. The costal cartilages of eighth to tenth ribs join each other and together with costal cartilage of seventh rib form the costal margin. The anterior ends of last two ribs tipped with costal cartilages are free.

The upper end of the thoracic cage is called **thoracic inlet**, which communicates the thoracic cavity with the root of the neck.

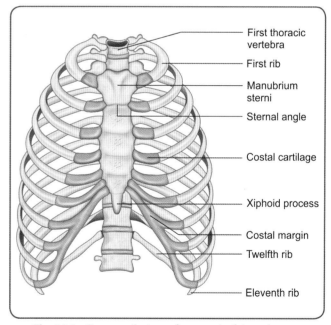

Fig. 34.1: Osseocartilaginous framework of thoracic cage

First thoracic vertebra
First rib
Manubrium sterni
Sternal angle
Costal cartilage
Xiphoid process
Costal margin
Twelfth rib
Eleventh rib

The lower end of the thoracic cage is called **thoracic outlet** (inferior thoracic aperture, which is closed in the living state by diaphragm).

The thoracic cavity provides protection to the main organs of respiration and circulation. As the lungs are constantly moving, the thoracic cage necessarily has to be resilient. The thoracic cage provides attachments to the muscles of respiration, which increase its volume during inspiration and decrease its volumes during expiration.

BONES OF THORAX

Sternum (Figs 34.2, 34.3A and B)

The sternum or the breast-bone is the axial bone located in the midline of the front of the chest. It is a flat bone consisting of rich red marrow. The sternum is easily palpable through the skin.

Parts of Sternum

The sternum consists of three parts. From above to downwards they are:
1. Manubrium sterni
2. Body
3. Pointed xiphoid process

Manubrium

The manubrium is the upper broadest and thickest part of the sternum. It has two surfaces and four margins.

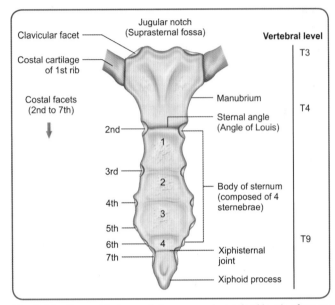

Fig. 34.2: General features of sternum and vertebral levels of upper margin of manubrium, sternal angle and xiphisternal joint

The anterior surface of manubrium is convex. It gives origin to pectoralis major and sternal head of sternomastoid muscles on each side.

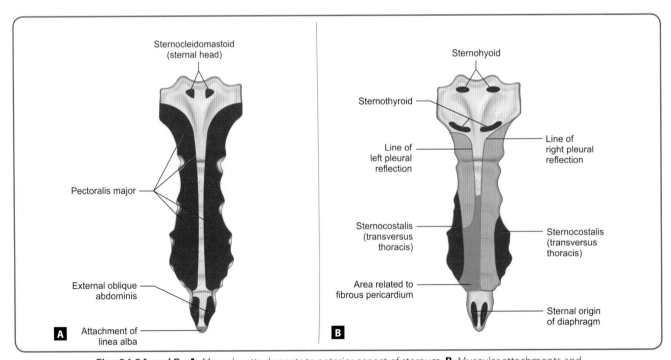

Figs 34.3A and B: **A.** Muscular attachments to anterior aspect of sternum; **B.** Muscular attachments and relations of posterior aspect of sternum

The posterior surface of manubrium forms the anterior boundary of superior mediastinum. This surface gives origin to two muscles of the neck, sternohyoid (at the level of clavicular notch) and sternothyroid (at the level of facet for first costal cartilage). The arch of aorta and its three branches are related to it. The left brachiocephalic vein crosses in front of the three branches, hence this vein is in danger of injury during sternal puncture. The anterior margins of lungs and anterior lines of pleural reflections are related to the lateral aspect of this surface.

 STUDENT INTEREST

> Note that two muscles (sternomastoid and pectoralis major) originate from the anterior surface of manubrium and two from its posterior surface (sternohyoid and sternothyroid). The sternohyoid muscle is attached above the sternothyroid as hyoid bone is above the thyroid cartilage in the neck.

The superior margin of manubrium is thick and rounded. The concavity in its middle is called **suprasternal notch** or **jugular notch**. The clavicular notch on each side of jugular notch articulates with sternal end of the clavicle to form sternoclavicular joint.

The inferior margin articulates with the body of sternum to form manubriosternal joint. There is a slight angulation of sternum at this joint. This angulation is called **sternal angle** or **angle of Louis**. The sternal angle articulates with the second costal cartilage on either side. The right and left lateral margins present a facet for articulation with first costal cartilage above and a demifacet for articulation with second costal cartilage below.

The muscles attached to the anterior and posterior surfaces of manubrium are shown in figures 34.3A and B.

Body

It is formed by the union of four sternebrae. It presents anterior and posterior surfaces and right and left lateral margins. Its upper end articulates with manubrium and lower end with xiphoid process.

The anterior surface of the body is marked by three ill defined transverse ridges indicating the fusion of the four sternebrae. It provides origin to pectoralis major muscle on either side (Fig. 34.3A).

The posterior surface of the body forms the anterior boundary of the anterior mediastinum. The lower part of the posterior surface gives origin to sternocostalis (transversus thoracis) on either side. The relations to lung and pleura and the pericardium are shown in figure 34.3B.

 CLINICAL CORRELATION

> In head-on collision, the steering wheel of the car may push through the body of sternum into the pericardium causing rupture of the heart and of ascending aorta of the driver. This is because of the close anatomical relation of the body of sternum to the fibrous pericardium.

Right and left margins

The right and left margins of the body are irregular due to presence of notches for the articulations with costal cartilages of second to seventh ribs.

Xiphoid process

It is the lower tapering part of sternum. It is cartilaginous in young age but by the age of forty it ossifies. It projects in the epigastrium of anterior abdominal wall. It gives attachments to some structures as shown in figures 34.3B and B.

Vertebral Levels of the Parts of Sternum

- **Upper margin of manubrium:** Third thoracic vertebra.
- **Lower margin of manubrium:** Lower margin of fourth thoracic vertebra.
- **Sternal body:** Fifth to ninth thoracic vertebrae.
- **Xiphisternal joint:** Ninth thoracic vertebra.

Joints of Sternum

- **Sternoclavicular joint** is a synovial joint between manubrium and medial end of the clavicle.
- **Manubriosternal joint** is a secondary cartilaginous joint or symphysis. It corresponds to angle of Louis or sternal angle, which is an important surface landmark for counting ribs in a patient.
- **Xiphisternal joint** is secondary cartilaginous joint, which turns into synostoses by 40th year.
- **Manubriocostal joint** (first sternocostal joint) is a synchondrosis or primary cartilaginous joint.
- **Sternocostal joints** (from second to seventh) between the costal cartilages and side of the body of sternum are synovial joints.

 STUDENT INTEREST

> Must know points about sternum—vertebral levels of parts, joints of sternum, anatomical and clinical importance of angle of Louis, muscle attachments and clinical insight.

Ossification

The sternum develops by fusion of two mesenchymal sternal plates in craniocaudal order. The cartilaginous sternal plate ossifies from multiple ossification centers. The centers for manubrium and four sternebrae appear before birth (1 or 2 centers in manubrium at 5th month, 1 in first sternebra in 6th month, 1 in second sternebra in 7th month, 1 in third sternebra in 8th month and 1 in fourth sternebra in 9the month). The center for xiphoid process appears in third year after birth. There is no bony union between manubrium and body. The second and third sternebrae unite by 17 to 25 years. The union between third and fourth sternebrae occurs by puberty and the xiphoid process unites with the lower end of the body by 40th year.

Non-union of the two sternal plate results in cleft sternum which may cause *ectopia cordis* (in which heart and pericardium are exposed to the surface).

Occasionally lower two sternebrae ossify by two centers which fail to fuse. In this situation lower part of body or xiphoid process is perforated by sternal foramen.

 CLINICAL CORRELATION

Sternal Puncture for Bone Marrow Sample

The bone marrow for histopathological examination can be obtained either from the manubrium or the body of sternum. Care is exercised not to injure the vital posterior relations of the manubrium and the body.

External Cardiac Massage

In a patient with cardiac arrest, the cardiopulmonary resuscitation (CPR) provides the basic life support. This is done by a technique called *external cardiac massage*. A firm pressure is applied to the chest vertically downwards on the lower part of the sternum, which should move posteriorly for 4–5 cm. This may force the blood out of the heart into the ascending aorta and may act as a stimulant for contraction of the heart.

Midline Sternotomy

The heart is usually approached for coronary bypass surgery by placing a midline sternum—splitting incision from the jugular notch to the xiphoid process. The split sternum is joined by steel wires after the surgery.

Ribs or Costae

The ribs are twelve pairs of arched bones in the thoracic cage. Eleven pairs of intercostal spaces are bounded by the adjacent margins of twelve pairs of ribs. The ribs extend from vertebral column posteriorly to the sternum and costal margin anteriorly. The rib and its cartilage are united to each other by the continuity of the periosteum of the rib with the perichondrium of its costal cartilage. The costal cartilages impart elasticity to the rib cage. The ribs contain spongy hemopoetic marrow.

There is increase in the length of the ribs from the first rib to the seventh and decrease from the seventh to the twelfth ribs. Therefore seventh rib is the longest.

CLASSIFICATIONS OF RIBS

Depending on Articulation with Sternum

- **True ribs** (first to seventh ribs are true ribs because they articulate with sternum directly).
- **False ribs** (eighth to twelfth ribs are false ribs because they do not articulate with sternum).

Depending on Anterior Attachments

- **Vertebrosternal ribs** are the ones that connect with the sternum through their costal cartilages. The first seven ribs are vertebrosternal ribs or true ribs.
- **Vertebrochondral ribs** or false ribs are connected to each other by cartilage (eight to tenth ribs).
- **Floating or vertebral ribs** (eleventh and twelfth ribs) present free anterior ends.

Depending on Morphological Features

- **Typical ribs** (third to ninth ribs, which have similar features).
- **Atypical ribs** (first, second, tenth, eleventh and twelfth ribs, which have special features).

Typical Rib (Fig. 34.4)

Each typical rib presents an anterior or sternal end, shaft and the posterior or vertebral end from before backward.

Anterior End

The anterior end of a typical rib is wider and bears a cup-shaped depression for articulation with its own costal cartilage.

Posterior End

The posterior end consists of head, neck and tubercle.

- The **head** has two articular facets separated by a crest. The upper smaller facet articulates with the body of the vertebra above and the lower larger one articulates with the body of numerically corresponding vertebra. The crest of the head is at the level of the intervertebral disc. The heads of the typical ribs are related anteriorly to the sympathetic chain.
- The **neck** is long and lies in front of the transverse process of the corresponding vertebra.
- The **tubercle** lies on the outer surface of the rib at the junction of the neck and shaft. The articular part of the tubercle articulates with facet on the transverse process of the numerically corresponding vertebra.

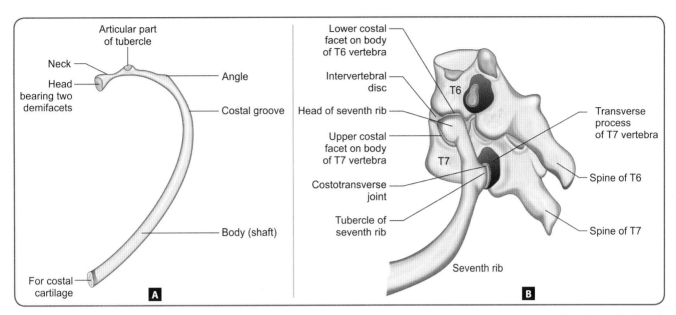

Figs 34.4A and B: A. Features of a typical rib as viewed from inferior aspect; **B.** Joints between rib and thoracic vertebrae (seventh rib and seventh and sixth thoracic vertebrae)
(Note the joints of the head of the rib with body of numerically corresponding vertebra and with the body of vertebra above. Also note the costotransverse joint between the facet on tubercle of the rib and the facet on the tip transverse process of numerically corresponding vertebra)

Shaft

The shaft is long and flat. It extends from posterior to anterior ends of the rib. It is angulated twisted and curved like a letter 'C'.

Angle of rib

A short distance (about 5 cm) in front of the tubercle, the rib shows a bend and is marked by a rough line. This point is the angle of the rib, where the rib is weakest and hence liable to fracture. The fractured rib may injure the pleura and the lungs. Injury to pleura may result in pneumothorax or hemothorax or both. Injury to the lower ribs may injure the abdominal organs. For example, fracture of the left tenth rib is likely to injure the spleen.

Features of shaft

The shaft presents outer and inner surfaces and upper and lower margins**.**

The **upper margin** has outer and inner lips. The outer lip receives insertion of external intercostal muscle and the inner lip receives the insertion of internal intercostal and intercostalis intimus muscles.

The **lower margin** is sharp and gives origin to external intercostal muscle.

The **outer surface** is smooth and convex. Closer to the anterior end the shafts of lower eight ribs provide origin to costal fibers of external oblique muscle of abdomen and

behind that to serratus anterior. In the case of upper eight rib. The serratus anterior originates from the lateral part of outer surface.

The **inner surface** is concave and smooth. Its lower part is marked by a costal groove, which houses three important structures—posterior intercostal vein, posterior intercostal artery and posterior intercostal nerve (**VAN**—from above downwards). The internal intercostal muscle originates from the floor of the groove whereas the intercostalis intimus arises from the upper rim of the groove.

 STUDENT INTEREST

The three intercostal muscles arise from floor, upper rim and sharp lower margin of costal groove of the upper rib and are inserted in to the upper margin of the lower rib. The upper and lower ribs bound the intercostal space containing the above three muscles. Out of 6 intercostal muscles attached to one rib, 3 inserted into upper margin belong to immediately upper intercostal space and 3 taking origin from costal groove belong to immediately lower intercostal space.

Articulations of Typical Rib (Fig. 34.4B)

- **Costovertebral joint** is the joint in which the head of the rib articulates with the body of numerically corresponding thoracic vertebra and with the body of the thoracic vertebra above.

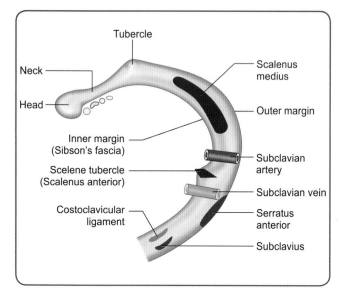

Fig. 34.5: Parts of typical rib, attachments and relations of its superior surface and relations of the anterior surface of its neck

- ***Costotransverse joint*** is the joint in which the tubercle of the rib and the transverse process of the numerically corresponding thoracic vertebra.
- ***Sternocostal joints*** of typical ribs are of synovial type.

Atypical Ribs

First Rib (Fig. 34.5)

The first rib is obliquely placed so that its posterior end is at a higher level compared to its anterior end. Its anterior end is very broad. The inner margins of the right and left ribs bound the thoracic inlet on either side.

Features

The first rib is the shortest, broadest and most curved.

Posterior end

- The ***head*** bears a single articular facet for articulation with first thoracic vertebra
- The ***neck*** is rounded and directed laterally, upwards and backwards. The anterior relations of the neck (Fig. 34.5) from medial to lateral side are the sympathetic chain, highest intercostal vein, superior intercostal artery and ventral ramus of first thoracic nerve
- The ***tubercle*** coincides with the angle of the rib and articulates with transverse process of first thoracic vertebra.

Anterior end

The anterior end is capped with costal cartilage, which articulates with the manubrium at first sternocostal joint.

Shaft

The shaft presents inner and outer margins and upper and lower surfaces.

The ***inner margin*** is concave and marked by scalene tubercle, which provides insertion to scalenus anterior. The inner margin gives attachment to Sibson's fascia (also called suprapleural membrane).

The ***outer margin*** is convex. It gives origin to first digitation of serratus anterior from its middle part.

The lower surface is smooth (as it is covered with costal pleura) and has no costal groove.

Relations of upper surface

The upper surface is rough and marked by two shallow vascular grooves (Fig. 34.5) separated by a ridge which continues medially with scalene tubercle on the inner margin. The vascular groove in front of the scalene tubercle is for subclavian vein and the one behind it is for subclavian artery and the lower trunk of brachial plexus. The subclavius takes origin from the anterior end of the upper surface. The scalenus medius is inserted behind the groove for subclavian artery (Fig. 34.5).

Second Rib

The length of second rib is twice that of first rib. The shaft is highly curved like the first rib. The shaft is not twisted, hence, both ends touch the surface when placed on the table top. The second costal cartilage articulates with sternal angle (which includes lowest part of manubrium and uppermost part of sternal body). There are two joint cavities due to presence of intra-articular ligament. During clinical examination of chest, the second rib is the guide in counting the other ribs and intercostal spaces.

Tenth Rib

This rib shows all the features of a typical rib except that it is shorter. Its head bears a single facet to articulate with the body of tenth thoracic vertebra near its pedicle.

Eleventh and Twelfth Ribs

These *floating ribs* are very short. Hence they are present only in the posterior abdominal wall. They have pointed ends, which are tipped with cartilage. The necks and tubercles of the ribs are absent. The angle and costal grooves are poorly marked in eleventh rib and absent in twelfth rib.

Both ribs are related posteriorly to the left kidney but only twelfth rib is related to the right kidney (Fig. 54.9). So, in operations on kidney by lumbar route the last two ribs are important landmarks.

Attachments and relations of twelfth rib

- *Costodiaphragmatic recess* is related to the medial three–fourth of costal surface.
- *Quadratus lumborum* muscle is inserted into the lower part of inner surface along with anterior layer of thoracolumbar fascia.
- Costal fibers of diaphragm arise from the inner surface of the rib closer to its costal cartilage.
- The lower margin gives attachment to middle layer of thoracolumbar fascia and the lateral *arcuate ligament*.
- The outer surface gives attachments to *latissimus dorsi, serratus posterior*—inferior and external oblique muscles.

Costal Cartilages

The costal cartilages are of hyaline variety. They represent the unossified anterior ends of the ribs. During inspiration they are twisted upwards. This movement of the costal cartilages stores energy, which is released during expiration. The costal cartilages provide external elastic recoil during normal quiet expiration so that the muscular effort is spared. The calcification of costal cartilages usually occurs in old age with resultant loss of elasticity of the rib cage.

♪ CLINICAL CORRELATION

- *The cervical rib* may arise from the seventh cervical vertebra. It may be unilateral or bilateral. It may be fully developed or just a fibrous strand reaching the first rib beyond the scalene tubercle. It may be symptomless but in some individuals it gives rise to pressure on the structures in relation to the upper surface of first rib (Fig. 34.5) causing neurovascular disturbances. In such cases surgical removal of the cervical rib along with its periosteum is undertaken in order to prevent regeneration of the cervical rib.
- *The lumbar rib* may arise from the first lumbar vertebra. When present, the lumbar rib may confuse the identification of vertebral levels in radiographs.
- The *subperiosteal resection of ribs* is performed to gain access to the thoracic cavity. In this procedure the rib segment is removed by incising the periosteum, which is left inside the body. In this way the lost rib regenerates in due course from the osteogenic layer of the periosteum.
- *Costochondritis* is the inflammation of the costal cartilages of the sternocostal joints. It causes severe pain in the chest wall.
- Flail chest is produced when there are multiple rib fractures at costochondral junctions and near the rib angles. As a result of this, a part of rib cage remains isolated without bony support. The isolated part undergoes paradoxical movements of chest wall (moves in during inspiration and moves out during expiration).
- Stove in chest condition develops from localized crushing injury with multiple rib fractures. The affected area is depressed and becomes relatively immobile.
- In the fracture of ribs, pleura and lung are in danger of injury. In fracture of lower ribs upper abdominal organs like spleen or liver are likely to be injured.

Thoracic Vertebrae

There are twelve thoracic vertebrae. They are of two types:
- Typical (second to eighth)
- Atypical (First and ninth to twelfth).

Features of Typical Thoracic Vertebra (Figs 34.6A and B)

- The *body* of the vertebra is heart-shaped. On each side of the body, there are two *demifacets* (superior and inferior). The superior demifacet is larger and articulates with the lower facet on the head of the numerically corresponding rib. The inferior demifacet is smaller and articulates with the upper facet on the head of the succeeding rib.

The posterior surface of the body is marked by *basivertebral foramen* through which the basivertebral vein comes out.

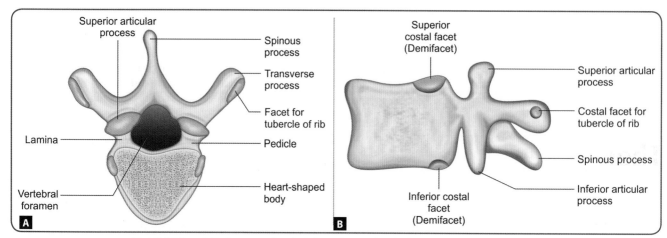

Figs 34.6A and B: Features of typical thoracic vertebra **A.** Superior view **B.** Lateral view

- The ***vertebral foramen*** is circular.
- The ***vertebral arch*** presents pedicles, laminae, superior articular processes, inferior articular processes, transverse processes and spinous process or spine.
- The ***large transverse processes*** extend posterolaterally from the junction of pedicles and laminae.
  The anterior surface of the transverse process near its tip bears a facet for articulation with the tubercle of the numerically corresponding rib.
- The ***spine*** is long and directed downwards and backwards. All thoracic spines give origin to trapezius and to latissimus dorsi from lower six spines. The spine of first thoracic vertebra gives origin to rhomboid minor and spines of second to fifth thoracic vertebrae to rhomboid major.

Features of Atypical Thoracic Vertebrae

- In the ***first thoracic vertebra***, the superior costal facet on the body is complete. It articulates with the first rib. The inferior demifacet is for articulating with second rib.
- In the ***tenth thoracic vertebra***, the body has a single complete costal facet.
- In the ***eleventh thoracic vertebra***, body has complete costal facet but the transverse process is devoid of the facet.
- In the ***twelfth thoracic vertebra***, the complete costal facet is located more on the pedicle. There is no facet on transverse process. The transverse process has superior, inferior lateral tubercles. The shape of the vertebra resembles that of a lumbar vertebra.

35

Thoracic Inlet and Thoracic Wall

Chapter Contents

THORACIC INLET

The thorax is the upper part of the trunk located between the neck and the abdomen. It consists of thoracic wall and thoracic cavity. In the lateral part of thoracic cavity on each side, the lung is enclosed in a serous sac called pleural cavity. The central part of the thoracic cavity between the two pleural cavities is called the *mediastinum*. The heart within the pericardial cavity is located inside the middle mediastinum.

BOUNDARIES OF THORACIC INLET

- *Posteriorly:* Body of first thoracic vertebra
- *Laterally:* Inner margins of the first ribs and their costal cartilages.
- *Anteriorly:* Upper margin of manubrium sterni.

Note: The first rib slopes downwards and forwards, hence, the first thoracic vertebral level is higher than that of the upper margin of the manubrium. Because of the inclination of the thoracic inlet, the apex of the lung with the overlying pleura appears to project into the base of the neck.

 ADDED INFORMATION

Details of structures passing through thoracic Inlet (Fig. 35.1)

The structures passing through the inlet are grouped into midline structures and those passing on either side of the midline.

Contd…

Contd…

 ADDED INFORMATION

Midline structures

In the midline, there are two strap muscles of the neck (sternothyroid and sternohyoid), inferior thyroid veins, trachea and the esophagus.

Structures on either side of midline

- The apex of lung and cervical pleura project upwards. The Sibson's fascia covers the cervical pleura
- Four structures (sympathetic chain, highest intercostal vein, first posterior intercostal artery and ventral ramus of the first thoracic nerve) forming close posterior relations of lung apex (Fig. 34.4A)
- The internal thoracic artery, vagus nerve and phrenic nerve descend in relation to the medial aspect of lung apex
- The subclavian vessels pass in front of the lung apex in lateral direction
- The scalenus anterior and medius muscles descend to gain insertion into the first rib
- The brachiocephalic artery and right brachiocephalic vein are seen on the right side of the midline and left common carotid artery, left brachiocephalic vein, left recurrent laryngeal nerve and the thoracic duct are seen on the left of the midline.

SCALENE TRIANGLE

The scalene triangle is a narrow triangular space bounded anteriorly by scalenus anterior, posteriorly by scalenus

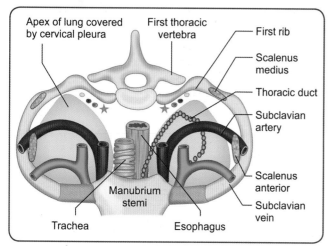

Fig. 35.1: Structures passing through the thoracic inlet (Note that the anterior relations of the neck of first rib are not labeled in the figure)

medius and inferiorly by upper surface of the first rib. Its contents are the lower trunk of the brachial plexus and the subclavian artery.

CLINICAL CORRELATION

Cervical Rib Syndrome (Fig. 35.2)

In the presence of a cervical rib or a congenitally hypertrophied scalenus anterior muscle, the scalene triangle is unduly narrowed resulting in compression of the subclavian artery and lower trunk of the brachial plexus. This causes neurovascular symptoms, which are collectively called cervical rib syndrome or scalenus anterior syndrome.

Contd…

Contd…

CLINICAL CORRELATION

Signs and Symptoms due to Compression of Subclavian Artery

- Pallor and coldness of the upper limb
- Reduction in the force or obliteration of the radial pulse on affected side, which is confirmed by Adson's test, which is done as follows—The patient sits on the stool and is asked to take deep breath in and to turn the face to the affected side. There is reduction in radial pulse in the presence of cervical rib.

Signs and Symptoms due to Compression of Lower Trunk of Brachial Plexus

- Numbness, tingling and pain along the medial side of the hand and little finger
- Weakness and wasting of interossei and lumbricals
- Advanced cases show flattening of hypothenar eminence and guttering of the interosseous spaces on the dorsum of the hand.

Surgical Treatment

To relieve the symptoms, the cervical rib is surgically removed. The periosteum of the rib is removed in order to prevent regeneration of the cervical rib.

THORACIC WALL

The thoracic wall or the chest wall consists of eleven intercostal spaces bounded by ribs and costal cartilages and composed of muscles, nerves and vessels.

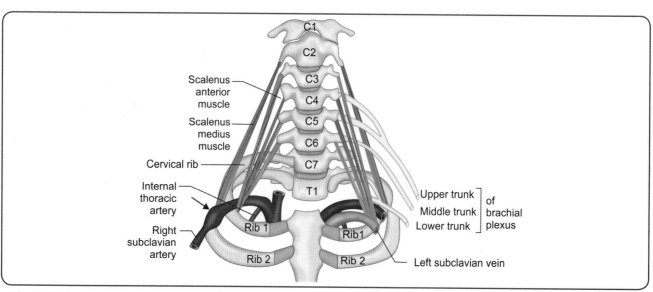

Fig. 35.2: Compression by the cervical rib of the neurovascular structures related to the superior surface of the first rib on the right side [Note the dilatation (marked by arrow) of the subclavian artery distal to the site of compression of the artery]

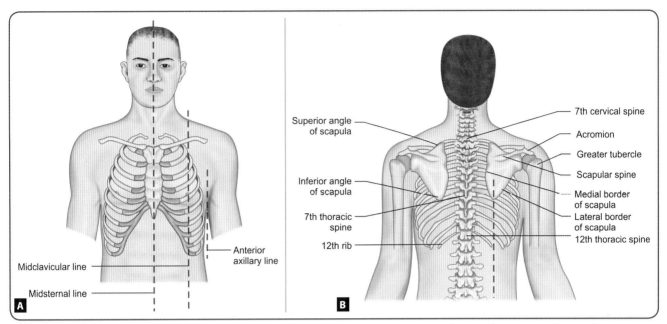

Figs 35.3A and B: A. Orientation lines on the anterior chest wall; **B.** Orientation lines on the posterior chest wall

Surface Landmarks on Anterior Aspect (Fig. 35.3A)

- The *suprasternal notch* is at the level of T2 vertebra. The trachea is felt through this notch.
- The *sternal angle or angle of Louis* is a palpable landmark. It lies at the level of the disc between fourth thoracic and fifth thoracic vertebrae. The second rib articulates with the costal notch at this level and hence sternal angle is a reference point to count the ribs and intercostal spaces downwards in a patient.
- The *xiphisternal joint* is at the level of disc between thoracic eighth and ninth vertebrae.
- The *lowest part of costal margin* corresponding to tenth rib in midaxillary line is at the level of third lumbar vertebra.

Surface Landmarks on Posterior Aspect (Fig. 35.3B)

- The spines of the thoracic vertebrae are palpable in the midline.
- The scapula is located in the upper part of the back of thorax. Its superior angle lies opposite second thoracic vertebra.
- The spine of the scapula is subcutaneous and its root is at the level of third thoracic vertebra.
- The inferior angle of scapula corresponds to seventh thoracic vertebra and seventh rib.

Orientation Lines

- The *midsternal line* passes through the midline of sternum.
- The *midclavicular line* passes through the midpoint of the clavicle.
- The *anterior axillary line* corresponds to the anterior axillary fold.
- The *midaxillary line passes* through the midpoint of the base of the axilla.
- The *posterior axillary line* corresponds to posterior axillary fold.
- The *scapular line* passes through the inferior angle of the scapula.

✎ CLINICAL CORRELATION

Thoracic wall in Clinical Examination
The pectoral region forms the front of the anterior chest wall and the scapular region forms part of the posterior chest wall. Deeper to these regions are the intercostal spaces, deeper to which are the heart and great vessels and the lungs inside the thoracic cavity.

The methods of clinical examination of thorax (to diagnose diseases of heart and lungs) are inspection, palpation, percussion and auscultation on the anterior and posterior chest walls. For this the anatomical knowledge of the skeletal and soft tissue landmarks and orientation lines is an essential prerequisite. It helps in delineating the internal structures on the thoracic wall. The clinician knows to identify sites for auscultation of heart and lungs. It also helps to identify safe sites for approaches to the pleural cavity, pericardial cavity etc.

INTERCOSTAL SPACE

The space between two adjacent ribs and their costal cartilages is called the *intercostal space.*

There are eleven intercostal spaces bounded by twelve ribs on each side. The upper nine spaces are closed anteriorly but the short tenth and eleventh spaces have open anterior ends, which reach up to the midaxillary line.

Contents (Figs 35.4A and B)

- Intercostal muscles
- Intercostal nerve
- Intercostal vessels.

Intercostal Muscles (Figs 35.4A and B)

From superficial to deep, the muscles are:
- External intercostal muscle
- Internal intercostal muscle
- Innermost intercostal or intercostalis intimus muscle.

External intercostal muscle

It takes origin from the lower sharp margin of the rib above and is inserted into the outer lip of the upper margin of the rib below.

Parts

- Fleshy interosseous part (between the shafts of the ribs)
- Membranous interchondral part (called anterior intercostal membrane located between the adjacent costal cartilages).

The direction of the muscle fibers is downwards and forwards.

Internal intercostal muscle

It takes origin from the costal groove of the rib above and is inserted into the inner lip of the upper margin of the rib below.

Parts

- Long and fleshy part extends from anterior end of intercostal space to the angle of the rib posteriorly. It is subdivided into intercartilaginous and interosseous parts.
- Short membranous part (called posterior intercostal membrane) is located beyond the angle of the rib.

The direction of the muscle fibers is downward and backward.

Innermost intercostal muscle (Fig. 35.4A)

It is a discontinuous muscle layer, which is separated from costal pleura by endothoracic fascia. It is divided into sternocostalis, intercostalis intimus and subcostalis from before backwards.

- ***Sternocostalis*** (transversus thoracis) lies behind sternum and costal cartilages (Fig 35.8). It takes origin from the posterior aspects of lower part of body of sternum, xiphoid process and also from adjacent fourth to seventh costal cartilages. From this wide origin the fibers pass upward and laterally to reach an equally wide insertion into the posterior aspect of costal cartilages of second to sixth ribs. It is related anteriorly to the internal thoracic artery.

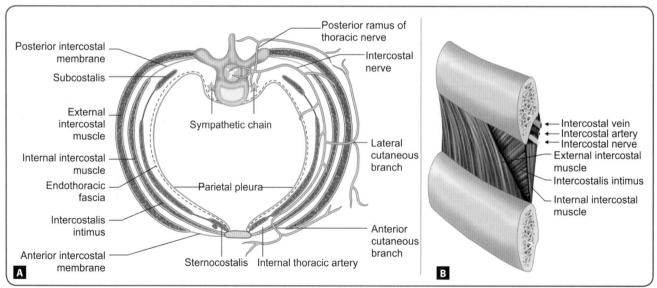

Figs 35.4A and B: A. Muscles of typical intercostal space on the right side and course of typical intercostal nerve in the neurovascular plane in the intercostal space on left side; **B.** Diagram of an intercostal space showing intercostal muscles and intercostal neurovascular bundle in the costal groove

- **Intercostalis intimus** originates from the ridge above the costal groove of the upper rib and is inserted into the inner lip of the upper margin of the lower rib.
- **Subcostalis muscles** are present in the posterior part of lower intercostal spaces only. The muscle arises from the inner surface of the rib above near its angle and is inserted in inner surface of the lower ribs after crossing one or two spaces.

Nerve supply

The intercostal muscles receive nerve supply from the corresponding intercostal nerves.

Actions

- The **external intercostal muscles** elevate the ribs to increase the anteroposterior and transverse diameters of the thorax during inspiration.
- The **internal intercostal muscles** have dual actions.
  - The intercartilaginous fleshy parts act synergistically with external intercostal muscles, and hence assist in inspiration.
  - The interosseous fleshy parts depress the ribs during forced expiration.

- The **sternocostalis muscles** assist in pulling the second to sixth ribs inferiorly.
- Collectively the intercostal muscles keep the intercostal spaces rigid. This action prevents indrawing of the spaces during inspiration and bulging out of the spaces during expiration.

Intercostal Nerves

The intercostal nerves are the anterior (ventral) primary rami of the thoracic spinal nerves. They are eleven in number on each side, being equal to the number of intercostal spaces (anterior or ventral primary ramus of twelfth thoracic spinal nerve is called subcostal nerve since it lies below the twelfth rib).

Unique feature

The intercostal nerves retain their segmental character, unlike the anterior primary rami from the other regions of the spinal cord, form nerve plexuses like cervical, brachial, lumbar and sacral.

Communications with sympathetic ganglion (Fig. 35.5)

Each intercostal nerve communicates with sympathetic ganglion by two communicating twigs.
- **White ramus communicans (WRC)** carries preganglionic fibers from the intercostal nerve to the sympathetic ganglion.

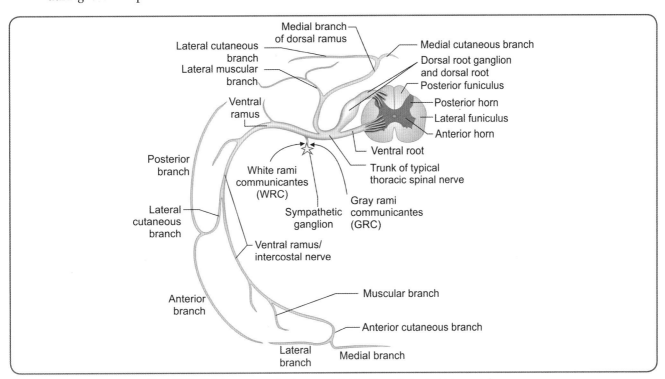

Fig. 35.5: Origin, communications and distribution of a typical intercostal nerve

- **Grey ramus communicans (GRC)** carries postganglionic fibers back to the intercostal nerve from the sympathetic ganglion.

The postganglionic sympathetic fibers supply pilomotor fibers to the arrector pilorum muscles, sudomotor fibers to the sweat glands and vasomotor fibers for the smooth muscle of the blood vessels in the skin of the area of sensory supply of the intercostal nerve.

 ADDED INFORMATION

Functional Components of Intercostal Nerve

The intercostal nerve is composed of four functionally different types of nerve fibers:
1. **General somatic efferent (GSE)** fibers supply the striated muscles derived from somites
2. **General somatic afferent. (GSA)** fibers bring cutaneous sensations to the spinal cord
3. **General visceral efferent (GVE)** fibers are the sympathetic fibres for the supply of the smooth muscle of the skin (arrector pilorum), sweat glands and the blood vessels of the skin
4. **General visceral afferent (GVA)** fibers bring visceral sensations to the spinal cord.

Classification of Intercostal Nerves

- **Typical Intercostal Nerves:** The typical intercostal nerves are the ones that are confined to their own intercostal spaces in the thoracic wall. The third, fourth, fifth and sixth intercostal nerves are the examples of typical intercostal nerve.
- **Atypical Intercostal Nerves:** The atypical intercostal nerves extend beyond the thoracic wall for distribution partly or entirely. The first, second, seventh to eleventh intercostal nerves are the example of atypical intercostal nerve.

Typical intercostal nerve

The typical intercostal nerve (Fig. 35.4 A and 35.5) enters the intercostal space at its vertebral end.

Course

At first the nerve turns laterally behind the sympathetic trunk. Then it travels towards the intercostal space between the parietal pleura and the posterior intercostal membrane.

Course in intercostal space

The nerve enters the costal groove of the corresponding rib to course laterally and forwards in the neurovascular plane (plane between internal intercostal and intercostalis intimus muscles), lying below the intercostal vessels (VAN). At the sternal end of the intercostal space the intercostal nerve crosses in front of the internal thoracic artery and pierces is succession the interchondral part of internal intercostal muscle, anterior intercostal membrane and sternocostal origin of pectoralis major muscle. It continues as its anterior cutaneous branch.

Branches

- The **collateral branch** arises from the posterior part of the intercostal nerve before it reaches the angle of the rib. This branch follows the inferior margin of the intercostal space in the neurovascular plane. The collateral nerve and the main trunk supply muscular branches to the intercostal muscles and additionally also supply the serratus posterior superior muscle in the back.
- The **lateral cutaneous branch** arises from the nerve along with the collateral branch and runs with the main trunk for a small distance and divides into anterior and posterior branches. The posterior branches supply the skin of back overlying the scapula and latissimus dorsi muscle and anterior branches supply the skin overlying the pectoralis major muscle.
- The **sensory branches** are given to the parietal pleura and the periosteum of the ribs.
- The **anterior cutaneous branch** supplies the skin of the pectoral region and gives sensory branches to the sternum.

🔖 **CLINICAL CORRELATION**

- The **intercostal nerve block** is given to produce local anesthesia in one or more intercostal spaces by injecting the anesthetic solution around the intercostal nerve near its origin, just lateral to the vertebra
- The diseases of the thoracic vertebrae may irritate the intercostal nerves and thereby cause radiating pain in the area of cutaneous distribution of the affected nerves
- The **pus from the tuberculous thoracic vertebrae** may track along the neurovascular plane of the space and point at the sites of emergence of the anterior and lateral cutaneous nerves (lateral margin of sternum and midaxillary line)
- In herpes zoster (shingles) of the thoracic spinal ganglion the cutaneous vesicles appear in the dermatome of the affected intercostal nerve
- In order to avoid the intercostal and collateral neurovascular bundles in an intercostal space (Fig. 36.19), it is safe to insert a needle midway between the two ribs or a little lower for approaching the pleural cavity to aspirate fluid.

Atypical intercostal nerves (Fig. 35.6)

First intercostal nerve

It is the smallest intercostal nerve because a large contribution of first thoracic nerve is given to the brachial

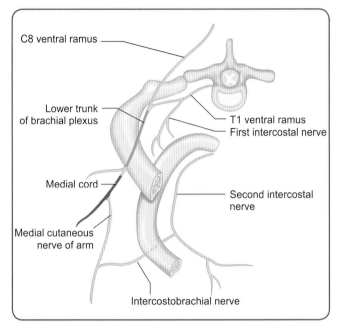

Fig. 35.6: Atypical features of first and second intercostal nerves

plexus. It gives no collateral or cutaneous branches. It courses along the lower surface of the first rib and the small neurovascular structures are arranged as nerve, artery and vein (NAV) from above downward (reverse of VAN arrangement). Due to absence of its cutaneous branches, T1 dermatome is absent on the chest wall. Hence T2 dermatome is placed adjacent to C4 dermatome at the level of the sternal angle (Fig. 11.3).

Second intercostal nerve

The lateral cutaneous branch of the second intercostal nerve (intercostobrachial nerve) joins the medial cutaneous nerve of arm and supplies the skin of the floor of axilla and of medial side of adjacent arm.

Seventh to eleventh intercostal nerves (Fig. 48.12)

The seventh to eleventh intercostal nerves are known as **thoracoabdominal nerves**. They are the lower five intercostal nerves (T7 to T11). They are called **thoracoabdominal** because they course first in thoracic wall and then after piercing the diaphragm, they course downwards in the anterior abdominal wall. During their thoracic course they supply the intercostal muscles of the respective spaces and also give sensory branches to the skin of the chest and to the parietal (costal) pleura. During their abdominal course, they supply the muscles and the skin of the anterior abdominal wall.

CLINICAL CORRELATION

Irritation of the thoracoabdominal nerves in **pleurisy** (inflammation of parietal pleura) may cause reflex spasm of anterior abdominal muscles and referred pain to the anterior abdominal wall. Therefore, when a patient comes with the complaint of pain in the abdominal wall the clinician advises radiograph of the chest to rule out pathology in the pleura.

Intercostal Arteries

- The upper nine intercostal spaces contain three arteries, one posterior intercostal and two anterior intercostal arteries, per space.
- The tenth and eleventh spaces are very short and have open anterior ends. They contain a single posterior intercostal artery in each space.

Posterior intercostal arteries

- In the first and second intercostal spaces, the posterior intercostal arteries are the branches of superior intercostal artery (which is a branch of the costocervical trunk of the subclavian artery as shown in (Fig. 35.7A)
- It the lower nine spaces, the posterior intercostal arteries arise directly from the descending thoracic aorta (Figs 35.7B and 43.11).

Course

Each posterior intercostal artery enters the vertebral end of the intercostal space and travels forward lying above the nerve and below the vein (VAN) in the neurovascular plane. Near the angle of the rib it gives off a collateral branch. At the costochondral junction, the main trunk of the posterior intercostal artery anastomoses with the upper anterior intercostal artery, whereas the collateral branch anastomoses with the lower anterior intercostal artery (Fig. 35.7B).

Anterior intercostal arteries

There are two anterior intercostal arteries (upper and lower) per space in upper nine spaces.
- In the first to six spaces, the anterior intercostal arteries are the branches of internal thoracic artery on each side (Fig 35.8).
- In the seventh to ninth spaces the anterior intercostal arteries are the branches of musculophrenic artery on each side.

Note: The tenth and eleventh spaces do not have anterior intercostal arteries).

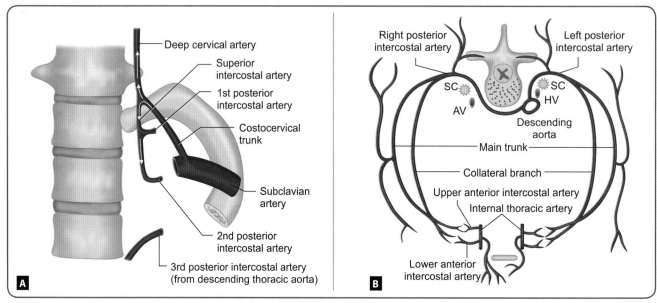

Figs 35.7A and B: A. Origin of first and second posterior intercostal arteries from the superior intercostal artery which descends from costocervical trunk of the subclavian artery; **B.** Arteries of typical intercostal spaces to show anastomoses between anterior and posterior intercostal arteries (Note that posterior intercostal artery takes origin from descending thoracic aorta and a pair of anterior intercostal arteries arises from internal thoracic artery) **Key:** SC- sympathetic chain, AV- azygos vein, HV- hemiazygos vein

Course

- The upper and lower anterior intercostal arteries in each of the upper nine spaces pass laterally and backwards along the upper and lower margins of the respective spaces.
- The upper anterior intercostal artery anastomoses with the main trunk of the posterior intercostal artery at the costochondral junction and the lower anterior intercostal artery anastomoses with the collateral branch (Fig. 35.7) at the same junction.
- The free anastomoses between anterior and posterior intercostal arteries connect the first part of subclavian artery and the descending thoracic aorta.

🎓 STUDENT INTEREST

Remember there are two anterior intercostal arteries (upper and lower) per intercostal space in upper nine spaces as against only one posterior intercostal artery per space. The posterior intercostal artery gives of a collateral branch. The upper anterior intercostal artery anastomoses with the main posterior intercostal artery and the lower anterior intercostal artery anastomoses with the collateral branch of posterior intercostal artery.

⚕ CLINICAL CORRELATION

In the condition of narrowing of the arch of aorta (coarctation of aorta distal to the origin of left subclavian artery as shown in figure 39.3), the blood is carried to the descending aorta by the enlarged and tortuous posterior intercostal arteries through the intercostal anastomoses. The enlarged posterior intercostal arteries erode the ribs which is seen in radiographs as '*rib notching*'.

Internal Thoracic Artery (Fig. 35.8)

The internal thoracic (mammary) artery supplies the anterior thoracic and anterior abdominal walls.

Origin

It is a branch of the first part of the subclavian artery in the root of the neck.

Course

It descends medially behind the sternal end of the clavicle and the first costal cartilage. Then it descends vertically behind the second to sixth costal cartilages lying about 2 cm from the margin of the sternum. Up to the level of

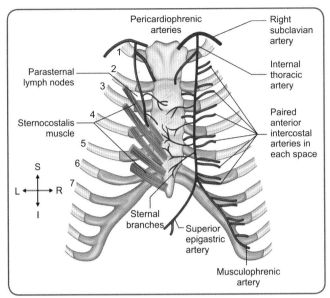

Fig. 35.8: Internal thoracic (mammary) artery viewed from the inner aspect of the anterior thoracic wall
(Note that sternocostalis muscle is shown only on the left side)

second costal cartilage, the artery is closely related to the costal pleura but below this the sternocostalis muscle intervenes between it and the pleura (Fig. 35.8).

Termination

It terminates in the sixth intercostal space by dividing into superior epigastric and musculophrenic arteries.

Venae comitantes accompany the artery upto the level of third costal cartilage, where the venae comitantes unite to form a single internal vein, which ascends on the medial side of the artery to open into the brachiocephalic vein of the corresponding side.

Branches

- Pericardiacophrenic branch accompanying phrenic nerve for supply of diaphragm.
- Mediastinal branches (for thymus, pericardium, lymph nodes etc).
- Perforating branches accompany the corresponding anterior cutaneous branches. In female the second, third and fourth perforating branches are large for the supply of the breast.
- One pair of anterior intercostal arteries per space in the upper six spaces.
- Sternal branches.
- Superior epigastric and musculophrenic arteries (terminal branches) supply the thoracic wall. They enter the anterior abdominal wall through the

diaphragm to supply the diaphragm and the anterior abdominal wall.

🐾 STUDENT INTEREST

Internal thoracic artery arises from lower side of first part of subclavian artery just above the sternal end of clavicle in the neck. It terminates in the sixth intercostal space by dividing into superior epigastric and musculophrenic arteries. Internal thoracic artery is an important artery since it supplies thorax, diaphragm and anterior abdominal wall. The artery is used as coronary artery graft.

⚕ CLINICAL CORRELATION

The internal mammary artery is favored over other vessels for coronary graft. It is observed that internal mammary artery is less prone to develop atherosclerosis due to presence of elastic tissue in its wall and the endothelial cells of its tunica intima secrete chemicals that prevent atherosclerosis. The left internal mammary artery (LIMA) is favored for anastomosing with left anterior descending branch (Fig. 35.9) of left coronary artery.

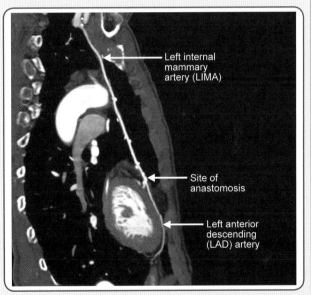

Fig. 35.9: Radiological image of the graft between left internal mammary artery (LIMA) and left anterior descending (LAD) artery after bypass surgery for blockage of LAD artery (a major branch of left coronary artery)

Intercostal Veins

Anterior intercostal veins

The anterior intercostal veins of the upper six spaces drain into the internal thoracic vein and those of seventh, eighth and ninth spaces drain into the musculophrenic vein.

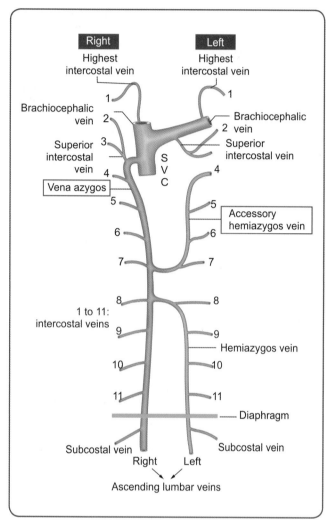

Fig. 35.10: Veins of thoracic wall (1 to11 are posterior intercostal veins)

Posterior intercostal veins (Fig. 35.10)

They reach the vertebral end of the intercostal spaces and receive intervertebral veins from the internal vertebral venous plexus.

- The first or highest posterior intercostal vein on the right side opens into right brachiocephalic vein and on the left side opens into the left brachiocephalic vein
- The veins of second, third and fourth right posterior intercostal veins unite to form the right superior intercostal vein, which opens into arch of azygos vein. The veins of second and third spaces (and sometimes the fourth space) unite to form left superior intercostal vein which ascends towards left to cross the left surface of arch of aorta between the left vagus and left phrenic nerves (Fig. 43.8) to open into the left brachiocephalic vein.
- The posterior intercostal veins of the remaining spaces open into the vertical part of azygos vein on the right side. However, on the left side the veins of the fourth to seventh spaces open into superior hemiazygos vein (accessory hemiazygos vein) and those from the eighth to eleventh spaces open into inferior hemiazygos vein (hemiazygos vein).

Lymph Nodes

The internal mammary lymph nodes (parasternal nodes) along the internal thoracic artery receive lymphatics from anterior part of intercostal space including the superficial and deep lymphatics from the breast. The posterior intercostal nodes located in the posterior part of the intercostal spaces near the heads of the ribs receive lymphatics from the posterior parts of the intercostal spaces.

Note: For further details of the lymph nodes refer to chapter 44.

36

Mediastinum, Pleural Cavities and Organs of Respiratory System

MEDIASTINUM

The thoracic cavity contains pleural cavities surrounding the lungs on either side of the midline partition called the **mediastinum**.

The mediastinum is a midline, narrow and elongated space (containing many structures including heart and great vessels) between the right and left pleural cavities. It is connected to the lung on each side by the root of the lung.

Boundaries of Mediastinum

The mediastinum is bounded by the sternum anteriorly. It is bounded by the thoracic vertebrae posteriorly and on either side by mediastinal pleura (Fig. 36.1).

Extent

The mediastinum extends from the inlet of thorax to the diaphragm (Fig. 36.2).

Subdivisions (Fig. 36.2)

The mediastinum is broadly divided into superior and inferior parts by means of an imaginary line passing

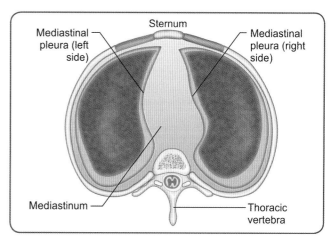

Fig. 36.1: Location of mediastinum in the thoracic cavity

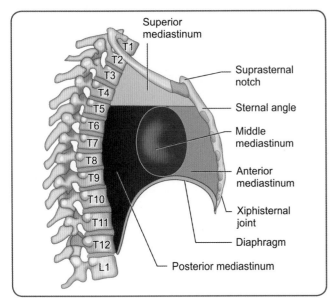

Fig. 36.2: Subdivisions of mediastinum into superior mediastinum, anterior mediastinum, middle mediastinum and posterior mediastinum

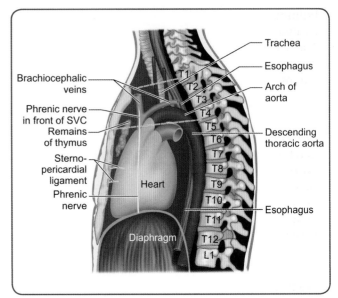

Fig. 36.3: Lateral view of thoracic cavity showing few contents of: **Superior mediastinum** (arch of aorta and its branches, superior vena cava, phrenic nerves, brachiocephalic veins, trachea, esophagus, etc.), **Anterior mediastinum** (thymus and sternopericardial ligaments), **Middle mediastinum** (heart, pericardium, phrenic nerves). **Posterior mediastinum** (descending thoracic aorta, esophagus, vagus nerves, vena azygos and thoracic duct)

through the manubriosternal joint and the disc between fourth and fifth thoracic vertebrae.

The inferior mediastinum is further subdivided into anterior, middle and posterior parts.

Boundaries of Superior Mediastinum

- **Anteriorly:** Posterior surface of manubrium sterni
- **Posteriorly:** Anterior surfaces of the bodies of upper four thoracic vertebrae.
- **Superiorly:** Plane of thoracic inlet
- **On each side:** Mediastinal pleura
- **Inferiorly:** Plane passing through the lower margin of the fourth thoracic vertebra and the sternal angle.

Contents (Fig. 36.3)

- **Muscles:** Origin of sternohyoid and sternothyroid muscles and the lower end of longus colli.
- **Arteries:** Arch of aorta and its branches (left subclavian, left common carotid and brachiocephalic).
- **Veins:** Superior vena cava, right and left brachiocephalic veins, terminal part of azygos vein and left superior intercostal vein.
- Remnant of the thymus
- Nerves on the right side: Right vagus and right phrenic and on the left side: Left vagus, left phrenic and left recurrent laryngeal.
- Esophagus and trachea and lymph nodes.

Boundaries of Anterior Mediastinum

The anterior mediastinum is a narrow space.
- **Anteriorly:** Body of sternum
- **Posteriorly:** Fibrous pericardium
- **Superiorly:** An imaginary plane passing through sternal angle
- **Inferiorly:** Diaphragm.

Contents

- Sternopericardial ligaments
- Remains of thymus, lymph nodes and areolar tissue.

Boundaries of Middle Mediastinum

- **Anteriorly:** Anterior mediastinum
- **Posteriorly:** Posterior mediastinum
- **Superiorly:** Superior mediastinum
- **Inferiorly:** Diaphragm
- **On each side:** Mediastinal pleura.

Contents

- Fibrous pericardium containing heart enveloped by serous pericardium.

- Pulmonary vessels and intrapericardial SVC and ascending aorta.
- Tracheal bifurcation and principal bronchi and deep cardiac plexus.
- Phrenic nerves.

Boundaries of Posterior Mediastinum

- *Anteriorly:* Tracheal bifurcation, pulmonary vessels and fibrous pericardium
- *Posteriorly:* Anterior surfaces of bodies of lower eight thoracic vertebrae
- *Inferiorly:* Diaphragm
- *Superiorly:* Lower limit of superior mediastinum
- *On each side:* Mediastinal pleura.

Contents

- Esophagus
- Descending thoracic aorta
- Azygos and hemiazygos veins
- Thoracic duct
- Vagus nerves
- Lymph nodes
- Splanchnic nerves (branches of sympathetic chain).

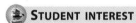

🐾 STUDENT INTEREST

The mediastinum, its subdivisions and contents are clinically relevant. A question on subdivisions and contents of mediastinum can be expected not only in anatomy but also in clinical subjects. Therefore, it is wiser to learn it when you can actually see the mediastinum in the specimen in dissection laboratory.

⚗️ CLINICAL CORRELATION

- *Mediastinal syndrome* is a condition in which the contents of superior mediastinum are compressed due to space-occupying lesion producing diverse signs and symptoms. For example, an enlarged lymph node in superior mediastinum may compress on the trachea, esophagus and left recurrent laryngeal nerve producing symptoms, like difficulty in breathing, difficulty in swallowing and hoarseness of voice respectively
- *The mediastinal shift* is an indication of lung pathology. The mediastinum shifts to the affected side due to lung collapse and decrease in intrapleural pressure. Mediastinal shift is detected by palpating the trachea in the suprasternal notch
- *Mediastinitis* is the inflammation of the loose connective tissue of the mediastinum. It occurs when deep infections of the neck spread downwards along the fascial continuity into the mediastinum (Fig. 36.9).

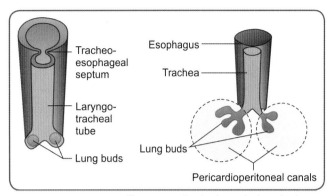

Fig. 36.4: Formation of laryngotracheal tube including the lung buds from endoderm of primitive pharynx

🔬 EMBRYOLOGIC INSIGHT

Development of Pleural Cavities and Respiratory Organs

The development of lungs is intimately associated with the development of the pleural cavities. In the embryonic life, the intraembryonic coelom is a horseshoe- shaped space enclosed in splanchnopleuric and somatopleuric layers of lateral plate mesoderm (Fig. 8.16A). It subdivides into pericardial, pleural and peritoneal cavities. Its median part is the future pericardial cavity and the two tubular parts are the forerunners of the peritoneal cavity. The narrow connections between the above two parts are called the pericardioperitoneal canals (future pleural cavities). The lung bud invaginates the pericardioperitoneal canal of its side and expands in all directions forming a double-layered pleural cavity. The splanchnopleuric layer forms the visceral pleura and the somatopleuric layer forms the parietal pleura.

Development of Laryngotracheal Tube from Endoderm

A laryngotracheal groove appears in the floor of the cranial end of foregut (Fig. 36.4). As this groove deepens and elongates in caudal direction, it is separated from the cranial end of the foregut by formation of a tracheoesophageal septum

Development of Larynx and Trachea

The cranial end of the laryngotracheal tube forms the larynx, the succeeding part develops into trachea and the caudal end bifurcates to develop into extrapulmonary bronchi and lung buds.

Development of Lungs

The lungs develop in three stages from lung buds:
- The glandular phase (Fig. 36.5) lasting from six to sixteen weeks is characterized by development of solid tubular outgrowths (like ducts) from the lung buds
- The canalicular phase (sixteen weeks to twenty-six weeks) is characterized by canalization of solid ducts, proliferation of blood vessels and differentiation of respiratory bronchioles and alveolar ducts

Contd...

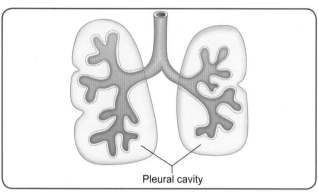

Fig. 36.5: Glandular phase of developing lung at 8 weeks of intrauterine life

Contd...

Contd...

 EMBRYOLOGIC INSIGHT

- The alveolar phase (twenty-six weeks until birth) is characterized by formation of alveoli including the cell types lining the alveoli. The developing lungs are now ready to perform normal function. Before birth, the alveoli are filled with amniotic fluid containing a small quantity of mucin and surfactant, due to which the lungs sink in water.
- With first breath, the fluid inside the alveoli is absorbed or expelled from respiratory passages and the lungs are filled with air. Hence, after the first breath, the lungs float in water. The alveoli are prevented from collapse by the surfactant.

STUDENT INTEREST

The laryngotracheal tube is formed from the endoderm of the cranial end foregut. It gives rise to larynx, trachea and it terminates into lung buds (which develop into intrapulmonary bronchial tree and respiratory portion of lungs.

TRACHEA (FIG. 36.7)

The trachea or windpipe is a tube that conducts air from the larynx to the principal bronchi.

Length

In the adult, the trachea is about 12 cm long.

Location

It is situated partly in the neck and partly in the superior mediastinum. The trachea lies in the midline in its cervical course but is deviated slightly to the right in its thoracic course.

Extent

It extends from the lower border of the cricoid cartilage (level with C6) to the upper border of the fifth thoracic

CLINICAL CORRELATION

Congenital Anomalies of Trachea and Lungs

- Tracheoesophageal fistula (TEF) is an anomaly, in which there is communication between trachea and esophagus. This is due to incomplete or defective tracheoesophageal septation accompanied by esophageal atresia. In about 90% of TEF, the lower segment of esophagus opens into the trachea (Fig. 36.6) closer to its termination. A newborn baby with this type of TEF will present with excessive frothing and choking with the first feed
- The respiratory distress syndrome is due to absence of, or inadequate secretion of, the surfactant resulting in collapse of alveoli after birth. This is one of the causes of death in neonatal period
- The apex of right lung may be divided by the pleural fold carrying the azygos vein in its bottom. The medial part of the divided apex is called lobe of the azygos vein. This may cast a shadow in the lung apex in a radiograph, which may be mistaken for a disease.

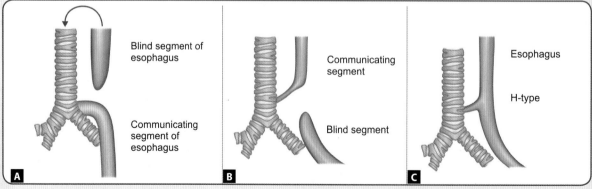

Figs 36.6A to C: Types of tracheoesophageal fistula. **A.** Lower segment of esophagus communicates with trachea near tracheal bifurcation (arrow showing); **B.** Upper segment of esophagus communicates with middle part of trachea by narrow passage; **C.** Middle portion of trachea communicates with trachea by a narrow passage (H-type of TEF)

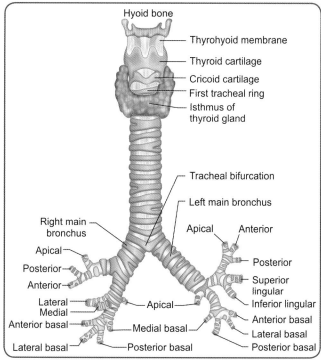

Fig. 36.7: Showing cervical and thoracic parts of trachea, its continuity with laryngeal cavity superiorly and tracheal bifurcation into right and left bronchi inferiorly

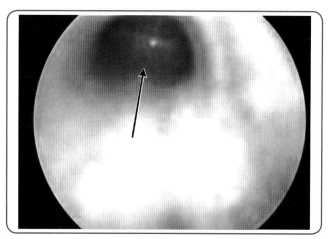

Fig. 36.8: Bronchoscopic view of carina at trachea bifurcation (arrow showing)

bronchoscopy. Hence, it is a useful landmark. It is located about 25 cm from the incisor teeth and 30 cm from the external nares. The mucosa of trachea is most sensitive at carina. If the tracheobronchial lymph nodes in the angle between the principal bronchi enlarge (due to spread from bronchogenic cancer), the carina becomes distorted and flattened. Therefore, changes in the appearance of carina are looked for during bronchoscopy (Fig. 36.8).

🐾 STUDENT INTEREST

Carina is present at tracheal bifurcation. Every student must learn this very important landmark and its clinical importance.

vertebra, where it divides into right and left principal bronchi.

Mobility

Its upper end moves with larynx and the lower end moves with respiration. During deep inspiration, the tracheal bifurcation may descend to the level of the sixth thoracic vertebra.

Patency

The walls of trachea are kept patent by 15 to 20 C-shaped cartilaginous rings. The posterior ends of the cartilaginous rings are held together by smooth muscle called trachealis, which flattens the posterior wall of the trachea. The soft posterior wall of the trachea allows for the expansion of the esophagus during swallowing.

Carina

At tracheal bifurcation, the lower margin of the lowest cartilaginous ring is called the **carina**, which is a hook-shaped or keel-shaped process curving downwards and backwards between the bronchi. The carina is visible as a sharp ridge at the tracheal bifurcation during

Relations

Relations of Cervical Part of Trachea (Fig 36.9 and 36.10A)

Anterior relation

The identification of anterior relations is essential in the operation of tracheostomy.

- The following layers are seen from superficial to deep aspect, skin, superficial fascia with platysma, investing layer of deep cervical fascia.
- The sternothyroid (deeper) and sternohyoid (superficial) muscles overlap the trachea.
- The isthmus of the thyroid gland and the arterial anastomosis along its upper margin, cross the second to fourth or second to third tracheal rings.
- The inferior thyroid veins descend from the isthmus into the superior mediastinum.
- The thyroidea ima artery, when present, is related below the isthmus.
- The jugular venous arch crosses the trachea in the suprasternal space.

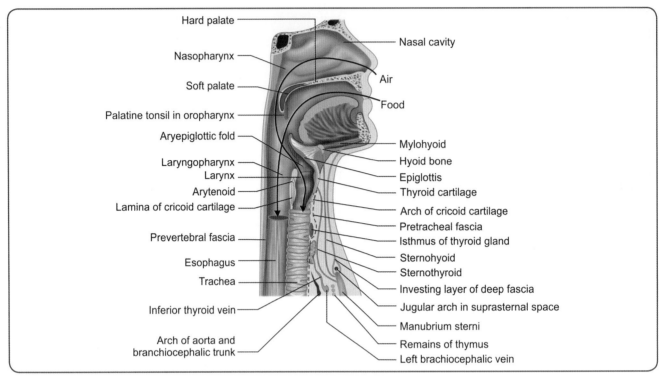

Fig. 36.9: Median section showing relations of trachea in the neck and in the superior mediastinum (Note the crossing of air and food paths in the oropharynx)

- The pretracheal lymph nodes are scattered on the anterior aspect.

Posterior relations

Posteriorly, the trachea lies on the esophagus with recurrent laryngeal nerve in the groove between trachea and esophagus.

Lateral relations

The trachea is related laterally to the lobes of the thyroid gland, inferior thyroid arteries and common carotid artery in the carotid sheath.

Relations of Thoracic Part of Trachea

Anterior relation

The vascular relations of trachea are very important in the superior mediastinum (Fig. 36.10B and 36.11).
- Arch of aorta and its two branches, brachiocephalic artery and left common carotid artery.
- Left brachiocephalic vein crosses the trachea from the left to the right side.
- Remains of thymus.
- Deep cardiac plexus and tracheobronchial lymph nodes at bifurcation.

Posterior relation

The trachea is in contact with the esophagus.

Left lateral relations

The trachea is related to the arch of aorta, left common carotid artery and left subclavian artery. It is also related to the left recurrent laryngeal nerve.

Right lateral relations

The trachea is in contact with the mediastinal surface of right lung and pleura. Its vascular relations on the right side are venous (right brachiocephalic vein, SVC and azygos arch). It is related to the right vagus nerve.

Surface Marking

The trachea is represented on the surface by a two cm wide midline band from the level of cricoid cartilage to the sternal angle with a slight inclination to the right at the lower end.

Blood Supply (Fig. 36.12)

- The cervical part of the trachea is mainly supplied by inferior thyroid arteries

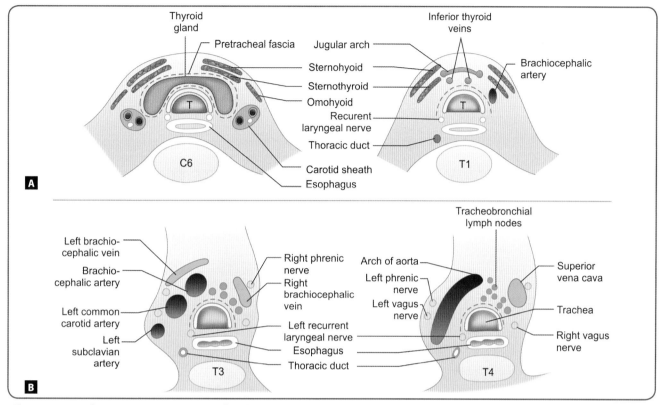

Figs 36.10A and B: A. Transverse sections of neck at C6 and T1 vertebral levels showing relations of cervical part of trachea; **B.** Transverse sections of superior mediastinum at T3 and T4 vertebral levels showing relations of thoracic part of trachea

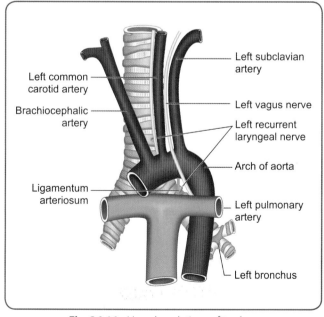

Fig. 36.11: Vascular relations of trachea

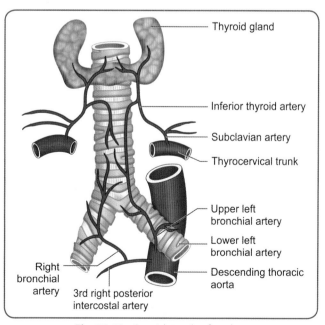

Fig. 36.12: Arterial supply of trachea

- The thoracic part of the trachea is additionally supplied by the bronchial arteries.
- The tracheal veins drain into the inferior thyroid venous plexus.

Lymphatic Drainage

Trachea drains into tracheobronchial, paratracheal and pretracheal lymph nodes (Fig. 36.30).

Nerve Supply

The nerve supply to the mucosa, tracheal glands and trachealis muscle is from the vagus nerves, recurrent laryngeal nerves and sympathetic ganglia.

⌀ CLINICAL CORRELATION

- Trachea is palpated in the suprasternal notch to confirm its position. Deviation to one side is suggestive of mediastinal shift. In aneurysm of arch of aorta, a tracheal tug can be felt in the suprasternal notch. This sign is elicited by palpating the trachea with the neck in extended position. A tug is felt coinciding with the pulsation of the aorta.
- The interior of the trachea is examined in a patient through the bronchoscope. The biopsies from tracheobronchial lymph nodes at the tracheal bifurcation are taken through the bronchoscope.
- In plain radiographs, the trachea appears as a translucent and dark tubular area in the neck because of the presence of air column in it.
- The insertion of endotracheal tube (*endotracheal intubation*) is necessary for giving general anesthesia. After positioning the head of the patient appropriately, an endotracheal tube is passed through the oral cavity or the nasal cavity and then guided through the laryngeal cavity with the help of a laryngoscope and pushed down till its tip reaches well above carina. The tube is guided keeping in mind the distance of the carina from the external nares or incisor teeth.
- *Tracheostomy* (Fig. 36.13) is making an artificial opening in the trachea if there is airway obstruction at laryngeal level. The site for the opening is in the cervical part of the trachea. The steps of the procedure are described along with structures in the midline of the neck in chapter 64.
- The commonest cause of tracheal compression in the neck is enlarged thyroid gland or thyroid swelling. The thoracic trachea may be compressed by enlarged lymph nodes or by aneurysm of arch of aorta in the superior mediastinum. Tracheal compression causes difficulty in breathing.

THE PLEURA AND PLEURAL CAVITY

The pleura is a smooth shining serous membrane that covers the lungs. It is divisible into the visceral (pulmonary)

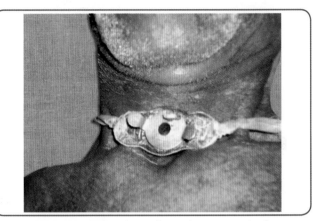

Fig. 36.13: Jackson's metallic tracheostomy tube for obstruction in laryngeal cavity

pleura and the parietal pleura. The visceral pleura covers the lung surface and gives it a glistening appearance. The parietal pleura lines the internal surfaces of the thoracic walls. The visceral and the parietal layers of the pleura are continuous with each other along the root of the lung and at the pulmonary ligament. The latter extends downwards from the hilum as a double-layered pleural fold. The pleural cavity is a potential space enclosed between the visceral and parietal pleura and contains a small amount of serous fluid.

Visceral or Pulmonary Pleura (Figs 36.14 and 36.15)

- The visceral pleura is inseparable from the lung.
- It dips into the fissures of the lungs.
- It shares the blood supply and nerve supply (autonomic nerves) with that of the lung.

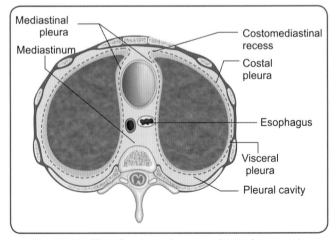

Fig. 36.14: Pleural cavity and costomediastinal recesses in transverse section

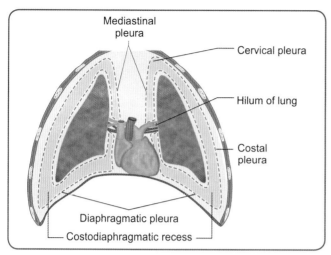

Fig. 36.15: Pleural cavity and costodiaphragmatic recesses (Note the continuity of mediastinal and visceral pleura at the hilum of lung)

- It is insensitive to pain
- It develops from splanchnopleuric mesoderm.

Parietal Pleura (Figs 36.14 and 36.15)

The parietal pleura is more extensive than the visceral pleura. It lines the walls of thoracic cavity internally and is supported on its external surface by a thick layer of endothoracic fascia. It develops from somatopleuric mesoderm, is supplied by somatic nerves and is pain-sensitive.

Subdivisions of Parietal Pleura (Fig. 36.15)

- Costal (costovertebral) pleura
- Mediastinal pleura
- Diaphragmatic pleura
- Cervical pleura or dome of pleura.

These different parts are continuous with each other along the lines of pleural reflection.

Costal pleura

The costal pleura lines the inner aspect of the thoracic wall, including ribs, intercostal spaces, sternum and sides of thoracic vertebral bodies. Anteriorly, the internal thoracic vessels directly rest on the pleura in the first and second intercostal spaces. It is loosely attached to the sternum, costal cartilages, ribs and intercostal muscles by endothoracic fascia. On the posterior aspect, the sympathetic chain on each side is located posterior to the costal pleura and the intercostal nerve travels between the costal pleura and the posterior intercostal membrane before entering the intercostal space (Fig. 35.4A).

Mediastinal pleura

The mediastinal pleura lines the medial surface of the lung and is in contact with the structures in the corresponding side of the mediastinum. It encloses the structures inside the lung root and becomes continuous with the visceral pleura around the hilum of the lung. It extends below the lung hilum as pulmonary ligament which is a connecting bond between the mediastinum and the medial surface of the lung below the hilum.

Diaphragmatic pleura

The diaphragmatic pleura lines the superior surface of the diaphragm. Superiorly, it is related to the base of the lung (costomediastinal recess of pleural cavity intervening between the two).

Cervical pleura

The cervical pleura is the continuation of costal pleura above the level of inner margin of the first rib (above the thoracic inlet). Here it covers the apex of the lung. It extends posteriorly up to the neck of the first rib, which is at a higher level. The suprapleural membrane or Sibson's fascia protects the cervical pleura. The cervical pleura is related anteriorly to subclavian artery and scalenus anterior muscle. Posteriorly, it is related to structures in close contact with front of the neck of first rib (Fig. 35.1).

Lines of Pleural Reflections

- Anteriorly, the costal pleura is continuous with the mediastinal pleura at the back of the sternum along the costomediastinal line of pleural reflection or anterior margin of pleura.
- Inferiorly, the costal pleura is continuous with the diaphragmatic pleura along the costodiaphragmatic line of pleural reflection or inferior margin of pleura.
- Posteriorly, the costal pleura is continuous with the mediastinal pleura by the side of the vertebral column along the costovertebral line of pleural reflection or posterior margin of pleura (Fig. 36.17).

Surface Marking

Costomediastinal Line (Fig. 36.16)

- On both sides, the costomediastinal lines begin behind the sternoclavicular joints and descend in medial direction to come closer to each other at the midpoint of sternal angle.
- On the right side, it runs vertically downward up to the midpoint of xiphisternal joint.

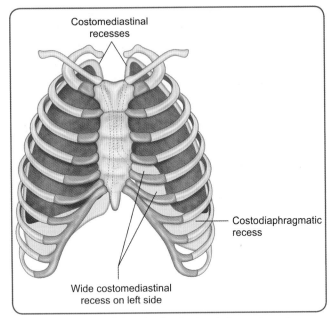

Fig. 36.16: Lines of pleural reflection in relation to thoracic cage from anterior aspect (Note that the inferior line of pleural reflection crosses the right costoxiphoid joint but not the left)

- On the left side, it descends vertically up to the level of fourth costal cartilage and then deviates laterally to the margin of the sternum and descends close to the sternum up to the left sixth costal cartilage.

Costodiaphragmatic Line (Figs 36.16 and 36.17)

- On the right side, the costodiaphragmatic line begins at the midpoint of xiphisternal joint and turns laterally along the seventh costal cartilage to reach the eighth rib in the midclavicular line, tenth rib in the midaxillary line, and twelfth rib in the scapular line to finally end at the level of spine of twelfth thoracic vertebra about 2 cm from the midline.
- On the left side, the line begins at the left sixth costosternal joint, beyond which it follows the course similar to that of right side.

Note: Inferior margin of pleura extends below the costoxiphoid angle on the right side only.

 STUDENT INTEREST

> For costodiaphragmatic line of reflection or inferior margin of pleura, remember 8th, 10th and 12th ribs.

Costovertebral Line

This line extends from a point 2 cm lateral to the seventh cervical spine to a point 2 cm lateral to the twelfth thoracic spine.

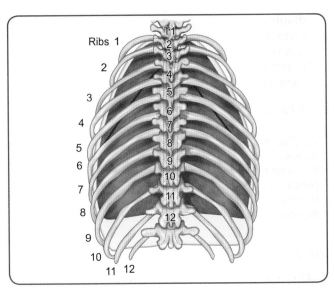

Fig. 36.17: Lines of pleural reflection in relation to thoracic cage from posterior aspect

Cervical Pleura

On the anterior aspect, the cervical pleura is represented by a curved line starting from the sternoclavicular joint and reaching a point 2.5 cm above the sternal end of clavicle. From here, the line curves down to meet a point at the junction of medial and middle third of clavicle.

Pleural Recesses

The pleural recesses are the extensions of the pleural cavities along the lines of pleural reflections The recesses are present because the pleural cavities are larger than the lung volumes. These spaces are unoccupied by lung during quiet breathing. They are present at two locations.

1. The ***costomediastinal recesses*** (Fig. 36.14) are present along the costomediastinal lines of pleural reflection. Thus, this recess is bounded by junctional parts of the costal and mediastinal pleurae. The right recess is very narrow and of uniform size. The left recess is wide at the level of fourth to sixth costal cartilages. The deviation of the anterior margin of the lung (due to the presence of cardiac notch) is much more compared to that of the pleural line at this site. The left costomediastinal recess is responsible for the presence of the area of superficial cardiac dullness. Except for the wider part of the left recess, the rest of the costomediastinal recesses are filled with lung during deep inspiration.

2. The ***costodiaphragmatic recesses*** (Fig. 36.15) are present along costodiaphragmatic lines of pleural reflection. Along this line, the lower margin of the pleura is two-rib distant below the lower margin of the lung. This recess is bounded by the costal and

diaphragmatic pleurae. In deep inspiration, the recesses of both sides are partially filled. The right recess is related to the liver and posterior surface of right kidney and the left recess to the fundus of stomach, spleen and posterior surface of left kidney.

STUDENT INTEREST

The pleural recesses are the extensions of pleural cavity along the lines of pleural reflections. They provide reserve space for the lungs to expand during deep inspiration. There are two pleural recesses on each side – costomediastinal anteriorly and costodiaphragmatic inferiorly. The pleural recesses are of importance to the radiologist and to the clinician.

Nerve Supply

- The visceral pleura receives innervation from autonomic nerves, hence, it is pain, insensitive.

- The parietal pleura is supplied by somatic nerves; hence, it is pain-insensitive. The pain is referred to the thoracic and abdominal walls or to the neck and shoulder.
    - The costal pleura receives twigs from intercostal nerves.
    - The peripheral part of diaphragmatic pleura receives branches from the intercostal nerves whereas its central part from the phrenic nerves.
    - The mediastinal pleura is supplied by the phrenic nerve.

Arterial Supply

The visceral pleura is supplied by the bronchial arteries and the parietal pleura by the intercostal and internal mammary arteries.

CLINICAL CORRELATION

- **Pleurisy** (pleuritis) is inflammation of the parietal pleura. It gives rise to pain, which is aggravated by respiratory movements and is radiated to thoracic and abdominal walls
- **Pneumothorax** means air in the pleural space. Air may enter the pleural cavity as a result of penetrating injuries of thorax, tear of visceral or parietal pleura or inadvertent puncture of pleural cavity by the clinician while drawing fluid from the cavity. The primary effect of pneumothorax is the collapse of lung on the affected side. The collapsed lung is not able to oxygenate blood. The patient experiences shortness of breath and cyanosis because of reduced oxygen in the blood. The mediastinum shifts to the normal side compressing the normal lung also
- **Pleural effusion** means excess fluid in the pleural cavity. This condition gives rise to dullness on percussion and reduction in the intensity of the breath sounds. Due to the collapse of the lung on the affected side the mediastinum shifts to the normal side, which can be confirmed by shift of the trachea. Fluid level can be confirmed by radiographic examination. If there is watery fluid in the pleural cavity, it is called hydrothorax.

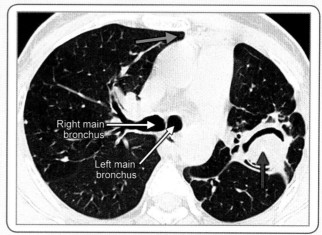

Fig. 36.18: Contrast CT of chest showing mediastinal shift to left side and compensatory hypertrophy on right side (red arrow shows lung pathology and green arrow shows mediastinal shift)

Accumulation of pus is called pyothorax, of blood is known as hemothorax and of lymph is called chylothorax
- Figure 36.18 shows mediastinal shift to the left due to collapse of left lung
- **Thoracocentesis** or pleural tap is done to remove excess fluid from the pleural cavity. This is performed with the patient in sitting position. Usually the needle is inserted in the posterior axillary line or the midaxillary line through the lower part of the sixth intercostal space. The needle passes in succession the skin, fasciae, serratus anterior, intercostal muscles, endothoracic fascia and the costal pleura before entering the pleural cavity **(Fig. 36.19).**

Contd...

Contd...

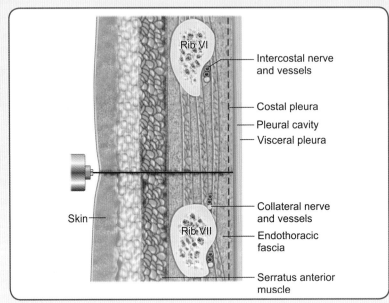

Fig. 36.19: Layers of chest wall pierced in succession by the needle inserted for pleural tapping along the posterior axillary line

- *Costodiaphragmatic recess* (being the most dependent part of the pleural cavity) shows widening in the radiograph, when a small quantity of fluid accumulates in it. This may be the first indication of fluid in the pleural cavity. Therefore, these recesses are examined routinely in the radiographs of the chest.
- In posterior surgical approach to the kidney while removing a section of the twelfth rib, care should be taken not to injure the inferior margin of pleura in relation to the twelfth rib.

LUNGS

The lungs are the seats of oxygenation of blood. Each lung lies free in its own pleural cavity, attached to the mediastinum only by its root and the pulmonary ligament. The lungs of the children are pink in color unlike in the adult, where deposition of carbon particles (inhaled from atmospheric air) imparts grayish black color to the lungs. During life, the lungs are soft, elastic and spongy. Being air-filled they float on water. The lungs of the newborn before the first breath sink in water.

Gross Features

The shape of each lung is conical with a rounded apex, a broad base or diaphragmatic surface (Fig. 36.20), costal surface and medial surface separated by three margins (borders).

Surfaces

There are three surfaces as follows:
- A large costal surface in contact with ribs and intercostal spaces.

- A base or diaphragmatic surface in contact with diaphragm.
- A medial surface facing mediastinum and vertebral column. The medial surface is subdivided into larger anterior mediastinal surface and smaller posterior vertebral surface. The mediastinal surface bears the hilum of the lung (Fig. 36.21).

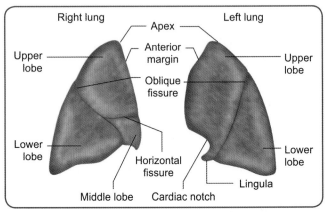

Fig. 36.20: Lobes and fissures of lungs viewed from anterior aspect (Note that lingula belongs to upper lobe of left lung)

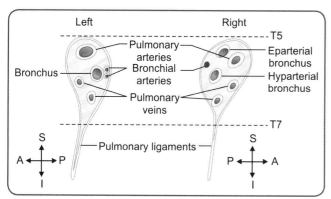

Fig. 36.21: Relationship of structures at hilum of right and left lungs (Note that the vertebral level of hilum is T5 to T7)

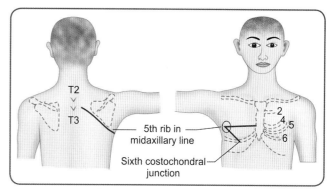

Fig. 36.22: Surface marking of oblique and transverse fissures of right lung (Note that oblique fissure extends from posterior to anterior aspect and its surface marking is similar on both sides)

Margins (Borders)

- The sharp anterior margin separates the mediastinal and costal surfaces. The anterior margin of left lung has a wide cardiac notch below the level of fourth costal cartilage.
- The rounded posterior margin separates the vertebral and costal surfaces.
- The inferior margin intervenes between the base (diaphragmatic surface) and other two surfaces.

Fissures

- There are two fissures (oblique and horizontal) in right lung, which divide the right lung into three lobes (upper, middle and lower).
- There is one fissure (oblique) in left lung, which divides the left lung into two lobes (upper and lower).

Surface marking of fissures (Fig. 36.22)

- The oblique fissure is marked by a line passing downward and forward from a point on the posterior chest wall about 2 cm lateral to the spine of third thoracic vertebra. The line crosses the fifth rib in the mid-axillary line and reaches the sixth costal cartilage 7 to 8 cm lateral to the mid-line (or at the sixth costochondral junction). Roughly the oblique fissure corresponds to the medial margin of the scapula in the fully abducted position of the arm.
- The horizontal fissure runs along the level of the right fourth costal cartilage and rib to meet the oblique fissure in the mid-axillary line.

External Features of Right and Left Lung

- The average weight in adult of right lung is 600 g and that of left lung is 550 g.

- The right lung is broader and shorter than the left lung because the massive liver pushes the right dome of the diaphragm upwards.
- The anterior margin of the right lung is sharp and straight. The anterior margin of left lung is sharp but not straight as it presents a cardiac notch and a projecting lingula below it.
- The right lung is divided into superior, middle and inferior lobes. Due to oblique plane of oblique fissure the inferior lobe is more posterior and the middle and superior lobes more anterior. The left lung is divided into superior and inferior lobes by the oblique fissure. The lingula is the tongue-shaped projection of superior lobe below the cardiac notch on anterior margin.
- The relations of the structures at the hilum on the two lungs are different (Fig. 36.21). The structures from above downwards in the right lung are eparterial bronchus, pulmonary artery, hyparterial bronchus and inferior pulmonary vein and in the left lung, pulmonary artery, principal bronchus and inferior pulmonary vein.
- However, none of these differences is reliable in assigning side to an isolated lung. For identification of the side of the lung, it is held in anatomical position (as if it belongs to the holder's own body). The apex points upwards, the base points downwards, sharp margin faces anteriorly and surface bearing the hilum faces medially.

🐾 STUDENT INTEREST

Mnemonic

To remember the order of structures from above downwards: Left lung asks question—**Are Beasts Violent**?—ABV, Right lung replies—**Beasts Are Born Violent**—BABV.

Surface Marking

- The apex of the lung is represented by a curved line forming a dome, the summit of which rises 2.5 cm above the medial one-third of the clavicle.
- The anterior margin of right lung coincides with the costomediastinal line of pleural reflection. The anterior margin of left lung coincides with the costomediastinal line of pleural reflection up to the level of fourth costal cartilage. Below this level, it deviates from the midline for a distance of 3.5 cm between the fourth and sixth costal cartilages.
- The inferior margin of lung is indicated by a line starting at the level of sixth costal cartilage on the left side and midpoint of the xiphisternum on the right side. Traced further, it cuts the sixth rib in the mid-clavicular line, eighth rib in the mid-axillary line and tenth rib in the scapular line.
- The posterior margin of lung extends vertically upwards from the transverse process of the tenth thoracic vertebra to a point lateral to the spine of the seventh cervical vertebra.

🎓 STUDENT INTEREST

For surface marking of inferior margin of lung remember 6th, 8th and 10th ribs (exactly two ribs above the surface marking of inferior margin of pleura).

♂ CLINICAL CORRELATION

Auscultation Sites

In order to find out the disease or normalcy of the pleura or lung, the clinician hears the breath sounds with the help of a stethoscope (auscultation). The knowledge of the surface marking of the lung is of use in delineating lung lobes on the surface of the chest wall.
- The apex of the lung is auscultated above the medial third of the clavicle anteriorly and in the upper part of suprascapular region posteriorly
- The upper lobe of the right lung is heard anteriorly in the area extending from the clavicle to the level of fourth costal cartilage
- The upper lobe of left lung is heard anteriorly in the area extending from the clavicle to the level of sixth costal cartilage
- The middle lobe of right lung is heard anteriorly between the right fourth and sixth ribs in front of the midaxillary line
- The apical or superior segment of the lower lobe (on both sides) is heard posteriorly in the interval between the medial border of the scapula and the vertebral spines. The basal segments of the lower lobe (on both sides) are heard posteriorly in the infrascapular region up to the level of tenth rib.

Apex of Lung

The relations of the apex of the lung (Fig. 36.23) are very important.

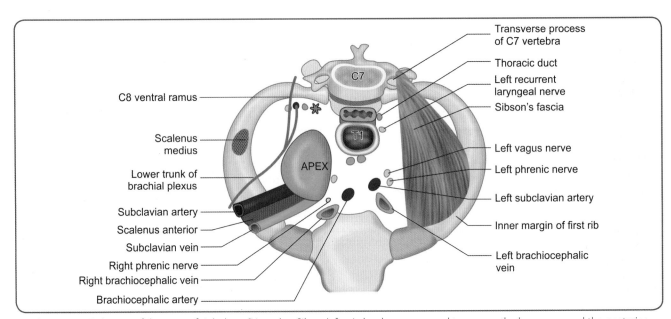

Fig. 36.23: Relations of the apex of right lung [Note that Sibson's fascia has been removed to expose the lung apex and the posterior relations of lung apex are the anterior relations of the neck of first rib (not labeled in the diagram)]

The apex is covered with the dome of the cervical pleura. The suprapleural membrane or Sibson's fascia protects the apex and the covering pleura in the root of the neck.

Relations

- **Anteriorly:** Subclavian artery, subclavian vein and scalenus anterior muscle
- **Posteriorly:** Sympathetic chain, highest intercostal vein, superior intercostal artery and ascending branch of the ventral ramus of the first thoracic nerve (from medial to lateral side).
- **Laterally:** Scalenus medius muscle
- **Medially:** On the right side, from anterior to posterior, the structures are right brachiocephalic vein, right phrenic nerve, brachiocephalic artery, right vagus and trachea.

On the left side from anterior to posterior, the structures are: left brachiocephalic vein, left subclavian artery, left recurrent laryngeal nerve, esophagus and thoracic duct.

 STUDENT INTEREST

Surface marking and relations of lung apex must be revised again and again because of its clinical relevance.

 CLINICAL CORRELATION

Malignancy of Lung Apex

The malignancy of the apex of the lung may present as symptoms and signs produced due to spread of cancer to neighboring structures.
- Spread of cancer in subclavian or brachiocephalic vein results in venous engorgement and edema in the arm or neck and face
- Pressure on the subclavian artery results in diminished pulse in the upper limb on the affected side
- Infiltration in the phrenic nerve results in paralysis of hemidiaphragm.

Pancoast Syndrome

When the structures in posterior relation of lung apex are involved due to cancer of lung apex, it produces symptoms and signs, which are collectively called Pancoast syndrome.
- Pain in ulnar distribution and wasting of small muscles of hand (due to injury to ventral ramus of T1 or lower trunk of brachial plexus)
- Horner's syndrome (due to injury to sympathetic chain)
- Erosion of first and second ribs.

Medial Surface of Lung

This surface has a larger mediastinal surface, which is characterised by hilum of the lung and pulmonary ligament. This surface presents markings and grooves produced by the structures in the mediastinum. The smaller and convex vertebral surface is devoid of markings.

Impressions on Mediastinal Surface of Right Lung (Fig. 36.24)

- The right subclavian artery produces grooves upper end of the anterior margin and the apex. The right first rib produces a notch on the anterior nmargin below that of right subclavian artery.
- A large cardiac impression (due to right atrium and right ventricle) is present in front of and below the hilum.
- Superiorly, cardiac impression is continuous with the groove for superior vena cava, which is located in front of the hilum and is prolonged upwards as the groove for right brachiocephalic vein.
- A deep groove for the arch of azygos vein begins from the posterior margin of the groove for SVC and arches backwards over the hilum of the lung.
- Above the hilum, trachea and right vagus nerve are related posterior to the groove for SVC.
- The right phrenic nerve descends in front of the hilum.
- The esophagus makes a wide shallow groove behind the trachea, the hilum and the pulmonary ligament. This groove stops short of the lower margin of the lung
- The inferior vena cava is related to the lung postero-inferior to the cardiac impression.

 STUDENT INTEREST

Identify following impressions on the specimen of right lung – groove for arch of azygos vein above the hilum, groove for superior ven cava, cardiac impression, wide shallow and long groove for esophagus, groove for right subclavian artery and first rib near the apex. Study features of mediastinal surfaces of both lungs with the help of diagrams.

Vertebral Surface of Right Lung

This surface is in contact with the right aspect of thoracic vertebrae and intervertebral discs, posterior intercostal vessels and splanchnic nerves (branches of thoracic sympathetic chain).

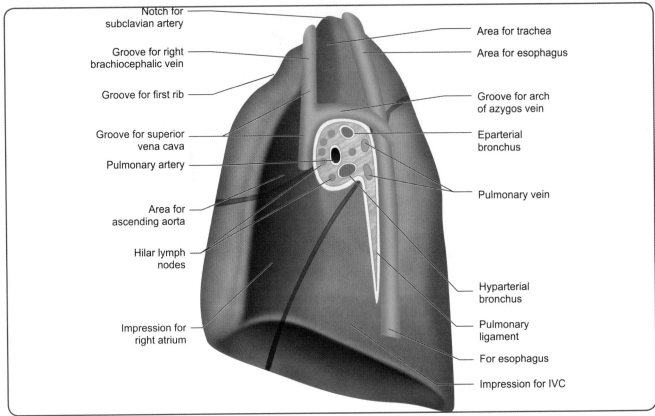

Fig. 36.24: Relations of medial (mediastinal and vertebral) surface of right lung

Impressions on Mediastinal Surface of Left Lung (Fig. 36.25)

- There is a large cardiac impression in front of and below the hilum. The left ventricle is mainly related to this area. The anterior part however, is related to the infundibulum of right ventricle.
- The pulmonary trunk lies in front of the hilum in continuation of the area for infundibulum.
- The arch of aorta produces a deep and wide groove immediately above the hilum.
- In continuation of groove for arch of aorta, there is a groove for descending thoracic aorta behind the hilum and pulmonary ligament. It reaches up to the lower margin of the lung.
- The grooves for left subclavian artery and for left common carotid artery course upwards from the groove for arch of aorta. The left common carotid artery produces an anteriorly located short groove. The groove for left subclavian artery runs upwards to cut the anterior margin just below the apex.
- The first rib comes in contact with this surface below that of left subclavian artery.

- The thoracic duct and esophagus are related behind the groove for left subclavian artery.
- The left brachiocephalic vein lies in a faint linear depression in front of the left subclavian artery.
- The left phrenic nerve descends in front of the hilum and crosses the cardiac impression.
- The lower esophageal impression lies in front of the groove for descending aorta and behind and below the lower end of the pulmonary ligament.

🐘 STUDENT INTEREST

Identify following impressions on left lung—groove for arch of aorta above the hilum, a long groove for descending aorta behind the hilum and pulmonary ligament, cardiac impression in front of hilum, groove for left subclavian artery and for first rib, upper esophageal impression, lower esophageal impression and structures at the hilum.

Vertebral Surface of Left Lung

This surface is related to the left aspects of thoracic vertebrae and intervening discs, posterior intercostal

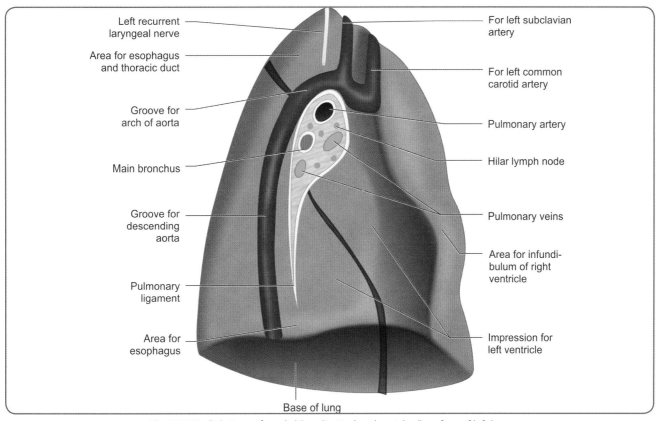

Fig. 36.25: Relations of medial (mediastinal and vertebral) surface of left lung

vessels and splanchnic nerves (branches of thoracic sympathetic chain).

Root of Lung (Fig. 36.26)

The root of lung connects the mediastinum to the lung. All the structures, which enter and leave the hilum of the lung, are enclosed in a tubular sheath of mediastinal pleura. This tubular sheath with its enclosed contents is called the root of the lung.

Vertebral Level

The lung root lies opposite T5 to T7 vertebrae.

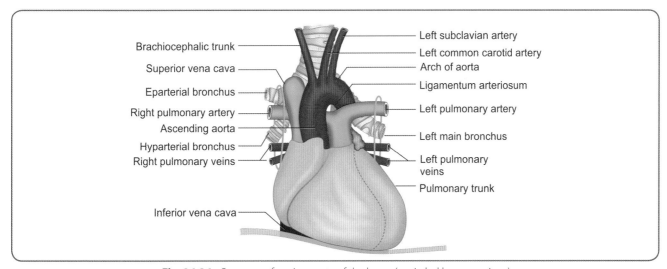

Fig. 36.26: Structures forming roots of the lungs (encircled by green rings)

Contents

- Single bronchus (principal bronchus on the left side) and two bronchi (eparterial and hyparterial) on the right side.
- A pair of pulmonary veins
- Pulmonary artery
- Bronchial vessels
- Lymph vessels and hilar or bronchopulmonary lymph nodes.
- Pulmonary nerve plexuses.

All the above structures are seen at the hilum also.

Pulmonary Ligament

It is a double fold of mediastinal pleura below the level of pulmonary hilum. It connects the mediastinal surface below the lung root to the side of posterior mediastinum. The layers of the pulmonary ligament are continuous medially with mediastinal pleura, laterally with the visceral pleura and superiorly with the pleura covering the lung root. Its lower border is free. There is a potential space between the two layers of the pulmonary ligament, which provides a dead space for expansion of inferior pulmonary veins during increased venous return and for the descent of lung root during inspiration.

Bronchial Tree (Fig. 36.27)

The principal bronchus passes inferolateral from the bifurcation of the trachea to the hilum of each lung. The right bronchus divides into eparterial and hyparterial bronchi before entering the hilum while left bronchus enters as such.

Right Main Bronchus

This is wider, shorter (length 2.5 cm) and more vertical than the left bronchus. Therefore, an aspirated foreign body is more likely to enter the right lung.

- The eparterial bronchus continues as the right superior lobar bronchus inside the lung and divides into three segmental bronchi namely, apical, anterior and posterior.

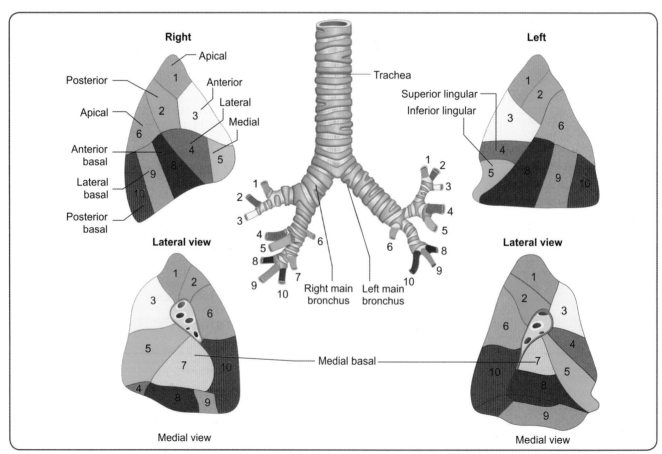

Fig. 36.27: Bronchopulmonary segments of lungs as seen in lateral and medial views (Note that the name of the segment is equivalent to the name of the segmental bronchus)

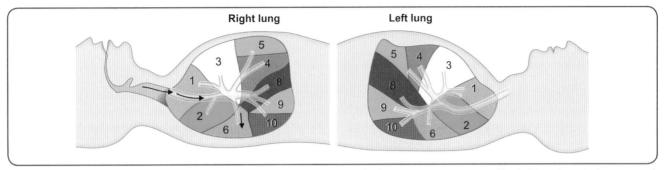

Fig. 36.28: Lateral view of bronchopulmonary segments and tracheobronchial tree in supine position of body (Note the apical segment of lower lobe is the most dependent in both the lungs in supine position of the body)

- The hyparterial bronchus divides into middle and right inferior lobar bronchi inside the lung. The middle lobar bronchus divides into two segmental bronchi called medial and lateral. The right inferior lobar bronchus divides into five segmental bronchi for the inferior lobe (superior or apical, medial basal, anterior basal, posterior basal and lateral basal.

Note: The superior or apical segmental bronchus is given off from the posterior aspect and goes directly backwards to the superior segment of the inferior lobe. In the supine position of the body, this segmental bronchus projects directly posteriorly and since it is the first branch to arise, foreign body is inhaled into it. The superior bronchopulmonary segment of lower lobe is the most dependent in supine position and hence secretions tend to collect in it (Fig. 36.28).

Left Main Bronchus

The left main bronchus is narrower, less vertical and longer (length 5 cm) than the right. Passing to the left from its origin, it lies inferior to the aortic arch and crosses the esophagus anteriorly (producing esophageal constriction). It enters the hilum of the lung and divides into superior and inferior lobar bronchi.

- The left superior lobar bronchus divides into superior and inferior stems. The superior stem gives off an anterior segmental bronchus and is then called apicoposterior segmental bronchus, which soon divides into apical and posterior segmental bronchi. The inferior stem descends towards the lingula and divides into superior and inferior lingular segmental bronchi
- The left inferior lobar bronchus gives off the superior (apical) segmental bronchus for the upper part of the inferior lobe. Similar to the right side, this bronchus projects directly posteriorly and in the supine position tends to collect secretions. Then the inferior lobar bronchus divides into antero-medial and postero-lateral stems. The antero-medial stem divides into medial basal and anterior basal segmental bronchi

while the postero-lateral stem divides into lateral and posterior basal segmental bronchi.

STUDENT INTEREST

Take a note of the differences between right and left main bronchi. Study the bronchial tree with the help of a diagram (Fig. 36.27).

Bronchopulmonary Segments

The bronchopulmonary segment is defined as a structural and functional unit of the lung parenchyma ventilated or aerated by a segmental or a tertiary bronchus. The names of the bronchopulmonary segments in right and left lungs are shown in Table 36.1.

TABLE 36.1: Names of Bronchopulmonary Segments

Lobes	Right lung	Left lung
Upper or superior	Apical, posterior anterior	Apical, posterior anterior, superior lingular, inferior lingular
Middle	Lateral, medial	NIL
Lower or inferior	Apical or superior Medial basal Anterior basal Lateral basal Posterior basal	Apical or superior Medial basal Anterior basal Lateral basal Posterior basal

Characteristic Features (Fig. 36.29)

- The shape of the bronchopulmonary segment is pyramidal with apex pointing towards the hilum and the base towards the lung surface
- Each segment has a covering of loose connective tissue
- Each segment contains segmental bronchus and its further subdivisions, segmental branches of pulmonary artery and of bronchial artery. Air and impure blood pass in the centre of each segment.

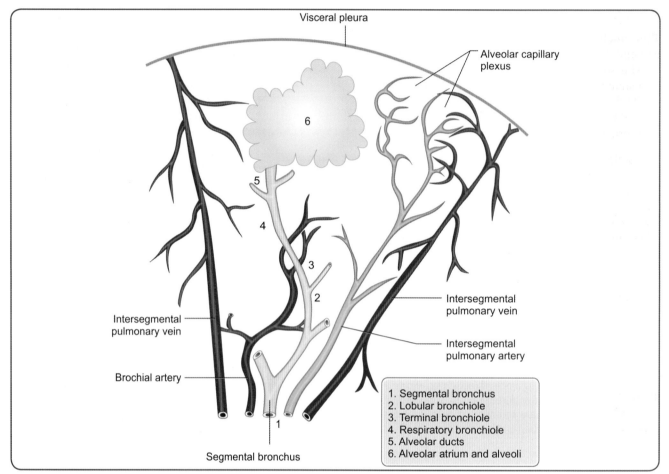

Visceral pleura

Alveolar capillary plexus

6

5

4

3

2

Intersegmental pulmonary vein

Intersegmental pulmonary artery

Intersegmental pulmonary vein

Brochial artery

Segmental bronchus

1

1. Segmental bronchus
2. Lobular bronchiole
3. Terminal bronchiole
4. Respiratory bronchiole
5. Alveolar ducts
6. Alveolar atrium and alveoli

Fig. 36.29: Bronchopulmonary segment showing its blood vessels, pulmonary vascular bed, ramifications of segmental bronchus inside the segment, lung parenchyma

- The tributaries of pulmonary veins supported in loose connective tissue are located in the intersegmental planes. Thus, the pure blood passes along the periphery of each segment.
- Each segment can be delineated radiologically (bronchography).
- Segmental resection is surgical removal of a diseased bronchopulmonary segment. During surgery the segmental bronchus of the diseased segment is located by dissection and it is clamped along with the blood vessels. This enables to delineate the segment, as the surface of that segment will darken due to loss of blood supply and air.

STUDENT INTEREST

Definition of bronchopulmonary segment, its characteristic features and nomenclature (Table 36.1) on right and left lungs are the must know topics. Note that lingula along with its 2 bronchopulmonary segments belongs to superior lobe of left lung.

Blood Supply

- The pulmonary arteries carry deoxygenated blood to the lung from the right ventricle. After entering the hilum the pulmonary arteries follow the divisions of the segmental bronchi. The arterioles accompanying the terminal and respiratory bronchioles are thin walled (without muscle fibers). These end up forming capillaries, which are in close proximity to the alveoli. The venous ends of the capillary beds join to form veins, which travel in the intersegmental planes. The intersegmental veins finally unite to form two pulmonary veins in each lung.
- The pulmonary veins carry oxygenated blood from the lungs to the left atrium.
- The bronchial arteries provide nutrition to the bronchial tree up to the level of terminal bronchioles (which means to the non-respiratory portions of the lungs).
- The respiratory portions of the lungs are nourished from pulmonary capillary beds and directly from atmospheric air contained inside the alveoli.

Bronchial Arteries (Figs 36.12 and 32.10)

The bronchial arteries supply the intrapulmonary bronchial tree and the connective tissue of lung parenchyma.

- The single right bronchial artery takes origin from usually from right third posterior intercostal artery.
- On the left side there are two bronchial arteries, upper and lower. Both are the direct branches of descending thoracic aorta at the level of tracheal bifurcation.

🏛 STUDENT INTEREST

Note the difference in the number and origin of bronchial arteries on the right and left sides. Single right bronchial artery arises from right third intercostal artery and two left bronchial arteries arise directly from descending aorta.

Bronchial Veins

- Right bronchial vein opens into the azygos vein
- Left bronchial vein opens either into left superior intercostal vein or into accessory hemiazygos vein.

Lymphatic Drainage (Fig. 36.30)

The lymphatic drainage of the lung is important because the nodes are enlarged in lung cancer and in pulmonary tuberculosis.

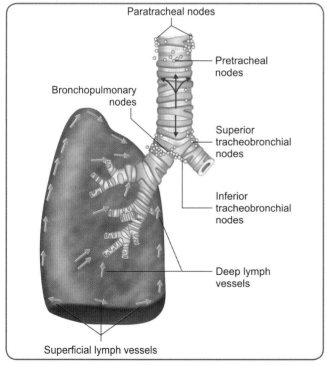

Fig. 36.30: Lymphatic drainage of lung, bronchi and trachea (Arrows indicate flow of lymph from superficial and deep lymph draining the lung)

- There are two sets of lymphatic plexuses, superficial and deep. The superficial plexus is subpleural in location and the deep plexus is seen along the bronchi and blood vessels. These two sets communicate with each other at the hilum and drain into the bronchopulmonary lymph nodes, which are also called hilar lymph nodes. These nodes are black in color due to the carbon particles drained into them from lungs.
- The efferent lymph vessels from the hilar nodes pass through tracheobronchial and paratracheal nodes. The tracheobronchial nodes communicate with the nodes in the base of the neck. The enlarged nodes may obstruct a lobar bronchus causing collapse (atelectasis) of the entire lobe.

Nerve Supply

The lungs receive both sympathetic and parasympathetic nerves from the pulmonary plexuses.

- The afferent fibers from the lung originate in endings sensitive to stretch, which are involved in reflex control of respiration and coughing.
- The parasympathetic fibers are cholinergic. The parasympathetic stimulation causes bronchoconstriction and increased secretion of the bronchial glands. The attack of bronchial asthma is produced due to spasm of smooth muscles in the wall of bronchioles. This may be precipitated by excessive vagal stimulation (due to exposure to pollen dust, cold air, ordinary dust, smoke, etc.).
- The sympathetic fibers are adrenergic. The sympathetic stimulation causes bronchodilatation, vasoconstriction and decreased secretion.

💡 ADDED INFORMATION

Radiological Anatomy

- In a plain radiograph, first the soft tissue shadows are examined. The trachea is identified in the midline in the superior mediastinum as a translucent air column. The lung fields are translucent, but the bronchovascular markings are seen as branching opacities throughout the lungs. The hilum is recognized as an opaque area because it contains large blood vessels and lymph nodes. The costodiaphragmatic recesses are visible and always examined for presence of fluid
- The CT scans and MRI of the thorax are also useful to study internal anatomy
- Bronchography is done to visualize the bronchial tree by injecting contrast medium.

CLINICAL CORRELATION

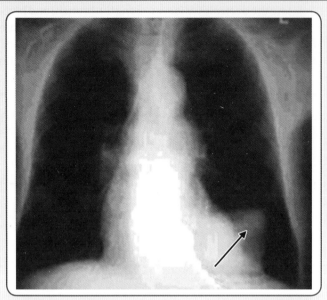

Fig. 36.31: Radiograph of the chest showing dense shadow in left lung (due to cancer) (arrow showing)

- In bronchoscopy (Fig. 36.8), the interior of trachea and the bronchi is inspected using a bronchoscope. Carina at tracheal bifurcation is an important landmark visible through the bronchoscope.
- Mendelson's syndrome is the aspiration pneumonia in the superior (apical) segment of the lower lobe. The anatomical reason for this is that in the supine position of the body, the superior segmental bronchus is the most dependent. Hence, it tends to collect the secretions, which may obstruct the bronchus leading to collapse of the superior segment of the lower lobe (atelectasis) and pneumonia.
- The bronchiectasis is the condition in which bronchi and bronchioles are dilated. The segmental bronchi to the basal segments of the lower lobe are prone to this condition in which the smaller divisions of the bronchi become permanently dilated and filled with pus. Postural drainage is performed to remove pus by giving appropriate position to the patient.
- The bronchogenic carcinoma originates from the epithelium of the bronchi. Cigarette smoke and automobile smoke increase the risk of this cancer. The presence of circular shadow (coin lesion) or an irregular shadow in a plain X-ray of chest may be the only finding in an otherwise asymptomatic patient. Carcinoma of left lung is detectable in plain radiograph of chest (Fig. 36.31).
- Figure 36.18 shows a pathological condition in which there is myceloma (fungal colony) in the preexisting tuberculous cavity in the left lung.

Thoracic Diaphragm and Phrenic Nerves

DIAPHRAGM

The diaphragm is a movable partition between the thoracic and abdominal cavities. It is partly muscular and partly tendinous. It is the chief muscle of inspiration. The diaphragm descends during inspiration and ascends during expiration. During quiet breathing it descends for a distance of 1.5 cm.

Parts and Relations (Fig. 37.1)

- The superior surface of the diaphragm projects as two domes or cupola into the thoracic cavity. The domes are covered with diaphragmatic pleura. The base of each lung fits into the corresponding dome.
- The central tendon is a depressed area between the two domes of diaphragm. The central tendon is fused with the base of the fibrous pericardium.
- The deeply concave inferior surface of the diaphragm forms the roof of the abdominal cavity. It is covered with parietal peritoneum. The right side of this surface is related to the right lobe of the liver, right kidney and right suprarenal gland. The left side of this surface is related to the left lobe of the liver, fundus of stomach, spleen, left kidney and left suprarenal gland.

Attachments

The diaphragm is attached circumferentially to the margins of inferior aperture of thoracic cavity or thoracic outlet (Fig. 37.1).

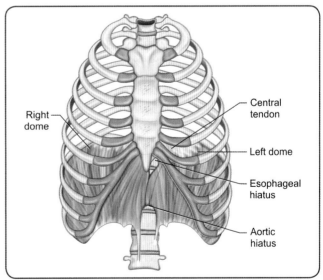

Fig. 37.1: Location of diaphragm in relation to the thoracic cage (Note that the diaphragm is a movable partition between the thorax and abdomen)

Right dome

Central tendon

Left dome

Esophageal hiatus

Aortic hiatus

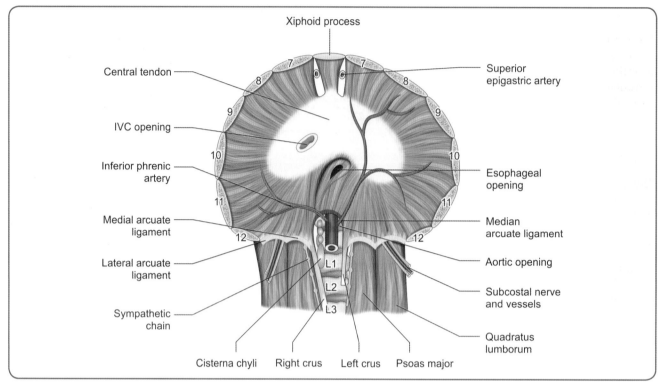

Fig. 37.2: Showing the vertebral, costal and sternal origins of the muscle of diaphragm as seen from abdominal aspect (numbers 7 to 12 indicate corresponding ribs)
Key: (IVC: inferior vena cava)

Origin (Fig. 37.2)

According to the site of origin, the diaphragm is subdivided into three parts (sternal, costal and vertebral or lumbar).

Sternal part

The sternal part arises as two muscular slips from the back of the xiphoid process.

Costal part

The costal part arises as six muscular slips from the inner surfaces of the costal cartilages and adjacent parts of the lower six ribs (seventh to twelfth ribs).

Vertebral or lumbar part

The vertebral or lumbar part arises from right and left crura and from medial and lateral arcuate ligaments (medial and lateral lumbocostal arches) on each side.

- The right crus arises from the anterolateral surface of the bodies of the upper three lumbar vertebrae and the intervening intervertebral discs. The right crus is longer and stronger on account of the fact that it pulls down the heavy liver during inspiration.

💡 **ADDED INFORMATION**

A few medial fibers of the right crus deviate to the left of the midline to encircle the lower end of the esophagus. These encircling fibers form the lower esophageal sphincter. Some fibers of the right crus are attached to the duodenojejunal flexure as suspensory ligament of duodenum (muscle of Treitz).

- The left crus arises from the anterolateral surface of the bodies of the upper two lumbar vertebrae and the intervening disc.
- Each medial arcuate ligament is a thickening of the fascia covering the upper part of psoas major muscle. It extends from the side of the body of the first lumbar vertebra to the middle of the front of the transverse process of the same vertebra.
- Each lateral arcuate ligament is the thickening of the upper margin of the anterior layer of thoracolumbar fascia in front of the quadratus lumborum muscle. It extends from the transverse process of first lumbar vertebra to the lower margin of twelfth rib.

Insertion

From the circumferential origin, the muscle fibers of diaphragm converge toward the central tendon for insertion. The central tendon has no bony attachments. It is trifoliate in shape and is inseparably fused with the base of the fibrous pericardium.

Apertures (Openings) in Diaphragm (Fig. 37.3)

There are three major apertures and a number of minor apertures in the diaphragm for the passage of structures between thorax and abdomen.

Major Apertures

- The vena caval aperture (for inferior vena cava) lies at the level of *T8 vertebra*. It is located in the central tendon to the right of the midline. The wall of the inferior vena cava is fused with the margins of the opening. The contraction of the diaphragm enlarges the caval opening, thereby dilating the vein and promoting the venous return. The branches of the right phrenic nerve pass through this opening along with IVC.
- The esophageal hiatus is located at the level of *T10 vertebra* in the muscular part of the diaphragm just posterior to the central tendon and to the left of the midline. The fibers of the right crus encircle it. The contraction of the diaphragm has a sphincteric effect on the hiatus (pinchcock effect). The vagal trunks and the esophageal branches of left gastric vessels pass through the hiatus along with esophagus.
- The aortic opening lies at the level of *T12 vertebra* posterior to the median arcuate ligament. The contraction of the diaphragm has no effect on this opening. The thoracic duct and vena azygos pass through the opening along with the aorta.

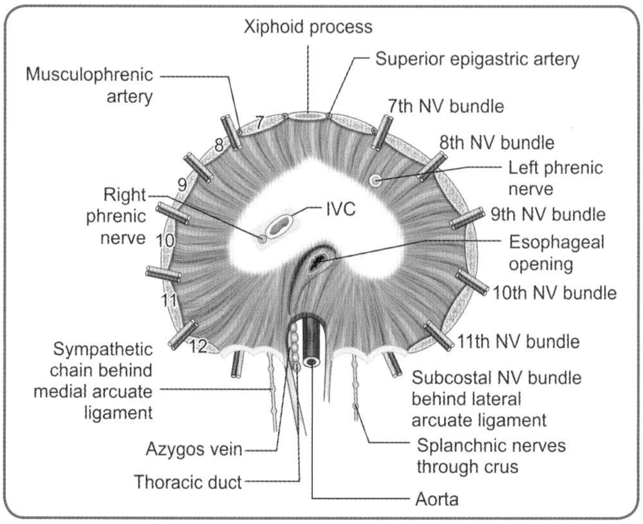

Minor Apertures (Openings)

- Superior epigastric vessels pass through a gap (space of Larry) between sternal and costal slips of origin of diaphragm from seventh costal cartilage.
- Musculophrenic vessels pass through the interval between slips of origin of diaphragm from the seventh and eighth ribs. The seventh intercostal nerve and vessels also pass through this interval.
- The eighth to eleventh intercostal nerves and vessels pass through intervals between the adjacent costal origins from subsequent ribs.
- Subcostal nerves and vessels pass behind the lateral arcuate ligament.
- Sympathetic chains pass behind the medial arcuate ligaments.
- Greater, lesser and least splanchnic nerves pierce the crus of the corresponding side.
- Hemiazygos vein pierces the left crus.
- Right phrenic nerve passes usually through the IVC opening and the left phrenic nerve through the muscular part in front of the central tendon.

Nerve Supply

Motor Nerve Supply

The phrenic nerves supply the muscle of the diaphragm. They pierce the diaphragm and ramify on its abdominal surface before entering the muscle (Fig. 37.10). The right phrenic nerve supplies the right half of the diaphragm up to the right margin of the esophageal opening. The left phrenic nerve supplies the left half of the diaphragm up to the left margin of the esophageal opening. Since the fibers of the right crus encircle the esophageal opening, it receives branches from both phrenic nerves.

Sensory Nerve Supply

- The central part of diaphragm and related pleura and peritoneum are supplied by phrenic nerves.
- The peripheral part of diaphragm and related pleura and peritoneum are supplied by lower intercostal nerves.

Fig. 37.3: Schematic diagram of the structures passing through the diaphragm (Note that aorta passes behind the diaphragm at T12 vertebral level)
Key: (IVC: inferior vena cava)

Arterial Supply

- Superior phrenic arteries (also called ***phrenic arteries***), which are the last branches of thoracic aorta, are distributed to the posterior part of the superior surface of the diaphragm.
- The musculophrenic and pericardiophrenic branches of the internal thoracic artery supply anterior part of the superior surface of diaphragm.
- Inferior phrenic arteries, which are the first branches of abdominal aorta, supply the inferior surface of the diaphragm.

Actions

- The diaphragm is the chief muscle of inspiration. When the diaphragm contracts, the domes of the diaphragm along with the central tendon descend, thereby increasing the vertical diameter of the thoracic cavity.
- The contraction of the diaphragm raises the intra-abdominal pressure, which is useful in all expulsive activities, like micturition, defecation and parturition. It also helps in weight-lifting when the raised intra-abdominal pressure is kept sustained by closure of the glottis and the vertebral column is kept in extended position by contraction of the trunk muscles.
- The contraction of the diaphragm facilitates venous return and lymph return. The rise in the intra-abdominal pressure and decrease in the intrathoracic pressure compress the blood in the inferior vena cava and lymph in the cisterna chyli (thus facilitating upward movement of the blood towards the right atrium and of the lymph towards the thoracic duct).

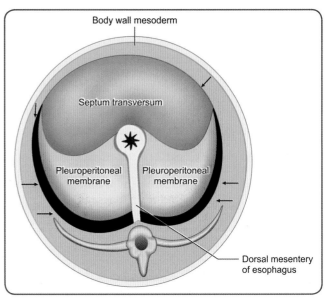

Fig. 37.4: Developmental sources of diaphragm (arrows indicate contribution of body wall mesoderm). The muscle of the diaphragm develops from cervical myotomes; hence the nerve supply by phrenic nerve

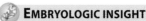 **EMBRYOLOGIC INSIGHT**

Development (Fig. 37.4)
The diaphragm is entirely mesodermal. It develops in the neck of the embryo from four different sources as follows:
- Septum transversum
- Right and left pleuroperitoneal membranes
- Dorsal mesentery of the esophagus
- Body wall mesoderm.

The muscle of the diaphragm develops from third, fourth and fifth cervical myotomes and, hence, its motor innervation is from the phrenic nerve. When the diaphragm descends from the neck to its definitive position, its nerve supply is dragged down.

CLINICAL CORRELATION

- **Congenital diaphragmatic hernia (CDH)**
  - The ***retrosternal hernia*** occurs through ***foramen of Morgagni*** (an enlarged ***space of Larry***)
  - The ***posterolateral hernia*** occurs through the vertebrocostal triangle (or ***foramen of Bochdalek***). It is a gap between the costal and vertebral origins of the diaphragm.
    This gap results due to failure of closure of the pleuroperitoneal canal. This hernia occurs more commonly on the left side. The abdominal viscera may herniate through this defect into the thorax producing hypoplastic lung (Fig. 37.5) and respiratory distress soon after birth. (Fig. 37.6) shows a child with CDH with typical scaphoid abdomen. The radiograph of chest shows herniated intestines and hypoplastic lung and shift of mediastinum to the right (Fig. 37.7). The surgical repair of hernia is shown in figure 37.8.

Contd...

Contd…

♪ CLINICAL CORRELATION

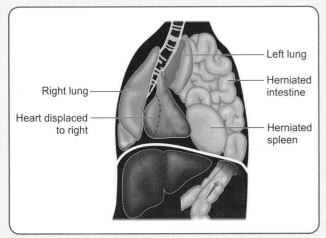

Fig. 37.5: Schematic diagram of congenital diaphragmatic hernia (CDH) (Note that the arrow indicates path of herniated intestine into the thorax and the spleen and intestine are crowding the left side, the thoracic cavity compressing the left lung)

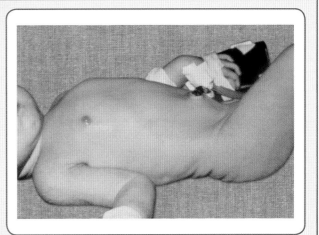

Fig. 37.6: Sunken abdomen of a child with CDH

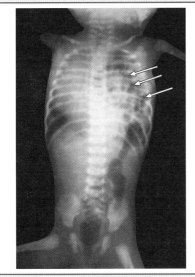

Fig. 37.7: Multiple air-filled areas in the thoracic cavity denoting air in the herniated intestine (arrows showing)

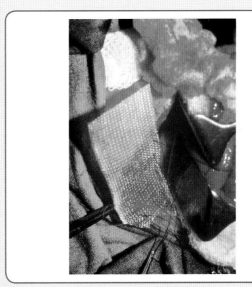

Fig. 37.8: Surgical repair of the defect in the diaphragm using synthetic mesh

- **Diaphragmatic paralysis**
  - Unilateral diaphragmatic paralysis is caused by damage to the phrenic nerve. The condition is diagnosed when an elevated hemidiaphragm as seen on fluoroscopy moves paradoxically.
  - Bilateral diaphragmatic paralysis is a fatal condition as it leads to respiratory failure.
- **Referred pain from diaphragm:** Irritation of the pleura or the peritoneum of the central part of diaphragm gives rise to referred pain in front of and at the tip of the shoulder, which is the area of cutaneous supply of supraclavicular nerves (C3, C4). In irritation of peripheral region the pain is referred to skin over anterolateral abdominal wall.

Contd…

Contd…

🎵 **CLINICAL CORRELATION**

- **Hiatal or hiatus hernia**

  The acquired diaphragmatic hernia (hiatus hernia) occurs through the esophageal opening (hiatus). It is of two types (Figs 37.9A and B).

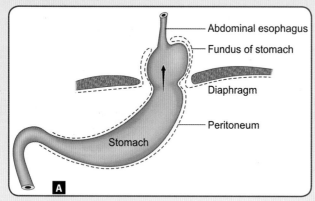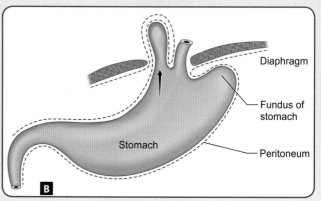

Figs 37.9A and B: A. Sliding type of hiatus hernia (Note that arrow incidicates the upward shift of stomach fundus and of cardio-esophageal junction in the posterior mediastinum); **B.** Paraesophageal or rolling type of hiatus hernia (Arrow indicates the upward shift of upper end of body of stomach but not of cardioesophageal junction)

- In the sliding hernia, the cardio-esophageal junction and the cardiac end of the stomach pass through the esophageal opening to enter the posterior mediastinum. This is caused due to weakness of the diaphragmatic muscle surrounding the esophageal opening and increased intra-abdominal pressure due to any cause. There is regurgitation of acid contents of the stomach into the esophagus causing peptic esophagitis (heartburn is the main symptom)
- In the rolling hiatus hernia, a part of the stomach passes through the esophageal opening into the posterior mediastinum. There is no reflux of gastric contents into the esophagus as the cardioesophageal junction is in normal position.

💡 **ADDED INFORMATION**

Mechanism of Respiration

The respiration rate in a healthy adult is 18–20 per minute. Each respiratory cycle consists of an inspiratory phase and an expiratory phase. Inspiration increases the thoracic volume with a simultaneous decrease in the intrapulmonary pressure. This ensures the inflow of air into the lungs until the pressures equalize. The expiration decreases thoracic volume with a simultaneous increase in the intrapulmonary pressure. This causes the air to flow out of the lungs until the pressures equalize.

Quiet Inspiration

- The movements of the ribs take place at costovertebral and costotransverse joints (Fig. 34.3B).
  - In the pump-handle movement, the upper ribs (2–6) bring about upward and forward movements of the anterior ends of the ribs along with the sternum. The lower ribs (7–10) are elevated as a unit thereby lifting the lower end of the sternum upward and forward. The net result is the increase in the anteroposterior diameter of the thoracic cavity.
  - In bucket-handle movement, the middle parts of the ribs are lifted in lateral direction so as to increase the transverse diameter of the thoracic cavity.
- The diaphragm forms a mobile floor of the thoracic cavity. Its contraction results in the descent of the diaphragm by about 1–1.5 cm in quiet inspiration. The contraction of the diaphragm is accompanied by the reciprocal relaxation of the anterior abdominal muscles. The descent of the diaphragm results in increase in the vertical dimension of the thoracic cavity. The diaphragm can also act on the lower ribs at the end of its vertical descent. Keeping the central tendon as a fixed point, the diaphragmatic contraction elevates the lower ribs, thereby increasing the anteroposterior and transverse diameters of the thorax.

Contd…

Contd…

Muscles of Inspiration

- The diaphragm is the chief muscle of inspiration
- The external intercostal muscles and interchondral portion of the internal intercostal muscles assist in inspiration.

Forced Inspiration

Additional muscles are brought into play to increase the volume of the thoracic cavity.

- The first two ribs are elevated along with the manubrium sterni by active contraction of scalenus anterior and sternomastoid muscles.
- The pectoral muscles, serratus anterior and serratus posterior muscles elevate the ribs.
- The power of the diaphragmatic contraction is increased by fixing the twelfth rib with the help of active contraction of quadratus lumborum.

Quiet Expiration

Quiet expiration is largely a passive process [by elastic recoil of the lungs (intrinsic elastic recoil) and of costal cartilage (extrinsic elastic recoil) accompanied by the relaxation of the diaphragm].

Forced Expiration

Forced expiration is an active process. It is brought about by active contraction of the muscles of anterior abdominal wall assisted by erector spinae, serratus posterior inferior and latissimus dorsi.

Phrenic Nerves

The right and left phrenic nerves are the only motor supply to the muscle of the corresponding half of the diaphragm. They are mixed nerves with 2:1 proportion of motor and sensory fibers. They suppling proprioceptive fibers to the central part of diaphragm and additionally supplies the diaphragmatic and mediastinal pleura, fibrous and parietal pericardium and diaphragmatic peritoneum of its side.

Origin

The phrenic nerve arises in the neck from the cervical plexus. It mainly carries fibers of ventral ramus of the fourth cervical nerve but receives contribution from the third and fifth cervical nerves as well. Hence, the root value of phrenic nerve is C3, C4, C5 (Fig. 37.10). C5 contribution may occasionally be received from accessory phrenic nerve. When present, the accessory phrenic nerve arises from the nerve to subclavius (carrying C5 fibers) and joins the phrenic nerve in the thorax.

Course and Relations

The phrenic nerve has a long course, which can be divided into cervical and thoracic parts.

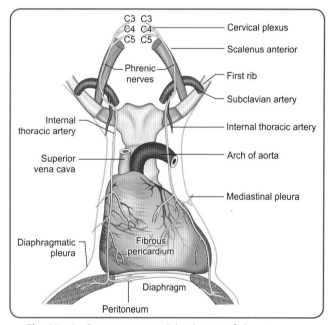

Fig. 37.10: Origin, course and distribution of phrenic nerves

Cervical course of phrenic nerves

The phrenic nerve begins from the cervical plexus. Three roots of the phrenic nerve unite at the lateral margin of scalenus anterior muscle and then the nerve courses downwards and medially on the anterior surface of the scalenus anterior muscle behind the prevertebral fascia.

Anterior relations

Anteriorly, the phrenic nerve is overlapped by internal jugular vein and sternomastoid muscle and is crossed by intermediate tendon of omohyoid and by transverse cervical and suprascapular arteries. The left phrenic nerve is crossed by the thoracic duct.

Posterior relations

The scalenus anterior muscle is the posterior relation of the phrenic nerve on each side. At the lower part of the neck, the left phrenic nerve leaves the medial margin of left scalenus anterior above the left subclavian artery. Therefore, the left phrenic directly crosses the left subclavian artery anteriorly. The right phrenic nerve lies in front of the right scalenus anterior muscle until the muscle crosses the subclavian artery. Therefore, it leaves the medial margin of right scalenus muscle below the level of right subclavian artery. Then the phrenic nerve crosses the internal thoracic artery from lateral to medial (either in front or behind) to enter the superior mediastinum behind the first costal cartilage.

Thoracic course of phrenic nerves

The left phrenic nerve is longer than the right and the right phrenic nerve is shorter and more vertical in the thoracic course. Both the nerves at first pass through the superior mediastinum and then anterior to the hilum of the respective lung to enter the middle mediastinum. Both descend in close relation to the respective lateral surfaces of fibrous pericardium. The pericardiophrenic vessels accompany the phrenic nerves in their thoracic course (Fig. 37.10).

Right Phrenic Nerve

The right phrenic nerve passes down along the right side of right brachiocephalic vein, superior vena cava, right atrium (which is inside right side of fibrous pericardium) and lastly the thoracic part of inferior vena cava. It leaves the thorax by passing through the vena caval opening or by piercing the central tendon in the vicinity of the caval opening.

Left Phrenic Nerve

The left phrenic nerve passes between the left common carotid and left subclavian arteries. Initially, it is laterally related to the left vagus nerve. Next, it crosses the left vagus nerve superficially and comes to lie medial to it. Then the phrenic nerve crosses the arch of aorta on its left and anterior aspect. Then it descends in front of left ventricle (which is inside the fibrous pericardium). It leaves the thorax by piercing the muscular part of diaphragm to the left of the anterior folium of the central tendon.

Distribution

The phrenic nerves divide into branches, which ramify in the substance of the diaphragm or on its inferior surface and supply motor branches to the muscle of diaphragm. The sensory branches supply the peritoneum lining the inferior surface of diaphragm, diaphragmatic pleura, and mediastinal pleura and to the parietal and fibrous pericardium.

⚕ CLINICAL CORRELATION

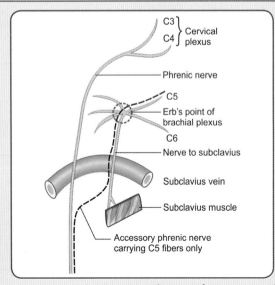

Fig. 37.11: Accessory phrenic nerve and its origin from nerve to subclavius

Injury to Phrenic Nerve

The phrenic nerve may be injured either in the neck or in the thorax. This results in unilateral paralysis of hemidiaphragm, which can be detected by X-ray screening. The paralyzed half of the diaphragm moves paradoxically during respiration and is pushed up into the thorax.

Phrenic Nerve Avulsion

The avulsion of phrenic nerve is sometimes necessary in treating certain diseases of lung. The phrenic nerve is approached via the base of the posterior triangle of the neck. It is freed from the prevertebral fascia in front of the scalenus anterior muscle and raised on a hook and then divided. The distal end of the nerve is grasped and twisted around the forceps and pulled upwards to tear out as much of the nerve as possible. If the accessory phrenic nerve is present, it is also avulsed (Fig. 37.11).

38

Development of Heart and Congenital Anomalies

Chapter Contents

INTRODUCTION

The heart is the first organ to start function in the human embryo (by the end of 25 to 27 days the heart begins rhythmic beating). The heart begins to develop during the third week of intrauterine life (IUL) as right and left endothelial cardiac tubes in the splanchnopleuric mesoderm (in the floor of pericardial coelom) in the cardiogenic area at the cranial end of the embryonic disc. Soon, a single straight cardiac tube is formed by the fusion of original two tubes. With the formation of the head fold of the embryonic disc, the pericardial coelom undergoes 180^0 rotation due to which the cardiac tube and the splanchnopleuric mesoderm come to lie in roof of the pericardial coelom. The cardiac tube surrounded by the myoepicardial mantle of splanchnopleuric mesoderm soon bulges more and more into the pericardial coelom from dorsal side. The endothelium of cardiac tube forms endocardium, myoepicardial mantle forms myocardium and epicardium (visceral layer of serous pericardium). The somatopleuric layer of pericardial coelom forms parietal layer of pericardial cavity. The cardiac tube is suspended in the pericardial cavity by means of dorsal mesocardium.

FATE OF DORSAL MESOCARDIUM

The dorsal mesocardium is short lived. It breaks down to form a communication between right and left halves of the pericardial cavity. This communication is the site of the transverse sinus of pericardium.

SUBDIVISIONS OF CARDIAC TUBE

The cardiac tube is divisible into five chambers (Fig 38.1) in craniocaudal order as follows.
1. Truncus arteriosus
2. Bulbus cordis
3. Common ventricle
4. Common atrium
5. Sinus venosus

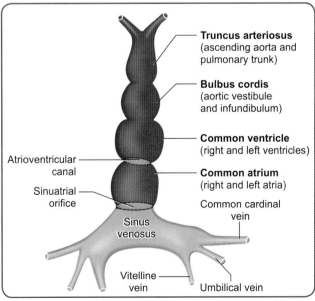

Fig. 38.1: Subdivisions of embryonic cardiac tube and the derivatives of each subdivision given in the bracket

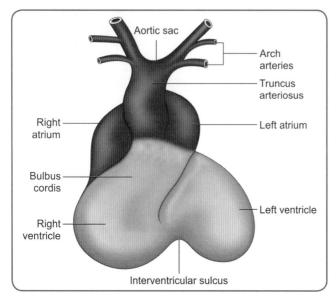

Fig. 38.2: S-shaped embryonic heart after folding of cardiac tube

The *truncus arteriosus* is the cranial or arterial end of cardiac tube. It projects out as ventral aortic sac, which is connected by the arch arteries to the dorsal aorta on each side.

The sinus venosus is the caudal or venous end of cardiac tube. Its two sides are drawn out as two horns which receive three pairs of veins on each side as shown in Figure 38.1.

 STUDENT INTEREST

You must remember the names of subdivisions of cardiac tube and the derivatives of each subdivision (Fig. 38.1).

FOLDING OF CARDIAC TUBE

The folding of the cardiac tube changes the tubular heart into a U-shaped bulboventricular loop. The sinus venosus moves upwards along with atrial chamber to lie behind and above the ventricle. The shape of the heart now changes to S-configuration (Fig 38.2) as the bulbus cordis and the common ventricle form a bulboventricular cavity in continuation with truncus arteriosus. The contour of the embryonic heart now resembles that of the adult heart.

SINUS VENOSUS (FIG. 38.3)

The sinus venosus is in communication with the atrial chamber by a midline sinuatrial orifice guarded by right and left venous valves.

It undergoes following changes:

- Left horn starts shrinking in size so that it is reduced to a tributary of the right horn
- Right horn grows very large (Fig. 38.3B)
- Position of sinuatrial orifice is shifted to the right.

Fate of Sinus Venosus (Figs 38.3 and 38.4)

- The enlarged right horn is absorbed into the right half of the primitive atrial chamber to form the smooth part of the right atrium.
- The shrunken left horn along with part of left common cardinal vein becomes coronary sinus.
- The right venous valve develops into crista terminalis, valve of opening of inferior vena cava (IVC) into right atrium and valve of opening of coronary sinus into right atrium.
- The left venous valve fuses with the interatrial septum.

 STUDENT INTEREST

Sinus venosus is an important topic. It receives 6 embryonic veins (3 veins per horn). This symmetry is abolished when the left horn starts shrinking. The right horn enlarges and is absorbed inside right part of common atrial chamber to subsequently become the rough part of right atrium. Learn what happens to right and left venous valves that guard the sinuatrial orifice. Only on knowing embryology of sinus venosus will you understand internal features of right atrium.

SEPTATION OF EMBRYONIC HEART

During 4–8 weeks of embryonic life, septation simultaneously takes place in atrioventricular canal, common atrium, common ventricle, bulbus cordis and truncus arteriosus. The partition of a single heart tube in a four chambered pump, which contains four valves and gives rise to two blood vessels, is achieved by formation of seven septa, the septum intermedium, septum primum, septum secundum, aorticopulmonary septum, proximal bulbar septum, distal bulbar septum and interventricular septum.

- Septum intermedium divides the atrioventricular canal into right and left halves. It is formed by fusion of dorsal and ventral endocardial cushions in the respective walls of the canal.
- Interatrial septum is a valvular septum between the developing right and left atria.

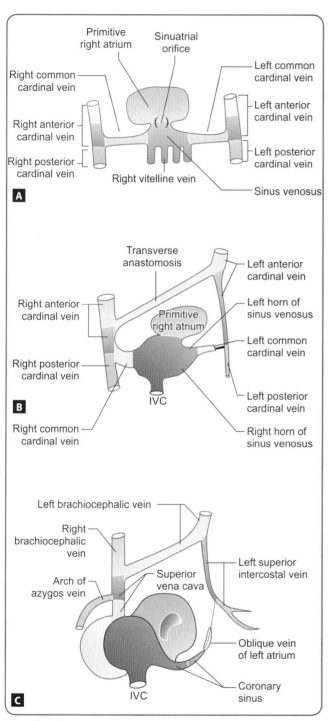

Figs 38.3A to C: Fate of sinus venosus (absorption of right horn and body of sinus venosus into right half of primitive atrium and formation of coronary sinus from left horn and left common cardinal vein)

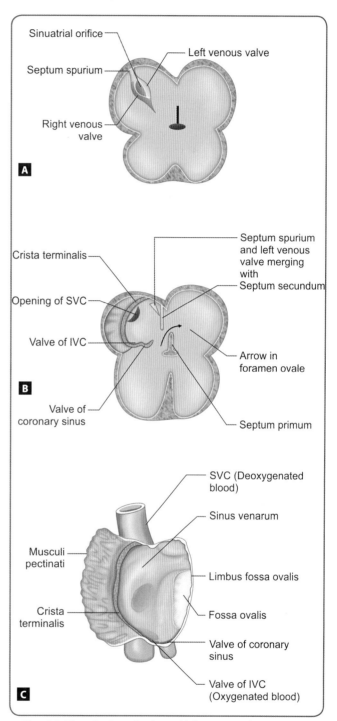

Figs 38.4A to C: Fate of right and left venous valves guarding sinuatrial orifice (Note that right venous valve becomes crista terminalis, valve of opening of IVC into right atrium and valve of opening of coronary sinus into right atrium. Also note that left venous valve merges with the interatrial septum)

Stages in Development of Interatrial Septum

- A thin septum primum, grows down gradually (towards the septum intermedium) from the roof of the common atrium near the midline. The steadily narrowing gap between the septum primum and septum intermedium is called foramen primum or ostium primum (Fig. 38.5 A)
- Before the fusion of septum primum with septum intermedium (and consequent closure of the foramen primum), the upper part of the septum primum breaks down to form foramen secundum or ostium secundum
- A thick septum secundum (to the right of the septum primum) grows from the roof of the atrial chamber, in the downward direction until it covers the foramen secundum on its right side (Fig. 38.4B)
- The lower margin of septum secundum is free and concave. The oblique gap between the lower margin of septum secundum and the upper margin of septum primum is called foramen ovale. This foramen short-circuits the inferior vena caval blood to the left atrium. The flow of blood is unidirectional from the right atrium to the left. The septum primum acts as a flap valve since the pressure is greater in the right atrium than in the left, in fetal life
- Foramen ovale closes after birth. This is accomplished as follows. The rise in the left atrial pressure soon after establishment of pulmonary circulation keeps the septum primum pressed against the septum secundum until they fuse. The septum primum becomes the floor of fossa ovalis and the lower margin of the septum secundum forms the limbus fossa ovalis
- The functional closure of the foramen ovale occurs immediately after birth while the anatomical closure occurs 6 to 12 months after birth. In 15–20 % of persons probe patency remains (which is symptom free).

STUDENT INTEREST

The gross features, embryology and defects in the interatrial septum (ASD) are the must know topics

DEVELOPMENT OF PULMONARY VEINS (FIGS 38.5A TO C)

A single primary or common pulmonary vein develops from the dorsal wall of the left half of the common atrial chamber. It divides into right and left pulmonary veins, which again divide and enter the lung bud. The common trunk of the single pulmonary vein and its right and left divisions until the bifurcation are absorbed inside the left half of common atrium. The result of this absorption is that four separate pulmonary veins establish communication with the left half of common atrium (future left atrium).

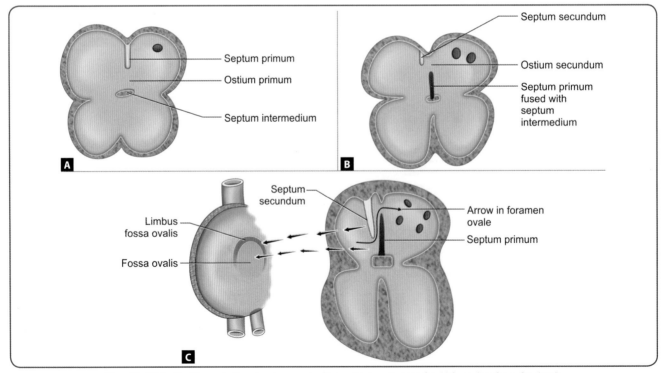

Figs 38.5A to C: Stages in the development of interatrial septum in fetal life and its fate after birth

EMBRYOLOGIC INSIGHT

Developmental Sources of Atria

- The **right atrium** develops from three sources as follows:
  - **Rough part:** From right half of common atrium
  - **Smooth part or sinus venarum:** From right horn of sinus venosus
  - **Vestibule of the atrioventricular orifice:** From right half of A-V canal.
- The **left atrium** develops from three sources as follows:
  - **Rough part:** From the left half of common atrium
  - **Smooth part:** From the absorbed divisions and stem of pulmonary vein
  - **Vestibule of the atrioventricular orifice:** From the left half of the A-V canal.

Derivatives of Truncus Arteriosus

- Ascending aorta
- Pulmonary trunk

(Spiral aorticopulmonary septum (Fig. 38.7) divides the truncus arteriosus into ascending aorta and pulmonary trunk).

Derivatives of Bulbus Cordis

- Infundibulum (outflow tract of right ventricle)
- Aortic vestibule (outflow tract of left ventricle).

Development of Interventricular Septum (Fig. 38.8)

The interventricular septum is of composite origin because its muscular and membranous parts develop from separate sources.
- The muscular part is the first to develop from the floor of the bulboventricular cavity
- The membranous part develops from right and left bulbar ridges from above and by proliferation from the right end of endocardial cushion tissue of septum intermedium.

Developmental Sources of Right Ventricle

- **Inflow part:** From right half of common ventricle
- **Outflow part (infundibulum):** From bulbus cordis.

Developmental Sources of Left Ventricle

- **Inflow part:** From left half of the common ventricle
- **Outflow part (aortic vestibule):** From bulbus cordis.

ADDED INFORMATION

Development of Semilunar Valves

At the truncoconal junction a distal bulbar septum is formed by the fusion of right and left endocardial cushions. The spiral septum fuses with the distal bulbar septum and divides it into anterior and posterior parts. The anterior part forms the pulmonary valve at the origin of pulmonary trunk. The posterior part forms the aortic valve at the origin of ascending aorta. In each part one more cushion develops, as a result of which each part comes to have three endocardial cushions.

Pulmonary and Aortic Cushions

- The pulmonary cushions, before rotation of heart are, anterior, right posterior and left posterior
- The aortic cushions, before rotation of heart are posterior, right anterior and left anterior.

After laevorotation of heart, the position of valves changes according to adult pattern.

The pulmonary cusps are posterior, right anterior and left anterior.

The aortic cusps are anterior, right posterior and left posterior (corresponding to aortic sinuses at the root of ascending aorta).

Development of Conducting Tissue

The nodal tissue develops from the sinus venosus close to the opening of the common cardinal vein. The right nodal tissue becomes the SA node around third month of intrauterine life. The AV node develops from the left nodal tissue in the sinus venosus as well as in the endocardial cushions in the A-V canal around 6 weeks of IUL.

Congenital Anomalies of Heart

Dextrocardia

In this defect, the heart rotates to the right so it is on the right side of chest and its apex is in the right fifth intercostal space.

Ectopia Cordis

In this defect, the heart is exposed on the chest wall due to defective formation of anterior thoracic wall with cleft sternum.

Atrial Septal Defect (ASD) (Figs 38.6A and B)

Atrial septal defect is the congenital anomaly, which becomes manifest in adult life. There are three types of ASD resulting in left to right shunt.

- The ostium secundum defect is one of the most common congenital heart defects. There is persistence of foramen secundum in this defect (Fig. 38.6A).
- In ostium primum defect there is persistence of foramen primum (Fig. 38.6B).
- Patent foramen ovale is due to failure of the septum primum and septum secundum to fuse after birth. This is extremely rare.

In ASD, there is increased load on the right side of the heart leading to progressive enlargement of right atrium, right ventricle and the pulmonary trunk. The patient begins to experience fatigue and breathlessness on exertion in the third or fourth decade of life and thereafter. The atrial septal defects can be corrected by surgery.

Ventricular Septal Defect (VSD)

The membranous septum is more often defective. Large VSD may lead to pulmonary hypertension and congestive cardiac failure in infancy. VSD may occur singly or in combination with other cardiac defects.

Tetralogy of Fallot (TOF)

Tetralogy of fallot TOF shows combination of four defects (Fig. 38.9) as listed below.

- Ventricular septal defect
- Over-riding of aorta (ascending aorta having connection to both ventricles)

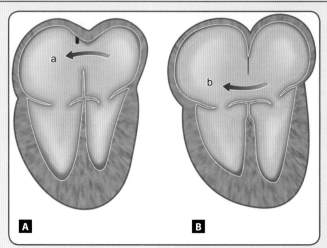

Figs 38.6A and B: Atrial septal defects; **A.** Ostium secundum defect; **B.** Ostium primum defect (Note that simultaneously common ventricle is subdivided by formation of interventricular septum)

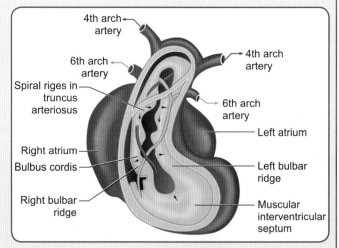

Fig. 38.7: Septation of truncus arteriosus and bulbus cordis by formation of spiral aorticopulmonary septum (Note that simultaneously common ventricle is subdivided by formation of interventricular septum)

Contd...

Contd…

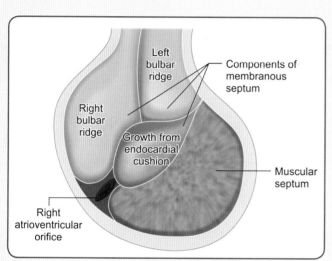

Fig. 38.8: Development of muscular and membranous parts of interventricular septum

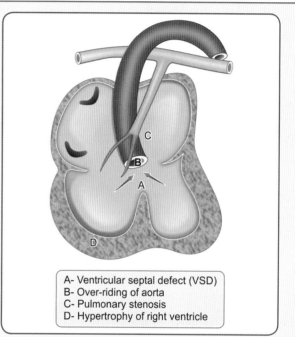

A- Ventricular septal defect (VSD)
B- Over-riding of aorta
C- Pulmonary stenosis
D- Hypertrophy of right ventricle

Fig. 38.9: Fallot's tetralogy (Note the narrowed pulmonary trunk and biventricular flow into the ascending aorta)

(Note the narrowed pulmonary trunk and biventricular flow into the ascending aorta)

- Pulmonary stenosis (narrowing of pulmonary trunk due to pulmonary stenosis)
- Right ventricular hypertrophy.

In this defect, the aorta carries mixed blood, which results in cyanosis. The child may have cyanotic spells especially during crying. There is shortness of breath or dyspnoea on exertion.

39

Pharyngeal Arch Arteries and Fetal Circulation

PHARYNGEAL ARCH ARTERIES

The basic arterial pattern of an embryo at the end of 4th week of development is like that of fishes as given as follows:

- On the dorsal body wall of embryo, a pair of dorsal aortae is present. The dorsal aortae fuse below the level of the seventh intersegmental arteries to form a single dorsal aorta.
- On the ventral body wall, there is an aortic sac, which is the dilated upper end of the truncus arteriosus of cardiac tube. The aortic sac is drawn out cranially as right and left horns (limbs). These horns are equivalent to the ventral aorta of fishes.
- The ventral and dorsal aortae are connected through a series of six aortic arch arteries that pass through the pharyngeal arches (equivalent to gills).
- The cranial arch arteries degenerate as the caudal ones make their appearance. Therefore, at any given time all of the six arch arteries are never present in human being. The fifth arch artery is rudimentary.

The third, fourth and sixth arch arteries along with the aortic sac and dorsal aorta gives rise to the definitive arteries of the thorax and neck.

Transformation of Arch Arteries (Fig. 39.1)

The symmetrical pattern of arch arteries and dorsal aorta undergoes changes during 6th to 8th weeks.

- The ductus caroticus is a segment of dorsal aorta between the third and fourth arch arteries. It degenerates on both sides. This creates a break in the dorsal aorta on each side.
- The sixth arch arteries are divided into dorsal and ventral segments due to the appearance of a vessel that establishes connection to the lung bud on each side.
- The dorsal segment of the right sixth arch artery degenerates.
- The right dorsal aorta degenerates between the origin of right seventh intersegmental artery and the point of its fusion with left dorsal aorta. This breaks the connection between right and left dorsal aorta.

Derivatives of Arch Arteries

- The right pulmonary artery develops from ventral segment of right sixth arch artery.
- The left pulmonary artery develops from ventral segment of left sixth arch artery.
- The ductus arteriosus develops from the dorsal segment of left sixth arch artery.
- The arch of aorta develops from four sources as follows—1. aortic sac, 2. left horn of aortic sac, 3. left fourth arch artery, and 4. part of left dorsal aorta.

Note: Some texts mention three developmental sources of the arch. This is probably because the aortic sac and its left horn are counted as one source.

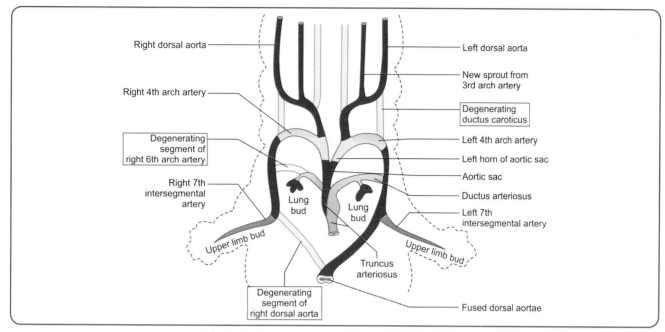

Fig. 39.1: Pharyngeal arch arteries and their derivatives

- The brachiocephalic artery develops from right horn of aortic sac between sixth and fourth arch arteries.
- The common carotid artery develops from the right horn of aortic sac between fourth and third arch arteries and a small contribution from the proximal part of third arch artery of its side.
- The internal carotid artery develops from the distal part of third arch artery and the dorsal aorta above ductus caroticus.
- The external carotid artery is a new sprout from the proximal part of third arch artery.
- The left subclavian artery develops from the left seventh intersegmental artery.
- The right subclavian artery develops from three sources—1. Right fourth arch artery, 2. Part of right dorsal aorta and 3. right seventh intersegmental artery.
- The descending thoracic aorta and abdominal aorta are derived from the fused dorsal aortae.

Relation to Recurrent Laryngeal Nerves

The recurrent laryngeal nerves are related to the dorsal segments of the sixth arch arteries. When the heart and the arch arteries descend from the neck to the thorax, the nerves are pulled down. Since the recurrent laryngeal nerves supply the larynx they retrace their course upwards. In this process, the nerves hook round the sixth arch arteries on both sides.

- ***On the right side***, the dorsal segment of the sixth arch artery involutes and the fifth arch artery is rudimentary. Therefore, the right recurrent laryngeal nerve recurs around the lowest persisting arch artery on the right side, namely ***the right subclavian artery***
- ***On the left side***, the dorsal segment of the sixth arch artery becomes the ductus arteriosus, which in postnatal life is modified into the ligamentum arteriosum. Therefore, the left recurrent laryngeal nerve hooks round the remnant of lowest persisting arch artery on the left side, namely ***ligamentum arteriosum***.

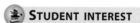 **STUDENT INTEREST**

Developmental sources of arch of aorta, right subclavian artery, left subclavian artery, descending aorta, pulmonary arteries are to be at the tip of the tongue of every student.

Contd...

⚕ **CLINICAL CORRELATION**

CONGENITAL ANOMALIES

Coarctation of Aorta (Figs 39.2 and 39.4)

Coarctation of aorta means narrowing of lumen of the arch of aorta. There are two types of coarctation in which the method of filling of the descending aorta distal to the narrowing is different.

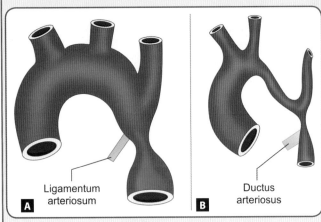

Figs 39.2A and B: Types of coarctation of aorta. **A.** Postductal; **B.** Preductal

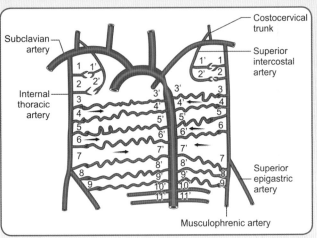

Fig. 39.3: Collateral circulation in postductal type of coarctation of aorta (Note that numbers 1 to 9 are the anterior intercostal arteries and 1′ to 9′ are the posterior intercostal arteries. Also note the tortuosity of and reversal of blood flow in 1′ to 9′ arteries)

Postductal Coarctation (Fig. 39.2A)

In postductal type, the narrowing is distal to the attachment of ligamentum arteriosus. The postductal coarctation is more common. The descending aorta is filled with blood through posterior intercostal arteries (Fig 39.3). Its characteristic signs are the radio-femoral delay and difference in the blood pressure in the upper and lower extremities. Radiological sign of rib notching may be present. Rib notching is due to erosion of the lower borders of the ribs by the enlarged and tortuous posterior intercostal arteries. These arteries carry blood from the anterior intercostal arteries to fill the descending aorta. Thus, there is reversal of blood flow in the posterior intercostal arteries (Fig. 39.4).

Preductal Coarctation (Fig. 39.2B)

In preductal type, the narrowing is proximal to the attachment of ductus arteriosus and ductus is invariably patent. The descending aorta receives deoxygenated blood through the patent ductus arteriosus.

Aberrant Right Subclavian Artery (Fig 39.5)

When the right subclavian artery takes origin from the arch of the aorta beyond the left subclavian artery, it is called *aberrant artery*. The embryologic basis of this anomaly

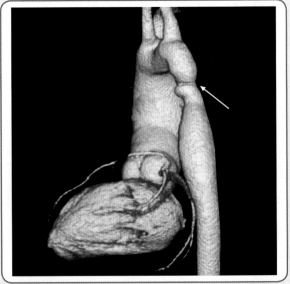

Fig. 39.4: Volume rendered 3-D reconstruction showing postductal coarctation of aorta (arrow showing)

Contd...

Contd...

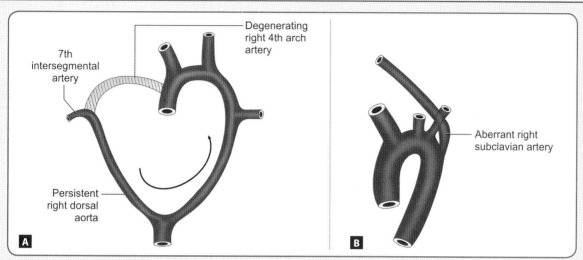

Figs 39.5A and B: Showing embryological basis of aberrant right subclavian artery

is the involution of the right fourth arch artery and the persistence of the normally disintegrating segment of right dorsal aorta. In the absence of right fourth arch artery the right recurrent artery does not recur. Hence it is called ***nonrecurrent right recurrent laryngeal nerve*** and it arises from the vertical part of the right vagus in the neck (Fig. 39.6).

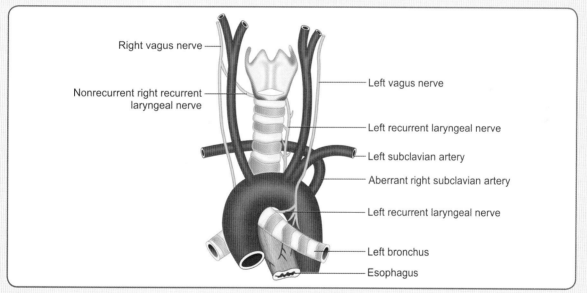

Fig. 39.6: Course of aberrant right subclavian artery and its association with nonrecurrent right recurrent laryngeal nerve

FETAL CIRCULATION (FIG. 39.7)

The circulation of blood in the prenatal life is different from that of postnatal life, primarily because the lungs of the fetus are not functional.

Unique Features of Fetal Circulation

- There are three shunts or bypass channels: (1) ductus venosus, (2) foramen ovale, and (3) ductus arteriosus.

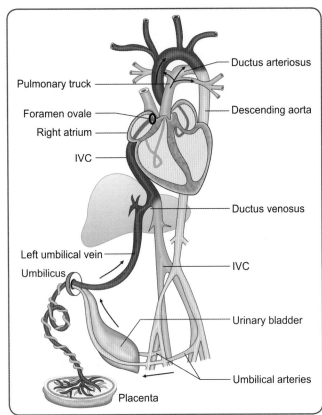

Fig. 39.7: Fetal circulation (Note the short circuiting channels of fetal circulation- ductus venosus in liver, foramen ovale in interatrial septum in heart and ductus arteriosus connecting aorta and left pulmonary artery)
Key: (IVC–inferior vena cava)

- There are three blood vessels connected to placenta 1. left umbilical vein, 2. umbilical artery left, and 3. right umbilical artery.
- The placenta acts as fetal lungs.

Blood Circulation in Fetus

- The left umbilical vein supplies oxygenated blood. It originates in the placenta. It enters the fetus through the umbilical cord and umbilicus and reaches the liver via falciform ligament and joins the left branch of portal vein.
- The blood is diverted from the left branch of portal vein to the inferior vena cava by the ductus venosus (bypassing liver). The inferior vena cava brings this oxygenated blood to the right atrium.

- From the right atrium, the oxygenated blood is directed through the foramen ovale to the left atrium. From the left atrium the blood enters the left ventricle and then into the ascending aorta.
- The venous blood from right ventricle reaches the arch of aorta (instead of reaching lungs) via a shunt called **ductus arteriosus**, which connects the aorta and the left pulmonary artery. Thus, the upper part of the body receives more oxygenated blood compared to the lower part because of mixing of venous blood in the aorta distal to the connection with the ductus arteriosus.
- The right and left umbilical arteries carry the deoxygenated blood from the lower end of abdominal aorta for purification back to the placenta.

Postnatal Changes in Fetal Circulation

The physiological closure of the three shunts and three blood vessels mentioned above occurs as immediately after birth. In the case of ductus arteriosus, the physiological closure is facilitated by release of bradykinin in lungs after first breath. The bradykinin stimulates the smooth muscle in the wall of ductus to contract.

Time of Anatomical Closure

- **Umbilical vessels and ductus venosus:** Two to three months after birth.
- **Ductus arteriosus:** One to three months after birth.
- **Foramen ovale:** Six months after birth.

Fate of Fetal Shunts and Umbilical Blood Vessels

- The left umbilical vein becomes the ligamentum teres of liver.
- The ductus venosus becomes the ligamentum venosum inside liver.
- The foramen ovale is indicated by fossa ovalis and limbus fossa ovalis (in the interatrial septum).
- The ductus arteriosus becomes the ligamentum arteriosum.
- The umbilical arteries undergo changes as follows: Their proximal patent parts are called the **superior vesical arteries** and distal obliterated parts become the lateral umbilical ligaments.

CLINICAL CORRELATION

Patent Ductus Arteriosus (PDA)

The patent ductus arteriosus (PDA) is commonly seen in the rubella syndrome, which occurs in children whose mothers suffer from German measles during the first two months of pregnancy. PDA may occur singly or in combination with other cardiac defects. In PDA, the ductus arteriosus fails to obliterate postnatally. So a communication exists between the arch of aorta and left pulmonary artery even after birth (Fig. 39.8). Since the pulmonary arterial pressure is lower than that in the aorta, there is a continuous flow of blood from the aorta to the pulmonary artery. This is the reason for the presence of characteristic continuous murmur (called *machinery murmur or rail in tunnel murmur*). There is overloading of pulmonary circulation. The symptoms of overload of pulmonary circulation are recurrent respiratory infections, shortness of breath on exertion and palpitation. Surgical correction can be undertaken in three to six months after birth.

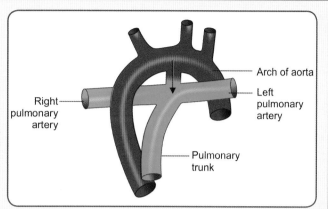

Fig. 39.8: Patent ductus arteriosus (PDA). The arrow in the patent ductus arteriosus indicates flow of blood from aorta into the pulmonary trunk.

STUDENT INTEREST

Fetal circulation tells us the story of how the maternal blood reaches the fetus via placenta and how the fetal blood after circulation in the body of fetus is returned to mother via the placenta. Pay attention particularly to the following structures: left umbilical vein, ductus venosus, foramen ovale, ductus arteriosus and umbilical arteries. Don't skip PDA.

40

Pericardium and Heart

Chapter Contents

- Pericardium
  - Subdivisions
  - Pericardial Cavity
- Heart
  - Orientation of Heart in Thorax

- External Features
- Margins
- Surfaces
- Surface Marking
- Chambers of Heart

- Surface Markings of Cardiac Valves
- Surface Markings of Cardiac Auscultation Areas
- Radiological Anatomy of Heart

PERICARDIUM

The pericardium is a fibroserous sac that covers the heart and the roots of great vessels in the middle mediastinum (Fig. 40.1). It is located behind the body of the sternum.

Subdivisions

- Outer fibrous pericardium

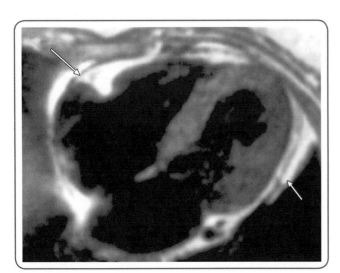

Fig. 40.1: MRI image showing pericardium surrounding the heart (arrows showing)

- Inner serous pericardium consisting of inner visceral layer of pericardium (epicardium) and outer parietal layer of pericardium.

Pericardial Cavity

It is a potential space enclosed between the parietal and visceral layers of serous pericardium. It contains a small quantity of serous fluid. This facilitates the sliding of the two serous layers over each other during cardiac movements.

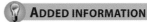

ADDED INFORMATION

Development of Pericardium

- The pericardial cavity develops from cranial part of the intraembryonic coelom
- The visceral layer of pericardium (epicardium) is derived from myoepicardial mantle (splanchnopleuric mesoderm) that envelops the cardiac tube
- The parietal layer of pericardium is derived from somatopleuric mesoderm of pericardial cavity
- The fibrous pericardium is derived from pericardiopleural membranes and septum transversum.

Fibrous Pericardium (Fig. 37.10)

It is a tough fibrous sac, which is shaped like a cone with an apex directed superiorly and a wide base inferiorly.

- The apex is continuous with the adventitia of great vessels at the level of sternal angle.

- The base blends with the central tendon of diaphragm. Inferior vena cava pierces the base posteriorly on the right side.
- Anteriorly, the fibrous pericardium is related to the structures in the anterior mediastinum. It is connected to upper and lower ends of the body of sternum by upper and lower sternopericardial ligaments. The anterior margins of lungs and pleurae overlap this surface except over the bare area of the pericardium (opposite fourth and fifth costal cartilages on the left side), where the anterior margins of left lung and pleura deviate and the pericardium comes in direct contact with the thoracic wall. The thymus (located in anterior mediastinum) is related to the upper part of pericardium in childhood.
- Posteriorly, it is related to the principal bronchi, the descending thoracic aorta and esophagus. This aspect is pierced by four pulmonary veins.
- Laterally, it is related to the mediastinal pleura and through it to the mediastinal surface of respective lung. Phrenic nerve and pericardiophrenic vessels descend on the left and right lateral surfaces of the fibrous pericardium. Incisions in the pericardium are always vertically placed to avoid injury to the phrenic nerves.

Functions

- The fibrous pericardium retains the heart in the middle mediastinum and prevents its overdistension.
- In external cardiac massage, the heart is squeezed inside the firm fibrous pericardium between the fixed vertebral column and somewhat resilient sternum and costal cartilages by applying rhythmic pressure to the lower sternum.

Blood supply

The pericardial branches of the internal thoracic artery and of descending thoracic aorta provide arterial blood. The pericardial veins drain into the azygos and hemiazygos veins.

Nerve supply

The phrenic nerves supply sensory branches to the fibrous pericardium.

Serous Pericardium

The visceral layer (epicardium) covers the myocardium and the intrapericardial parts of the great vessels closely. It is reflected at the points, where the great vessels pierce the fibrous pericardium, onto the parietal layer, which lines the internal surface of the fibrous pericardium. Along

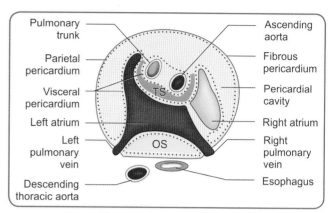

Fig. 40.2: Pericardial sinuses
Key: TS–Transverse sinus and OS-Oblique sinus)

the lines of pericardial reflection there are two pericardial sinuses, namely transverse and oblique.

Boundaries of transverse sinus (Fig 40.2)

Anteriorly, it is limited by the visceral pericardium covering the ascending aorta and pulmonary trunk and posteriorly by the visceral pericardium covering anterior surface of left atrium. The transverse sinus is open on either side and thus communicates the two halves of the pericardial cavity to each other.

CLINICAL CORRELATION

Surgical Importance of Transverse Sinus

The transverse sinus provides space during cardiac surgery to clamp the ascending aorta and pulmonary trunk in order to insert tubes of heart lung machine in these vessels.

EMBRYOLOGIC INSIGHT

Development of Transverse Sinus

The transverse sinus develops as result of degeneration of dorsal mesocardium. After the folding of the cardiac tube its venous and arterial ends come close to each other and the space enclosed between them (space at the site of dorsal mesocardium) becomes the transverse sinus.

Boundaries of oblique sinus (Fig. 40. 3)

Its anterior boundary is the visceral pericardium covering the posterior surface of left atrium. Its posterior boundary is the parietal pericardium lining the posterior surface of fibrous pericardium. On the right, it is bounded by the pericardial reflection from IVC (inferior vena cava) and right pulmonary veins. On the left, it is limited by the

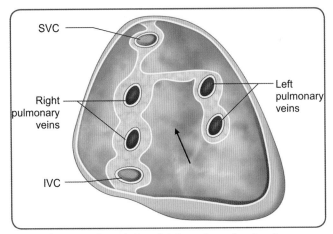

Fig. 40.3: Boundaries of oblique sinus of pericardium (indicated by arrow)
Key: SVC–Superior vena cava; IVC – Inferior vena cava)

pericardial reflection from left pulmonary veins. Superiorly there is pericardial reflection along the superior margins of the left atrium. The sinus is open inferiorly. The oblique sinus intervenes between the left atrium anteriorly and the esophagus posteriorly. It is believed to act as a bursa for the left atrium to expand during filling.

🧬 EMBRYOLOGIC INSIGHT

Development of Oblique Sinus

The atria receive six veins, two in the right atrium and four in the left atrium. When these veins separate from each other (due to increase in size of the atria) the line of pericardial reflection becomes irregular. Along this irregular line a small recess of pericardial cavity is trapped. This recess is called the *oblique sinus*, which lies posterior to the left atrium.

Blood supply and nerve supply of serous pericardium

- The parietal layer shares its blood supply and nerve supply with the fibrous pericardium.
- The visceral layer shares its blood supply and nerve supply with the myocardium.

🔖 CLINICAL CORRELATION

- Inflammation of serous pericardium is called *pericarditis*. Pain of pericarditis is felt in the precordium (front of chest) or epigastrium.
- Accumulation of fluid in pericardial cavity is known as *pericardial effusion*. The heart sounds are faintly audible on auscultation in pericardial effusion. X ray chest shows globular heart shadow.

Contd…

Contd…

🔖 CLINICAL CORRELATION

- Excess fluid in pericardial effusion is removed by one of the two routes. In parasternal route, the needle is inserted in the left fourth or fifth intercostal space close to the sternum avoiding injury to the internal thoracic vessels. Since the line of pleural reflection deviates in 4th and 5th intercostal spaces the needle does not pierce the pleura. This route is also preferred for giving intracardiac injections. In the subcostal (costoxiphoid) route (Fig. 40.4) the needle is inserted at the left costoxiphoid angle in an upward and backward direction through the rectus sheath and the central tendon of diaphragm (Fig. 36.15).
- Cardiac tamponade is a condition in which there is rapid accumulation of fluid in the pericardial cavity. This interferes with the atrial filling during diastole and causes decrease in cardiac output, increase in heart rate and increase in venous pressure. Immediate aspiration of fluid is necessary to restore normal cardiac output.

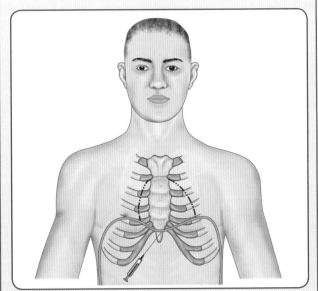

Fig. 40.4: Pericardiocentesis through left costoxiphoid angle

🐾 STUDENT INTEREST

Pericardium is a must know topic

HEART

The heart is a four chambered muscular pump. It is covered with double-layered serous membrane (pericardium) enclosing a potential pericardial cavity. The muscle of the heart is known as **myocardium**, which contracts non-stop throughout life. The right side of the heart consisting of right atrium and ventricle receives venous blood, which is pumped to the lungs for oxygenation by the pulmonary trunk and pulmonary arteries. The left side of the heart consisting of left atrium and ventricle receives oxygenated blood, which is pumped to the entire body by the aorta and its branches. The interatrial septum and the interventricular septum are the partitions between atria and ventricles respectively. There are four cardiac orifices, two atrioventricular orifices (mitral and tricuspid) and two semilunar orifices (pulmonary and aortic).

Orientation of Heart in Thorax

The heart is placed obliquely in the middle mediastinum. Approximately two-thirds of the heart lies to the left and one-third to the right of the midline (Fig. 40.5). The heart makes an angle of 45^0 with the sagittal plane. Therefore, the terms right and left used in reference to relationship of cardiac chambers to each other are not strictly true. The correct perspective regarding the position and relations of the cardiac chambers is depicted in (Figs 40.6 and 40.7), in which one can observe that the right chambers of the heart (right atrium and right ventricle) are anterior to left ventricle and left atrium respectively. This is due to levorotation of heart (rotation of the heart to the left). Since the major part of right ventricle is anterior to the left ventricle, a knife pushed into the chest by the side of the sternum in the left fifth or sixth intercostal space will enter the right ventricle. The pulmonary orifice of right ventricle is actually to the left, superior and anterior to the aortic orifice of the left ventricle. The average size of the heart is

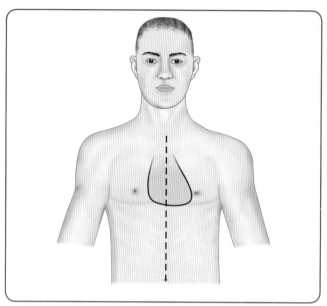

Fig. 40.5: Outline of normally positioned heart in relation to sagittal plane

that of a clenched fist of the person. The average weight of the adult heart is 250 to 300 g.

External Features

- The atrioventricular or AV sulcus (coronary sulcus or groove) separates the atria and the ventricles. The anterior part of this sulcus is masked by ascending aorta and pulmonary trunk on the sternocostal surface (Fig. 40.8). Its oblique right part is between right auricle and right ventricle while its small left part is between

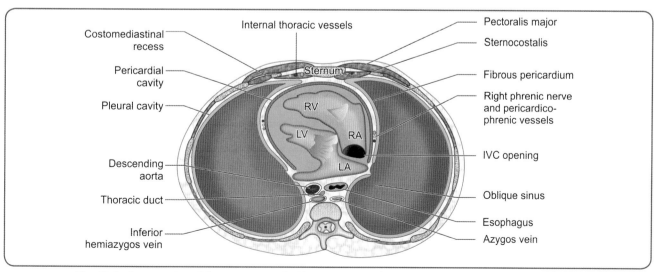

Fig. 40.6: Cross section of thorax at T8 vertebral level positions of chambers of heart in relation to each other
Key: RV – Right ventricle; RA – Right atrium; LV – Left ventricle; LA – Left atrium)

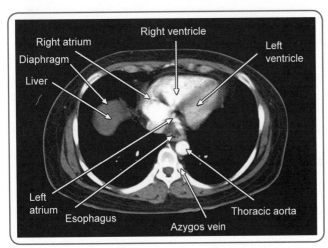

Fig. 40.7: CT scan of thorax at T7 to T8 vertebral level to show heart and other structures

left auricle and left ventricle. The posterior part of the AV sulcus is between the diaphragmatic surface and the left atrium (Fig. 40.1).

- The interatrial sulcus is faintly visible on the posterior surface between the two ventricles.
- It is visible on the posterior aspect of the base of the heart.
- The interventricular sulci or grooves are present on the sternocostal and inferior or diaphragmatic surfaces respectively, separating the right and left ventricles.

Crux of Heart

The point of junction of the posterior atrioventricular, interatrial and posterior interventricular sulci is termed the crux of the heart.

Margins (Borders)

The heart has a pointed apex directed inferiorly and to the left and a broad base directed posterosuperiorly. There are four margins limiting four surfaces. The margins are, superior, inferior (acute), right and left (obtuse).

Surfaces

The surfaces are, anterior or sternocostal, inferior or diaphragmatic, left and right.

Apex of Heart

The apex is the most mobile part of the heart. It is directed downward, forward and to the left. It is formed by left ventricle only. The apex is located at the junction of inferior and left borders of the heart. It is separated from the anterior thoracic wall by left lung and pleura. The apex beat is the impulse produced by the apex when it impinges

on the chest wall during systole. It may be visible in thin individuals or is felt in the left fifth intercostal space 9 cm away from the midline.

> **CLINICAL CORRELATION**
>
> **Shift of Apex**
>
> In hypertrophy of left ventricle the apex shifts in downward and lateral direction. A few causes of downward and lateral shift of the apex are systemic hypertension, mitral regurgitation and aortic regurgitation.

Margins

- The right margin is entirely formed by the right atrium and is almost vertical.
- The inferior or acute margin is formed by right ventricle mainly with a very small contribution of the left ventricle. The right marginal branch of right coronary artery courses along this margin.
- The left or obtuse margin is formed by left ventricle mainly with a small contribution of left auricle superiorly.
- The superior margin is formed by the upper margins of the atria and is hidden from the sternocostal surface by the ascending aorta and pulmonary trunk.

Surfaces

The heart presents sternocostal, diaphragmatic, posterior, right and left surfaces.

Sternocostal Surface (Figs 40.8 and 40.9)

The sternocostal surface faces upwards, forwards and to the left. The chambers contributing to this surface are— right atrium, right auricle, right ventricle, small strip of left ventricle and left auricle.

- The oblique part of atrioventricular (coronary) sulcus seen to the right of the roots of ascending aorta and pulmonary trunk, extends upto the junction of the right and inferior margins. It contains right coronary artery embedded in the fat. The anterior cardiac veins cross over the sulcus to reach the right atrium. A smaller left of coronary sulcus lying between left auricle and left ventricle contains circumflex branch of left coronary artery.
- The anterior interventricular groove (sulcus) demarcates the two ventricles on this surface. It contains anterior interventricular branch of left coronary artery and the great cardiac vein embedded in fat.

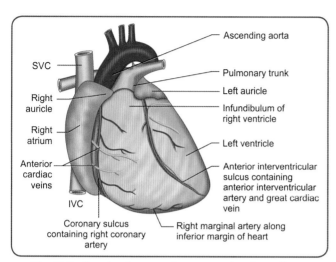

Fig. 40.8: Showing features of sternocostal surface of heart
Key: (SVC – Superior vena cava; IVC – Inferior vena cava)

- Superiorly and to the left, the right ventricle is prolonged as the infundibulum, which continues as the pulmonary trunk.
- Inferiorly and to the left, the left ventricle forms the apex of the heart.
- A finger -shaped left auricle projects on the sternocostal surface to overlap the left aspect of the pulmonary trunk.
- Anteriorly, the sternocostal surface is related (from within outwards) to the pericardium, anterior mediastinum, anterior margins of the lungs and pleura (including the left costomediastinal recess), the body of sternum and the third to sixth costal cartilages. the appearance of sternocostal surface after incising the pericardium during by pass surgery is depicted in figure 40.9.

Diaphragmatic or Inferior Surface (Fig. 40.10)

The diaphragmatic surface is flat and rests on the central tendon of diaphragm. The left ventricle (left two-thirds) and the right ventricle (right one-third) contribute to this surface. The demarcating line between the two ventricles is the posterior interventricular groove, which contains posterior interventricular branch of right coronary artery and middle cardiac vein. The posterior part of the coronary sulcus is between the base and the diaphragmatic surface. Its left part contains circumflex artery and coronary sinus. One notable peculiarity here is that blood flow in both venous and arterial vessels is towards the right (it means unidirectional). The right part of the coronary sulcus extending from to the right side of the crux contains the stem of right coronary artery.

Posterior Surface or Base (Fig. 40.10)

This surface is quadrilateral in outline and faces backwards and to the right. It lies at the level of fifth to eighth thoracic vertebrae in supine position. In standing position, it descends by one vertebra.

- The left atrium forms the left two-thirds of the base and the right atrium forms the right one-third. A faint interatrial groove marks the demarcation between the two atria.
- Six large veins open into the base four pulmonary veins (one pair on each side) open into left atrium and two great veins (SVC and IVC) open into the right atrium.
- The base is related anteriorly to the transverse sinus of pericardium and the roots of ascending aorta and pulmonary trunk. Posteriorly, the oblique sinus

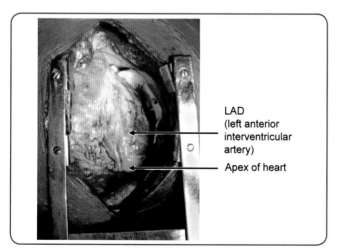

Fig. 40.9: Exposure of sternocostal surface of heart by incising the pericardium during surgery for CABG (coronary artery bypass graft)

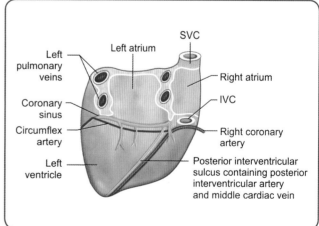

Fig. 40.10: Showing posterior surface or base of heart and diaphragmatic or inferior surface of heart (**Key:** SVC–Superior vena cava; IVC–Inferior vena cava)

intervenes between it and the posterior part of fibrous pericardium (Fig. 40.2). The esophagus in the posterior mediastinum is an immediate posterior relation of fibrous pericardium. It is to be noted that the thickness of tissue between the base of heart and esophagus is only 0.5 cm.

- The left surface or left pulmonary surface is in contact with mediastinal pleura and mediastinal surface of left lung. This surface is widest above, where it is crossed by the left part of the atrioventricular sulcus (containing left circumflex artery and great cardiac vein). It is related to left phrenic nerve and accompanying artery.
- The rounded right surface or the right pulmonary surface is formed by right atrial wall. The sulcus terminalis is visible on this surface.

Surface Marking (Fig 40.11)

- The apex of the heart is marked by a point 9 cm away from the midline in the left fifth intercostal space.

- The right margin is represented by a line joining a point on the lower part of the second right intercostal space (close to the sternum)to a point on the right sixth costal cartilage 1–2 cm from the sternal margin.
- The inferior margin is represented by a line joining a point on the right sixth costal cartilage 1–2 cm from the margin of the sternum to a point coinciding with the apex.
- The left margin is represented by a line joining the point of the apex to a point on the second left intercostal space 1–2 cm from the sternal margin.
- The superior margin is indicated by a line from a point on the upper part on the left second intercostal space 1–2 cm lateral to the sternal margin to a point close to the margin of the sternum in the lower part of right second intercostal space.
- The anterior part of the atrioventricular sulcus is indicated by an oblique line extending from the sternal end of the left third costal cartilage to the sternal end of right sixth costal cartilage.

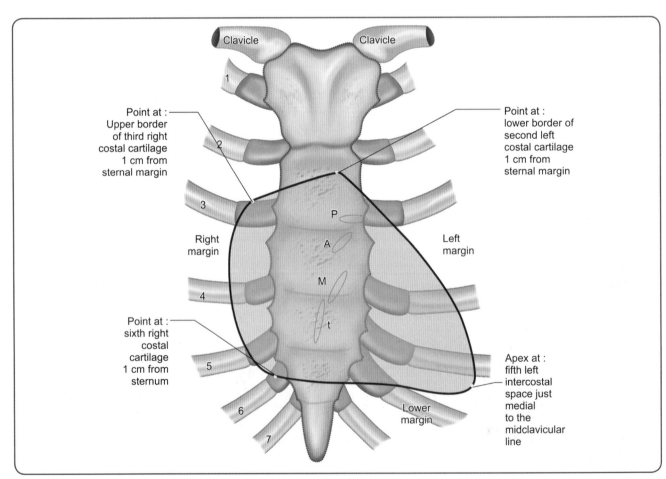

Fig. 40.11: Surface marking of cardiac margins and apex of heart
Key: P – Pulmonary; A – Aortic; M – Mitral; T – Tricuspid)

Learn to hold the specimen of heart in anatomical position. This way you will become familiar with the margins, surfaces and apex of the heart. Apex is directed downwards and to the left. Anterior interventricular sulcus containing anterior interventricular artery and great cardiac vein is on the sternocostal surface. Right margin is straight and entirely formed by right atrium. Major part of inferior or acute margin is formed by right ventricle. Left margin formed by left ventricle is obtuse. The base of heart or superior margin is hidden from sternocostal surface. Left auricle is seen of the left of base of ascending aorta and right auricle is seen on the right of base of pulmonary trunk. The inferior or diaphragmatic surface shows the posterior interventricular groove carrying posterior interventricular artery and middle cardiac vein. Identify the coronary sinus on posterior part of coronary sulcus and 4 pulmonary veins opening into posterior wall of left atrium. Surface marking of the apex and margins of heart is very important and hence the must know topic.

Chambers of Heart

The heart has four chambers—right atrium, left atrium, right ventricle and left ventricle

Right Atrium

The right atrium receives the venous blood from the entire body via SVC (superior vena cave) and IV and from the myocardium via coronary sinus and other cardiac veins. The venous blood goes out of right atrium into the right ventricle via the tricuspid orifice. The right atrium has the thinnest wall. It forms part of the sternocostal surface, base and right lateral surface of the heart. The right auricle projects from it to overlap the right side of the base of the pulmonary trunk. The sulcus terminalis is a visible groove that extends along the right lateral surface from the right side of the superior vena cava (SVC) above to the right side of the inferior vena cava (IVC) below. The upper end of the sulcus terminalis lodges the SA (sinoatrial) node of conducting tissue of heart in subepicardial position.

Interior of right atrium (Fig. 40.12)

The cavity of the right atrium is divisible into three parts:
1. The sinus venarum or smooth part is located posteriorly (derived from right horn of sinus venosus)
2. Right atrium proper along with right auricle forms the rough part (derived from common atrial chamber of cardiac tube)
3. The vestibule of tricuspid valve forms the floor or anteroinferior part.

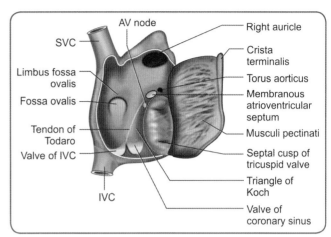

Fig. 40.12: Right lateral view of opened right atrium to depict internal features
Key: AV node – atrioventricular node; SVC – Superior vena cava; IVC – Inferior vena cava

Features of sinus venarum or smooth part

- The opening of the superior vena cava is located at the roof of the right atrium. An intervenous tubercle located below this opening, directs the superior vena caval blood to the tricuspid orifice in fetal life.
- The opening of inferior vena cava is guarded by a small Eustachian valve. It is located at the lowest and posterior part of the atrium near the interatrial septum.
- The opening of coronary sinus is guarded by a thin Thebesian valve. It is located between the opening of IVC and the tricuspid orifice.
- The multiple small openings of venae cordis minimae (smallest cardiac veins, also called Thebesian veins) draining the myocardial capillary bed are seen in all chambers of heart.

Features of right atrium proper and auricle (rough part)

- The crista terminalis demarcates the rough and smooth parts of right atrium. It corresponds to the sulcus terminalis on the external surface of atrium. It is a C-shaped muscular ridge. It starts at the upper end of the interatrial septum, passes in front of the SVC opening and then turns along its lateral margin downward to reach the opening of the IVC.
- The musculi pectinati (so called because of their resemblance to comb) are the parallel muscular ridges extending from the crista into the right auricle. The dense trabeculations of musculi pectinati inside the right auricle makes it a potential site for thrombi formation. The thrombi dislodged from the right atrium enter the pulmonary circulation and may produce pulmonary embolism.
- The anterior cardiac veins open into this part.

Vestibule of tricuspid valve

This is the anteroinferior part (floor) of the right atrium. It leads into the tricuspid orifice.

Interatrial septum (Fig. 40.12)

The interatrial septum forms the septal or posteromedial wall of the right atrium.

It presents fossa ovalis, which is an ovoid, membranous and depressed portion. A curved ridge called the limbus fossa ovalis forms the superior, right and left margins of the fossa ovalis. The floor of the fossa ovalis represents the septum primum and the limbus fossa ovalis is the remnant of the lower margin of the septum secundum of the fetal heart (Fig. 38.5). So the fossa ovalis with its limbus indicates the site of the valvular foramen ovale of fetal circulation. This foramen is normally completely obliterated after birth. A small slit (probe patency) may be found along the upper margin of the fossa ovalis in one-third of normal hearts.

(For developmental sources of right atrium, development of interatrial septum and its congenital anomalies refer to chapter 38).

Right Ventricle

The right ventricle receives venous blood from the right atrium through the tricuspid orifice and pumps it through the pulmonary orifice into the pulmonary trunk. It takes a large share in the formation of sternocostal surface and a small share in the formation of diaphragmatic surface. It forms almost the entire inferior or acute margin of heart.

Thickness of right and left ventricles

The thickness of right ventricular wall varies in fetal and adult. In fetus, the right ventricle pumps blood into the arch of aorta through the pulmonary artery and ductus arteriosus. Hence its wall is thicker than that of left ventricle. In postnatal stage, the right ventricle pumps blood into pulmonary circulation, where systolic arterial pressure is 25–35 mm Hg. Hence the thickness of its walls is much less compared to that of left ventricle.

Interior of right ventricle (Fig. 40.13)

The shape of the cavity of the right ventricle is crescentic. The cavity of the right ventricle is divisible broadly into two parts.

- The trabecular body (ventricle proper) is the rough inflow part.
- The infundibulum or conus arteriosus is the smooth outflow part.

The inflow and outflow parts make an angle of 90^0 to each other. The supraventricular crest, which is the largest muscular ridge, separates ridged wall of inflow part from the smooth wall of the outflow part. The inflow

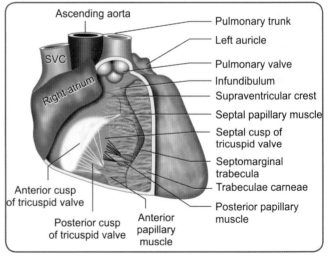

Fig. 40.13: Anterior view of opened right ventricle to depict internal features
Key: SVC – Superior vena cava

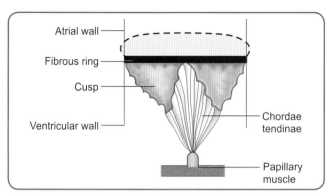

Fig. 40.14: Components of atrioventricular valve (fibrous ring, cusps, chordae tendineae and papillary muscles)

part receives blood through tricuspid orifice from right atrium and outflow part ejects blood into pulmonary trunk through pulmonary orifice. These two orifices are guarded by respective valves.

Components of atrioventricular valve (Fig. 40.14)

- Annulus or collagenous ring encircling the orifice.
- Cusps or valve leaflets attached to the annulus.
- Chordae tendineae or tendinous cords.
- Papillary muscles (2 on left side and 3 on right side).

Tricuspid orifice and valve (Fig. 40.15)

The tricuspid valve is the right atrioventricular valve. It allows the blood to flow from right atrium to the inflow part of right ventricle. The tricuspid orifice accommodates the tips of three fingers.

- An annulus of the tricuspid valve is a ring of collagenous (fibrous) tissue for attachment to the cusps of the valve.
- There are three cusps in tricuspid valve named anterior, posterior (or inferior) and septal. Each cusp is formed by a duplication of endocardium enclosing collagenous tissue. It presents an attached margin and a free margin and ventricular surface and an atrial surface.

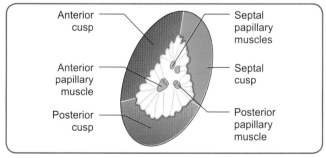

Fig. 40.15: Simplified diagram of three cusps, three papillary muscles and chordae tendineae connecting the cusps and papillary muscles

- The chordae tendineae connect apices of the papillary muscles to the free margins and ventricular surfaces of the cusps.
- The papillary muscles are conical muscular projections (numbering three) and are named anterior, posterior and septal. They arise from the corresponding wall of the ventricle. The chordae tendineae arising from the anterior papillary muscle are attached to the anterior and posterior cusps; those from posterior papillary muscle to the posterior and septal cusps; and those from the septal papillary muscle to the anterior and septal cusps.

Right ventricle proper

The cavity of right ventricle proper (trabecular body) is characterized by the presence of muscular projections, which are collectively called the trabeculae carneae. There are three types of trabeculae in the right ventricle named, ridges, bridges and papillary muscles.

- The ridges are found all over the cavity in large numbers.
- The bridges are the elevations, which are fixed at the two ends but remain free in between. The septomarginal trabecula (moderator band) is the best example of this type. This trabecula passes from the interventricular septum to the base of the anterior papillary muscle. It carries the right branch of atrioventricular bundle (RBB) in its substance. This ensures early contraction of papillary muscles so that chordae tendineae are already taut before ventricular contraction begins.
- The papillary muscles are conical muscular projections. Depending on their attachment to the ventricular wall, the papillary muscles are described as anterior, posterior and septal. The large anterior papillary muscle is attached to the right anterolateral wall, where it blends with the right end of the septomarginal trabecula. The posterior papillary muscle is attached to the inferior wall. The septal papillary muscles are several small muscles attached to the septal limb of the septomarginal trabecula.

Infundibulum (Outflow Tract)

Superiorly, the right ventricle tapers into the infundibulum or conus arteriosus that leads into pulmonary trunk (the two being separated by pulmonary valve). The infundibulum is funnel shaped. Unlike the rest of ventricular cavity, it is smooth. The supraventricular crest constitutes its posterior and right lateral walls and the membranous interventricular septum separates it from the aortic vestibule of the left ventricle.

(For developmental sources of right ventricle refer to chapter 38).

Pulmonary valve

The pulmonary valve and aortic valve are grouped as semilunar valves since each of the three cusps is semilunar in shape. The pulmonary valve is the most superior and anterior of the cardiac valves. In normal individuals, it lies anterior and to the left of the aortic valve. Its cusps are named, right anterior, left anterior and posterior. The free margin of each cusp presents a localized thickening (called the nodule of Arantius) and the thin margin called the lunule. The pulmonary sinuses are the dilatations in the wall of the pulmonary trunk just above the cusps.

Note: The cusps in semilunar valves are directly attached to the wall of the blood vessel due to absence of collagenous ring.

Left Atrium

The left atrium receives oxygenated blood from the lungs by two pairs of pulmonary veins. It communicates with left ventricle through bicuspid or mitral orifice. It is positioned behind and to the left of the right atrium. It forms left two-thirds of the base or posterior surface of heart. The pulmonary trunk and the ascending aorta conceal its anterior surface. The left auricle projects anterosuperiorly from it to overlap the left aspect of the pulmonary trunk.

(For relations of the left atrium refer to base of the heart in chapter 40).

Interior of left atrium

The interior of left atrium is divided into three parts.
1. The smooth part presents at the openings of the pulmonary veins, two on either side on its posterior wall.

2. The rough part is confined to the left auricle, which is characterized by musculi pectinati. The left auricle is a potential site of formation of thrombi, which if dislodged, can result in embolism in the systemic arteries (for example, renal, internal carotid, common iliac, femoral, brachial etc.).
3. The vestibule of the mitral valve is a narrow passage just preceding the mitral orifice.

(For developmental sources of left atrium refer to chapter 38).

Left Ventricle

The left ventricle is a powerful pump, which propels blood into the systemic circulation against the peripheral vascular resistance of 80/120 mm of Hg. In keeping with this workload, the wall of the left ventricle is three times thicker than that of the right ventricle. The left ventricle forms the cardiac apex, one-third of the sternocostal surface, two-thirds of the inferior surface and left surface of the heart. The left ventricle receives the blood from the left atrium and pumps the same into the ascending aorta via the aortic orifice.

Interior of left ventricle

The cavity of the left ventricle is circular on cross section. The left ventricle is divisible into two parts:
1. The inflow part or trabeculated body or ventricle proper.
2. The outflow part or aortic vestibule.

The inflow part is trabeculated and receives oxygenated blood from mitral orifice guarded by mitral valve. The outflow part is aortic vestibule. It is smooth and leads into aortic orifice guarded by aortic valves.

Mitral orifice and mitral valves

The mitral valve is the left atrioventricular valve lying posteroinferior and slightly to the left of the aortic valve. The mitral orifice can admit the tips of two fingers. The orifice has two cusps hence the name bicuspid valve. The mitral cusps resemble in shape the bishop's miter (crown).

Components of mitral valve

- Annulus or collagenous ring of the orifice.
- The anterior and posterior cusps.
- Chordae tendineae or tendinous cords.
- Papillary muscles.

The anterior cusp or leaflet is attached to anteromedial part of collagenous ring. It separates the aortic vestibule from the mitral orifice. It is larger than the posterior cusp. The smaller posterior or mural cusp is attached to the posterolateral part of the collagenous ring.

The chordae tendineae are attached only to the free margin of anterior cusp but are attached to the free margin and ventricular surface of the posterior cusp. The anterior and posterior papillary muscles arise from the anterior and inferior or diaphragmatic walls respectively and control the cusps via chordae tendineae.

Left ventricle proper

The left ventricle proper has rough walls due muscular projections called trabeculae carneae, which form a fine meshwork. The trabeculae are especially rich at the apex and on the inferior wall. There are two papillary muscles. The anterior papillary muscle originates from the anterior wall and its chordae tendineae are attached to both the cusps of the mitral valve. The posterior papillary muscle originates from the inferior wall and its chordae tendineae are attached to both the cusps of the mitral valve.

Aortic vestibule (outflow part)

This is the smooth part of the left ventricle. It is situated a little in front and to the right of the mitral valve. The anterior cusp of the mitral valve and the adjacent part of fibrous skeleton of the heart (subaortic curtain) form its posterior wall. The membranous part of the interventricular septum forms its anterior and right walls and separates it from the right ventricle and right atrium.

(For developmental sources of left ventricle refer to chapter 38)

Aortic orifice and aortic valves

The aortic valve is a semilunar valve like the pulmonary valve. It presents three cusps or leaflets and is stronger in structure than the pulmonary valve. The free margins of the cusps project into the ascending aorta and present nodule (of Arantius) at the midpoint and lunule on either side.

Like the pulmonary sinuses, there are three aortic sinuses of Valsalva above the aortic cusps at the root of ascending aorta.

According to the position of the cusps, the sinuses are described as:
- Anterior aortic sinus (giving originto right coronary artery).
- Right posterior aortic sinus (or noncoronary sinus).
- Left posterior aortic sinus (giving originto left coronary artery).

Note: The right posterior aortic sinus (non-coronary sinus) projects in the right atrium to produce torus aorticus.

Interventricular septum (Fig. 40.16)

The interventricular septum is a partition between the two ventricles. The septum is 0. Its attachment to the anterior

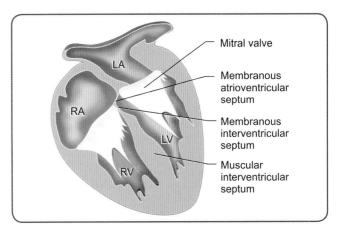

Fig. 40.16: Showing muscular and membranous parts of interventricular septum (Note that membranous part is subdivided into interventricular and atrioventricular components)
Key: LA – Left atrium; RA – Right atrium; LV – Left ventricle; RV – Right ventricle

wall is indicated by the anterior interventricular groove on the sternocostal surface and to the inferior surface by the posterior interventricular groove. The right surface of the septum faces forwards and bulges into the right ventricle, while the left surface looks backwards and is concave towards the left ventricle.

Parts of interventricular septum

It has two parts, muscular and membranous.
- The muscular part is very large and thick.
- The membranous part is located posterosuperior to the muscular part. It appears as a small oval transparent area, which is in continuity with the central fibrous body (part of fibrous skeleton of heart). The attachment of the septal cusp of the tricuspid valve divides the membranous part into anterior interventricular part and posterior atrioventricular part. The interventricular part separates the aortic vestibule of the left ventricle from the infundibulum of the right ventricle. The atrioventricular part separates the aortic vestibule from the floor of the right atrium.

Conducting tissue in interventricular septum

- The membranous septum is pierced by the left branch of the atrioventricular bundle near its junction with the muscular part.
- The left surface of the muscular septum carries the left branch of atrioventricular bundle in the sub-endocardial position. The right branch of the atrioventricular bundle (also called right bundle branch or RBB) passes along the right surface of the septum in the subendocardial position. The RBB is further carried inside the septomarginal trabecula to the anterior papillary muscle.

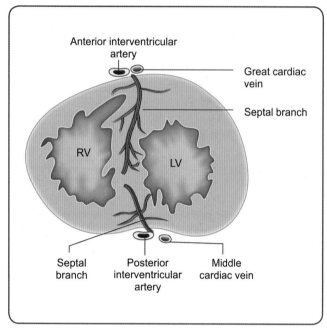

Fig. 40.17: Arterial supply of interventricular septum
Key: RV – Right ventricle; LV – Left ventricle

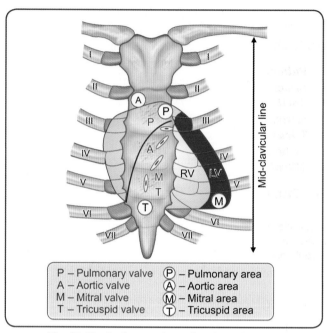

P – Pulmonary valve   Ⓟ – Pulmonary area
A – Aortic valve   Ⓐ – Aortic area
M – Mitral valve   Ⓜ – Mitral area
T – Tricuspid valve   Ⓣ – Tricuspid area

Fig. 40.18: Surface marking of cardiac valves and auscultation areas (Note the pink colour is used to denote surface marking of cardiac valves in PAMT order from above downwards and capital letters inside circles denote auscultation areas)

Arterial supply of interventricular septum (Fig 40.17)

- The anterior two-third of the septum receives anterior septal branches of the anterior interventricular artery (a branch of left coronary artery).
- Small posterior septal branches of the anterior interventricular and short septal branches of posterior interventricular artery (a branch of right coronary artery) supply the posterior one-third of the septum.

The thrombosis of the septal branches results in septal infarction and heart block.

Note: In right dominance the left coronary artery takes a larger share in the arterial supply of the interventricular septum. In "left dominance" the entire supply is derived from the left coronary artery.

🎓 STUDENT INTEREST

Observe the interventricular septum in the sectioned heart in the dissection laboratory. On its surface facing the right ventricle observe the septal papillary muscle and moderator band (septomarginal trabecula). You must feel the interventricular part of membranous septum between your fingers high up between the two ventricles but to feel the atrioventricular part of membranous septum you have to put one finger in right atrium and other in left ventricle. Remember that it is the membranous septum that shows congenital defects called ventricular septal defects (VSDs). You should be aware of the fact that interventricular septum is a pet topic of examiners in theory and practical examinations.

Surface Markings of Cardiac Valves (Fig. 40.18)

- The pulmonary orifice is indicated by a 2.5 cm long transverse line partly behind the left third costal cartilage and partly behind the adjacent left half of sternum.
- The aortic orifice is denoted by an oblique line 2.5 cm long behind the left half of the body of sternum at the level of third left intercostal space.
- A 3 cm long oblique line behind the left half of the sternum opposite the fourth left costal cartilage marks the mitral orifice.
- A 4 cm long line placed vertically behind the right half of the sternum opposite the fourth intercostal space.

🎓 STUDENT INTEREST

Mnemonic for remembering level of cardiac valves—PA3MT4 (pulmonary valve-left third costal cartilage and aortic valve at the level of left third intercostal space, mitral valve – behind left half of sternum at the level of left fourth costal cartilage and tricuspid valve behind right half of sternum at the level of fourth intercostal space).

Surface Markings of Cardiac Auscultation Areas (Fig 40.18)

- *Pulmonary valve:* Second intercostal space to the left of sternum.
- *Aortic valve:* Second intercostal space to the right of sternum.
- *Tricuspid valve:* Fifth intercostal space over the centre of the body of sternum.
- *Mitral valve:* Near the cardiac apex.

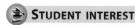

STUDENT INTEREST

The closure of atrioventricular valves (mitral and tricuspid) produces first heart sound. The closure of semilunar valves (pulmonary and aortic) produces second heart sound.

Radiological Anatomy of Heart

- In the posteroanterior (PA) X-ray of chest (Fig. 40.19), the transverse diameter of the cardiac shadow of normal sized heart is equal to half the diameter of the chest (1:2).
- The right margin of the cardiac shadow is formed by SVC, right atrium and IVC from above downward.
- The left margin of cardiac shadow is formed by aortic knuckle or aortic knob (prominence due to arch of aorta), pulmonary trunk, left auricle and left ventricle from above downward.
- The inferior margin of cardiac shadow merges with the shadow of the diaphragm and liver.

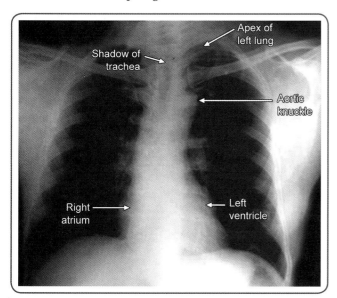

Fig. 40.19: Plain radiograph of chest showing heart, blood vessels, trachea and lungs

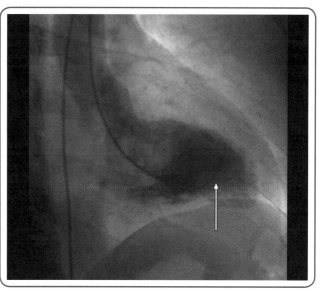

Fig. 40.20: Showing angiographic appearance of left ventricle (arrow showing) (Note the tip of the catheter carrying the dye entering the left ventricle via aortic orifice)

- The serial CT scans of the thorax is the best way to study the anatomical relations of the heart and the surrounding structures to each other.
- In cardiac catheterization and angiography, the cardiac chambers are delineated with the help of the contrast medium. A special cardiac catheter is passed through the femoral vein to reach the right side of heart. The left side of the heart (Fig. 40.20) is approached through the brachial or femoral artery.
- Echocardiography (ECHO) is a modified ultrasound imaging of the heart. It shows the details of internal anatomy of the heart. The usual approach for this procedure is transthoracic. One drawback of this route is that it is not possible to properly see the structures at the base of the heart. This drawback is overcome by the transesophageal echography, which improves the imaging of the base considerably because the esophagus is very close to the base of the heart.

CLINICAL CORRELATION

Diseases of the valves of the heart are very common. Depending on the extent of the damage to the valve components, the orifice of the valve may be narrowed causing stenosis or the valves may become incompetent causing regurgitation.

Disorders of Cardiac Valves

- *Mitral stenosis:* Due to narrowing of mitral orifice, there is obstruction to the left atrial blood during ventricular filling.

Contd...

Contd…

This may lead to accumulation of blood in left atrium leading to dilatation of left atrium (Fig. 40.21), which may press on the esophagus causing dysphagia and on left recurrent laryngeal nerve causing hoarseness of voice (Ortner's syndrome). The passage of blood through narrowed mitral orifice produces a typical sound which on auscultation is heard as mid-diastolic murmur.

- **Mitral regurgitation:** The incompetent mitral valve fails to close during systole leading to regurgitation of blood into the left atrium. So during diastole there is overfilling of the left ventricle. This increases the workload of the left ventricle leading to gross dilatation and hypertrophy of left ventricle.
- **Aortic stenosis:** In narrowing of aortic orifice, the blood accumulates inside the left ventricle causing its hypertrophy and dilatation. There is low cardiac output, which may manifest as angina pectoris and syncope (fainting) on exertion.
- **Aortic regurgitation:** The incompetent aortic valve fails to close the aortic orifice completely during diastole. There is overfilling of left ventricle during diastole because it receives blood not only from left atrium but also from ascending aorta. The left ventricle undergoes dilatation and hypertrophy.
- **Tricuspid stenosis:** Due to narrowing of tricuspid orifice, the blood flow from right atrium to right ventricle is reduced. This results in reduction of blood in the pulmonary circulation. The

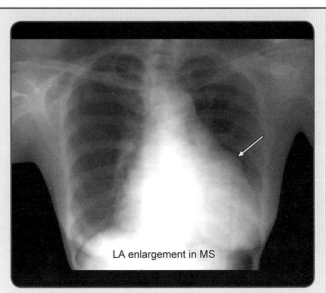

LA enlargement in MS

Fig. 40.21: Dilatation of left atrium in mitral stenosis (MS) (arrow showing)
Key: LA–Left atrial

net result is decreased cardiac output and elevation of right atrial pressure leading to systemic venous congestion.
- **Tricuspid regurgitation:** The incompetent tricuspid valve fails to close during systole leading to regurgitation of blood into right atrium. Ultimately the right side of the heart dilates and gives rise to systemic venous congestion.
- **Pulmonary stenosis:** The pulmonary stenosis is almost always congenital, either isolated or as part of Fallot's tetralogy. The stenosis of the pulmonary orifice results in hypertrophy of the right ventricle and reduction in the cardiac output.

41

Blood Supply of Heart

Chapter Contents

ARTERIAL BLOOD SUPPLY

The myocardium beats nonstop throughout life and is capable of working harder during times of increased physical activities. Therefore, the oxygen demand of the myocardium is very high. The right and left coronary arteries supply blood to the heart. The stems of the two arteries and their major anastomosing branches (located in the subepicardial fat) encircle the heart like an obliquely inverted crown.

Unique Features of Coronary Arteries

- The coronary arteries are the biggest vasa vasora (plural of vasa vasorum) in the body because the heart is considered to be a modified blood vessel.
- The coronary arteries are functionally end arteries but anatomically they are not. The branches of the two coronary arteries anastomose at arteriolar level, but the caliber of the anastomosing arteries is not sufficient to maintain normal circulation, if one of the arteries is suddenly blocked.
- Unlike other arteries of the body, the coronary arteries fill during diastole of the ventricles. Duration of the systole in a cardiac cycle is constant irrespective of the rate of heart. Therefore, in response to increase in the heart rate (tachycardia), diastole is shortened, thus reducing the coronary filling. So, in patients with coronary artery disease, increase in heart rate due to any cause may precipitate ischemia (reduction in arterial supply to heart).

- The coronary arteries are more prone to atherosclerosis (subendothelial deposition of fatty material) compared to other arteries. Atherosclerosis in coronary arteries is the number one cause of ischemic heart diseases.

 STUDENT INTEREST

Right coronary artery arises from anterior aortic sinus and left coronary artery arises from left posterior aortic sinus at the root of ascending aorta. So, the coronary arteries are branches of ascending aorta and fill during diastole.

Right Coronary Artery

Origin (Fig. 41.1)

The right coronary artery takes origin from the anterior aortic sinus at the root of the ascending aorta.

Course (Figs 41.2 and 41.3)

The artery is divided into three segments to understand its course easily.

- The first segment extends from the aortic root to the coronary sulcus on the sternocostal surface. It courses between the pulmonary trunk and the auricle of right atrium in anterior direction to appear on the sternocostal surface.
- The second segment lies in right part of the coronary sulcus on the sternocostal surface, where it runs almost vertically downward to reach the lower end of the right at its junction with inferior margin. This segment is

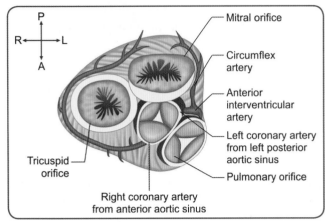

Fig. 41.1: Showing origin of coronary arteries from the sinuses at the base of ascending aorta

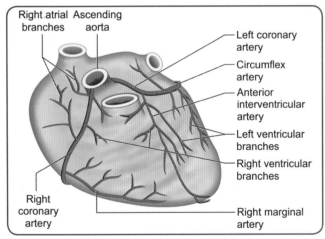

Fig. 41.2: Course and branches of right and left coronary arteries on sternocostal surface (Note the anastomosis of conus arteries on the surface of infundibulum of right ventricle)

covered by subepicardial fat and is crossed by anterior cardiac veins.

- The third segment occupies the right portion of coronary sulcus on the posterior aspect (Fig. 41.4). It runs upwards and to the left with small cardiac vein up to the crux of heart.

Modes of Termination

- In 60% of subjects, the right coronary artery ends a little to the left of the crux by anastomosing with circumflex branch of the left coronary artery.
- In 10% of subjects, it terminates at the lower end of the right margin.
- In 10% of subjects, it terminates between the right border and the crux.

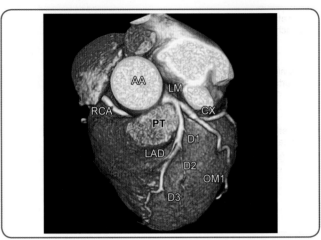

Fig. 41.3: 3D reconstruction from CT serial sections of anterior aspect of heart showing origin of coronary arteries and branches of left anterior descending (LAD) branch of left coronary artery **Key:** (AA—ascending aorta, RCA—right coronary artery, LM—main trunk of left coronary artery, PT—pulmonary trunk, LAD—left anterior descending, CX—circumflex artery, D1, D2, D3—diagonal arteries, OM—obtuse marginal artery)

- In 20% of subjects, it reaches the left border by coursing the entire coronary sulcus, thus replacing posterior part of circumflex artery.

Branches of First Segment

Right conus artery, which supplies the base of the pulmonary trunk. If the conus artery arises independently from the anterior aortic sinus, it is called the third coronary artery.

Branches of Second Segment

- Right anterior atrial branch (supplying the anterior part of the right atrium and the SA node through a nodal branch).
- Right anterior ventricular branches (supplying the anterior part of the right ventricle).
- Right marginal artery (supplying both the ventricles).

Branches of Third Segment

- Right posterior ventricular branches (supplying the diaphragmatic surface of right ventricle).
- Right posterior atrial branches and AV nodal branches.
- Posterior interventricular artery (posterior descending artery or PDA) supplying diaphragmatic surfaces of both ventricles and posterior one-third of the interventricular septum.

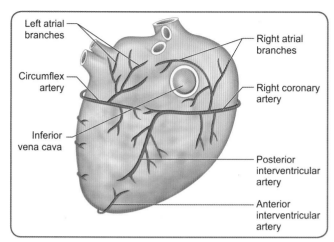

Fig. 41.4: Branches of right coronary artery and of circumflex branch of left coronary artery on the posterior and inferior surfaces of heart

Area of Supply

The right coronary artery supplies right atrium, right ventricle, posterior one third of interventricular septum and sinoatrial node, atrioventricular node and atrioventricular bundle,

Left Coronary Artery (Fig. 41.1)

Origin

The left coronary artery takes origin from the left posterior aortic sinus at the root of the ascending aorta. It is larger in size and much shorter than the right coronary artery. It supplies a greater volume of myocardium.

Course

Its short stem courses anteriorly between pulmonary trunk and left auricle to emerge on the sternocostal surface, where it divides into terminal branches of equal size, namely anterior interventricular artery (left anterior descending artery or LAD) and circumflex artery.

Branches

Anterior interventricular artery or left anterior descending artery

The anterior interventricular artery (left anterior descending or LAD artery) descends in the anterior interventricular groove or sulcus on the sternocostal surface accompanied by great cardiac vein. It terminates by meeting the end of the posterior interventricular artery near the apex of the heart or in the posterior interventricular groove after winding round the apex.

Branches

- Right ventricular and left ventricular branches
- Left conus artery
- Anterior septal branches
- Diagonal artery (a large left anterior ventricular branch) running down between LAD and circumflex artery.

Thus, it is evident that the anterior interventricular artery supplies a large area of left ventricle and of the interventricular septum.

Circumflex artery

The circumflex artery continues in the short left part of the coronary sulcus on the sternocostal surface (Figs 41.2 and 41.3) along with great cardiac vein and curves round the upper end of the left margin of the heart to appear in the left portion of the coronary sulcus on the posterior aspect (Fig. 41.4). Usually it terminates to the left of the crux by anastomozing with the right coronary artery but at times it continues as the posterior interventricular artery.

Branches

- Left marginal artery (obtuse marginal as shown in figure 41.2B).
- Ventricular branches to inferior surface of left ventricle.
- Left atrial branches.

Area of Supply

The left coronary artery supplies most of the left ventricle, a narrow strip of right ventricle, anterior two-thirds of the interventricular septum and the left atrium.

 STUDENT INTEREST

The stem of right coronary artery is much longer than the stem of left coronary as the latter divides into anterior interventricular and circumflex arteries as soon as it reaches the sternocostal surface on the left side of pulmonary trunk as seen in (Figures 41.2 and 41.3).

Coronary Dominance

In the right dominance, the posterior interventricular artery arises from the right coronary artery while in the left dominance, the posterior interventricular artery is a branch of the left coronary artery. In balanced pattern, both coronary arteries give rise to posterior interventricular branches, which run parallel in the posterior interventricular sulcus.

 STUDENT INTEREST

The topic on 'Coronary arteries' is the MUST KNOW in Anatomy, Physiology, Pathology, Surgery, Medicine, Cardiology and Cardiovascular surgery.

- The coronary angiography is a radiological procedure by which coronary arteries are visualized after injecting a contrast medium into them. Angiography is useful in localizing the sites of the blocks in the coronary arteries or their branches. In this procedure a special catheter is passed usually through the femoral artery up into the aorta till the base of the ascending aorta. The contrast material is injected into the coronary ostia located at this site and then the radiographs are taken. Figure 41.5 shows normal right coronary artery whereas Figure 41.6 shows block in LAD.
- In angina pectoris due to narrowing of coronary artery or arteries, there is reduction in blood supply and lack of sufficient oxygen to the myocardium (ischemia). On physical exertion, the patient experiences pain in the chest. The typical anginal pain is of gripping or constricting type of retrosternal pain, which radiates to the inner side of left arm or shoulder or to the neck. The anginal pain is accompanied by weakness, dizziness and perspiration. It is relieved after rest.
- In myocardial infarction (MI), there is a complete block in the stem of coronary artery or in the major branch either due to thrombus or embolus formation on the atheromatous patch. This results in complete loss of blood supply to the myocardium and consequent infarction. Massive myocardial infarction is usually fatal. LAD is very much prone to atherosclerosis and narrowing in men in middle age. Hence, its block is the reason of massive and fatal infarction. On account of this LAD has been popularly called the 'widow maker'.

Restoration of Arterial Supply of Ischemic Myocardium

There are two methods by which the blood supply to the myocardium can be restored if the main coronary arteries or their main branches are blocked.

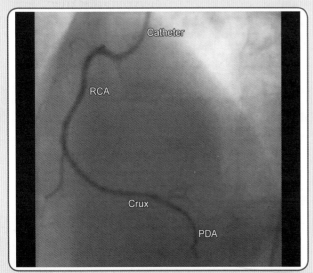

Fig. 41.5: Angiographic appearance of right coronary artery (RCA—Right coronary artery; PDA—Posterior descending artery)

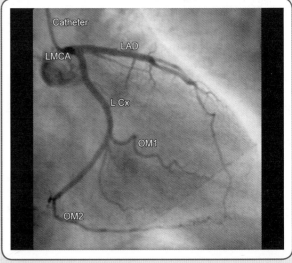

Fig. 41.6: Angiographic appearance of left coronary artery and its branches (LMCA—Left main coronary artery; LAD—Left anterior descending artery; OM—Obtuse marginal artery)

Percutaneous Transluminal Coronary Angioplasty

- The percutaneous transluminal coronary angioplasty (PTCA) is done for increasing the inside diameter of the narrowed coronary artery. A balloon catheter is passed into the coronary artery and the balloon is inflated at the site of the block in order to squash the atheromatous plaque against the wall of the artery. Nowadays stenting of blocked artery is a preferred method (Fig. 41.7).

Contd…

Contd...

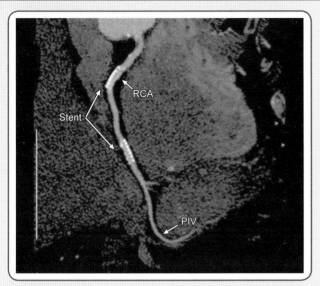

Fig. 41.7: Stents in right coronary artery to dilate sites of blocks (RCA—Right Coronary Artery; PIV—Posterior Inter-ventricular Artery)

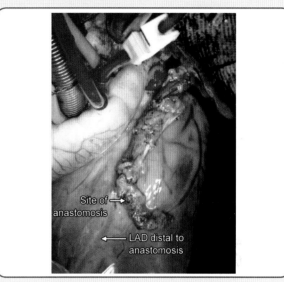

Fig. 41.8: Operative view of LIMA to LAD (Left anterior descending artery) graft

- The coronary artery bypass graft (CABG) is a major surgical procedure (Fig. 41.8). The patient's own vessels are used for the graft. The commonly used vessels are the great saphenous vein, the internal mammary artery and the radial artery. Amongst these options, internal mammary artery graft is the most favored. This graft has the greatest success rate because the wall of the internal mammary artery has elastic tissue in it and chances of re-stenosis are far less. In patients with multiple blocks (three or four) all the three blood vessels can be used (Fig. 41.9). Before taking the radial artery graft, the patency of the ulnar artery is always ascertained by Allen's test (Fig. 19.8A and B).

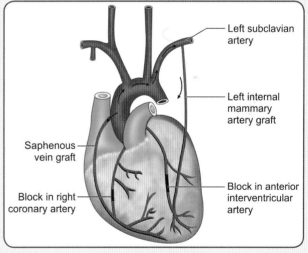

Fig. 41.9: Schematic depiction of saphenous vein graft and internal mammary graft

Veins of Heart (Fig. 41.10)

There are three major veins which drain blood from the myocardium:

- The coronary sinus is the chief vein of the heart. It collects venous blood from the myocardium and empties it into the right atrium.
- There are three or four anterior cardiac veins, which directly open into the rough part of the right atrium.
- The venae cordis minimae (Thebesian veins) are scattered all over the myocardium and open directly into all the cardiac chambers.

Corosnary Sinus

This is a short (2.5 cm long) and wide venous channel located in the posterior part of the atrioventricular sulcus (coronary sulcus) between the left atrium and left ventricle.

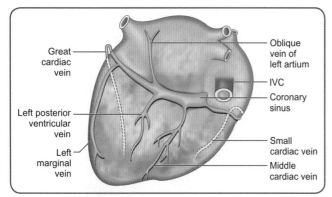

Fig. 41.10: Coronary sinus (continuation of great cardiac vein) and its tributaries viewed from posterior aspect of heart
Key: (IVC—Inferior vena cava)

Origin and Termination

The coronary sinus begins as the continuation of the great cardiac vein at the left end of the coronary sulcus. From here it courses downward and to the right lying initially between the left atrium and left ventricle and opens into the smooth part of the right atrium. The opening of the coronary sinus is guarded by a small valve (Thebesian) and is located between the opening of inferior vena cava and the tricuspid orifice.

Tributaries

- The great cardiac vein begins at the cardiac apex. It ascends in the anterior interventricular groove to enter the coronary sulcus and follows this to reach the left border of the heart, where it joins the left end of the coronary sinus.
- The middle cardiac vein begins at the cardiac apex, ascends in the posterior interventricular groove and joins the coronary sinus at its right end.
- The small cardiac vein has a variable course. It may follow the right coronary artery and open into the right end of the coronary sinus. It may take the place of right marginal vein so that it accompanies the right marginal artery as well as the right coronary artery in its posterior course.
- The posterior vein of left ventricle lies parallel to the middle cardiac vein.
- The oblique vein of left atrium or oblique vein of Marshall opens near the left end of the coronary sinus (Fig. 41.10). The oblique vein of left atrium is the remnant of left common cardinal vein.

Developmental Source

The coronary sinus develops from the left horn of the sinus venosus and part of left common cardinal vein (Fig. 38.3C).

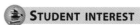 **STUDENT INTEREST**

The coronary sinus is the main vein of the heart. It is a continuation of the great cardiac vein and terminates directly into the right atrium. It is easy to remember if its diagram is practiced while reading its description.

42

Fibrous Skeleton, Conducting Tissue and Nerve Supply of Heart

FIBROUS SKELETON OF HEART

The fibrous skeleton (Fig. 42.1) of the heart gives support to the cardiac valves and the myocardium. It is described as a dynamically deformable tissue. The fibrous skeleton gives origin to the myocardium of atria and ventricles and ensures electrophysiological discontinuity between the atria and ventricle except where the bundle of His penetrates the central fibrous body.

Component Parts

The atrioventricular valves and the aortic valve are located close to each other and share a common fibrous ring (annulus) while the pulmonary valve has a separate fibrous ring. The pulmonary annulus is connected to the aortic annulus by the tendon of conus or infundibulum.

A large mass of common fibrous tissue between the annulus of atrioventricular valves behind and the aortic orifice in front is divisible into:
- Left fibrous trigone, where the aortic and mitral valves meet.
- Subaortic curtain between the aortic valve and the mitral valve annulus.
- Right fibrous trigone, where the aortic, mitral and tricuspid rings meet and which is continuous with the membranous part of the interventricular septum.

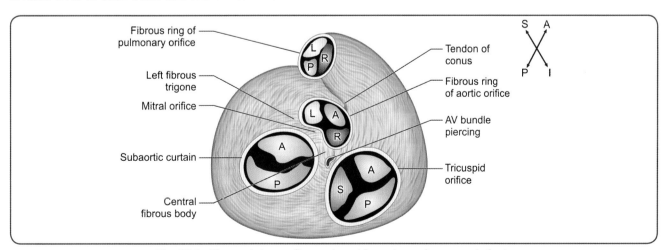

Fig. 42.1: Fibrous skeleton of heart viewed from above after removal of atria
Key: (AV–atrioventricular)

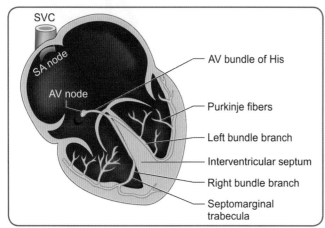

Fig. 42.2: Parts of conducting tissue of heart
Key: (SVC–superior vena cava; SA–sinoatrial; AV–atrioventricular)

The central fibrous body is the combination of right fibrous trigone and the membranous part of interventricular septum. The bundle of His penetrates this important structure.

The tendon of Todaro is the collagenous connection between the central fibrous body and the valve of the inferior vena cava.

Injury to central fibrous body results in injury to AV bundle causing atrioventricular dehiscence (a serious condition).

CONDUCTING TISSUE OF HEART

The conducting tissue (Fig. 42.2) consists of excitable tissue, which consists of modified myofibers. This specialized tissue is responsible for maintaining the heart rate at 70–90 per minute in the adult.

Components

The conducting tissue consists of:
- Sinuatrial (SA) node
- Internodal pathways
- Atrioventricular (AV) node
- Atrioventricular bundle of His
- Right and left bundle branches
- Purkinje fibers (conduction myofibers).

Sinoatrial (SA) Node

The SA node is situated in the wall of the right atrium at the upper end of the crista terminalis partially surrounding the opening of the superior vena cava. It is subepicardial in position. It is capable of generating electrical impulses; hence, it is called the pacemaker of the heart. The SA node is a very vascular area of the heart.

Internodal Pathways

It is believed that three internodal pathways exist across the atrial wall and they connect the SA node to the AV node. Similarly, a path (Bachmann's bundle) connecting right and left atria is also believed to exist. But for want of histological evidence of these paths, it is assumed that the internodal and interatrial conduction occurs through ordinary working myocardium.

Atrioventricular (AV) Node

The AV node is located in the triangle of Koch in the lower part of the right atrium to the left of the coronary sinus opening. It extends downwards up to the junction of interatrial septum and the central fibrous trigone. In this way the AV node is related to, mitral and tricuspid valves, interatrial septum, membranous part of interventricular septum and the aortic valve. The AV node initiates the ventricular systole. The impulse is carried in the atrioventricular bundle to the ventricles. In case of damage to SA node, the AV node takes over the function of the pacemaker.

Atrioventricular Bundle of His

The atrioventricular bundle of His is the only muscular connection between the myocardium of atria and of ventricles. It passes through the central fibrous body and along the posterior margin of the membranous interventricular septum to the junction of the muscular and membranous parts of the interventricular septum. At this level, it divides into two bundle branches, one for each ventricle.

Right and Left Bundle Branches

The right bundle branch (RBB) passes down on the right side of the interventricular septum. A part of this bundle enters the septomarginal trabecula, which carries it to the anterior papillary muscle, and the remainder breaks up into fine fibers, which supply the, rest of the right ventricle. The left bundle branch (LBB) pierces the septum and passes down in a superficial position on the left aspect of the septum. It divides into fibers that enter the ventricular musculature. The fibers of the bundle of His are in continuity with Purkinje fibers in the ventricular wall.

Arterial Supply of Conducting Tissue (Fig. 42.3)

- SA node is supplied by the nodal branch of right coronary artery near its origin in 60 percent of people.

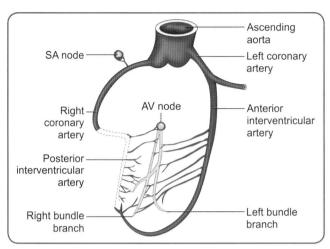

Fig. 42.3: Arterial supply of conducting tissue of heart
Key: (SA–sinoatrial; AV–atrioventricular)

In the remaining 40 percent the circumflex branch of left coronary supplies it.

- AV node is supplied by the branch of right coronary artery at the crux of heart in 90 percent of people. In 10% the circumflex branch of left coronary artery supplies it.
- The atrioventricular bundle of His is supplied by septal branches of right coronary artery.
- The right bundle branch (moderator band) is supplied by septal branches of left coronary artery.
- The left bundle branch is supplied largely by septal branches from anterior interventricular branch of left coronary artery and its posterior subdivision is supplied additionally by septal branches of posterior interventricular branch of right coronary artery.

⚲ CLINICAL CORRELATION

Injury to AV Node and AV Bundle

Injury to AV node results in heart block which results in asynchronous beating of atria and ventricles. A pace-maker which artificially regulates the heart may have to be installed.

Artificial Cardiac Pacemaker (Fig. 42.4)

In patients who have suffered from heart block, a pacemaker is installed subcutaneously to restore the normal cardiac rhythm. The pacemaker consists of a pulse generator and a lead or wire tipped with electrode. The pulse generator is a tiny computer powered by battery. It is inserted under the clavicle in the pectoral region. The lead is inserted via the venous route (right subclavian vein, right brachiocephalic vein and SVC) first in to right atrium and then into right ventricle through tricuspid orifice. Inside the right ventricle it is firmly fixed to trabeculae carneae. The artificial pacemaker initiates ventricular contractions at pre-determined rate.

NERVE SUPPLY OF HEART

Both sympathetic and parasympathetic nerves control the action of heart through the cardiac plexuses and the coronary plexuses.

Efferent Nerve Supply

- Parasympathetic efferent supply is via the cervical cardiac branches of vagus and cardiac branches of recurrent laryngeal nerves. The parasympathetic is cardioinhibitor.
- The sympathetic supply is via the three cervical cardiac branches and a few thoracic cardiac branches of the sympathetic chain. The sympathetic is cardioaccelerator.

Afferent Nerve Supply

The heart is insensitive to touch, cutting; cold or heat but ischemia and resultant accumulation of metabolic products stimulate pain nerve endings in the myocardium. The pain sensation is carried in the middle and inferior cervical cardiac branches and thoracic cardiac branches of the sympathetic chain to the thoracic ganglia of the sympathetic chain (Fig. 42.4). From here the impulse passes via the white rami to the thoracic spinal nerves (T1-T5) and to the dorsal root ganglia. The central processes

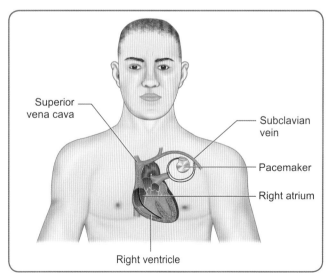

Fig. 42.4: Location of pacemaker in a patient

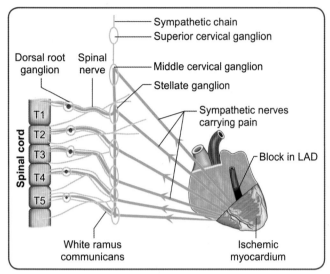

Fig. 42.5: Path of pain from ischemic myocardium to the spinal cord
Key: (LAD–Left anterior descending artery)

of the neurons in the dorsal root ganglia carry the impulses to the posterior horns of T1 to T5 spinal segments (mostly of the left side).

The afferent fibers in the vagus nerves reach the medulla oblongata and are concerned with reflexes controlling the cardiovascular activity.

✆ CLINICAL CORRELATION

Referred Pain in Angina Pectoris

When the pain impulses from ischemic myocardium reach the spinal cord, they stimulate the somatic sensory neurons of the corresponding segments of the spinal cord, usually on the left side. Thus, pain is felt in the cutaneous area of T1 and T2 dermatomes (along the inner border of the left upper limb). The pain may also be felt in the precordium and back, which are supplied by T2 to T5 spinal nerves (Fig. 42.5).

43

Major Blood Vessels of Thorax

Chapter Contents

INTRODUCTION

The major blood vessels of thorax are listed below:
- Pulmonary vessels (pulmonary trunk, pulmonary arteries, pulmonary veins)
- Ascending aorta
- Arch of aorta
- Descending thoracic aorta
- Superior vena cava
- Azygos system of veins

Pulmonary Vessels

The pulmonary vessels consist of pulmonary trunk and its terminal branches, the right and left pulmonary arteries, and one pair of pulmonary veins on each side. The pulmonary arteries and veins communicate with each other at the pulmonary capillary bed in the lungs. The pulmonary arteries carry deoxygenated blood from the right ventricle to the lungs and the pulmonary veins bring oxygenated blood from the lungs to the left atrium.

Pulmonary Trunk

This vessel begins as the continuation of infundibulum of the right ventricle at the pulmonary valve (Fig. 43.1). It is five cm long and three cm wide. It systolic pressure is 15–20 mm of Hg. The pulmonary trunk bifurcates into right and left pulmonary arteries inside the fibrous pericardium. Its bifurcation is at the level of the superior margin of the atria (level with fifth thoracic vertebra).

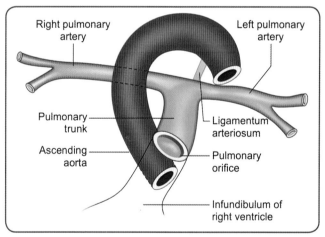

Fig. 43.1: Pulmonary trunk and its division into right and left pulmonary arteries

Relations

The pulmonary trunk is intimately related to the ascending aorta. Both the vessels are covered in a common sleeve of visceral pericardium due to their common development from the truncus arteriosus. The pulmonary trunk is anterior to the ascending aorta at its beginning but soon it comes to lie on the left of the ascending aorta. Both vessels form the anterior boundary of transverse sinus of pericardium and hence lie in front of the left atrium. At its origin, the pulmonary trunk is flanked by the corresponding coronary artery and auricle.

Course and Distribution of Pulmonary Arteries

- The ***right pulmonary artery,*** has a longer intrapericardial course than the left pulmonary artery. During its intrapericardial course it is related anteriorly (in succession) to the ascending aorta, superior vena cava (SVC) and the upper right pulmonary vein. It pierces the fibrous pericardium and reaches the hilum of right lung, where it divides into two unequal branches. The smaller branch enters the upper lobe of the lung while the larger branch soon divides into lobar branches for the middle and the lower lobes. The lobar branches divide into segmental branches for individual bronchopulmonary segment. Thus, the arterial divisions follow the pattern of bronchial tree.

- The ***left pulmonary artery,*** has a very short intrapericardial course. After it pierces the fibrous pericardium, the ligamentum arteriosum connects it to arch of aorta. At the hilum of the left lung, it divides into two equal branches for the two lobes of the left lung. Each lobar branch gives off segmental branches corresponding to the number of bronchopulmonary segments. The arterial divisions follow the bronchial pattern.

Radiology

The pulmonary arteries are visualized by radiological methods like plain radiograph of chest, pulmonary angiography (arteriography), computed tomography (CT scan) chest (Fig. 43.2), transesophageal echocardiography, 3D image reconstruction from serial cross sections of CT chest (Fig. 43.3) etc;

Pulmonary Veins (Fig. 43.4)

The pulmonary veins originate as small venous tributaries from the pulmonary capillaries. The veins lie in the planes separating the adjacent bronchopulmonary segments. The intersegmental veins unite to form lobar veins. A pair of pulmonary veins emerges on each side from the hilum of the lung. The veins proceed transversely to pierce the fibrous pericardium and open into the posterior wall of the left atrium. They are valveless veins.

> **CLINICAL CORRELATION**
>
> - Pulmonary arterial hypertension develops in several conditions. Some common causes include pulmonary stenosis, right ventricular failure etc.
> - Pulmonary embolism or pulmonary thromboembolism (PTE) means occlusion of pulmonary artery or its branches by emboli. The emboli usually originate from thrombosis in distant peripheral veins like calf veins or pelvic veins or from the right auricle. Massive pulmonary embolism is a cause of sudden death. Symptoms of pulmonary embolism include sudden dyspnoea, anginal pain, hemoptysis (blood in sputum) and cyanosis. Radiological investigations like pulmonary angiography are essential in confirming the diagnosis.
> - Pulmonary edema is a condition in which there is an accumulation of tissue fluid in the lung alveoli due to rise in the hydrostatic pressure in the capillaries.

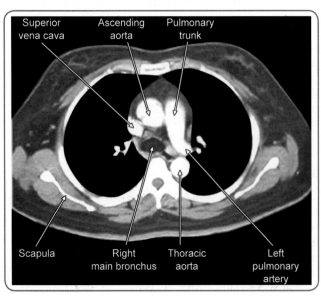

Fig. 43.2: Cross section of thorax at T5 vertebral level obtained by computed tomography (CT scan) to show pulmonary trunk, ascending aorta and tracheal bifurcation

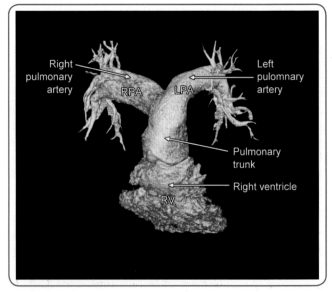

Fig. 43.3: 3 D reconstruction image (from serial sections of CT scan) of right ventricle, pulmonary trunk and pulmonary arteries

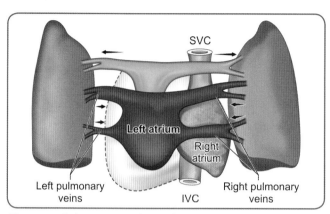

Fig. 43.4: Pulmonary vessels (4 pulmonary veins and 2 pulmonary arteries) seen from posterior aspect (SVC—Superior vena cava; IVC—Inferior vena cava)

Ascending Aorta (Figs 43.5 and 43.6)

The ascending aorta begins from the left ventricle at the level of aortic valve. It continues as the arch of aorta at the level of sternal angle. Its length is five cm and diameter is three cm. It lies in the middle mediastinum and is entirely intrapericardial. The ascending aorta pierces the apex of fibrous pericardium at the level of sternal angle. It is enclosed with the pulmonary trunk in a common sleeve of visceral pericardium.

Surface Marking

The aortic valve is drawn on the left half of the body of sternum at the level of 3rd intercostal space by a line 2.5 cm broad. From the ends of this line two parallel lines

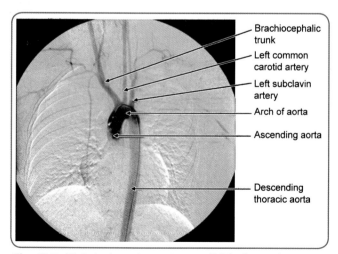

Fig. 43.5: Digital subtraction angiogram (DSA) of ascending aorta, arch of aorta and descending aorta

are drawn in upward direction to reach the right half of sternum at the sternal angle.

Sinuses of Valsalva

Just above the aortic valves the wall of the ascending aorta shows dilatations, called *aortic sinuses of Valsalva.* Their positions are anterior, right posterior and left posterior. The anterior aortic sinus is called the *right coronary sinus* because it gives origin to right coronary artery.

- The left posterior sinus is called the *left coronary sinus* because it gives origin to left coronary artery.
- The right posterior sinus is called the *non-coronary sinus* since it does not give origin to coronary artery.

> **ADDED INFORMATION**
>
> The bulb of ascending aorta is a dilatation on the right side of the ascending aorta, which is subjected to constant thrust of the forceful blood current ejected from the left ventricle. This site is prone to aneurysm.

Relations

Anterior relations

- The lower part of ascending aorta is related to infundibulum of right ventricle and the auricle of right atrium.
- Its middle part is related to the pulmonary trunk and auricle of right atrium.
- Its upper part is related to the right lung and pleura.
- The entire ascending aorta anteriorly is very close to the body of sternum.

Posterior relations

The transverse sinus of pericardium separates the ascending aorta from the left atrium. Its upper end is related posteriorly to right pulmonary artery.

Right relations

The superior vena cava (SVC) and the right atrium form close relation on the right side.

Left relation

The pulmonary trunk is related on the left side in its middle part.

Note: The pulmonary trunk is first related anteriorly and then comes on the left side.

Branches

- Right coronary artesry
- Left coronary artery

Pulmonary trunk and ascending aorta are inside the pericardium. Both develop from truncus arteriosus. Ascending aorta has two branches arising from sinuses at its base—right and left coronary arteries.

CLINICAL CORRELATION

Aneurysm of Ascending Aorta

The aneurysm occurs at the bulb of the aorta. It may compress the pulmonary trunk, superior vena cava (SVC), right atrium or right main bronchus (through the pericardium). It may cause anginal pain. Its serious complication is rupture, which results in rapid accumulation of blood in the pericardial cavity (hemopericardium).

Rupture of Ascending Aorta

In view of the close anterior relation of ascending aorta to the body of sternum, in car accidents the steering wheel may push through the body of sternum into the pericardium causing rupture of the ascending aorta and heart of the driver. Massive bleeding in pericardial cavity may lead to fatal hemopericardium.

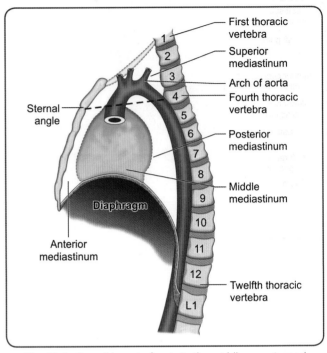

Fig. 43.6: Overall layout of aorta in the middle, superior and posterior mediastinum

Arch of Aorta (Fig. 43.6)

The arch of aorta (aortic arch) is located in the superior mediastinum. It is the continuation of ascending aorta and it continues as the descending thoracic aorta, both events take place at the level of sternal angle (Fig. 43.6). The arch begins anteriorly while it ends posteriorly (very close to the left side of the fourth thoracic vertebra). The arch reaches the level of mid-manubrium, as it spans the distance between its two ends.

Surface Marking (Fig. 43.7)

The arch of aorta is represented by a curved and wide (2.5 cm) band, which connects the right second costal cartilage close to the sternum to the left second costo-sternal junction. The most convex point of this band reaches the midpoint of the manubrium sterni.

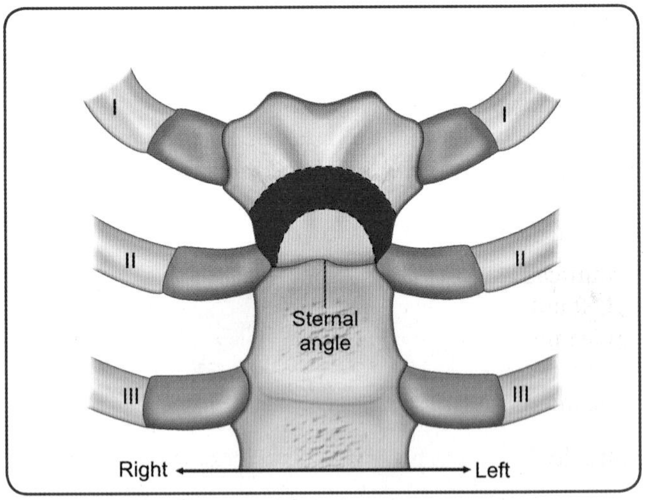

Course

- The arch of aorta begins at the level of upper margin of right second costal cartilage.
- It describes two convexities during its course, the first convexity being upwards and the second to the left. It turns upwards, backwards and to the left side of the

Fig. 43.7: Surface marking of arch of aorta

trachea. It passes downward on the body of the fourth thoracic vertebra and arches over the hilum of the left lung.

- It continues as the descending aorta at the lower margin of the body of fourth thoracic vertebra.

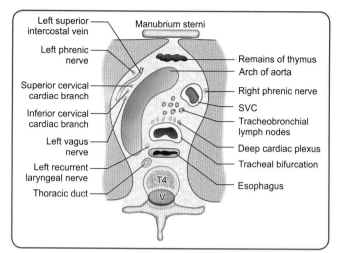

Fig. 43.8: Transverse section of thorax at T 4 vertebral level to show relations of arch of aorta (SVC—Superior vena cava)

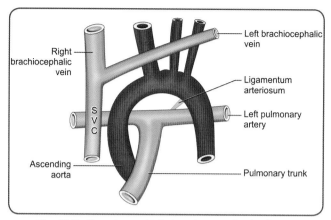

Fig. 43.9: Superior and inferior relations of arch of aorta

Relations (Fig. 43.8)

Anteriorly and to the left (from anterior to posterior)

- Left phrenic nerve
- Inferior cervical cardiac branch of left vagus nerve
- Superior cervical cardiac branch of left sympathetic chain
- Left vagus nerve
- Left superior intercostal vein crosses the arch between phrenic and vagus nerves.

Other structures include left lung, pleura and the remains of thymus

Inferior

- Bifurcation of pulmonary trunk
- Left pulmonary artery and the left main bronchus
- Ligamentum arteriosum and superficial cardiac plexus
- Left recurrent laryngeal nerve winding round the ligamentum arteriosum.

Posteriorly and to the right (from before backward)

- Lower end of trachea with deep cardiac plexus
- Left recurrent laryngeal nerve
- Left side of esophagus
- Thoracic duct
- Left side of fourth thoracic vertebra.

Superior

- Three branches the arch aorta (Brachiocephalic artery, Left common carotid artery and Left subclavian artery).
- The left brachiocephalic vein crosses from left to right, anterior to these three branches very close to their origin from arch of aorta (Fig. 43.9).

Branches

- Brachiocephalic (Innominate) artery
- Left common carotid
- Left subclavian artery.

Occasionally a fourth branch called ***thyroidea ima*** may arise from the arch of aorta.

Arterial Supply

- The vasa vasora (small twigs from the branches of the aortic arch) enter its wall from outside. These branches supply outer part of aortic wall.
- The inner part of the aortic wall is nourished from the blood inside the lumen of the arch.

 EMBRYOLOGIC INSIGHT

Development (Fig. 43.10)
The arch of aorta develops from four sources as given below:
1. Aortic sac
2. Left horn of aortic sac
3. Left fourth arch artery
4. Left dorsal aorta.

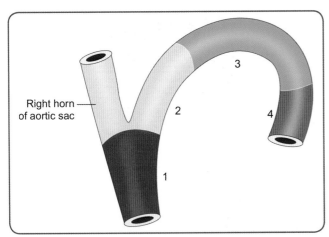

Fig. 43.10: Showing developmental sources of arch of aorta

- **Congenital anomalies of arch of aorta**
  - Patent ductus arteriosus (Fig. 39.8)
  - Coarctation of aorta (Figs 39.2A and B, and 39.3)
  - Aberrant right subclavian artery (Figs 39.5A and B)
  - Double aortic arch.

For details of the development and anomalies of the arch of aorta refer to chapter 39 on pharyngeal arch arteries.

- **Aneurysm of aortic arch (Figs 39.2A and B, and 39.4)**

The aneurysm of aortic arch is a localized dilatation of the vessel. A characteristic clinical sign of this condition is the tracheal tug, which is a tugging sensation felt in the suprasternal notch, where trachea is palpated in extended position of the neck. The aneurysm usually causes compression of neighboring structures in the superior mediastinum producing diverse signs and symptoms.

  - Pressure on esophagus causes dysphagia
  - Pressure on trachea causes stridor (high pitched sound during inspiration) and dry cough
  - Pressure on left recurrent laryngeal nerve produces hoarseness of voice
  - Pressure on sympathetic chain causes Horner's syndrome
  - Compression of veins in superior mediastinum causes venous congestion in the neck and upper limb leading to swelling in upper limb and face.

Radiological Appearance

- In the P–A view of X-ray chest, the arch of aorta appears as a small projection at the upper end of the left margin of the cardiac shadow. It is called *aortic knuckle* or *knob*.
- In left anterior oblique(LAO) view of X-ray chest, a translucent space enclosed by the arch of aorta is identifiable. It is called *aortic window* in which faint shadows of pulmonary arteries are seen.

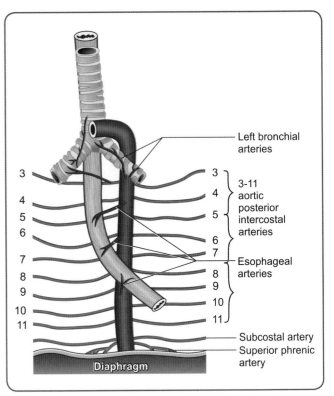

Fig. 43.11: Extent and branches of descending thoracic aorta

Location, extent, branches, relations and development of arch of aorta are very important in examinations. Therefore 'arch of aorta' is a must known topic.

Descending Thoracic Aorta (Fig. 43.11)

Location

The descending thoracic aorta is located in the posterior mediastinum.

Extent

It extends from the left side of the lower border of fourth thoracic vertebra to the lower border of the front of the twelfth thoracic vertebra.

At its upper end it is continuous with the arch of aorta. At its lower end it passes through the aortic opening of the diaphragm to become continuous with the abdominal aorta.

At its commencement the aorta is to the left of the vertebral column. During its descent it gradually inclines towards the midline till it lies directly anterior to the vertebral column at its entry point into the abdomen.

Relations

Anterior (from above downwards to)
- Left lung root
- Pericardium (with left atrium inside it)
- Esophagus
- Diaphragm.

Posterior

Vertebral column and hemiazygos veins

Right

- In its upper part to esophagus, thoracic duct and vena azygos.
- In its lower part to the right lung and pleura.

Left

Produces a deep vertical groove on mediastinal surface of left lung.

Branches

The branches of descending thoracic aorta are given in Table 43.1.

TABLE 43.1: Branches of Descending Thoracic Aorta	
Visceral branches	• Pericardial • Esophageal • Mediastinal • Left bronchial
Parietal branches	• Posterior intercostal arteries of third to eleventh spaces • Subcostal arteries • Superior phrenic arteries

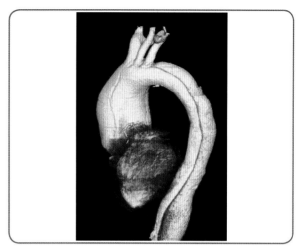

Fig. 43.12: 3D reconstruction image of dissecting aneurysm of descending aorta

🎼 CLINICAL CORRELATION

Dissecting aneurysm (Fig. 43.12)

The aortic dissection (dissecting aneurysm) is a condition that mostly affects the descending thoracic aorta. There is a tear in the intima of aorta through which blood from aortic lumen enters its wall. This causes dilatation of the aorta. The patient usually experiences pain in the back due to compression of intercostal nerves. Occasionally the aorta may rupture into the left pleural cavity. Replacement of diseased segment with prosthetic vascular graft is one method of surgical treatment.

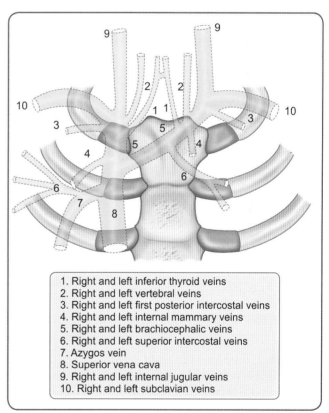

1. Right and left inferior thyroid veins
2. Right and left vertebral veins
3. Right and left first posterior intercostal veins
4. Right and left internal mammary veins
5. Right and left brachiocephalic veins
6. Right and left superior intercostal veins
7. Azygos vein
8. Superior vena cava
9. Right and left internal jugular veins
10. Right and left subclavian veins

Fig. 43.13: Formation, tributaries and termination of brachiocephalic veins

MAJOR VEINS OF THORAX (FIG. 43.13)

Superior Vena Cava (SVC)

The superior vena cava (SVC) drains blood from the head and neck, upper limbs, walls of thorax and upper abdomen into the right atrium of the heart. The superior vena cava is without valves since gravity facilitates the flow of blood inside it.

Length

It is seven 7 cm long.

Parts

- Extrapericardial part in the superior mediastinum
- Intrapericardial part in the middle mediastinum.

Formation

The superior vena cava is formed by the union of the right and left brachiocephalic veins behind the lower border of right first costal cartilage close to the sternum.

Course

It passes vertically downwards behind the first and second right intercostal spaces and pierces the fibrous pericardium to open into the upper posterior part of the right atrium at the level of the third costal cartilage. The arch of the azygos vein opens into it just before the superior vena cava pierces the fibrous pericardium. The intrapericardial part is closely related to the ascending aorta and the right pulmonary artery.

Relations of Extrapericardial Part

- **Anteriorly:** Right pleura and lung
- **Posteriorly:** Right vagus nerve and trachea
- **Medially:** Brachiocephalic artery
- **Right side:** Right phrenic nerve, right pleura and lung

Relations of Intrapericardial Part

- **Anteriorly:** Pericardium
- **Posteriorly:** Right pulmonary artery
- **Medially:** Ascending aorta
- **Right side:** Pericardium

Tributaries

Azygos vein is the only large tributary. Smaller mediastinal and pericardial veins open into it.

Surface Marking

Superior vena cava (SVC) is represented by two parallel and vertical lines two cm apart starting from the lower border of the first costal cartilage to the upper border of the third costal cartilage close to the right side of sternum.

 STUDENT INTEREST

Remember the numbers 1, 2, 3. Superior vena cava (SVC) is formed at the level of **1st right costal cartilage** (by union of right and left brachiocephalic veins), is joined by azygos vein at the level of **2nd right costal cartilage** and opens into right atrium at the level of **3rd right costal cartilage**. It has extrapericardial part in superior mediastinum and intrapericardial part in middle mediastinum. Its biggest tributary is vena azygos.

Brachiocephalic Veins (Fig. 43.13)

There are two brachiocephalic veins,—right brachiocephalic vein and left brachiocephalic vein.

Formation

Each vein is formed behind the respective sternoclavicular joint by the union of the internal jugular and subclavian veins.

Termination

The right and left brachiocephalic veins unite to form the superior vena cava at the lower margin of the right first costal cartilage close to the margin of sternum. Both veins are devoid of valves.

Right Brachiocephalic Vein

The right brachiocephalic vein is short (2.5 cm) and extends from the right sternoclavicular joint to the lower margin of first costal cartilage. Its tributaries are right vertebral vein, right internal thoracic vein, right inferior thyroid vein and the first right posterior intercostal vein.

Left Brachiocephalic Vein

The left brachiocephalic vein is about twice the length of the right vein (6 cm). It runs obliquely across the superior mediastinum from the left sternoclavicular joint to the lower margin of first right costal cartilage, where it unites with the right vein. It is closely related to the posterior surface of the manubrium sterni. Posteriorly, it is related to the three branches of the arch of aorta and two nerves (left vagus and left phrenic). This vein receives left vertebral vein, left internal thoracic vein, left inferior thyroid vein (sometimes both inferior thyroid veins), first left posterior intercostal vein, left superior intercostal vein, thymic veins and pericardial veins.

Azygos Vein or Vena Azygos (Fig. 35.10)

The name azygos means single or without a companion. The azygos vein is present on the right side only. It is provided with valves. It presents a tortuous appearance. It passes through two regions—(1) posterior abdominal wall, (2) posterior mediastinum.

Formation in Abdomen

The azygos vein begins on posterior abdominal wall usually as a continuation of lumbar azygos vein (which arises from posterior aspect of IVC) or is formed by the union of right ascending lumbar and right subcostal veins (Fig. 44.2).

Exit from Abdomen

The azygos vein leaves the abdomen through the aortic opening of the diaphragm to enter the posterior mediastinum.

Course in Posterior Mediastinum

The azygos vein ascends vertically upwards lying in front of the vertebral column up to the level of the fourth thoracic vertebra, where it arches forwards superior to the hilum of the right lung (which it grooves) to open into the posterior aspect of superior vena cava (SVC) just before the latter pierces the fibrous pericardium.

Tributaries

- Right superior intercostal vein
- Right posterior intercostal veins from the fourth space downwards
- Right subcostal vein
- Right ascending lumbar vein
- Hemiazygos vein
- Accessory hemiazygos vein (superior hemiazygos vein)
- Right bronchial vein
- Esophageal veins
- Pericardial veins
- Mediastinal veins.

Hemiazygos Vein (Inferior Hemiazygos Vein)

The hemiazygos vein is present on the left side. It is formed like the azygos vein in the abdomen from either the continuation of left lumbar azygos vein that arises from the posterior surface of the left renal vein or by the union of left ascending lumbar and the left subcostal veins. The hemiazygos vein pierces the left crus of the diaphragm and enters the posterior mediastinum. It passes vertically upward lying on the front of the vertebral bodies and crosses over to the right side in front of the eighth thoracic vertebra to open into the azygos vein. This vein receives, left ascending lumbar vein, left subcostal vein and the left posterior intercostal veins of the ninth to eleventh intercostal spaces.

Accessory Hemiazygos Vein (Superior Azygos Vein)

The accessory hemiazygos vein begins as the continuation of usually the fifth posterior intercostal vein and descends on the left side of the vertebral column. At the level of the seventh thoracic vertebra, it crosses over to the right side behind the descending aorta and the thoracic duct to open into the azygos vein. This vein receives the fifth to seventh left posterior intercostal veins and the left bronchial vein.

Posterior Intercostal Veins (Fig. 35.10)

There are eleven pairs of posterior intercostal veins.
- The vein of the first space (the highest intercostal vein) ascends in front of the neck of the first rib and then arches over the cervical pleura in anterior direction to open into the corresponding brachiocephalic vein.
- The right superior intercostal vein begins by the union of right posterior intercostal veins of the second, third and often the fourth spaces. It opens into the arch of azygos vein.
- The left superior intercostal vein begins by the union of left posterior intercostal veins of the second, third and often the fourth spaces. It descends to the level of the vertebral end of the aortic arch and then crosses the left and anterior surfaces of the arch of aorta. It terminates in the left brachiocephalic vein. Its tributaries are the left bronchial vein, and sometimes the left pericardiacophrenic vein.
- The posterior intercostal veins of the remaining spaces (from fourth to eleventh) on the right side drain into the vertical part of azygos vein. The corresponding veins on the left side drain into hemiazygos veins as mentioned above.

Venous Communications

The posterior intercostal veins communicate with anterior intercostal veins, which are the tributaries of internal thoracic veins. They also communicate with the vertebral venous plexuses. This communication is responsible for venous spread of cancer cells in the vertebrae and skull bones from primary cancer in breast, prostate and thyroid gland.

 ADDED INFORMATION

Collateral Venous Circulation

The superior vena cava (SVC) may be compressed at two sites given below:
1. In the superior mediastinum (above the entry of azygos vein)
2. In the middle mediastinum (below the entry of azygos vein).

Contd…

Contd…

 ADDED INFORMATION

Depending on the site of obstruction the different collateral pathways are developed.
- In the obstruction above the entry of azygos vein, the following two venous routes drain the blood from the upper part of the body into right atrium
  - The blood from the internal thoracic veins reaches the azygos vein via the anastomoses between the anterior and posterior intercostal veins. The azygos vein brings the blood to superior vena cava, which brings it to the right atrium
- If the obstruction is below the entry of the azygos vein, venous blood from the upper part of the body reaches the right atrium via the inferior vena cava as follows
  - There is reversal of blood flow in the azygos vein. As a result of this the blood from azygos vein reaches the inferior vena cava via the lumbar azygos or ascending lumbar vein (formative tributaries of vena azygos, which have connections with inferior vena cava IVC)
  - There are other devious routes to reach the inferior vena cava as follows. ***One route*** is via the communication of superior and inferior epigastric veins to the external iliac vein and finally to IVC. ***Another route*** is by communications of superficial veins of thorax and anterior abdominal wall. The lateral thoracic vein (a tributary of axillary vein) communicates with superficial epigastric vein of anterior abdominal wall by thoraco-epigastric veins. The superficial epigastric vein is a tributary of femoral vein (note that in this alternate path venous blood from subclavian vein travels via the axillary vein into the lateral thoracic vein, thoraco-epigastric vein to the superficial epigastric vein to reach the femoral vein). As a result, the superficial venous collateral channels are dilated along the lateral thoracic and abdominal walls.

Development of Veins of Thorax

During the fourth week of embryonic life there is a symmetrical pattern of venous channels. There are three pairs of cardinal veins.

Cardinal Veins

- ***Anterior cardinal veins***, drain the cephalic half of the embryo
- ***Posterior cardinal veins***, drain the caudal half of the embryo
- ***Common cardinal veins***, or the ***ducts of Cuvier*** (formed by the union of anterior and posterior cardinal veins) enter the respective horns of the sinus venosus.

Loss of Symmetry of Cardinal Veins

During the fifth to seventh weeks the symmetry a transverse anastomotic channel develops between right and left anterior cardinal veins. This channel diverts the venous blood from the left to the right side, consequent to which the veins on the left side shrink in size.

Developmental Sources of Individual Veins

- The right brachiocephalic vein develops from the part of right anterior cardinal vein, which is cranial to the transverse anastomosis as given follows:
- The left brachiocephalic vein develops from following two sources
  1. Left anterior cardinal vein cranial to the transverse anastomosis
  2. Transverse anastomosis
- The superior vena cava develops from two sources as follows:
  1. Extrapericardial part from right anterior cardinal vein caudal to the transverse anastomosis
  2. Intrapericardial part from right common cardinal vein (right duct of Cuvier)
- The left superior intercostal vein develops from two sources as follows:
  1. Left anterior cardinal vein
  2. Terminal part of left posterior cardinal vein
- The oblique vein of Marshall is a remnant of left common cardinal vein. It is connected to the left superior intercostal vein by means of a ligament (ligament of left vena cava), which is also a remnant of left common cardinal vein
- The arch of azygos vein develops from the terminal part of right posterior cardinal vein.

44

Lymphatic Organs and Autonomic Nerves of Thorax

Chapter Contents

LYMPHATIC ORGANS IN THORAX

The thymus, thoracic lymph nodes and the thoracic duct are the lymphatic organs in the thorax.

THYMUS

The thymus is the primary lymphoid organ. It is the only lymphoid organ that is responsible for the differentiation of T lymphocytes. The thymic secretory products are indispensable for the development and maintenance of immunologically competent T lymphocyte pool for the entire body.

Location (Fig. 44.1)

The thymus mainly lies in superior mediastinum with extension in anterior mediastinum in front of the pericardium.

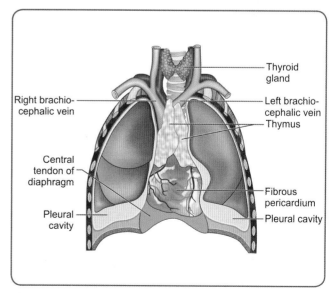

Fig. 44.1: Location and appearance of thymus during adolescence

Shape

It is roughly pyramidal with the base pointed inferiorly. The thymus is often bilobed but the two lobes are joined in the midline by connective tissue.

Age Changes

- At birth, the thymus is well developed and weighs about 30 g.
- At puberty, it reaches maximum size and weighs about 40 g.
- During adulthood, there is a gradual reduction in the weight as the lymphatic tissue is replaced by fatty tissue.
- In old age, it is much reduced in size and turns into a fibro-fatty mass. The number of lymphocytes inside the thymus is greatly reduced. However, lymphocyte production and differentiation persist throughout life.

Relations in Superior Mediastinum

- *Anteriorly:* To manubrium sterni, sternohyoid and sternothyroid muscles.
- *Posteriorly:* To left brachiocephalic vein, arch of aorta and its three branches.

Relations in Anterior Mediastinum

- *Anteriorly:* To body of sternum and upper four costal cartilages.
- *Posteriorly:* To fibrous pericardium.

Blood Supply

The branches of internal thoracic artery and inferior thyroid artery supply the thymus.

The thymic veins usually drain into the left brachiocephalic vein, though drainage into internal thoracic and inferior thyroid veins is also possible.

Lymphatic Drainage

The efferent lymphatic vessels drain into the brachiocephalic, tracheobronchial and parasternal lymph nodes. The thymus receives no afferent lymphatics.

EMBRYOLOGIC INSIGHT

The thymic epitheliocytes develop from endoderm of third pharyngeal pouches of both sides. The lymphocytes, connective tissue and blood vessels of thymus develop from embryonic mesenchyme.

Function

- Undifferentiated lymphocytes from the bone marrow enter the thymus from circulating blood. The lymphocyte-processing takes place within the thymus.
- The T-cells committed to the production of cell-mediated immunity are released into the circulation.
- Only when T-cells start circulating through the lymph nodes and spleen, the lymphocytes within these structures become B-lymphocytes, which are committed to the production of specific antibodies.

CLINICAL CORRELATION

- Patients with thymic aplasia, agenesis or hypoplasia, as occurs in DiGeorge syndrome (embryologic insight box in chapter 66) have lymphopenia, decreased immunity and die early from infection. DiGeorge syndrome presents with severest form of deficient T-cell immunity
- In hyperplasia of thymus, there are lymphatic follicles in the thymic lobules. The patient may develop myasthenia gravis
- Epithelial cell tumor of thymus called *thymoma* may present as myasthenia gravis. When the thymoma is large in size it may compress on trachea, esophagus and large veins in the superior mediastinum
- Myasthenia gravis is a chronic autoimmune disease of adults, in which there is reduction in the power of certain voluntary muscles for repetitive contractions. The muscles commonly involved are the levator palpebrae superioris (causing bilateral ptosis) and the extraocular muscles (causing diplopia).

LYMPH NODES OF THORAX

The lymph nodes that drain the thoracic walls are superficial lymph nodes and those that drain the thoracic viscera belong to the deep group.

Superficial Lymph Nodes

- The parasternal or internal mammary lymph nodes are located along each internal thoracic artery. These nodes receive lymph vessels from mammary gland, structures of supraumbilical anterior abdominal wall, superior hepatic surface and the deeper parts of anterior thoracic wall. The efferent lymphatic vessels from the parasternal nodes unite with the efferents from tracheobronchial and brachiocephalic nodes to form the bronchomediastinal trunk.
- The intercostal lymph nodes are placed at the posterior end of the intercostal spaces. They receive deep lymph vessels from mammary gland and the posterolateral

aspect of thoracic wall. Efferents from the nodes in lower four to seven intercostal spaces on both sides unite to form the descending thoracic lymph trunk which descends into the abdomen through aortic orifice and may join the thoracic duct. Efferents from the nodes in the upper left intercostal spaces form the upper intercostal lymph trunk, which ends in the thoracic duct, and the corresponding ones on the right side join the right lymph trunk.

Deep Lymph Nodes

- The brachiocephalic nodes lie in the superior mediastinum anterior to the brachiocephalic veins. They receive lymph from thymus, thyroid, pericardium, heart and the lateral diaphragmatic nodes. Their efferents unite with those from tracheobronchial nodes to form right and left bronchomediastinal trunks.
- The posterior mediastinal nodes lie vertically in the posterior mediastinum along the descending aorta and the esophagus. They receive lymph from the contents of posterior mediastinum, diaphragm and the lateral and posterior diaphragmatic nodes. Their efferents join the thoracic duct.
- The tracheobronchial nodes (Fig. 36.30) consist of five subgroups. The paratracheal nodes are seen on the front and sides of the trachea. The superior tracheobronchial nodes lie in the angles between trachea and bronchi. The inferior tracheobronchial nodes are present in the angle between bronchi.
- The bronchopulmonary or hilar lymph nodes are present in the hilum of the lung.
- The pulmonary lymph nodes are inside the lung substance. These nodes drain lungs and bronchi, thoracic trachea, heart and receive lymph from posterior mediastinal nodes. Their efferents join the efferents of parasternal and brachiocephalic nodes to form right and left bronchomediastinal trunks.
  The right bronchomediastinal trunk opens independently at right jugulo-subclavian junction. The left bronchomediastinal trunk opens into thoracic duct.

THORACIC DUCT

The thoracic duct is a thin walled elongated lymph vessel about 45 cm long. It conveys the lymph from the body excluding right upper limb, right half of thorax and right half of head and neck (Fig. 4.5) into the venous stream. The lymph in the thoracic duct is milky white in color because it is loaded with fat globules.

Extent (Fig. 44.2)

The thoracic duct extends from the upper end of cisterna chyli on the posterior abdominal wall to the junction of left internal jugular and left subclavian veins, at the base of the neck.

Appearance

The thoracic duct is beaded in appearance due to the presence of numerous valves throughout its course. A constant valve guards the opening of the duct in the jugulo-subclavian junction to prevent regurgitation of blood into the duct.

Area of Drainage

The thoracic duct drains lymph from the entire body except the right half of thorax, right half of head and neck and the right upper limb (Fig 4.5).

Course and Relations (Fig. 44.2)

The course of thoracic duct can be divided into three parts—(1) abdominal, (2) thoracic, and (3) cervical.

Abdominal Course

The abdominal part of the thoracic duct extends from the lower border of the twelfth thoracic vertebra as a

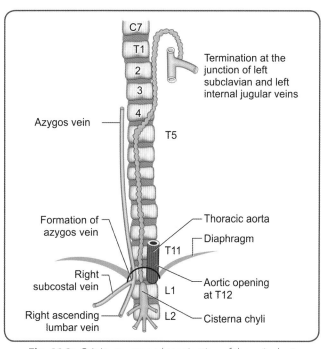

Fig. 44.2: Origin, course and termination of thoracic duct

continuation of cisterna chyli (a receptacle of lymph on the posterior abdominal wall) upto the aortic opening of the diaphragm. At the aortic opening it is related anteriorly to the median arcuate ligament and posteriorly to the twelfth thoracic vertebra. The azygos vein is on its right and the aorta on its left.

Course in Posterior Mediastinum

After passing through the aortic opening in the diaphragm, the thoracic duct enters the posterior mediastinum. It ascends in the posterior mediastinum lying on the vertebral bodies to the right of the midline. On reaching the level of the fifth thoracic vertebra, it gradually inclines to the left and enters the superior mediastinum at the left side of the sternal angle. The esophagus is related to it anteriorly. The azygos vein is on its right and thoracic aorta is on its left.

Course in Superior Mediastinum

In the superior mediastinum, the thoracic duct ascends along the left margin of esophagus to the thoracic inlet. Anteriorly, it is related to the arch of aorta and the left subclavian artery above it. Posteriorly, it lies on the bodies of upper four thoracic vertebrae. On its right, it is related to the esophagus and on its left it is related to the left lung and pleura.

Cervical Course

The cervical part of the thoracic duct (Fig. 44.3) arches laterally at the level of transverse process of the seventh cervical vertebra. The summit of the arch is 3–4 cm above the clavicle. Anteriorly, the arch is related to the carotid sheath and its contents. Its posterior relations are

important. The ascending limb of its arch is related to left vertebral artery and vein, left stellate ganglion and left thyrocervical trunk and its three branches. The descending limb of the arch is related to the medial margin of scalenus anterior muscle, left phrenic nerve and the first part of left subclavian artery.

Termination

In the usual mode of termination, the thoracic duct opens at the union of left subclavian and left internal jugular veins.

Tributaries

A large number of tributaries join the thoracic duct throughout its course.
- Descending thoracic lymph trunks (from lymph nodes of lower intercostal spaces)
- Ascending lumbar lymph trunks (in abdomen)
- Upper intercostal trunk of left side
- Mediastinal trunks (from mediastinum, diaphragm and diaphragmatic surface of liver)
- Left bronchomediastinal trunk (from lungs and mediastinum)
- Left jugular trunk (from head and neck)
- Left subclavian trunk (from upper limb).

🔹 STUDENT INTEREST

Thoracic duct is the major lymphatic channel that pours lymph collected from the major part of the body (Fig. 4.5) into venous circulation. It begins on posterior abdominal wall as cisterna chyli and enters the posterior mediastinum via aortic opening of diaphragm at T12 vertebral level. It crosses from right to left at the level of T5 vertebra to enter the superior mediastinum from where it enters the neck. It arches laterally at the level of C7 vertebra. Its ascending limb is related to structures in the scalenovertebral triangle and descending limb is related to the medial margin of scalenus anterior muscle (which is the lateral margin of scalenovertebral triangle). It terminates at the junction of left subclavian and left internal jugular veins.

⚙ CLINICAL CORRELATION

- Injury to thoracic part of the thoracic duct may cause chylothorax (lymph in the pleural cavity).
- Thoracic duct may be obstructed by microfilarial parasites in which case it produces widespread effects like, chylothorax, chyloperitoneum and even the accumulation of lymph in the tunica vaginalis testis (hydrocele).
- Cervical part of thoracic duct may be injured during removal of the left supraclavicular lymph nodes. This is a serious complication, which needs prompt treatment.

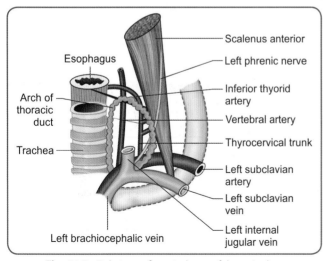

Fig. 44.3: Relations of cervical part of thoracic duct

Labels: Esophagus; Scalenus anterior; Left phrenic nerve; Arch of thoracic duct; Inferior thyroid artery; Vertebral artery; Thyrocervical trunk; Trachea; Left subclavian artery; Left subclavian vein; Left brachiocephalic vein; Left internal jugular vein

RIGHT LYMPHOVENOUS PORTAL

On the right side there are three lymph trunks that converge at the jugulo-subclavian junction. They are the right jugular trunk (draining the right half of head and neck), the right subclavian trunk (draining the right upper limb) and the right bronchomediastinal trunk from the right half of thorax. The termination of the three lymph trunks of right side is subject to variation. Usually the lymph trunks open independently in the jugulo-subclavian junction. Occasionally, the three trunks unite to form the right lymphatic duct, which has a similar course in the neck like that of thoracic duct.

NERVES OF THORAX

Autonomic Nerves of Thorax

The autonomic nervous system has sympathetic and parasympathetic components. The cervical and thoracic branches of vagus nerve (parasympathetic) and of the sympathetic chains form autonomic plexuses in the thorax, which supply the visceral musculature and secretory glands through post-ganglionic branches. The visceral afferent fibers are carried from the viscera via the plexuses to the spinal cord and brainstem.

Vagus Nerve (Parasympathetic Supply)

The vagus nerve (tenth cranial nerve) originates in the medulla oblongata and carries the pre-ganglionic parasympathetic fibers from the dorsal nucleus of vagus. These fibers leave the vagus nerve through its cervical and thoracic branches (superior and inferior cervical cardiac branches of vagus nerve). They take part in the formation of superficial and deep cardiac plexuses. The right recurrent laryngeal nerve is given off at the root of the neck from the right vagus. This nerve gives rise to thoracic cardiac branches.

Course in Thorax

In the superior mediastinum, the right vagus nerve lies on the right side of trachea. It is posteromedial to the superior vena cava and then passes deep to azygos arch to reach the posterior aspect of the hilum of the right lung. The left vagus nerve is positioned between left common carotid and left subclavian arteries. Then it crosses the left surface of the arch of aorta to reach the posterior side of the hilum of the left lung. At the hilum of the lung each vagus nerve divides into a number of branches, which join the sympathetic branches to form pulmonary plexuses. Below the hilum the vagal branches on both sides come

in relation to the esophagus. The right vagus nerve is located on the posterior side and the left vagus nerve on the anterior side of the esophagus. After taking part in the esophageal plexuses along with sympathetic branches, the vagus nerves leave the thorax through the esophageal opening as posterior vagal trunk (right vagus) and anterior vagal trunk (left vagus).

BRANCHES IN THORAX

- Thoracic cardiac branches (by both vagi)
- Pulmonary branches (by both vagi)
- Esophageal branches (by both vagi)
- Left recurrent laryngeal nerve (by left vagus nerve only)

As the left vagus nerve crosses in front of the left surface of the arch of aorta it gives off the left recurrent laryngeal branch, which winds round the ligamentum arteriosum and then passes upwards and medially deep to the arch of aorta. Similar to the right recurrent laryngeal nerve, the left recurrent laryngeal nerve gives thoracic cardiac branches.

VISCERAL AFFERENT FIBERS

There are visceral afferent fibers in these cervical and thoracic branches, which terminate in the sensory ganglia of the vagus nerve. The central processes of these ganglia carry the impulses to the medulla oblongata. The vagus nerves carry sensations from the heart, great blood vessels and respiratory organs. The visceral afferent fibers are involved in maintaining the reflex activity of these organs.

SYMPATHETIC CHAINS (FIG. 44.4)

Each sympathetic chain extends from the base of the cranium to the coccyx. It passes through the cervical, thoracic, lumbar and sacral (pelvic) regions. It bears a number of ganglia along its length, where majority of pre-ganglionic fibers synapse.

The sympathetic chain gives cervical cardiac and thoracic branches for the supply of the thoracic viscera.

Cardiac Branches of Cervical Sympathetic Chain

The cervical sympathetic chain presents three ganglia—superior, middle and inferior. There are three—cervical cardiac branches on each side. They are named as superior, middle and inferior cervical cardiac branches according to the ganglion from which they originate.

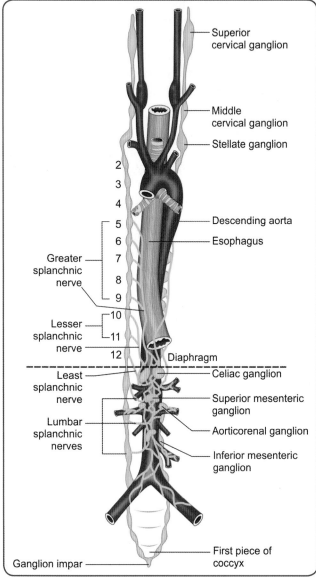

Superior
cervical ganglion

Middle
cervical ganglion

Stellate ganglion

2
3
4
5
6
7
8
9
10
11
12

Greater
splanchnic
nerve

Lesser
splanchnic
nerve

Least
splanchnic
nerve

Lumbar
splanchnic
nerves

Descending aorta

Esophagus

Diaphragm

Celiac ganglion

Superior mesenteric
ganglion

Aorticorenal ganglion

Inferior mesenteric
ganglion

First piece of
coccyx

Ganglion impar

Fig. 44.4: Extent of sympathetic chains
(Note the origin of greater, lesser and least splanchnic nerves from the thoracic sympathetic ganglia)

Thoracic Sympathetic Chain

The sympathetic on each side chain enters the thorax through the thoracic inlet. The thoracic part of the chain consists of eleven ganglia. The first thoracic ganglion is fused with inferior cervical ganglion to form cervicothoracic or stellate ganglion, which lies in front of the neck of the first rib. The thoracic sympathetic chain lies on the heads of the succeeding ribs, posterior to the costal pleura. It leaves the thorax behind the medial arcuate ligament to become continuous with lumbar part of the sympathetic chain.

Branches of Thoracic Sympathetic Chain

- Upper five ganglia supply the thoracic aorta and its branches.
- Pulmonary branches arise from second to sixth ganglia.
- Cardiac branches arise from second to fifth ganglia.
- Branches to esophagus and trachea reach either directly or indirectly from plexuses.
- Greater, lesser and least splanchnic nerves (Fig. 44.4) leave the thorax to supply the abdominal organs. They carry pre-ganglionic sympathetic fibers for relay in the celiac ganglion in the abdomen.

The greater splanchnic nerve arises from fifth to ninth ganglia and perforates the crus of diaphragm to enter the abdomen. The lesser splanchnic nerve arises from ninth to tenth ganglia and pierces the diaphragm along with greater splanchnic nerve. The least splanchnic nerve from the lowest ganglion enters the abdomen with the sympathetic chain.

VISCERAL AFFERENT FIBERS

The visceral afferent fibers (from thoracic viscera) accompany the pre-ganglionic and post-ganglionic sympathetic fibers and terminate in the dorsal root ganglia of the thoracic spinal nerves. They mediate pain and other nociceptive impulses to the spinal cord.

AUTONOMIC PLEXUSES IN THORAX

The autonomic plexuses are composed of the post-ganglionic sympathetic fibers, pre-ganglionic parasympathetic fibers and small parasympathetic ganglia. The pre-ganglionic parasympathetic fibers either synapse in these ganglia or synapse in the ganglia, which are located in the wall of the viscera. Besides these, the plexuses contain visceral fibers.

Superficial Cardiac Plexus

This plexus is located on the ligamentum arteriosum below the arch of aorta.

Nerves taking part in formation of superficial cardiac plexus are:
- Superior cervical cardiac branch of left sympathetic chain.
- Inferior cervical cardiac branch of left vagus nerve.
  This plexus is in communication with the deep cardiac plexus, right coronary plexus and left anterior pulmonary plexus.

Deep Cardiac Plexus

This plexus is located in front of the bifurcation of trachea. Symphathetic Contribution to deep cardiac plexus
- Middle and inferior cervical cardiac branches of left sympathetic chain.
- Superior, middle and inferior cervical cardiac branches of right sympathetic chain.
- Cardiac branches of upper five thoracic sympathetic ganglia from both sides.
  Parasympathetic contribution to deep cardiac plexus:
  - Superior cervical cardiac branch of left vagus.
  - Superior and inferior cervical cardiac branches of right vagus.
  - Cardiac branches of right and left recurrent laryngeal nerves.
  - Direct cardiac branches of right and left vagus nerves.
  - The deep cardiac plexus also contains pain fibers from the ischemic myocardium. The pain impulse is carried in the cardiac branches of middle and inferior cervical sympathetic ganglia and cardiac branches of the thoracic ganglia to the upper thoracic spinal nerves and finally to the spinal cord via the corresponding dorsal root ganglia.

Connections of Deep Cardiac Plexus

The right half of the deep cardiac plexus directly supplies branches to the right atrium and is in communication with right coronary plexus. The left half of the deep cardiac plexus is connected with superficial cardiac plexus and gives direct branches to the left atrium. It continues as the left coronary plexus.

Pulmonary Plexuses

The anterior and posterior pulmonary plexuses are located in respective relation to the hilum of the lungs. The thoracic branches of vagus and sympathetic trunk (upper four or five ganglia) take part in their formation. The two plexuses are interconnected. The network of nerves arising from the plexuses enters the lung along the bronchi, pulmonary and bronchial vessels. There are small ganglia on tracheobronchial tree, in which pre-ganglionic vagal fibers synapse.

Esophageal Plexus

This plexus is composed of esophageal branches of fifth to ninth sympathetic ganglia, esophageal branches of both vagi and branches of recurrent laryngeal nerves. The neurons in myenteric and Aurbach's plexuses in the wall of the esophagus are the relay stations for parasympathetic fibers. Congenital absence of these neurons results in achalasia or cardiospasm.

Esophagus

ESOPHAGUS

The esophagus is a muscular tube about 25 cm long. It transports food from laryngopharynx to the stomach by rapid peristaltic movements.

Extent

It is continuous above with the laryngopharynx at the lower border of cricoid cartilage at the level of sixth cervical vertebra (C6) in the neck, and below with the cardiac orifice of stomach in the abdomen at the level of eleventh thoracic vertebra (T11).

Course (Fig. 45.1)

The esophagus passes through three regions of the body namely, (1) neck, (2) thorax, and (3) abdomen. The thoracic esophagus is the longest and abdominal part is the shortest. During its course, the esophagus shows three curves. At the root of the neck, the esophagus inclines to the left by 0.5–1 cm from the midline. It comes back in the midline at the level of fifth thoracic vertebra. Again, it deviates to the left below the seventh thoracic vertebra and inclines anteriorly to pass through the muscular part of diaphragm at the level of tenth thoracic vertebra.

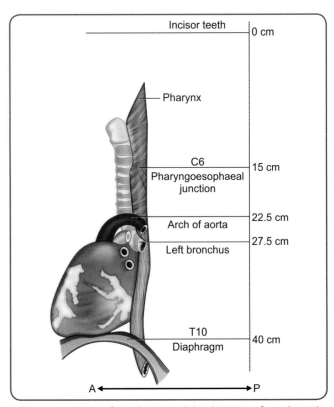

Fig. 45.1: Extent of esophagus and the distances of esophageal constrictions from incisor teeth

Constrictions (Fig. 45.1)

There are four sites of constrictions or narrowing in the esophagus. The distance of each constriction is measured from the upper incisor teeth as given follows:

1. **The first constriction** at a distance of 15 cm is the pharyngo-esophageal junction.
2. **The second constriction** at a distance of 22.5 cm is produced by the arch of aorta.
3. **The third constriction** at a distance of 27.5 cm is produced by left bronchus.
4. **The fourth constriction** at a distance of 40 cm is at the esophageal hiatus in the diaphragm.

The constrictions are the potential sites where swallowed foreign bodies can get stuck. These are the sites, where strictures develop after ingestion of caustic substances.

 STUDENT INTEREST

All sites of constriction in the esophagus are important. As an aid to memory one must tell one's mind to start from the commencement of esophagus and go down until diaphragm: The pharyngoesophageal junction in the neck is the first constriction, second constriction produced by arch of aorta is in superior mediastinum (where the left side of esophagus is closely related to the right and posterior surface of the arch as shown in Fig. 43.8), third constriction is just below the second and is produced by left bronchus which crosses the esophagus anteriorly to reach the hilum of left lung and the last constriction is at the esophageal hiatus in the diaphragm.

Relations

Relations of Cervical Esophagus

- **Anteriorly**, the esophagus is related to the trachea and to the recurrent laryngeal nerves.
- **Posteriorly**, it is related to the prevertebral fascia and vertebral column.
- The common carotid artery and lateral lobe of thyroid are its lateral relations. In addition, on the left side it is related to the thoracic duct at the root of the neck.

Relations of Thoracic Esophagus (Figs 45.2A to D)

- Anterior relations (from above downwards) are trachea, arch of aorta, right pulmonary artery, left principal bronchus, fibrous pericardium and oblique sinus (separating it from left atrium) and diaphragm. The close anterior relation of esophagus to left atrium is useful for trans-esophageal echography to examine the base of the heart.

- Left lateral relations are as follows:
  - In the upper part of the superior mediastinum it is related to left subclavian artery, thoracic duct, left recurrent laryngeal nerve and left pleura and upper lobe of left lung. In the lower part of the superior mediastinum, its left edge is related to the arch of aorta.
  - In the posterior mediastinum, the descending aorta is on the left side in the upper part. The esophagus once again makes an impression on the mediastinal surface of left lung behind the lower end of pulmonary ligament.
- Right lateral relations are as follows; The esophagus is related to mediastinal surface of right lung, arch of azygos vein and the descending thoracic aorta.
- Posterior relations are as follows:
  - In **superior mediastinum**, it is related to the thoracic vertebrae.
  - In **posterior mediastinum** at the level at T5 level, thoracic duct crosses behind the esophagus and below T5 level, descending thoracic aorta, thoracic duct and azygos vein are posterior relations.

 STUDENT INTEREST

The esophagus has triple relations with descending aorta because it crosses in front of the descending aorta. It has triple relations with the thoracic duct because the duct crosses behind the esophagus. The esophagus comes in contact with the left lung twice (Fig. 36.25) but with the right lung only once.

Relations to Vagus Nerves

Below the level of pulmonary hilum, the right vagus is in contact with the posterior surface and the left vagus in contact with the anterior surface of the esophagus. These branches unite to form esophageal plexus along with the sympathetic branches.

Relations at Esophageal Aperture in Diaphragm

The esophagus passes through the muscular part of right crus of diaphragm at the level of tenth thoracic vertebra. The left vagus (now called **anterior gastric nerve**) is related anteriorly and the right vagus (**now called posterior gastric nerve**) is related posteriorly to it. The esophagus is also related to the esophageal branches of left gastric vessels.

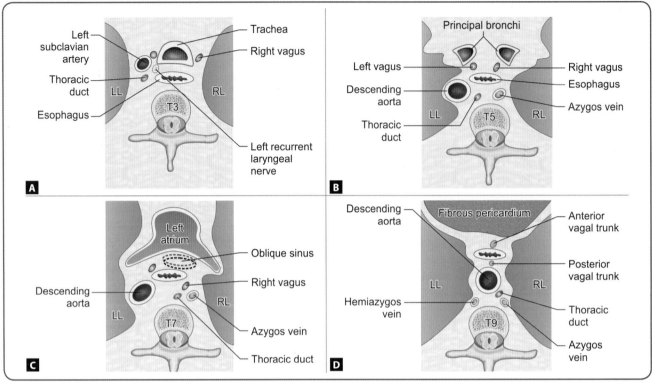

Figs 45.2A to D: Relations of thoracic part of esophagus at different vertebral levels
Key: (RL- right lung, LL- left lung)

Abdominal Part of Esophagus

This part is about two cm long and is the only part of esophagus covered with peritoneum. It is related to the posterior surface of left lobe of liver anteriorly and to the left crus of diaphragm posteriorly. The right and left gastric nerves enter the abdomen lying along the posterior and anterior surfaces respectively.

Lower Esophageal Sphincter

There is no anatomical sphincter at the gastroesophageal junction. There are two mechanisms that are believed to operate for preventing the gastroesophageal reflux.

- The lower esophageal sphincter shows a specialized area of circular smooth muscle, which possesses the physiological properties of the sphincter. The muscle in this area is maintained under tonic contractions by the intramural plexuses of enteric nervous system.
- The muscle fibers of the right crus of the diaphragm, which surround the terminal portion of the esophagus provide external sphincter.

This combination provides adequate antireflux barrier, which is lowered momentarily during swallowing under normal conditions. It is also lowered during vomiting.

If the intragastric pressure rises sufficiently, the acidic contents of the stomach regurgitate into the lower end of the esophagus, to be returned to the stomach by reflex peristalsis. The stratified squamous non-keratinized epithelium of the esophagus has no protective properties against gastric acid. This leads to reflux esophagitis, which causes burning pain behind the sternum (or heartburn).

Arterial Supply

Several arteries at various levels supply the esophagus through an anastomotic chain on its surface.

- Inferior thyroid arteries supply the cervical part of esophagus.
- Descending thoracic aorta and bronchial arteries supply the thoracic part of the esophagus.
- Left gastric and left inferior phrenic arteries supply the abdominal esophagus.

Venous Drainage

- The cervical part of esophagus drains into inferior thyroid veins.
- The thoracic part of esophagus drains into the azygos and hemiazygos veins.

- The abdominal part of esophagus is drained by left gastric vein, which is a tributary of portal vein. The veins of the lower thoracic part are systemic. Therefore, there is a potential portosystemic anastomosis between the two sets of veins at the lower end of esophagus in the submucosa. In patients with portal hypertension, the submucous venous plexuses are enlarged. Such dilated venous plexuses covered with mucosa are called **esophageal varices**. They protrude into the lumen of lower esophagus. They are asymptomatic until they rupture causing a large bout of blood vomiting (hematemesis).

Lymphatic Drainage

From cervical part lymph drains in deep cervical nodes. From thoracic part lymph drains in posterior mediastinal nodes and from abdominal part and adjacent thoracic parts lymph drains in left gastric nodes.

Nerve Supply

The sympathetic efferent fibers are vasoconstrictors. The parasympathetic efferent fibers are motor to the musculature of esophagus as well as to the esophageal glands. The striated muscle in the upper two thirds receives nerve supply from vagus while the smooth muscle in the lower part receives nerve supply through the esophageal plexus. The sympathetic afferent fibers carry pain sensations. The pain impulses reach T4 and T5 segments of the spinal cord along the afferent sympathetic paths. Hence, the esophageal pain is referred to the **lower thoracic region and epigastric region of abdomen**. In some cases, it is difficult to distinguish the esophageal pain from anginal pain.

 STUDENT INTEREST

The muscular tissue in muscularis externa of upper third of esophagus is striated like that of pharynx, that of middle third is the mixture of both striated and non-striated and that of the lower third is non-striated only. Esophagus is not covered with peritoneum except its abdominal part. The lower end of esophagus is a potential site of portosystemic anastomosis.

 EMBRYOLOGIC INSIGHT

The esophagus develops from the endoderm of cranial part of the foregut.

Congenital Anomalies

- Esophageal atresia is due to failure of recanalization of the esophagus. It is associated with hydramnios because the fetus is unable to swallow the amniotic fluid.
- Tracheo-esophageal fistula (TEF) (Figs 36.6A to C) is due to maldevelopment of the septum between the esophagus and the trachea. They are invariably associated with localized atresia of esophagus, and hence hydramnios is a constant feature.
- Anomalous blood vessels (aberrant right subclavian artery shown in Fig. 39.6) may cause dysphagia or may remain symptomless.

 CLINICAL CORRELATION

- Radiological examination of esophagus by barium swallow (Fig. 45.3) is a commonly used investigation to detect diseases of esophagus and to detect enlargement of left atrium.
- Esophagoscopy is performed to directly inspect the interior of the esophagus.
- Dysphagia means difficulty in swallowing. Extrinsic causes of dysphagia are, pressure from aneurysm of aortic arch, enlarged lymph nodes, aberrant right subclavian artery (passing posterior to the esophagus), retrosternal goiter and enlarged left atrium. Intrinsic causes are strictures and carcinoma is esophagus.
- Carcinoma of esophagus (Fig. 45.4) usually spread by lymphatics and involves posterior mediastinal nodes. The direct spread through the wall of the esophagus can lead to involvement of lung, bronchi and aorta. The cancer from lower third of esophagus spreads to the gastric and celiac nodes in the abdomen.

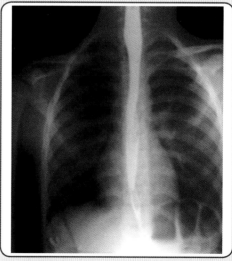

Fig. 45.3: Barium swallow radiograph of 8-year old child showing cervical, thoracic and abdominal parts of esophagus

Contd...

Contd…

- Hiatus hernia (Figs 37.9A and B) is an acquired condition in which the stomach herniates into the posterior mediastinum through the esophageal hiatus in the diaphragm. Refer to clinical insight box for further details in chapter 37.

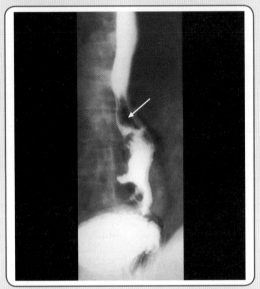 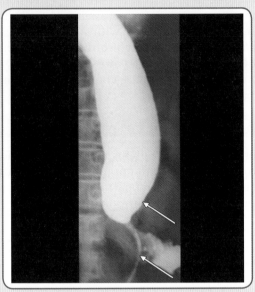

Fig. 45.4: Radiological appearance of esophageal cancer (arrow showing)

Fig. 45.5: Rat's tail appearance of esophagus in achalasia cardia (upper arrow shows dilated part of esophagus and lower arrow shows the narrowed part of esophagus)

- Achalasia cardia is primarily the disease in which lower esophageal sphincter fails to relax in response to swallowing. There is ineffective peristalsis or absence of peristalsis in the esophagus. This leads to impaired emptying and gradual dilation of proximal esophagus. The basic pathology is loss of parasympathetic ganglia in myenteric plexuses, formation of fibrous tissue in the wall of esophagus and thickening of lower esophageal sphincter. The symptoms consist of difficulty in swallowing solid foods and liquids, regurgitation of food and liquid during or after meals, feeling of fullness behind sternum after meals and retrosternal pain or heartburn.

  The barium swallow examination reveals the typical ***bird's beak*** appearance or ***rat tail*** appearance of esophagus (Fig. 45.5) in which the dilated proximal segment represents the bird's head and the tapered lower end its beak.

- Barrett's esophagus is characterized by metaplasia (abnormal change) of esophageal epithelium from non-keratinized stratified squamous type to simple columnar type of intestinal epithelium in the lower esophagus. The metaplastic changes are considered to be pre-malignant stage as there is a strong association between Barrett's esophagus and adenocarcinona (a lethal cancer) of esophagus.

Clinicoanatomical Problems and Solutions

CASE 1

A 35-year-old man came to the hospital with complaints of severe pain in the right side of chest. The pain radiated down to the anterior abdominal wall. Auscultation of chest revealed absent breath sounds over the inferior lobe of right lung and X-ray chest confirmed pleural effusion on the right side.

Questions and Solutions

1. Name the space in which there is accumulation of fluid around the lungs.

Ans. Pleural cavity

2. Give the boundaries of the space and its normal content.

Ans. The pleural cavity is a potential space that is bounded by visceral and parietal layers of pleura. Normally it contains very small quantity of serous fluid.

3. Enumerate the differences in parietal and visceral pleura.

Ans. The visceral pleura is adherent to the lung surface and dips into the fissures of the lung. It develops from splanchnopleuric mesoderm. Hence, it is supplied by autonomic nerves. It is pain-insensitive. It shares its arterial supply and lymph drainage with lung. The extensive parietal pleura lines the internal surface of thoracic wall, mediastinum and upper surface of diaphragm. It develops from somatopleuric mesoderm. Hence, it is supplied by somatic nerves (intercostal and phrenic nerves). It is pain-sensitive. It shares its arterial supply and lymph drainage with body wall.

4. What is the name of the intercostal nerves that supply both thoracic and anterior abdominal walls?

Ans. The nerves that supply both thoracic and abdominal walls are collectively called 'thoracoabdominal' nerves. They are lower five intercostal nerves (T7 to T11).

5. Name the pleural recesses giving their functions.

Ans. There are two pleural recesses, costomediastinal and costodiaphragmatic. They provide space for the expansion of lung during deep inspiration.

CASE 2

A 50-year-old man with a history of chronic smoking consulted the doctor because he had complaints of weight loss, persistent cough and blood in the sputum. He also noticed absence of sweating on the right side of face. On examination, partial ptosis and constriction of pupil were noted in the right eye. PA view of chest X-ray showed a lesion in the apex of right lung. The diagnosis of cancer of lung apex was confirmed.

Questions and Solutions

1. Name the posterior relations of apex of the lung in medial to lateral order.

Ans. Sympathetic chain, highest intercostal vein, superior intercostal artery and ascending branch of T1 ventral ramus are related from medial to lateral side to the apex of lung.

2. Which structure is affected due to cancer to cause partial ptosis and constricted pupil?

Ans. Sympathetic chain (producing Horner's syndrome)

3. Give the surface marking of lung apex.

Ans. The apex of the lung is represented by a curved line forming a dome, the summit of which rises 2.5 cm above the medial one-third of the clavicle.

4. Name the protective serous covering and fascial covering of the lung apex.

Ans. The serous covering is called cervical pleura and fascial covering is called Sibson's fascia or suprapleural membrane.

5. Which bronchopulmonary segment is most dependent in supine position?

Ans. Apical (superior) bronchopulmonary segment of the lower lobe is most dependent in supine position.

6. Where would you place the diaphragm of your stethoscope to hear breath sounds of the apical segment of lower lobe of right lung?

Ans. The superior or apical segment of lower lobe of the lung is auscultated in the area between the vertebral margin of scapula and the midline on the right side.

CASE 3

A 38-year-old man was brought to the casualty because of sudden onset of severe chest pain. On examination, his respiration and pulse were rapid. On auscultation, the heart sounds were faintly audible. X-ray chest showed a globular enlarged heart shadow suggestive of fluid around the heart.

Questions and Solutions

1. Name the space in which the fluid is accumulated giving its boundaries.

Ans. Pericardial cavity is bounded by parietal and visceral layers of pericardium

2. Name the outermost layer surrounding the heart and give its nerve supply.

Ans. The fibrous pericardium is the outermost layer surrounding the heart. The phrenic nerves supply it.

3. Name the sinus bounded by visceral layers of pericardium. Give its boundaries and surgical importance.

Ans. Transverse sinus is the space between the visceral pericardium covering the atria and the common sleeve of visceral pericardium surrounding ascending aorta and pulmonary trunk. It is a passage connecting the right and left halves of pericardial cavity hence lined by visceral pericardium only. It provides a space to the cardiac surgeon during ligation of ascending aorta and pulmonary trunk in the coronary artery bypass surgery.

4. What is the area of cardiac dullness?

Ans. The area of cardiac dullness is the bare area of pericardium, which is dull on percussion. It is located to the left of the sternal margin from 4th to 6th costal cartilages. This area is not covered with lung due to the presence of cardiac notch in the anterior margin of left lung. Hence, it is dull on percussion.

CASE 4

A 30-year-old woman with a history of rheumatic fever in childhood came to the hospital with complaints of dyspnea (shortness of breath) for three months. On auscultation, a prominent mid-diastolic murmur was heard. Echocardiography confirmed the narrowing of mitral orifice and dilatation of left atrium.

Questions and Solutions

1. Name the clinical condition involving the mitral valve?

Ans. Mitral stenosis

2. Give the surface marking of the mitral valve.

Ans. The mitral valve is marked on the left half of sternum at the level of fourth costal cartilage.

3. What is the posterior relation of left atrium?

Ans. Esophagus

4. What is the significance of this relationship in mitral stenosis?

Ans. The enlarged left atrium compresses the esophagus, which can be detected in barium swallow radiograph. It may cause dysphagia.

5. Explain how can a thrombus dislodged from left atrium block the left radial artery.

Ans. A thrombus dislodged from the left atrium first enters the left ventricle via mitral orifice and then systemic circulation via the aortic orifice. The clot can enter any of the systemic arteries in the body. The clot reaches the left radial artery via the arch of aorta and its direct branch—left subclavian artery, which becomes the left axillary artery at the outer margin of first rib. The left axillary artery continues as left brachial artery, which divides into left radial and left ulnar artery.

CASE 5

An elderly patient presented with a pulsating swelling protruding from the upper margin of the sternum. On examination, the sign of tracheal tug was positive. CT scan of chest and aortic angiography showed localized dilatation of aortic arch.

Questions and Solutions

1. Name the clinical condition.

Ans. Aneurysm of aortic arch

2. What is the location of arch of aorta in thoracic cavity?

Ans. Superior mediastinum

3. What are the boundaries of this location?

Ans. (i) Anteriorly: Manubrium sterni

(ii) Posteriorly: Upper four thoracic vertebrae.

(iii) Superiorly: Thoracic inlet

(iv) Inferiorly: Lower limit is the plane passing through the disc between the fourth and fifth thoracic vertebrae

(v) Laterally: Mediastinal pleura on both sides.

4. Name the structures that may be compressed by the dilated aortic arch.

Ans. Superior vena cava, trachea, esophagus, phrenic nerves, left recurrent laryngeal nerve

5. Name the connection between the arch of aorta and the left pulmonary artery in the fetus and in the adult.

Ans. In the fetus, the arch of aorta is connected to left pulmonary artery by means of ductus arteriosus and in the adult, the two are connected by ligamentum arteriosum, which is a remnant of the ductus arteriosus.

CASE 6

A 58-year-old woman complained of dysphagia (difficulty in swallowing) for the duration of one month. Ba-swallow and esophagoscopy were performed. A biopsy taken from the lesion in the lower third of esophagus confirmed the diagnosis of malignancy.

Questions and Solutions

1. What is the vertebral extent of esophagus?

Ans. Vertebral extent is from C6 to T11

2. Name the structures that produce constrictions in the esophagus.

Ans. First constriction located at upper end of esophagus is produced by cricopharyngeus muscle, second by arch of aorta, third by left bronchus and the lowest at the esophageal hiatus in diaphragm.

3. Describe the lymphatic drainage of esophagus.

Ans. Refer to Chapter 45.

4. Describe the arterial supply of esophagus.

Ans. The cervical part of esophagus receives branches from inferior thyroid arteries and the thoracic esophagus receives branches from bronchial arteries and from descending aorta. The lower part of esophagus receives branches from left gastric artery.

5. What is the length of abdominal esophagus?

Ans. 2 cm

6. Write a note on lower esophageal sphincter.

Ans. There is no anatomical lower esophageal sphincter at gastroesophageal junction but there are two mechanisms that are believed to operate for preventing the gastroesophageal reflux.

(i) The lower esophageal sphincter shows a specialized area of circular smooth muscle, which possesses the physiological properties of the sphincter. The muscle in this area is maintained under tonic contractions by the intramural plexuses of enteric nervous system.

(ii) The muscle fibers of the right crus of the diaphragm, which surround the terminal portion of the esophagus provide external sphincter.

The failure of LES to relax during swallowing results in achalasia cardia. There is ineffective peristalsis or absence of peristalsis in the esophagus. This leads to impaired emptying and gradual dilatation of proximal esophagus. The basic pathology is loss of parasympathetic ganglia in myenteric plexuses in the wall of esophagus. The symptoms include gradually increasing difficulty in swallowing solid foods and liquids, a feeling of fullness behind sternum after meals and retrosternal pain or heartburn. The barium swallow examination reveals the typical bird's beak appearance.

CASE 7

A newborn baby had difficulty in breathing. On examination, the child was cyanotic and breath sounds were feeble on left side. There was mediastinal shift towards right (causing compression of the right lung). The abdomen of the baby was concave (scaphoid shaped). X-ray chest showed intestinal shadows into the left half of thoracic cavity.

Questions and Solutions

1. Which anatomical structure showed congenital defect through which intestines herniated in chest?

Ans. Diaphragm

2. Which is the exact site of the defect?

Ans. Costovertebral triangle on left side (Bochdalek's foramen)

3. Explain the embryological basis of the above defect.

Ans. The diaphragm is composite since it develops from four different sources.

(i) Septum transversum

(ii) Pleuroperitoneal membranes (right and left)

(iii) Dorsal mesentery of esophagus

(iv) Body wall mesoderm

The muscle of diaphragm develops from third, fourth and fifth cervical myotomes. This is the reason why phrenic nerve with root value (C3, C4, C5) supplies the muscle of diaphragm.

The site of the defect is between the vertebral and costal origin of diaphragm. This is the site of pleuroperitoneal canal connecting the embryonic pleural and peritoneal cavities. During development of diaphragm, these canals are closed by development of pleuroperitoneal membranes. Failure of the pleuroperitoneal canal to close (failure of pleuroperitoneal membranes to develop, usually on the left side) leads to deficiency at this site and the herniation of abdominal contents into the thoracic cavity. This is known as posterolateral hernia.

4. Name the major openings in this structure giving their vertebral levels.

Ans. Inferior vena cava: Vertebral level T8

Esophageal: Vertebral level T10

Aortic: Vertebral level T12

5. Through which of the major openings herniation cannot occur and what is the reason for it?

Ans. Diaphragmatic herniation cannot occur through vena caval opening because this opening is in the central tendon of diaphragm and the wall of the vena cava is firmly attached to the central tendon.

CASE 8

A 53-year-old bank manager used to spend his evenings watching TV and eating fried delicacies and ice cream. One day while climbing the steps, he felt uneasiness in the left side of his chest. He was all right after resting. On consulting the doctor, he was adviced coronary angiogram.

Questions and Solutions

1. What is the origin of coronary arteries?

Ans. The coronary arteries are the branches of ascending aorta. The right coronary artery begins at anterior aortic sinus and left coronary artery begins at left posterior aortic sinus.

2. Mention the physiological peculiarity of these arteries.

Ans. Unlike other systemic arteries, coronary arteries fill during diastole.

3. What is the purpose of coronary angiography?

Ans. Coronary angiography is a radiological procedure by which dye is injected into them to locate blocks or narrowing in the main arteries and their branches.

4. Describe the commonly used anatomical path to reach the coronary arteries to inject the dye.

Ans. The femoral artery is relatively superficial in position in the thigh; hence, it is preferred for coronary angiography. The catheter is introduced into the femoral artery and then in succession it ascends in the external iliac artery, common iliac artery, abdominal aorta, descending thoracic aorta, arch of aorta and the ascending aorta to reach the aortic sinuses. Here the dye is injected into the coronary ostia. The radiographs are taken after this procedure to study the anatomy of coronary arteries.

5. Which blood vessels from patient's body can be used for coronary artery bypass?

Ans. Long saphenous vein, internal mammary artery and radial artery.

SINGLE BEST RESPONSE TYPE MULTIPLE CHOICE QUESTIONS

1. Which of the following is a typical intercostal nerve?
   a. First
   b. Second
   c. Third
   d. Seventh

2. A man was stabbed on the back with a knife. The tip of the knife pierced the left lung halfway between apex and base. Name the part of the lung that is pierced:
   a. Inferior lobe
   b. Superior lobe
   c. Hilum
   d. Lingula

3. Crista terminalis is a feature of:
   a. Right ventricle
   b. Right atrium
   c. Left ventricle
   d. Left atrium

4. The phrenic nerve supplies all the following except:
   a. Fibrous pericardium
   b. Parietal layer of pericardium
   c. Pulmonary pleura
   d. Mediastinal pleura

5. The most anterior valve of the heart is:
   a. Mitral
   b. Tricuspid
   c. Pulmonary
   d. Aortic

6. Conducting tissue of the heart is a modification of:
   a. Epicardium
   b. Myocardium
   c. Endocardium
   d. Nerve fibers

7. Which of the following is related to the arch of aorta on its right side?
   a. Left phrenic nerve
   b. Right phrenic nerve
   c. Right recurrent laryngeal nerve
   d. Left recurrent laryngeal nerve

8. The lower margin of the lung cuts the following rib in midaxillary line.
   a. Sixth
   b. Eighth
   c. Tenth
   d. Twelfth

9. The following structures pass along with aorta at aortic orifice of diaphragm.
   a. Vagus nerves and hemiazygos vein
   b. Vagus nerves and accessory hemiazygos vein
   c. Thoracic duct and azygos vein
   d. Thoracic duct and left phrenic nerve

10. The right margin of cardiac shadow in a radiograph is formed by all the following except:
    a. Superior vena cava
    b. Right brachiocephalic vein
    c. Right atrium
    d. Right ventricle

11. The ductus arteriosus develops from:
    a. Proximal segment of right sixth arch artery
    b. Proximal segment of left sixth arch artery
    c. Distal segment of right sixth arch artery
    d. Distal segment of left sixth arch artery

12. What is not true regarding the carina?
    a. Mucosa most sensitive
    b. Located at tracheal bifurcation
    c. Located at a distance of 15 cm from incisor teeth
    d. Visible in bronchoscopy

13. Which of the following is not related to superior surface of first rib?
    a. Ventral ramus of T1
    b. Lower trunk of brachial plexus
    c. Subclavian artery
    d. Subclavian vein

14. Foramen secundum is present in:
    a. Septum secundum
    b. Septum primum
    c. Septum intermedium
    d. Septum spurium

15. The thymus is located in the following part of mediastinum:
    a. Superior and anterior mediastinum
    b. Superior and middle mediastinum
    c. Anterior and middle mediastinum
    d. Middle mediastinum

16. An unconscious patient involved in a major car accident was brought to the casualty with an injury of sharp object on his chest in the middle of the sternum at the level of fourth costal cartilage. Which chamber of heart is likely to be punctured?
    a. Left atrium
    b. Left ventricle
    c. Right atrium
    d. Right ventricle

17. Lingula is a tongue-shaped projection from:
    a. Superior lobe of right lung
    b. Superior lobe of left lung
    c. Inferior lobe of right lung
    d. Inferior lobe of left lung

18. The greater splanchnic nerve carries the following fibers:
    a. Preganglionic parasympathetic
    b. Preganglionic sympathetic
    c. Postganglionic parasympathetic
    d. Postganglionic sympathetic

19. A stethoscope placed on the left second intercostal space just lateral to the sternal margin is best positioned to hear sounds of which cardiac valve?
   a. Mitral
   b. Tricuspid
   C. Pulmonary
   d. Aortic

20. Postoperatively, a 50-year-old woman suddenly developed respiratory distress and cyanosis. She had blood in sputum. These signs and symptoms are indicative of embolism in which blood vessel?
   a. Pulmonary artery
   b. Bronchial artery
   c. Bronchial vein
   d. Pulmonary vein

KEY TO MCQ

1. c	2. a	3. b	4. c	5. c	6. b	7. d	8. b
9. c	10. d	11. d	12. c	13. a	14. b	15. a	16. d
17. b	18. b	19. c	20. a.				